This book is based on the religious literature and works of L. Ron Hubbard, who developed Scientology applied religious philosophy and Dianetics spiritual healing technology. It is presented to the reader as Mr. Hubbard's ideas and expressions concerning his observations and research into the human mind and spirit, and not as a statement of claims made by the Church, the author or publisher. The benefits and goals of Scientology philosophy and Dianetics technology can be attained only by the dedicated efforts of the reader.

This material is not professed to provide a physical handling for bodies nor is any claim made to that effect. There are no medical recommendations or claims for the processes given in this book and those processes do not supplant, nor are they intended to dissuade anyone from seeking competent medical attention for any injury, illness or physical condition.

The Purification program is a religious service delivered by the Church of Scientology. There are no medical recommendations or claims for the Purification program or for any of the vitamin or mineral regimens described in this book.

The author and publisher make no warranties, express or implied, concerning the contents of this book. Accordingly, the reader assumes full responsibility for the use of the materials contained herein.

We hope the reading of this book is only the first stage of a personal voyage of discovery into this new and vital world religion.

The Church of Scientology International

THIS BOOK BELONGS TO:

____

THE SCIENTOLOGY HANDBOOK

A Practical Guide to Building a Better World

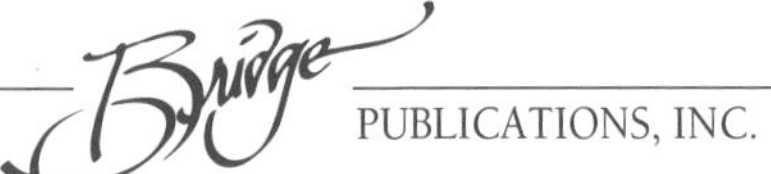
Bridge Publications, Inc.

The Scientology Handbook

Based on the Works of

L. Ron Hubbard

Compiled by
LRH Book Compilations staff
of the Church of Scientology International

Bridge Publications, Inc.
4751 Fountain Avenue
Los Angeles, California 90029

ISBN 0-88404-899-3

NEW ERA Publications International ApS
Store Kongensgade 53
1264 Copenhagen K, Denmark

ISBN 87-7336-999-3

Printed in the United States of America

Important Note

In reading this book, be very certain you never go past a word you do not fully understand.

The only reason a person gives up a study or becomes confused or unable to learn is because he or she has gone past a word that was not understood.

The confusion or inability to grasp or learn comes AFTER a word that the person did not have defined and understood.

It may not only be the new and unusual words that you will have to look up. Some commonly used words can often be misdefined and so cause confusion.

This datum about not going past an undefined word is the most important fact in the whole subject of study. Every subject you have taken up and abandoned had its words which you failed to get defined.

Therefore, in reading this book be very, very certain you never go past a word you do not fully understand. If the material becomes confusing or you can't seem to grasp it, there will be a word just earlier that you have not understood. Don't go any further, but go back to BEFORE you got into trouble, find the misunderstood word and get it defined.

As an aid to the reader, a glossary of Scientology terms is included at the back of this book.

The Aims of Scientology

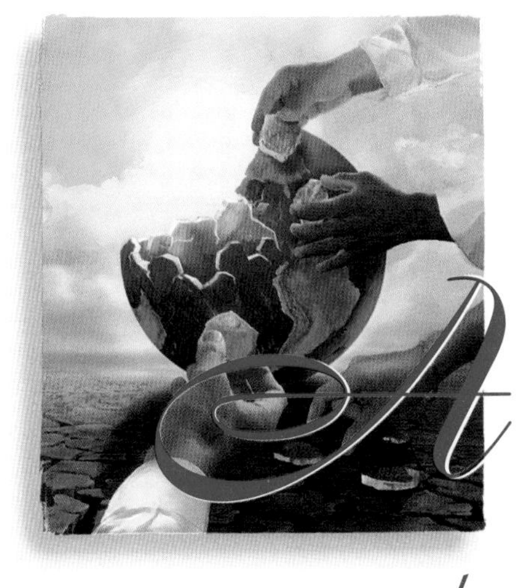

*A civilization without insanity,
without criminals and without war,
where the able can prosper
and honest beings can have rights,
and where man is free
to rise to greater heights,
are the aims of Scientology.*

L. Ron Hubbard

Table of Contents

About This Book

This book is a companion text to the encyclopedic reference work *What Is Scientology?* which provides a complete description of the religion—its religious philosophy, organizations and activities. *The Scientology Handbook* provides the broad panoply of breakthrough Scientology principles and technology for application to everyday living, resolving the conditions that prevent happiness and fulfillment for individuals and civilization itself.

Scientology is unique, not only in the answers it provides to questions man has pondered since the beginning of time, but also the manner these answers can be *applied* to actually *achieve* the long-sought goal of spiritual freedom.

When one understands all of life, and its very essence, there is no situation which cannot be resolved. For this reason, the application of Scientology breakthroughs—its *technology*—has unlimited use in the here and now. Hence, *The Scientology Handbook* provides basic procedures and processes to repair failing marriages, resolve human conflict, bring relief to those in pain or mental anguish and much, much more. Indeed, there is no aspect of life and no quarter of society that cannot be bettered with what one finds in this book.

Moreover, because Scientology is pan-denominational, the principles herein can and are being used by members of every faith to improve conditions and fulfill the responsibility of religion in bringing peace, compassion and decency to this world. In that regard, *The Scientology Handbook* is the text used to train Volunteer Ministers of all denominations. Churches of Scientology provide courses to bring about a full understanding and ability to apply the technology contained herein.

In this age of supermaterialism, nothing would be of greater benefit to mankind than an army of Volunteer Ministers restoring purpose, truth and spiritual values. The ability to accomplish that objective is precisely what this book provides. Men of goodwill who study and apply its principles are doing something effective about the crime, cruelty, injustice and violence permeating our civilization. And in so doing, they are making a difference.

Religious Influence in Society by L. Ron Hubbard

An early twentieth-century philosopher spoke of the impending decline of the West. What he failed to predict was that the West would export its culture to the rest of the world and thus grip the entire world in its death throes.

Today we are witnessing that decline and since we are involved in it, it is of utmost importance to us. At stake are whether the ideals we cherish will survive or some new abhorrent set of values win the day.

These are not idle statements. We are today at a watershed of history and our actions today will decide whether the world goes up from here or continues to slide into some new dark age.

It is important to understand bad conditions don't just happen. The cultural decay we see around us isn't haphazard. It was caused. Unless one understands this he won't be able to defend himself or reach out into the society with effectiveness.

A society is capable of surviving for thousands of years unless it is attacked from within or without by hostile forces. Where such an attack occurs, primary targets are its religious and national gods and heroes, its potential of leadership and the self-respect and integrity of its members.

Material points of attack are finance, communications, technology and a denial of resources.

Look around today and you will find countless examples of these points. They scream at us every day from the newspapers.

Probably the most critical point of attack on a culture is its religious experience. Where one can destroy or undermine religious institutions then the entire fabric of the society can be quickly subverted or brought to ruin.

Religion is the first sense of community. Your sense of community occurs by reason of mutual experience with others. Where the religious sense of community and with it real trust and integrity can be destroyed then that society is like a sandcastle unable to defend itself against the inexorable sea.

For the last hundred years or so religion has been beset with a relentless attack. You have been told it's the "opiate of the masses," that it's unscientific, that it is primitive; in short, that it is a delusion.

But beneath all these attacks on organized religion there was a more fundamental target: the spirituality of man, ***your own basic spiritual nature, self-respect and peace of mind.*** *This black propaganda may have been so successful that maybe you no longer believe you have a spiritual nature but I assure you you do.*

In fact, you don't have a soul, you **are** *your own soul. In other words, you are not this book, your social security card, your body or your mind. You are you.*

Convince a man that he is an animal, that his own dignity and self-respect are delusions, that there is no "beyond" to aspire to, no higher potential self to achieve, and you have a slave. Let a man know he is himself, a spiritual being, that he is capable of the power of choice and has the right to aspire to greater wisdom and you have started him up a higher road.

Of course, such attacks on religion run counter to man's **traditional** *aspirations to spiritual fulfillment and an ethical way of life.*

For thousands of years on this planet thinking man has upheld his own spirituality and considered the ultimate wisdom to be spiritual enlightenment.

The new radical thought that man is an animal without a spiritual nature has a name: totalitarian materialism. Materialism is the doctrine that "only matter matters." The apostles of this new thought are trying to sell everybody on the idea that people really down deep are just a mass and what the person wants to do is cohese with this mass and then be protected by the mass.

This philosophical position was very handy to militaristic and totalitarian governments and their advocates of the last hundred years who wished to justify their atrocities and subjugation of populaces.

One of the tricks of the game has been to attack religion as unscientific. Yet science itself is merely a tool by which the physical universe can be better controlled. The joke is that science itself can become a religion.

Gerhard Lenski on page 331 of his **The Religious Factor, a Sociologist's Inquiry**, *defines religion as "a system of beliefs about the nature of force(s),* *ultimately shaping man's destiny, and the practices associated therewith, shared by members of a group."*

Scientific activities can be as fanatical as religious ones. Scientific groups can themselves be religious "orthodox science" monopolies. The Einsteinian concept of space and time can itself become a holy writ, just as Aristotle's writings were converted into dogmas by the orthodoxy to squash any new ideas in the Middle Ages. (Einstein himself until late in his life was looked upon as a maverick and denied admittance into learned societies.)

Science in itself can become a new faith, a brave new way of overcoming anxiety by explaining things so there is no fear of God or the hereafter.

Thus science and religion are not a dichotomy (pair of opposites). Science itself was borrowed from ancient religious studies in India and Egypt.

Religion has also been attacked as primitive. Too much study of primitive cultures may lead one to believe religion is primitive as it is so dominant in them and that "modern" cultures can dispense with it. The truth of the matter is that at no time is religion more necessary as a civilizing force than in the presence of huge forces in the hands of man, who may have become very lacking in social abilities emphasized in religion.

The great religious civilizing forces of the past, Buddhism, Judaism, Christianity, and others, have all emphasized differentiation of good from evil and higher ethical values.

The lowering of church attendance in the United States coincided with a rise in pornography and general immorality, and an increase in crime which then caused a rise in numbers of police without a subsequent decline in actual moral aberration.

When religion is not influential in a society or has ceased to be, the state inherits the entire burden of public morality, crime and intolerance. It then must use punishment and police. Yet this is unsuccessful as morality, integrity and self-respect not already inherent in the individual, cannot be enforced with any great success. Only by a spiritual awareness and inculcation of the spiritual value of these attributes can they come about. There must be more reason and more emotional motivation to be moral, etc., than threat of human discipline.

When a culture has fallen totally away from spiritual pursuits into materialism, one must begin by demonstrating they are each a soul, not a material animal. From this realization of their own religious nature individuals can again come to an awareness of God and become more themselves.

Medicine, psychiatry and psychology "solved" the whole problem of "human nature" simply by dumping it into the classification of material nature—body, brain, force. As they politically insist on monopoly and use social and political propaganda to enforce their monopoly, they debar actual search for real answers to human nature.

Their failures are attested by lack of result in the field of human nature. They cannot change man—they can only degrade. While asserting dominance in the field of human nature they cannot demonstrate results—and nowhere do they demonstrate that lack more than in their own persons. They have the highest suicide rate and prefer the use of force on others. Under their tutelage the crime rate and antisocial forces have risen. But they are most condemned by their attacks on anyone who seeks answers and upon the civilizing influences of religion.

Of course, if one is going to find fault with something, it implies that he wishes to do something about it and would if he could. If one does not like the crime, cruelty, injustice and violence of this society, he **can** *do something about it. He can become a VOLUNTEER MINISTER and help civilize it, bring it conscience and kindness and love and freedom from travail by instilling into it trust, decency, honesty and tolerance.*

Briefly, a Volunteer Minister fulfills the definition of religion in this increasingly cynical and hopeless world.

Let's look again at the definition of religion.

*In a few words, religion can be defined as belief in spiritual beings. More broadly, religion can be defined as a system of beliefs and practices by means of which a group of people struggles with the ultimate problems of human life. The quality of being religious implies two things: first, a belief that evil, pain, bewilderment and injustice are fundamental facts of existence; second, a set of practices and related sanctified beliefs that express a conviction that man can ultimately be saved from those facts.**

*Reference: *A Scientific Study of Religion* by J. Milton Yunger, Oberlin College.

Thus, a Volunteer Minister is a person who helps his fellow man on a volunteer basis by restoring purpose, truth and spiritual values to the lives of others.

A Volunteer Minister does not shut his eyes to the pain, evil and injustice of existence. Rather, he is trained to handle these things and help others achieve relief from them and new personal strength as well.

How does a Volunteer Minister accomplish these miracles? Basically, he uses the technology of Scientology to change conditions for the better—for himself, his family, his groups, friends, associates and for mankind.

A society to survive well, needs at least as many Volunteer Ministers as it has policemen. A society gets what it concentrates upon. By concentrating on spiritual values instead of criminality a new day may yet dawn for man.

L. Ron Hubbard

A World in Need of Change

The past century has been the most turbulent in man's history. That is undeniable. Fifty million people died in the two World Wars alone. Additionally, there have been millions of deaths due to racially or politically motivated massacres in Africa and Asia. Violent revolutions subjected more than a third of the world's population to totalitarian political rule and, to this day, constant human rights abuses take place in many developing nations. It doesn't take much imagination to think that some change occurred in man, something that turned him into a violent, uncaring and dangerous being.

The lessons of history would question that premise, for man has often resorted to war and revolution to solve his problems. Yet never have the results of war been so destructive. And never have the consequences of man's other actions been so potentially disastrous.

Something about man has changed.

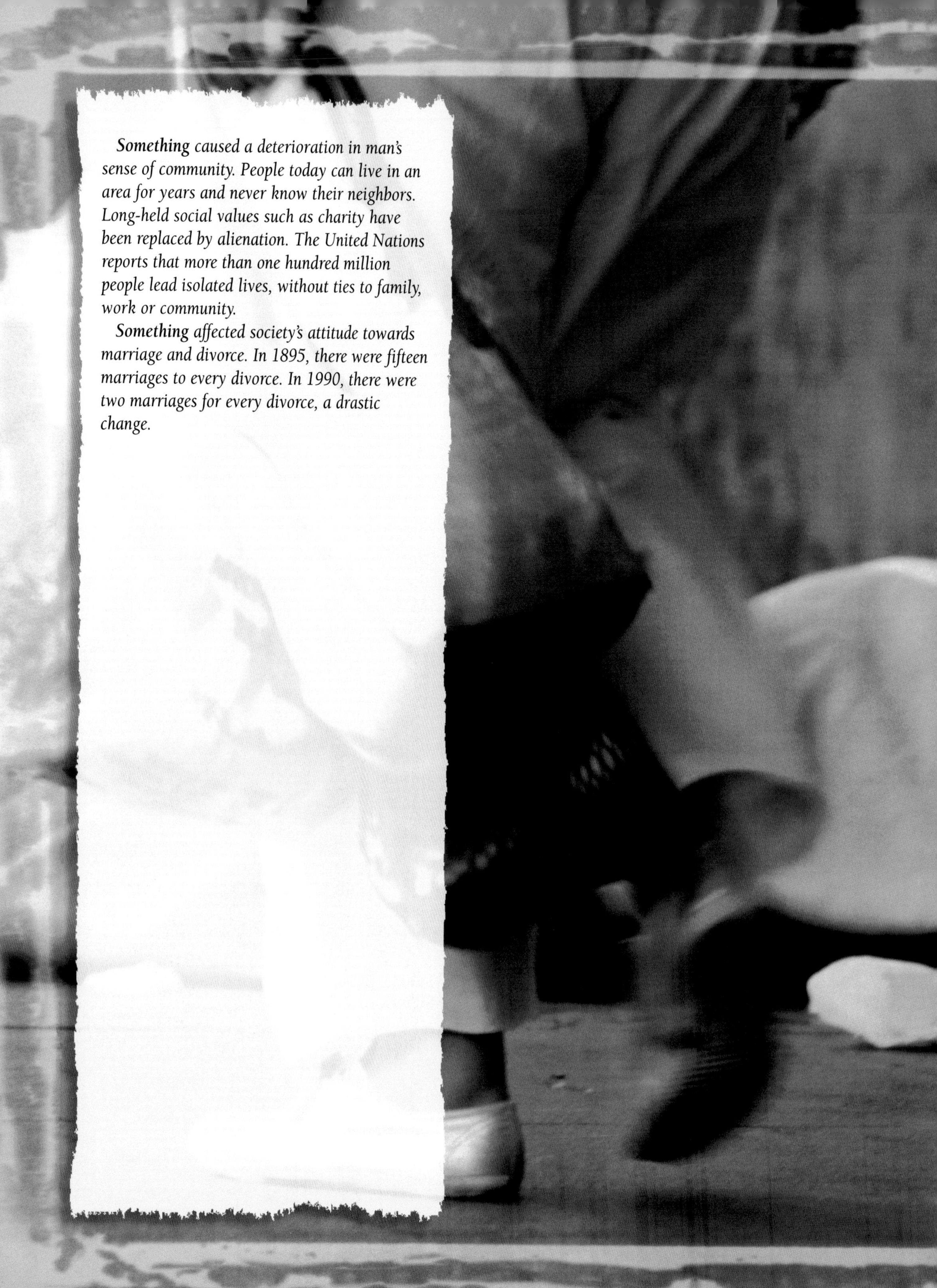

Something caused a deterioration in man's sense of community. People today can live in an area for years and never know their neighbors. Long-held social values such as charity have been replaced by alienation. The United Nations reports that more than one hundred million people lead isolated lives, without ties to family, work or community.

Something affected society's attitude towards marriage and divorce. In 1895, there were fifteen marriages to every divorce. In 1990, there were two marriages for every divorce, a drastic change.

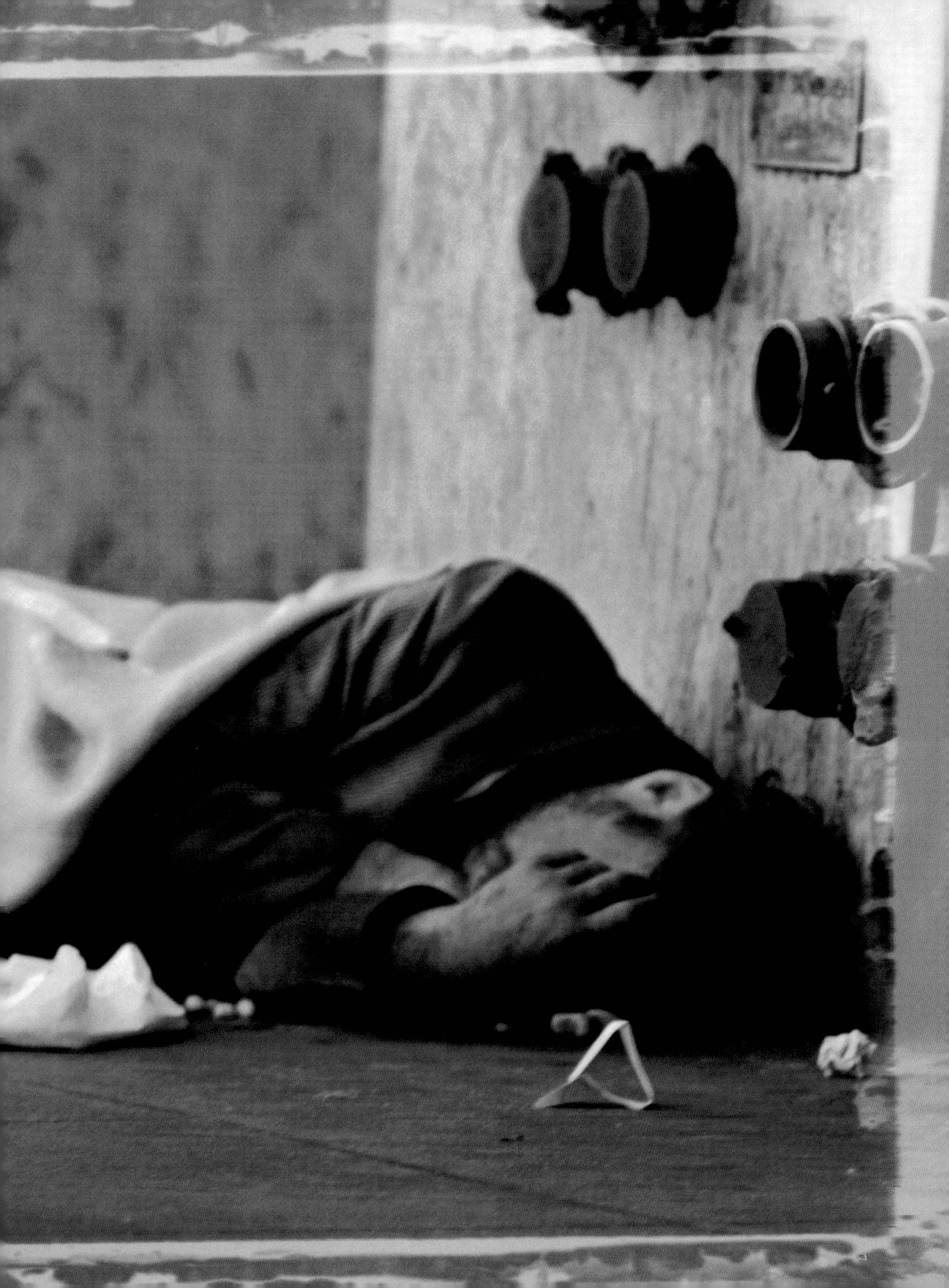

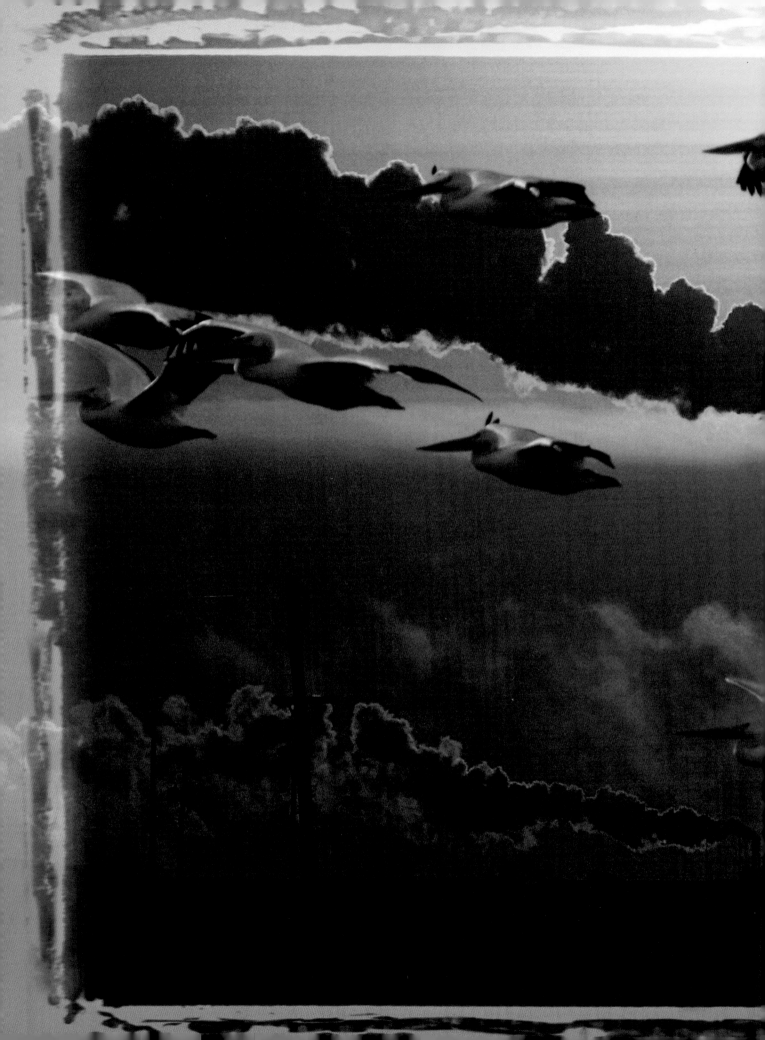

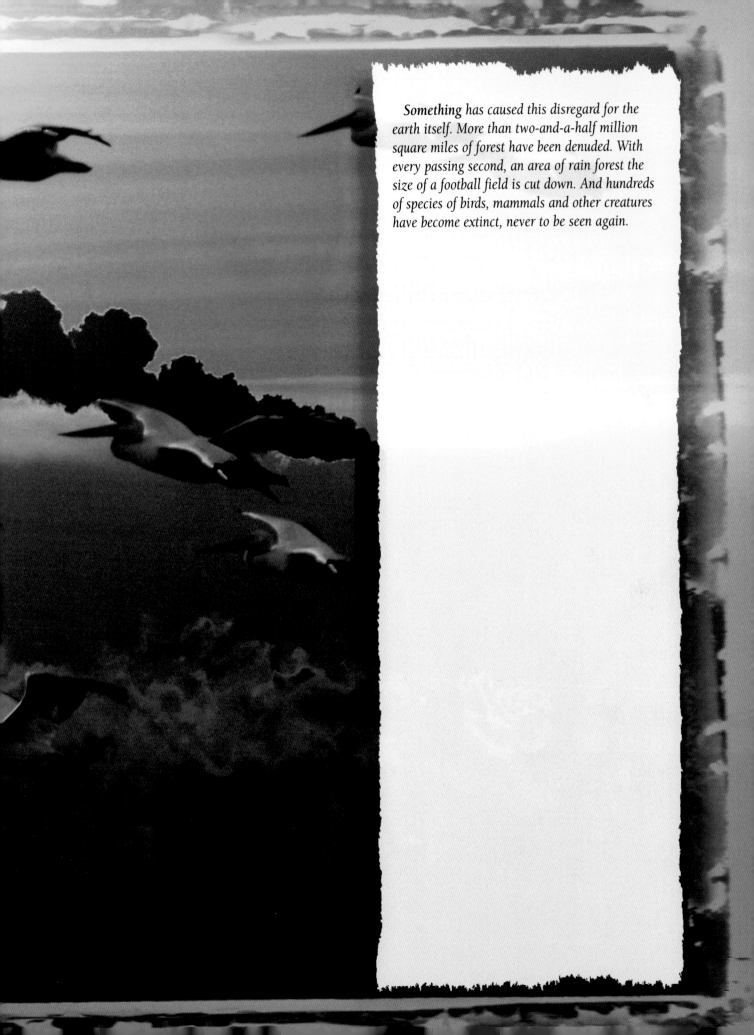

***Something** has caused this disregard for the earth itself. More than two-and-a-half million square miles of forest have been denuded. With every passing second, an area of rain forest the size of a football field is cut down. And hundreds of species of birds, mammals and other creatures have become extinct, never to be seen again.*

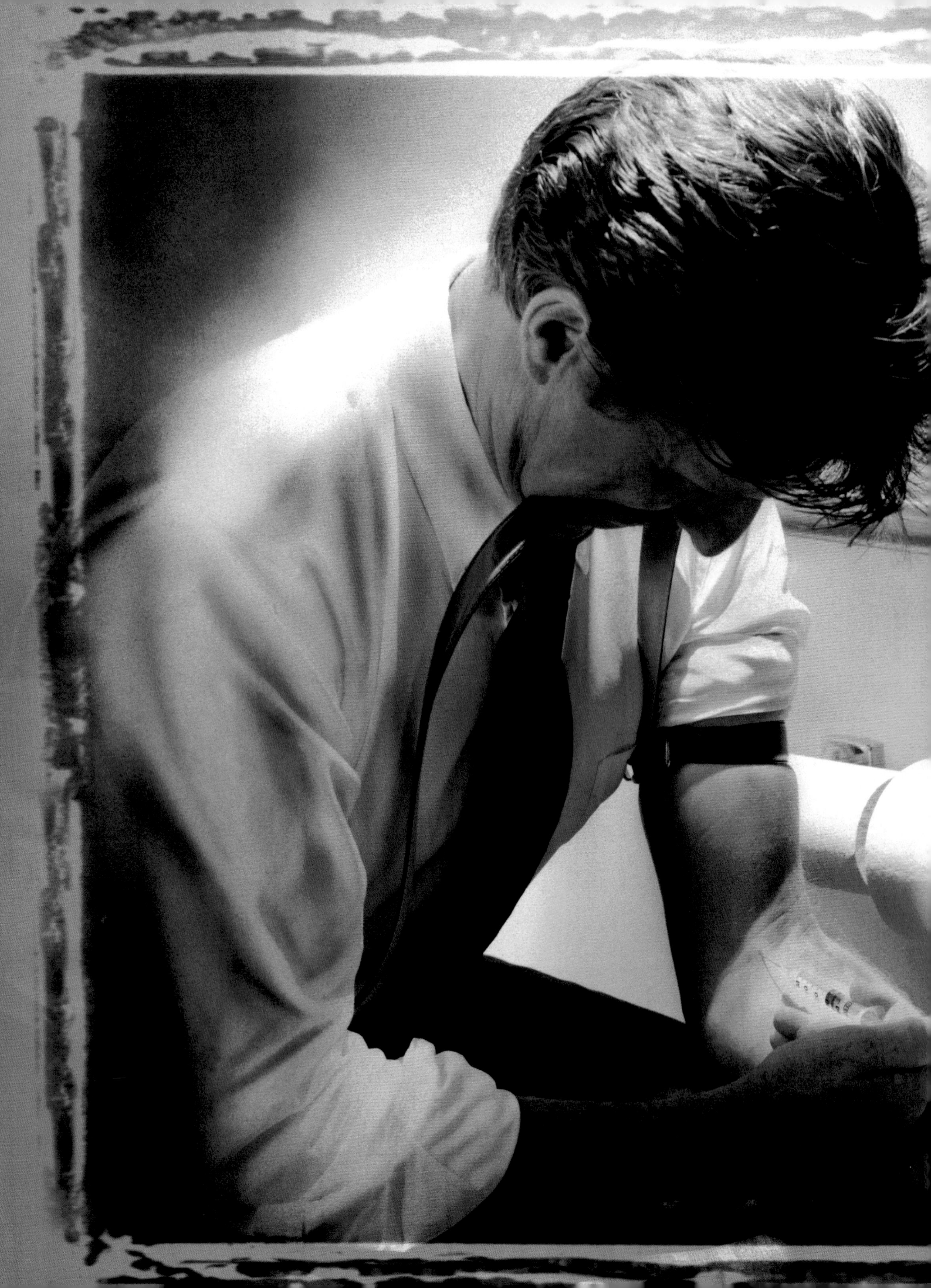

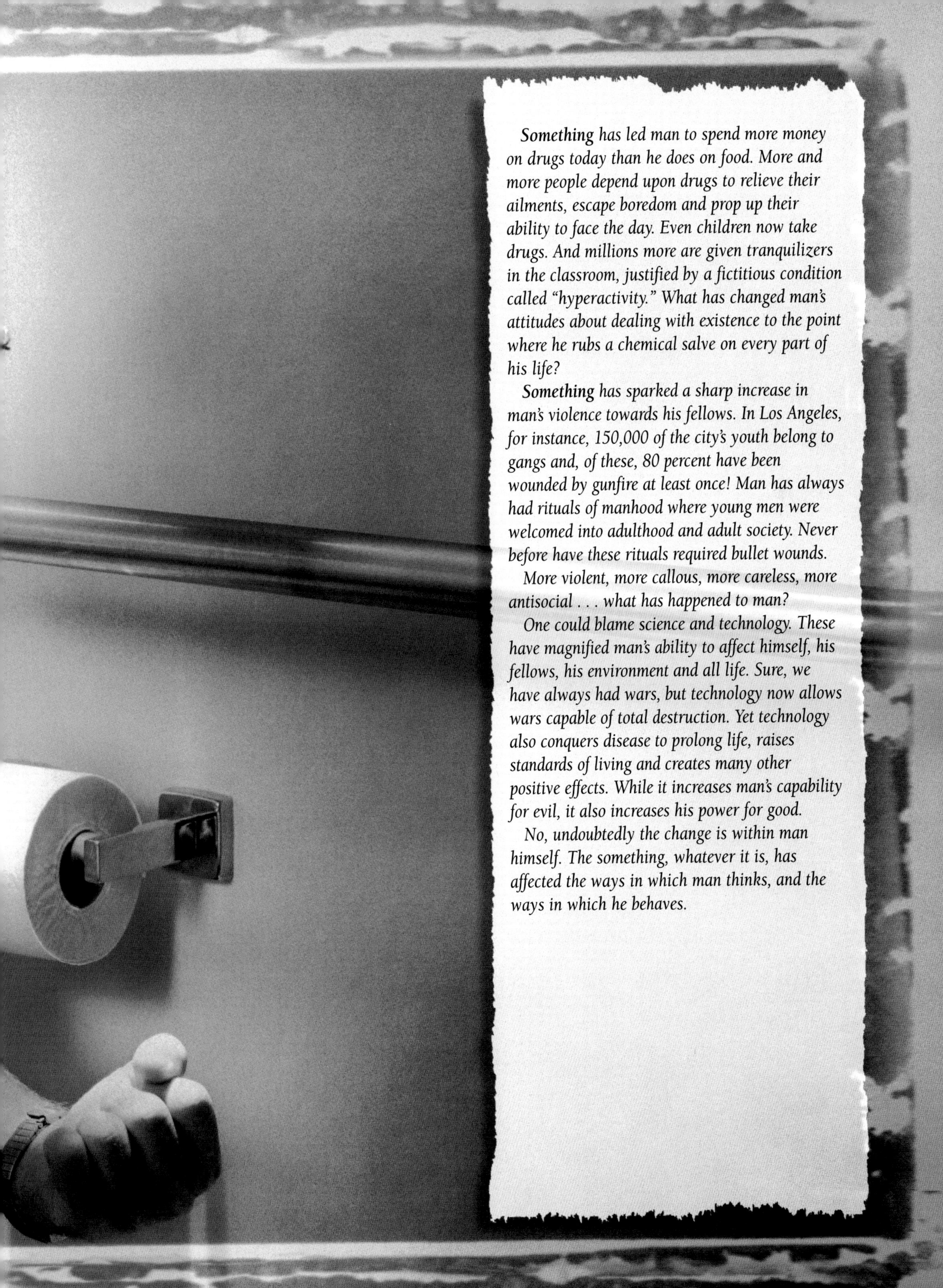

Something has led man to spend more money on drugs today than he does on food. More and more people depend upon drugs to relieve their ailments, escape boredom and prop up their ability to face the day. Even children now take drugs. And millions more are given tranquilizers in the classroom, justified by a fictitious condition called "hyperactivity." What has changed man's attitudes about dealing with existence to the point where he rubs a chemical salve on every part of his life?

Something has sparked a sharp increase in man's violence towards his fellows. In Los Angeles, for instance, 150,000 of the city's youth belong to gangs and, of these, 80 percent have been wounded by gunfire at least once! Man has always had rituals of manhood where young men were welcomed into adulthood and adult society. Never before have these rituals required bullet wounds.

More violent, more callous, more careless, more antisocial . . . what has happened to man?

One could blame science and technology. These have magnified man's ability to affect himself, his fellows, his environment and all life. Sure, we have always had wars, but technology now allows wars capable of total destruction. Yet technology also conquers disease to prolong life, raises standards of living and creates many other positive effects. While it increases man's capability for evil, it also increases his power for good.

No, undoubtedly the change is within man himself. The something, whatever it is, has affected the ways in which man thinks, and the ways in which he behaves.

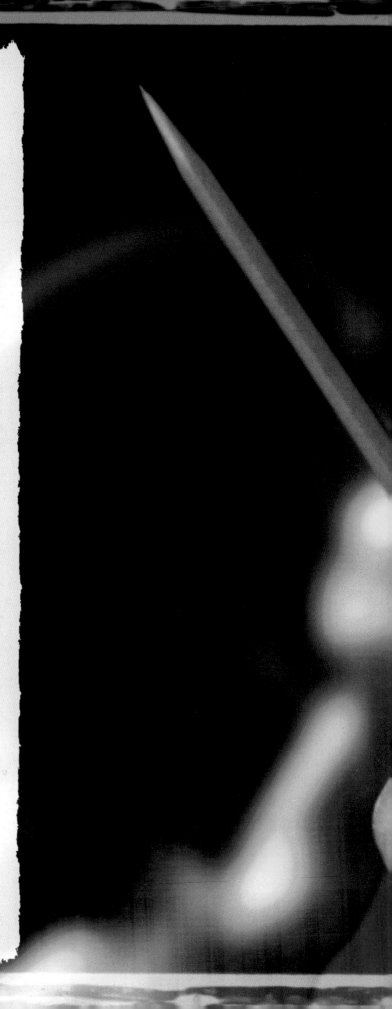

THE "MAN IS AN ANIMAL" THEORY

Along with the increased turbulence, the twentieth century saw the rise of another **view** *of man. From this came many repercussions in the way man looks at and treats himself and his fellows. And from this grew the most fundamental challenge facing man as he began the twenty-first century.*

The thing that most separates man from any life form is his ability to **understand** *and reason. And perhaps the thing he has most universally tried to understand is himself. How is it that, despite being able to act rationally, man could also act so* **irrationally***? Philosophers, religious leaders, scientists and scholars—the greatest minds among men—have wrestled with this riddle, but never arrived at a satisfactory explanation.*

Many great thinkers in history believed that life consisted of both the material and immaterial, that the mind was separate from matter. This idea is called "dualism." Other people throughout history, known as "materialists," believed that everything is made of matter.

In nineteenth-century Europe, the Industrial Revolution caused many changes in Western culture and materialistic theories became dominant in man's thinking.

And it is in **this** *view that we find the source of what troubles man and casts the longest shadows over his happiness and, indeed, his very survival.*

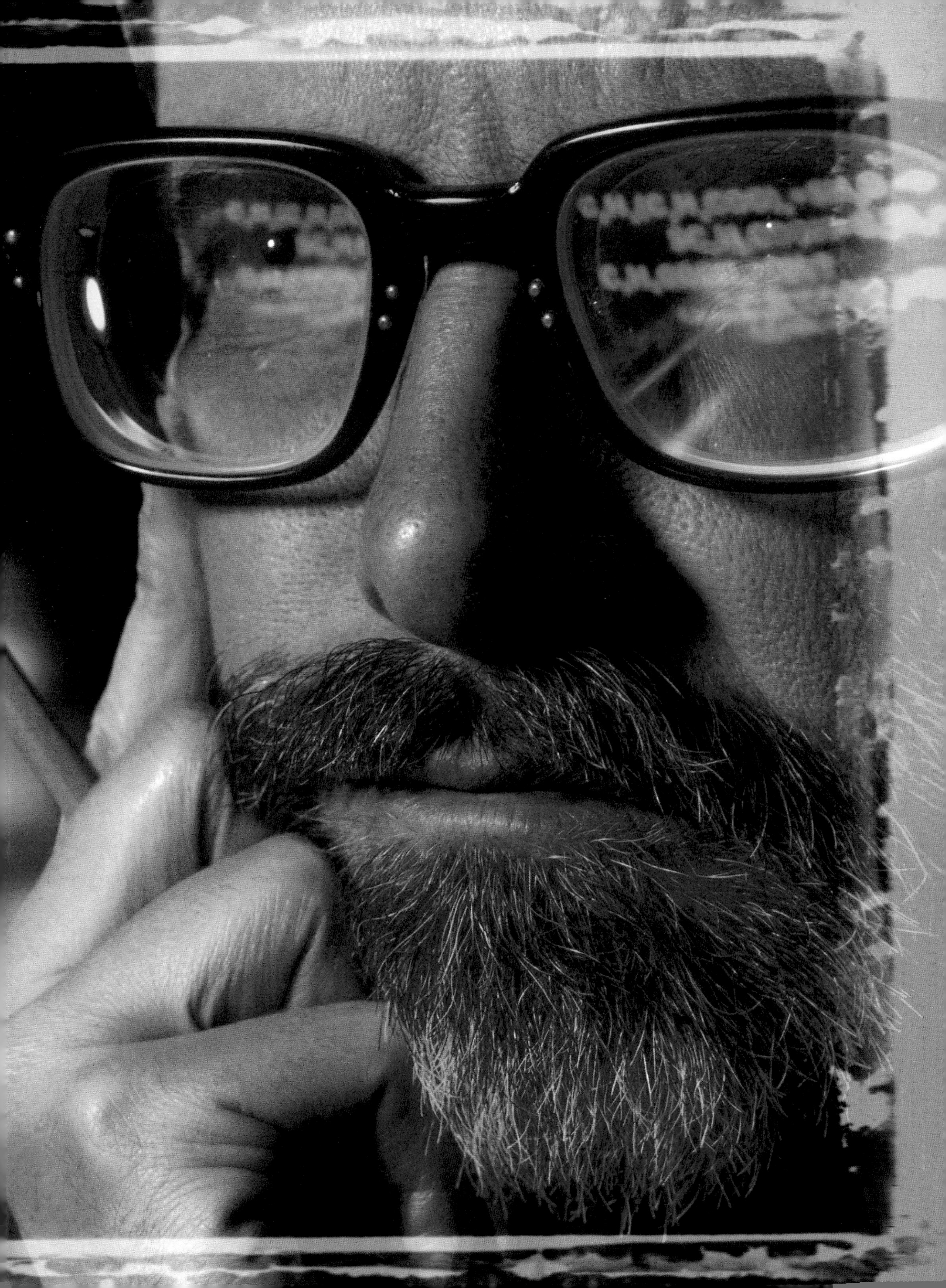

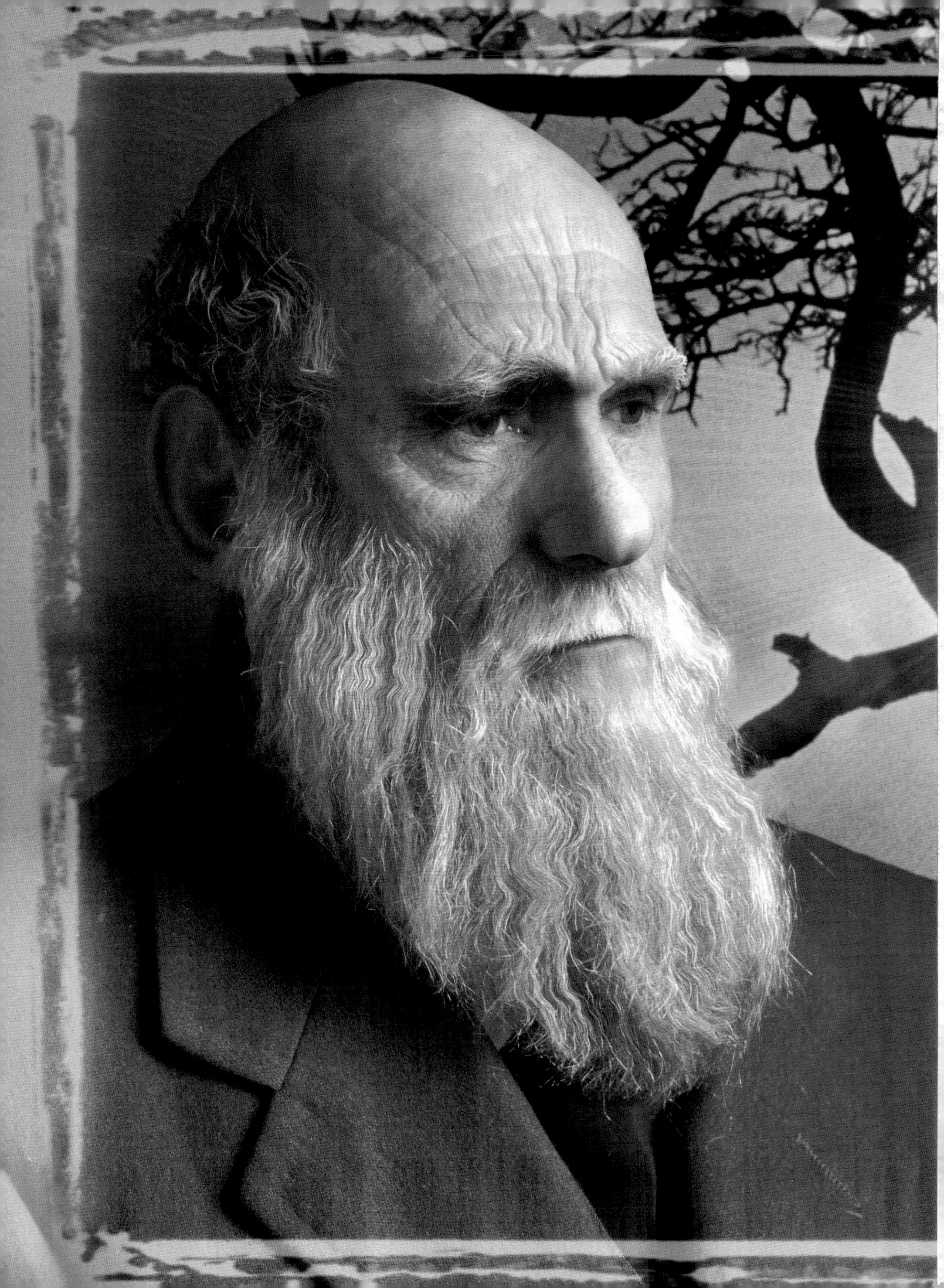

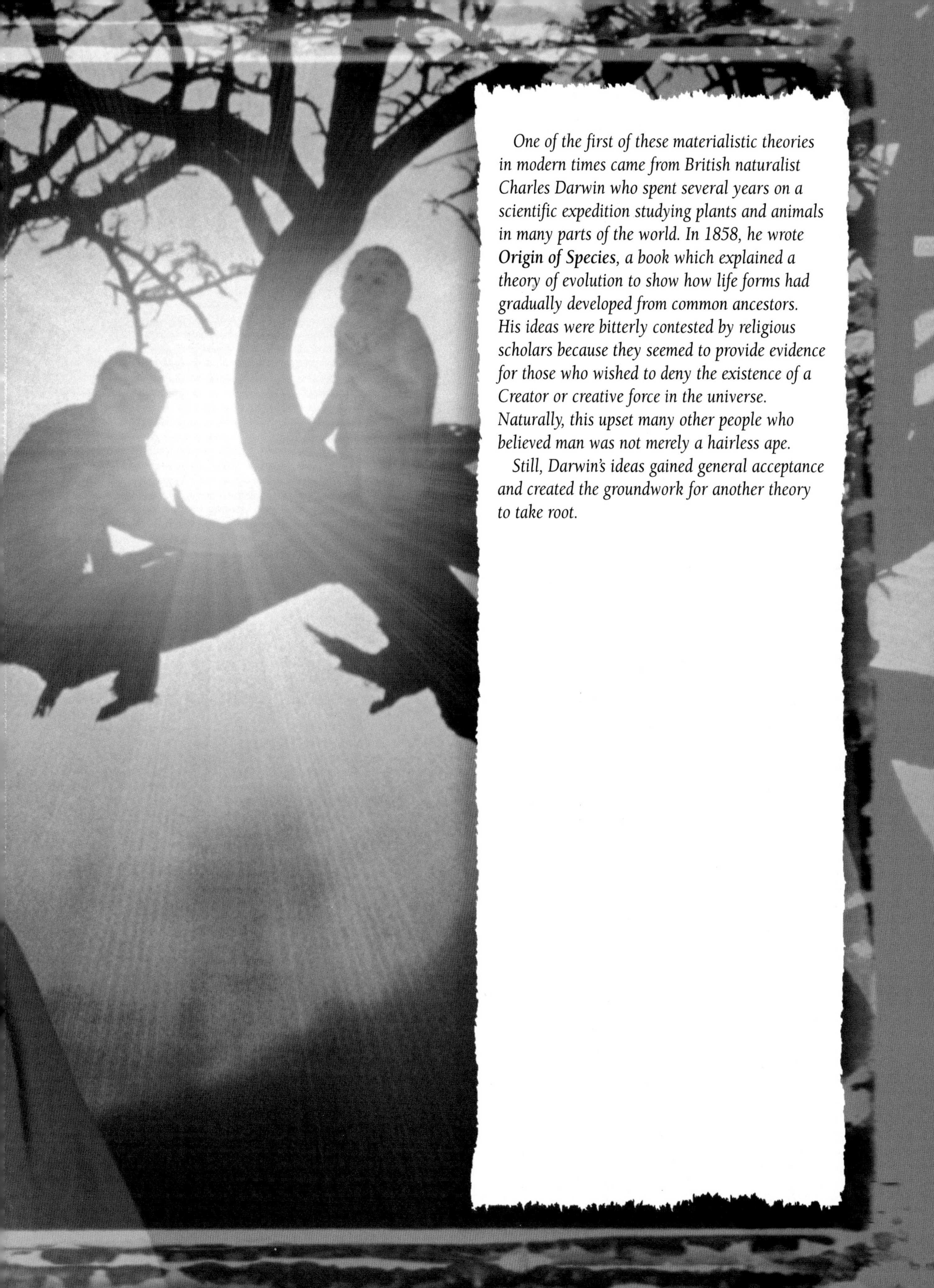

One of the first of these materialistic theories in modern times came from British naturalist Charles Darwin who spent several years on a scientific expedition studying plants and animals in many parts of the world. In 1858, he wrote **Origin of Species**, *a book which explained a theory of evolution to show how life forms had gradually developed from common ancestors. His ideas were bitterly contested by religious scholars because they seemed to provide evidence for those who wished to deny the existence of a Creator or creative force in the universe. Naturally, this upset many other people who believed man was not merely a hairless ape.*

Still, Darwin's ideas gained general acceptance and created the groundwork for another theory to take root.

It came from a German, a Professor Wilhelm Wundt of Leipzig University. In 1879, Wundt advanced the theory that man could be totally understood by studying material things only. Wundt had been trained in physiology, the study of physical structure and function in living things. Through his training, he arrived at the notion that investigating the soul or spirit was a waste of time because a man could be studied in the same way that a frog or a rat is studied. His teachings refuted the dualist idea that mind and matter were different. From this it was only a short hop to the conclusion that man was just another animal who had merely evolved to a higher level of intelligence than all the others. It was simply a matter of brain cells, the theory went.

In spite of the fact that Wundt never really proved any of his ideas, the school of experimental psychology was born.

The word **psychology** *means "study of the soul," from the Greek word "psyche," meaning "the soul." But today, psychologists proclaim that there is no soul and instead study human and animal behavior. This makes as much sense as a baker claiming there is no such thing as bread. The original definition of psychology died with the unproven idea that an individual's actions were simply a response to stimuli perceived by the organism and were not related to any nonmaterial part of a person. According to Wundt, there was no nonmaterial part of man, no mind, no soul.*

Ultimately, then, man was no more than a higher order animal. And if a person could be convinced of this, his ideas of personal responsibility could be changed.

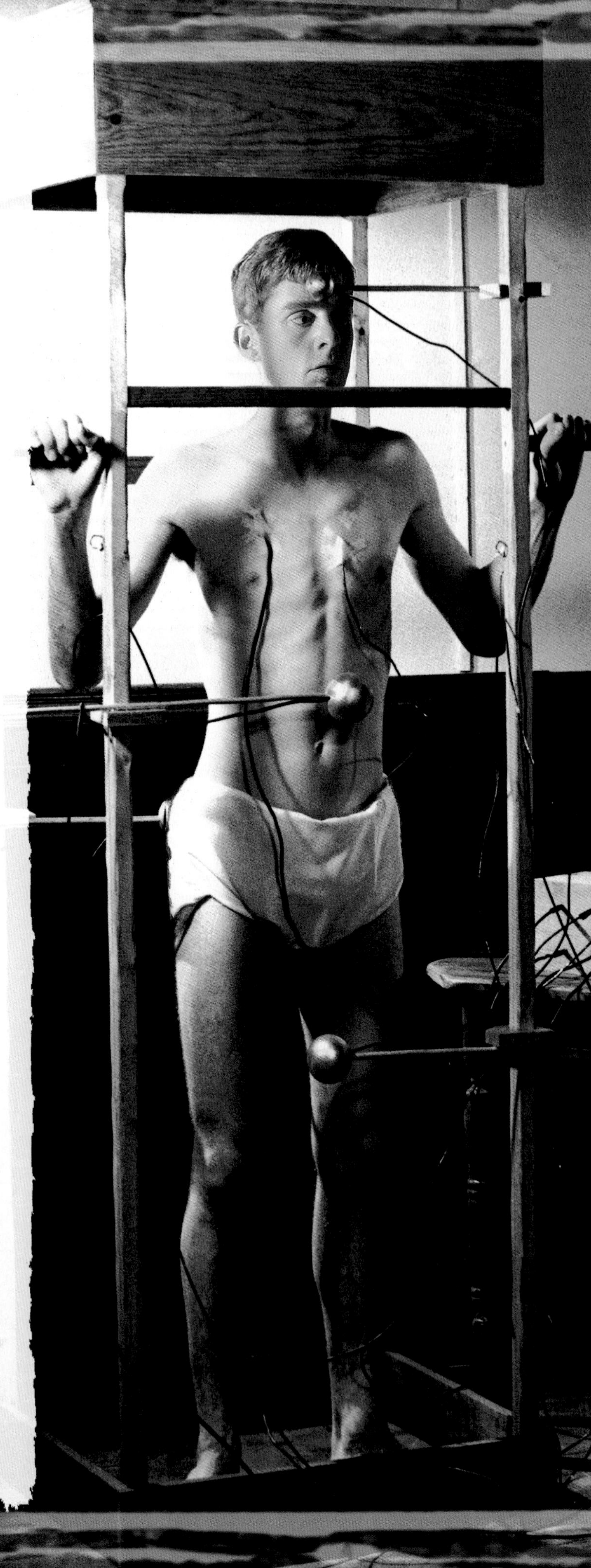

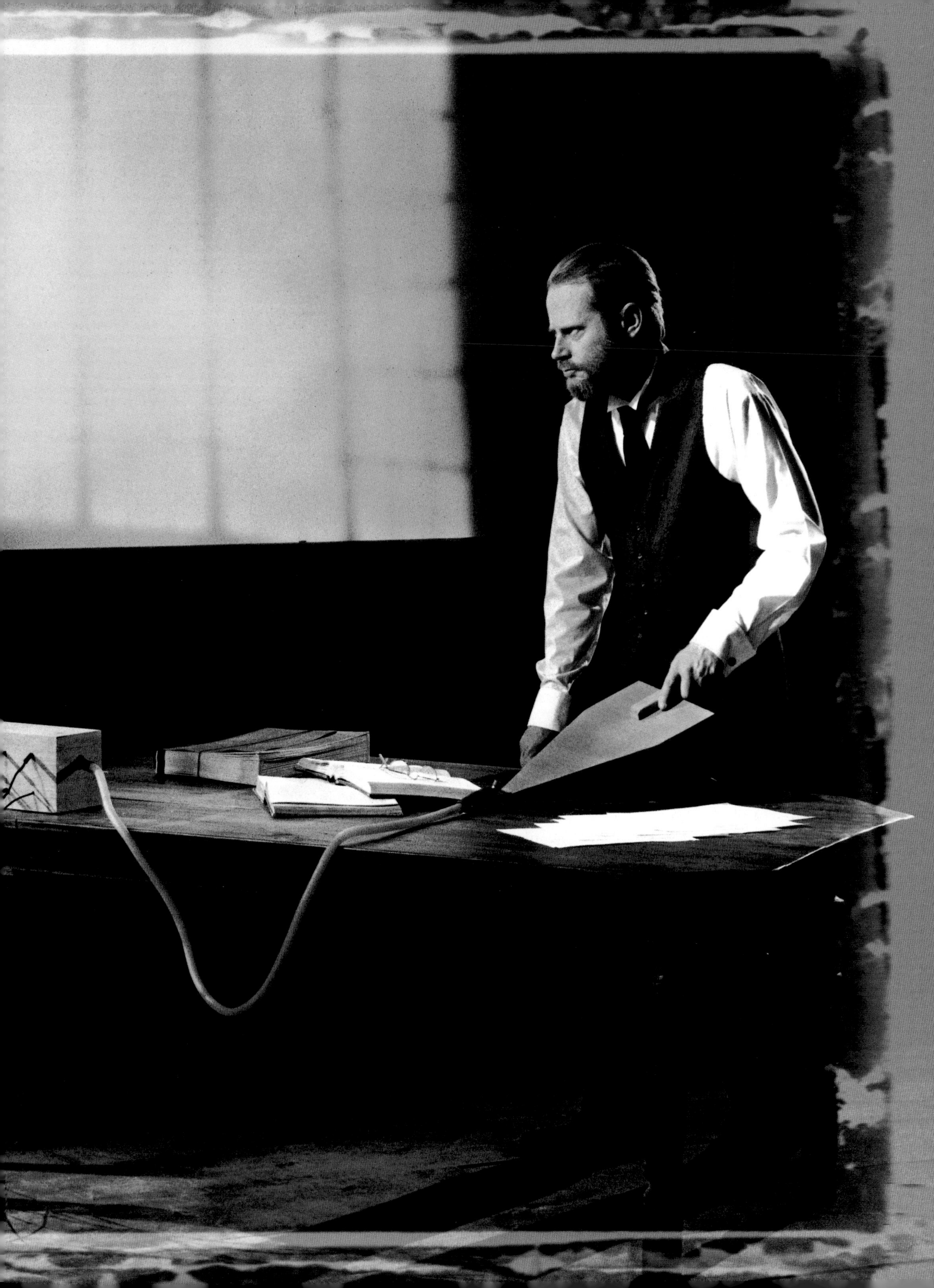

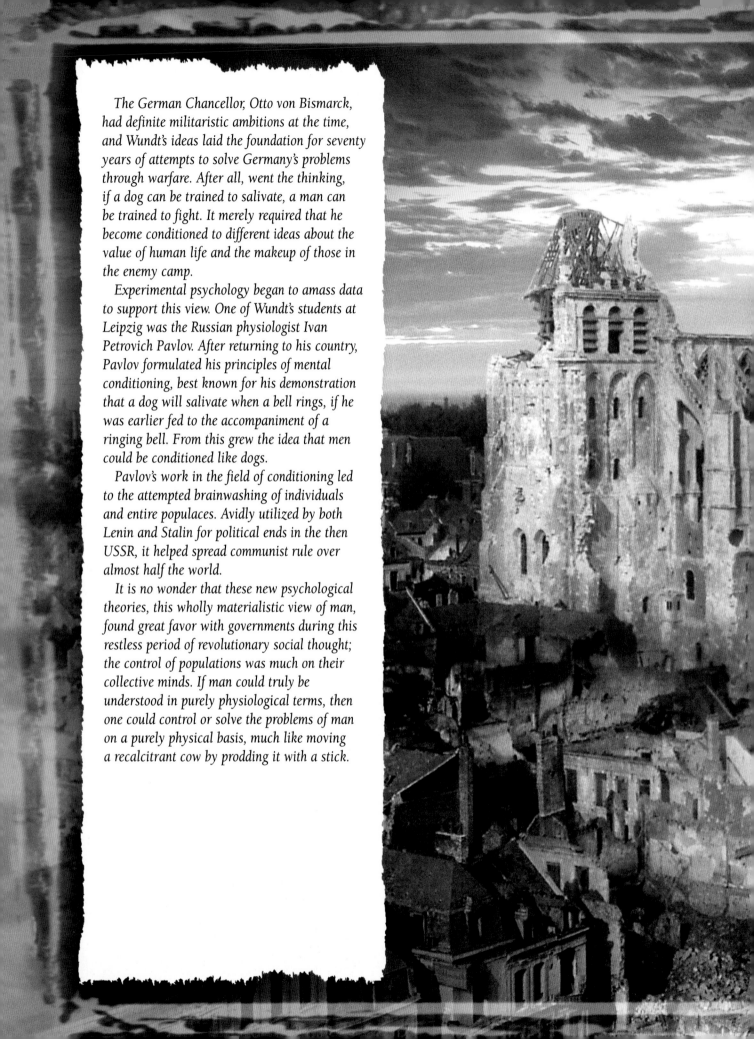

The German Chancellor, Otto von Bismarck, had definite militaristic ambitions at the time, and Wundt's ideas laid the foundation for seventy years of attempts to solve Germany's problems through warfare. After all, went the thinking, if a dog can be trained to salivate, a man can be trained to fight. It merely required that he become conditioned to different ideas about the value of human life and the makeup of those in the enemy camp.

Experimental psychology began to amass data to support this view. One of Wundt's students at Leipzig was the Russian physiologist Ivan Petrovich Pavlov. After returning to his country, Pavlov formulated his principles of mental conditioning, best known for his demonstration that a dog will salivate when a bell rings, if he was earlier fed to the accompaniment of a ringing bell. From this grew the idea that men could be conditioned like dogs.

Pavlov's work in the field of conditioning led to the attempted brainwashing of individuals and entire populaces. Avidly utilized by both Lenin and Stalin for political ends in the then USSR, it helped spread communist rule over almost half the world.

It is no wonder that these new psychological theories, this wholly materialistic view of man, found great favor with governments during this restless period of revolutionary social thought; the control of populations was much on their collective minds. If man could truly be understood in purely physiological terms, then one could control or solve the problems of man on a purely physical basis, much like moving a recalcitrant cow by prodding it with a stick.

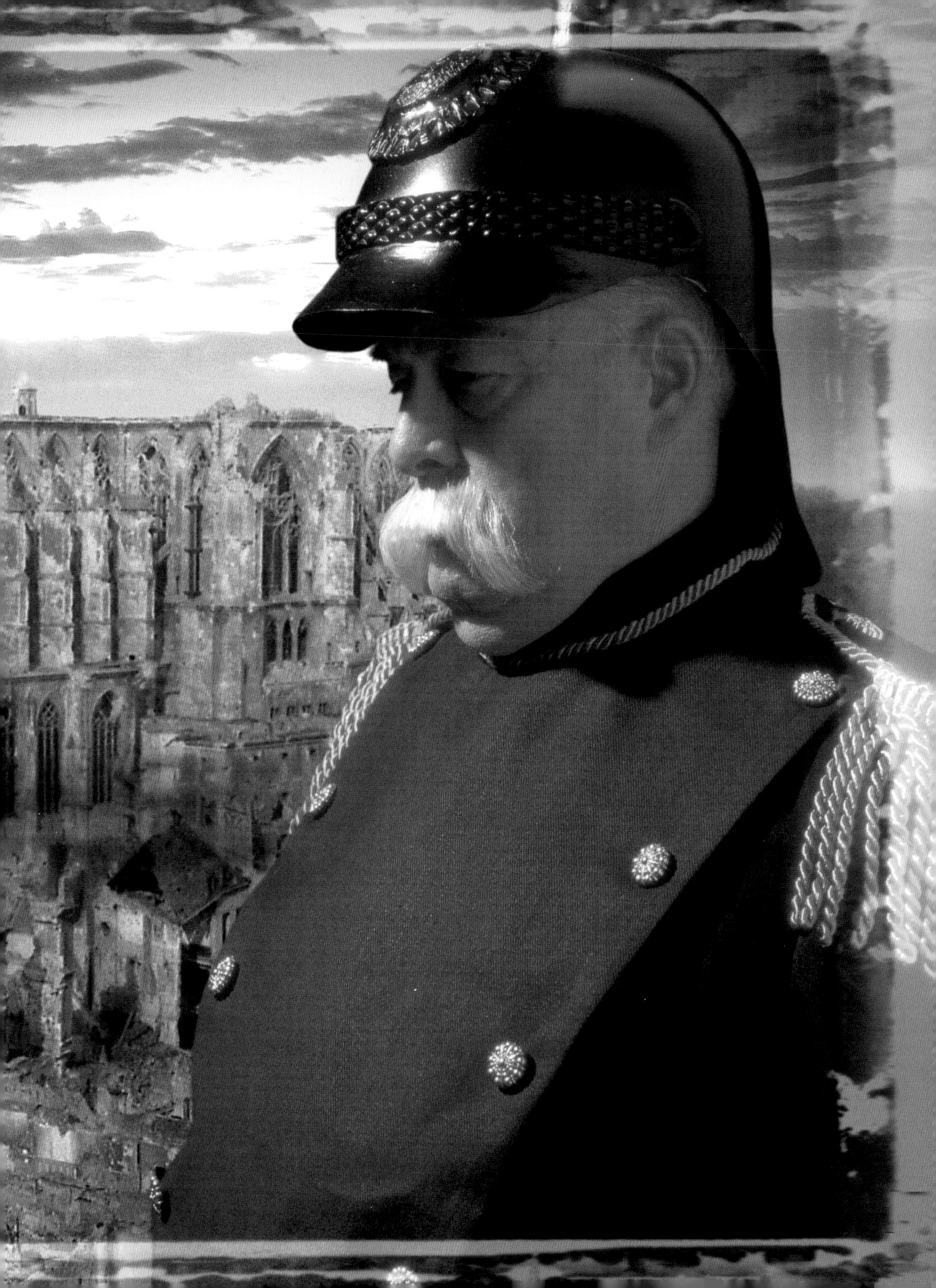

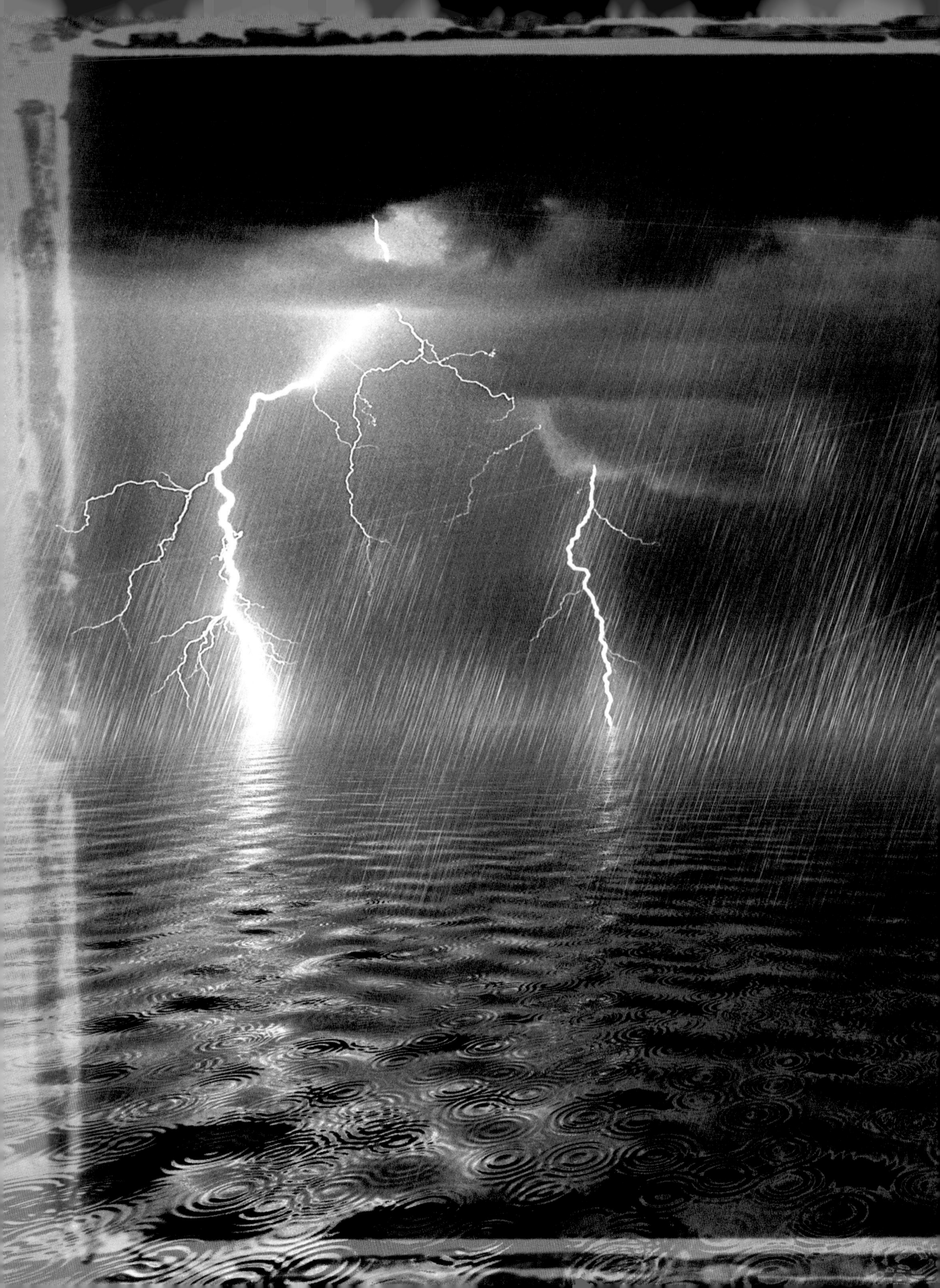

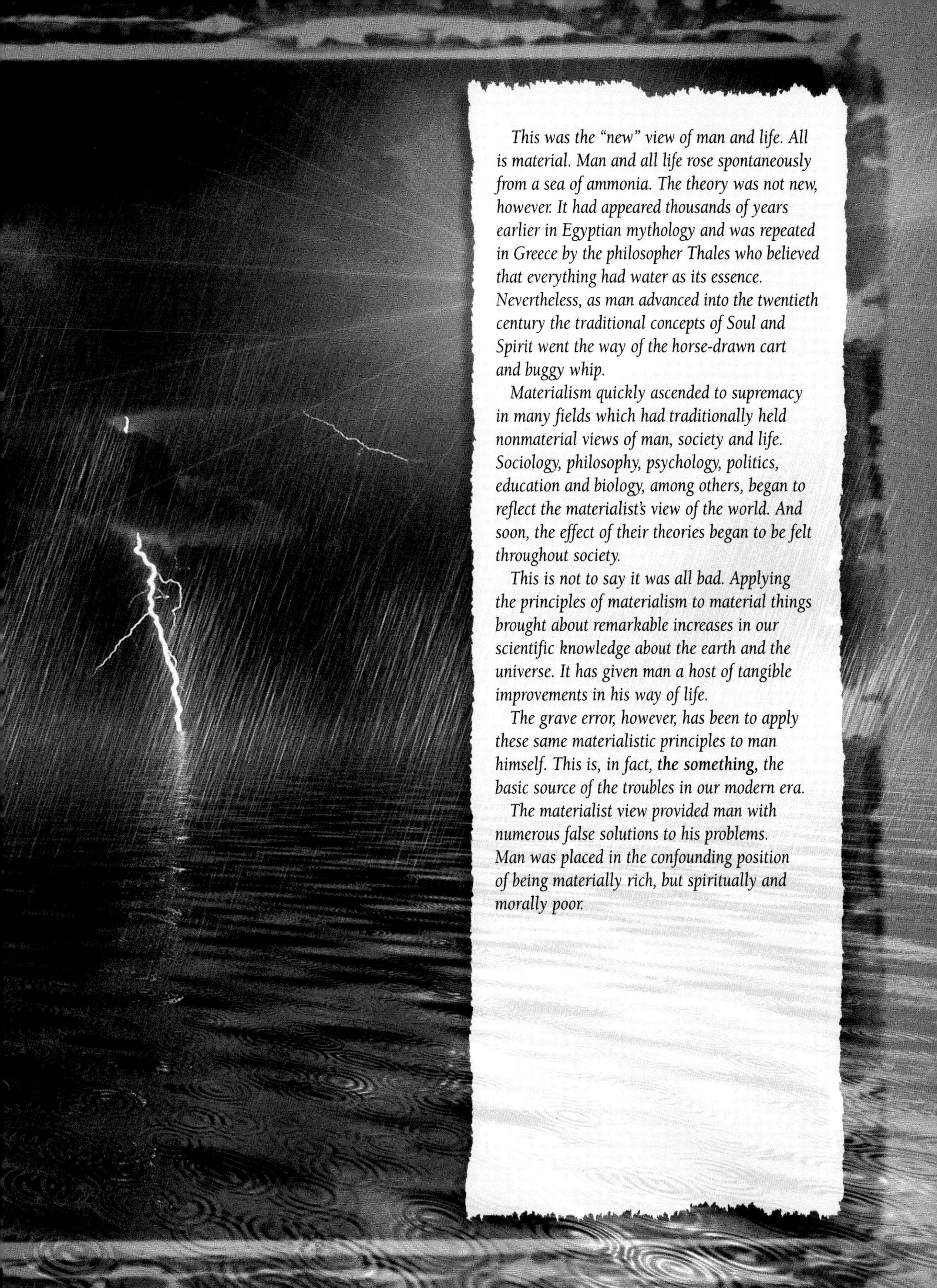

This was the "new" view of man and life. All is material. Man and all life rose spontaneously from a sea of ammonia. The theory was not new, however. It had appeared thousands of years earlier in Egyptian mythology and was repeated in Greece by the philosopher Thales who believed that everything had water as its essence. Nevertheless, as man advanced into the twentieth century the traditional concepts of Soul and Spirit went the way of the horse-drawn cart and buggy whip.

Materialism quickly ascended to supremacy in many fields which had traditionally held nonmaterial views of man, society and life. Sociology, philosophy, psychology, politics, education and biology, among others, began to reflect the materialist's view of the world. And soon, the effect of their theories began to be felt throughout society.

This is not to say it was all bad. Applying the principles of materialism to material things brought about remarkable increases in our scientific knowledge about the earth and the universe. It has given man a host of tangible improvements in his way of life.

The grave error, however, has been to apply these same materialistic principles to man himself. This is, in fact, ***the something,*** *the basic source of the troubles in our modern era.*

The materialist view provided man with numerous false solutions to his problems. Man was placed in the confounding position of being materially rich, but spiritually and morally poor.

The Results

Broad application of Wundt's "man is an animal" theory had disastrous and widespread consequences. And nowhere is this heritage more apparent than in the field of psychiatry.

Nineteenth-century psychiatry, with its long history of mistreatment of the insane, leaped onto the coattails of experimental psychology to enter the universities of Europe and America. Thus, in short order, the psychiatrist expanded his sphere of influence from insane asylums to the halls of political power and other institutions. Now, however, he carried with him not only the creed of materialism, but the attitudes of his heritage: that the insane needed to be controlled through any necessary means of force and duress. Applied to populations at large, these attitudes have had disastrous consequences for society.

The belief that force can monitor thinking, personality and behavior, laid the foundation for two world wars—the most destructive in mankind's history. Psychiatrists in Germany developed the pseudoscience of eugenics, with its ideas of "racial purity." "Super races," they claimed, could be bred to improve racial characteristics in the same way that farmers breed horses to get bigger, stronger animals. From this idiocy came Hitler's political ideology that the race could be improved by cleaning it of inferior stock. And thus resulted the wholesale slaughter of entire populations during the Nazi Holocaust. The German people were duped into believing their problems stemmed from the presence of genetically inferior races within its population. Their "solution" is forever imprinted upon human history.

The genocidal activity in the former Yugoslavia, euphemistically termed "ethnic cleansing," is but a continuation of this brutal mind-set. In the late 1980s, a psychiatrist traveled widely throughout the region and stirred up Serbian nationalism, inflaming long-buried ethnic hatreds. Another psychiatrist, a pupil of the first, became a Serbian political and military leader and it is his troops that initiated the bitter warfare which erupted in 1990 and conducted the campaign of terror to rid the area of "inferior" Muslims. It was psychiatrists who stirred up the hatreds that are so horrifying the world.

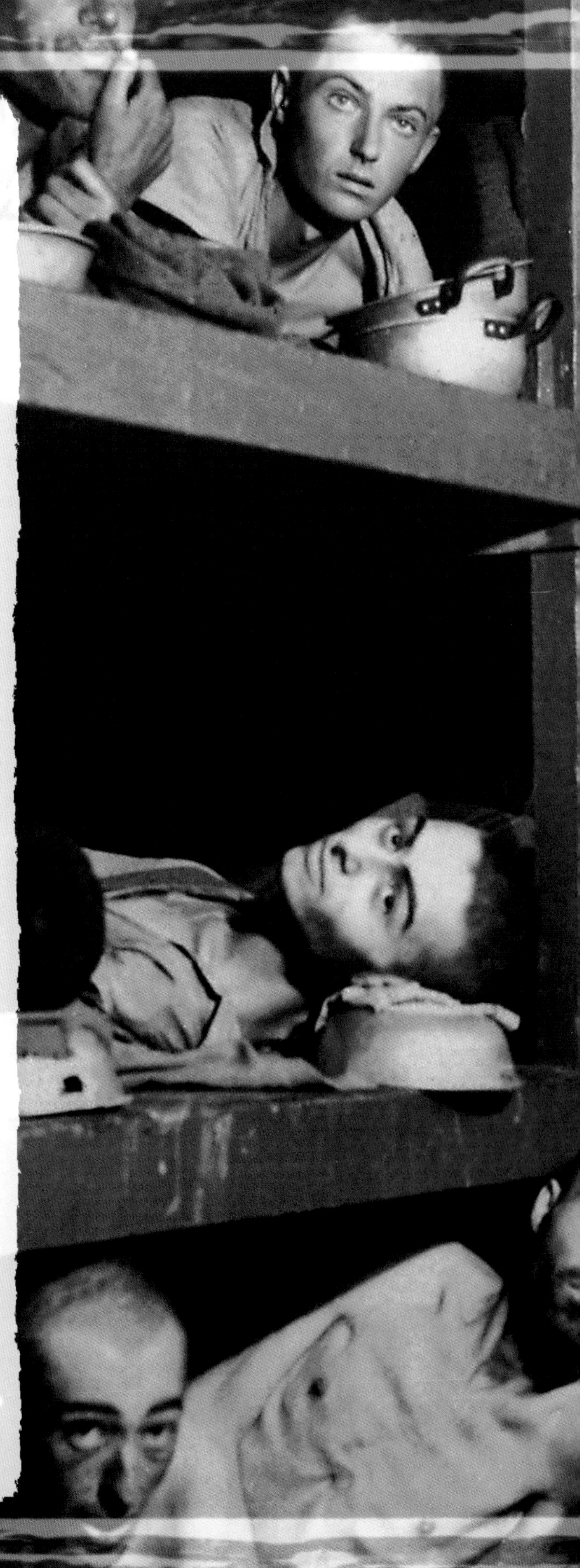

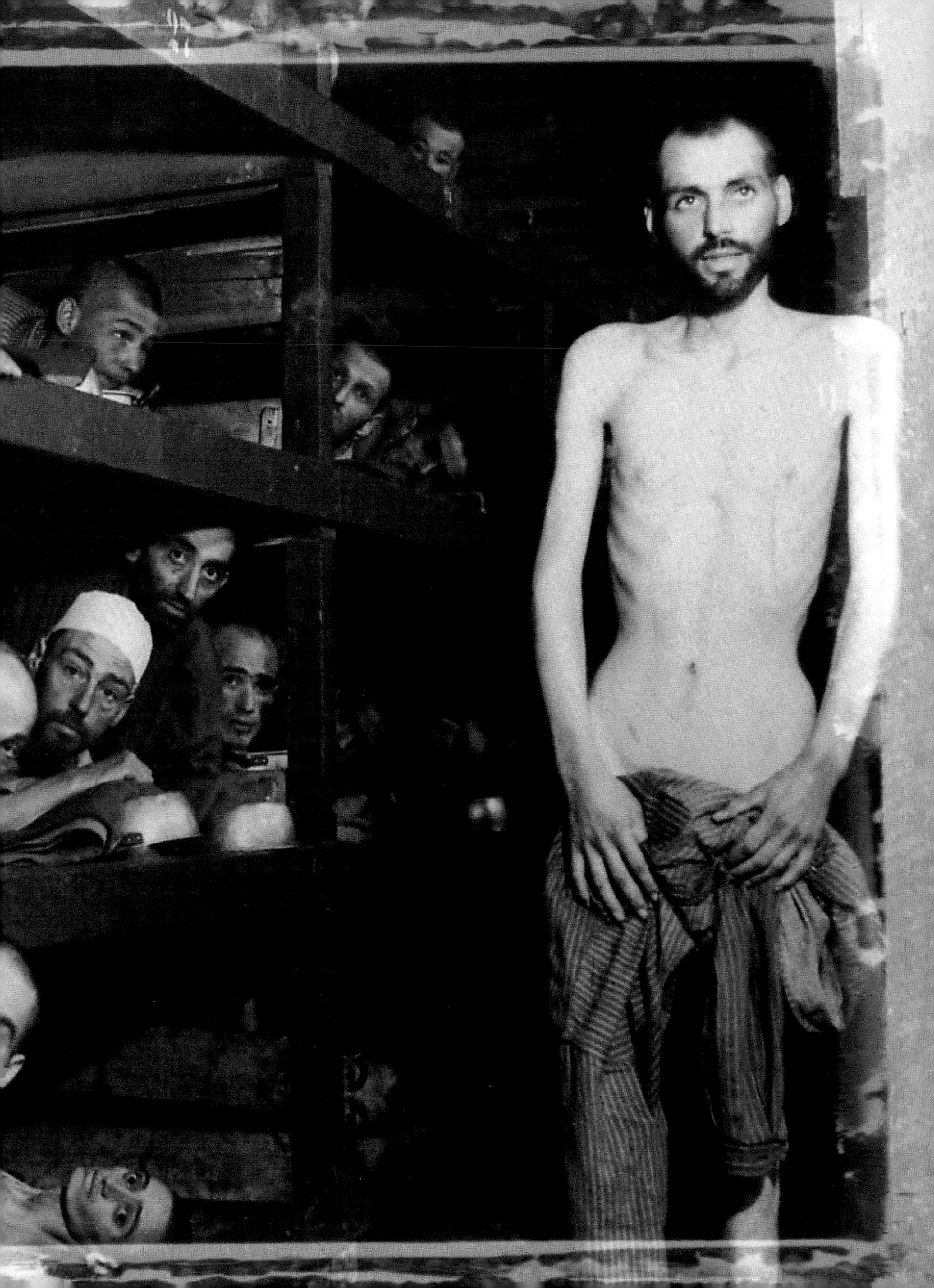

If this strikes one as outrageous, it is! Nevertheless, it is true. The facts speak for themselves. The materialist idea that some peoples are genetically inferior to others and need to be wiped out for the greater good of mankind is a lunacy created and perpetuated to this day by psychiatry.

And what of mental illness, the area psychiatry officially claimed expertise in?

Materialism decrees that any personality problem is physical in nature. Thus psychiatry treats it with physical means: drugs to tranquilize or shock the system; electricity to convulse the person out of his current patterns of behavior; and, operations to incapacitate the nervous system and make unacceptable behavior impossible. Today's extensive use of psychotropic drugs is simply an extension of this philosophy. After all, if a living being has no soul, it does not really matter what one does to it.

Psychiatry has had almost half a century in which to gauge the success of this approach. And governments the world over have poured money into its coffers, based upon its promises of a new world with a docile populace. The success of this grand experiment would be easily provable by improvements in apparent mental disorders, emotional problems and a general bettering of the quality of life. Instead we have exactly the opposite—a drastic deterioration in all the above.

Psychiatry has consistently invented more and more mental illnesses during the last fifty years, and the pharmaceutical industry has been quick to jump on the gravy train by inventing the chemical "cures." The effects of these drugs create yet more categories of mental illness profiting everyone but the patient.

In the mid-1800s, 1 in 1,000 individuals in the US was deemed mentally ill; today, psychiatrists claim that 20 percent of the population is in need of psychiatric treatment.

It is not just mental illness, however. All societal problems which existed before the rise of materialism have drastically worsened through the use of materialistic solutions. And, in particular, it is easily provable by statistics that any segment of society in which psychiatry has dabbled has considerably deteriorated.

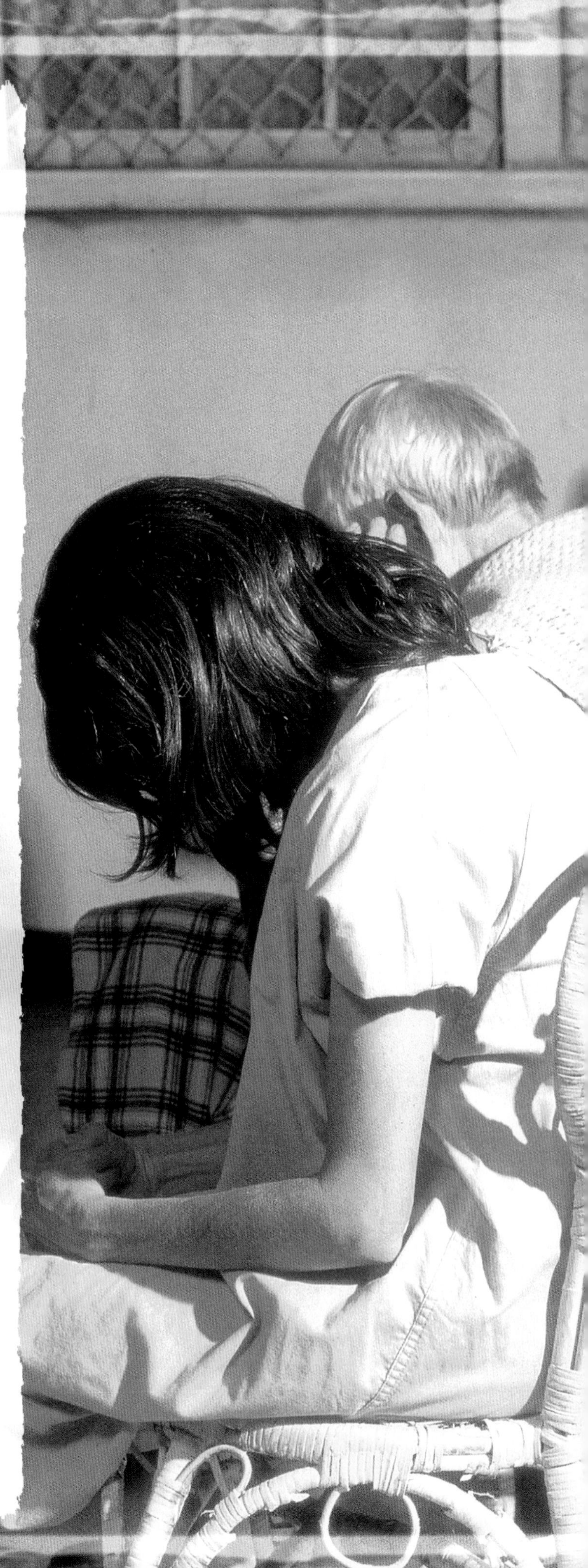

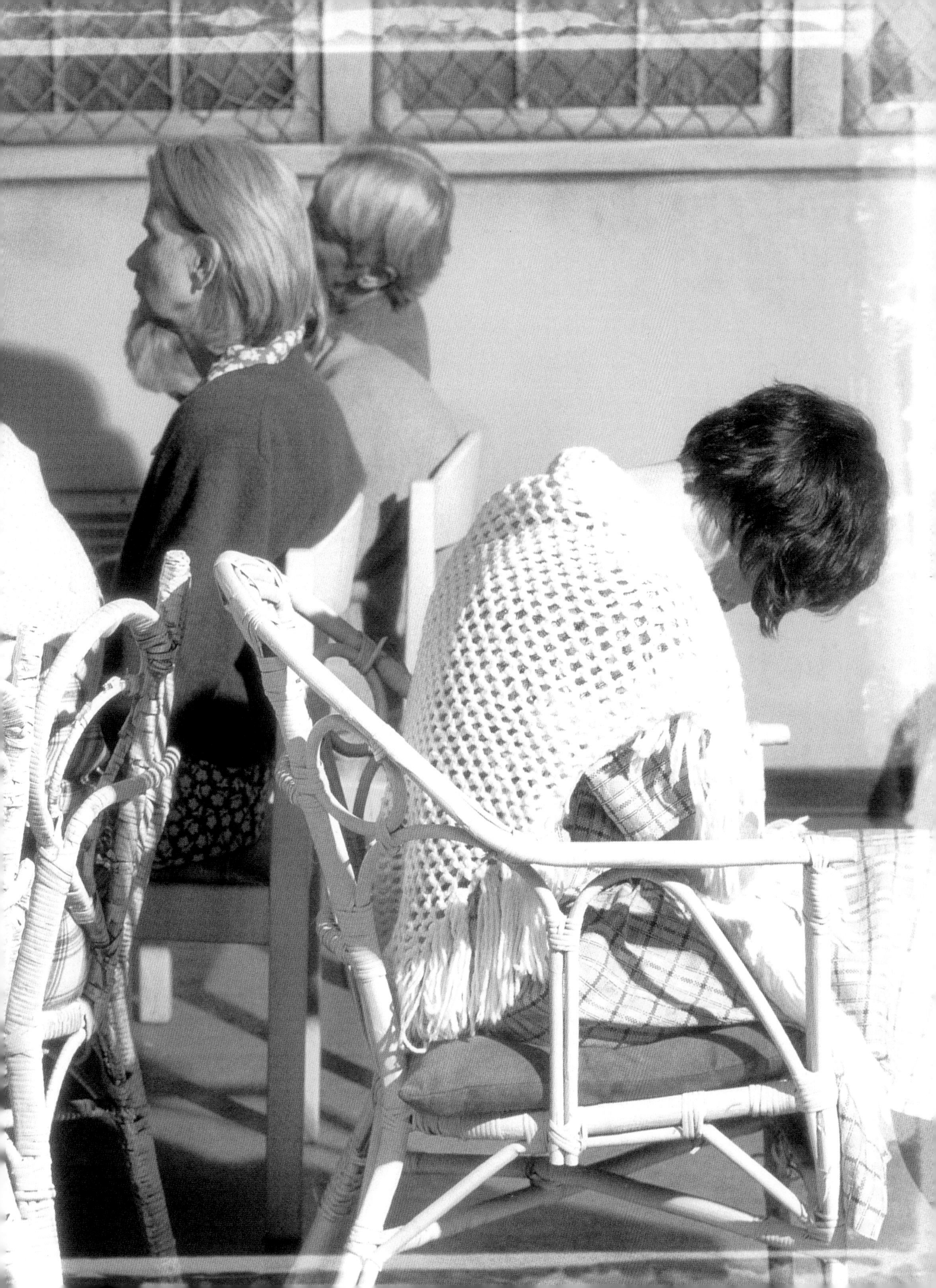

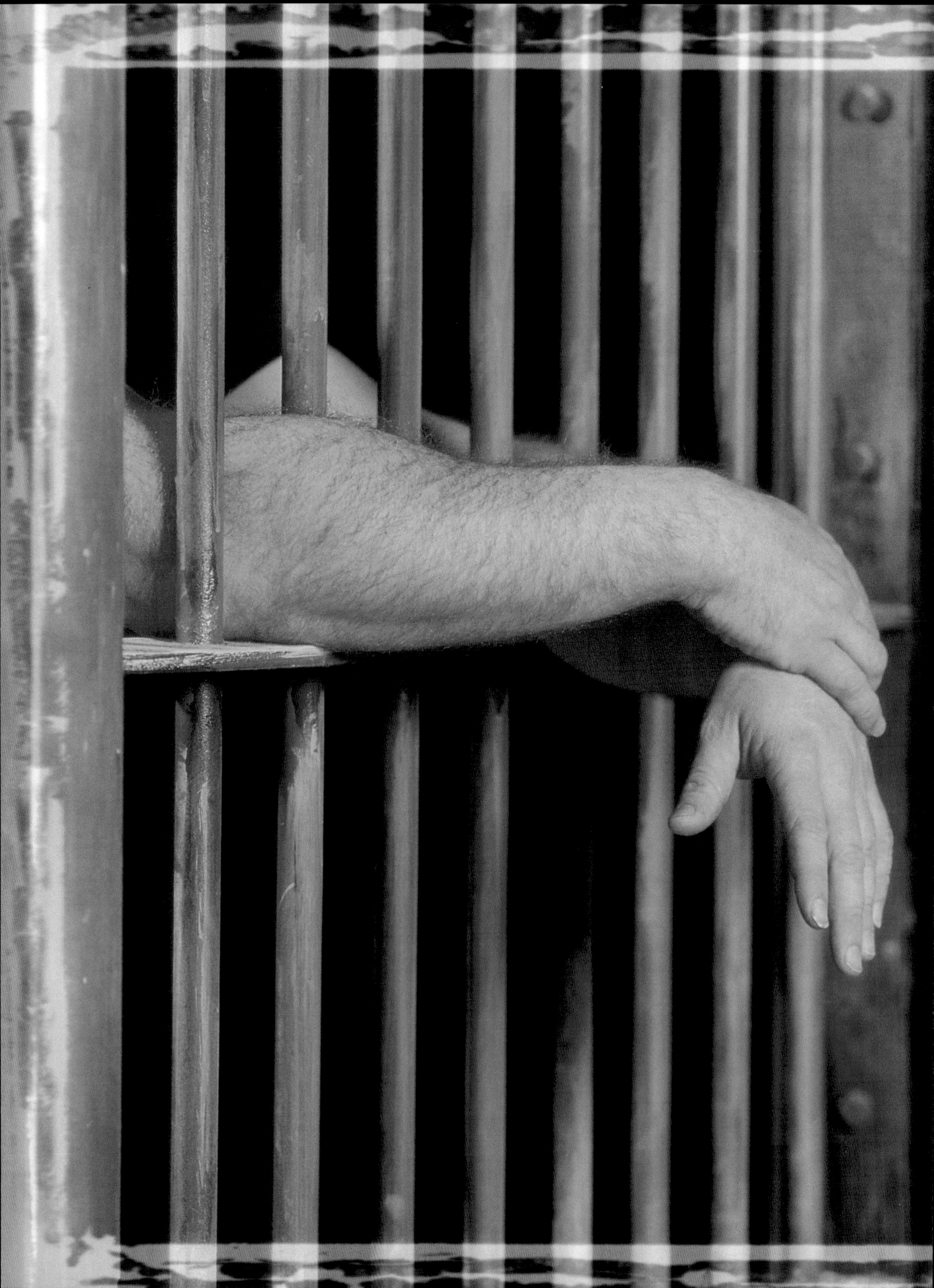

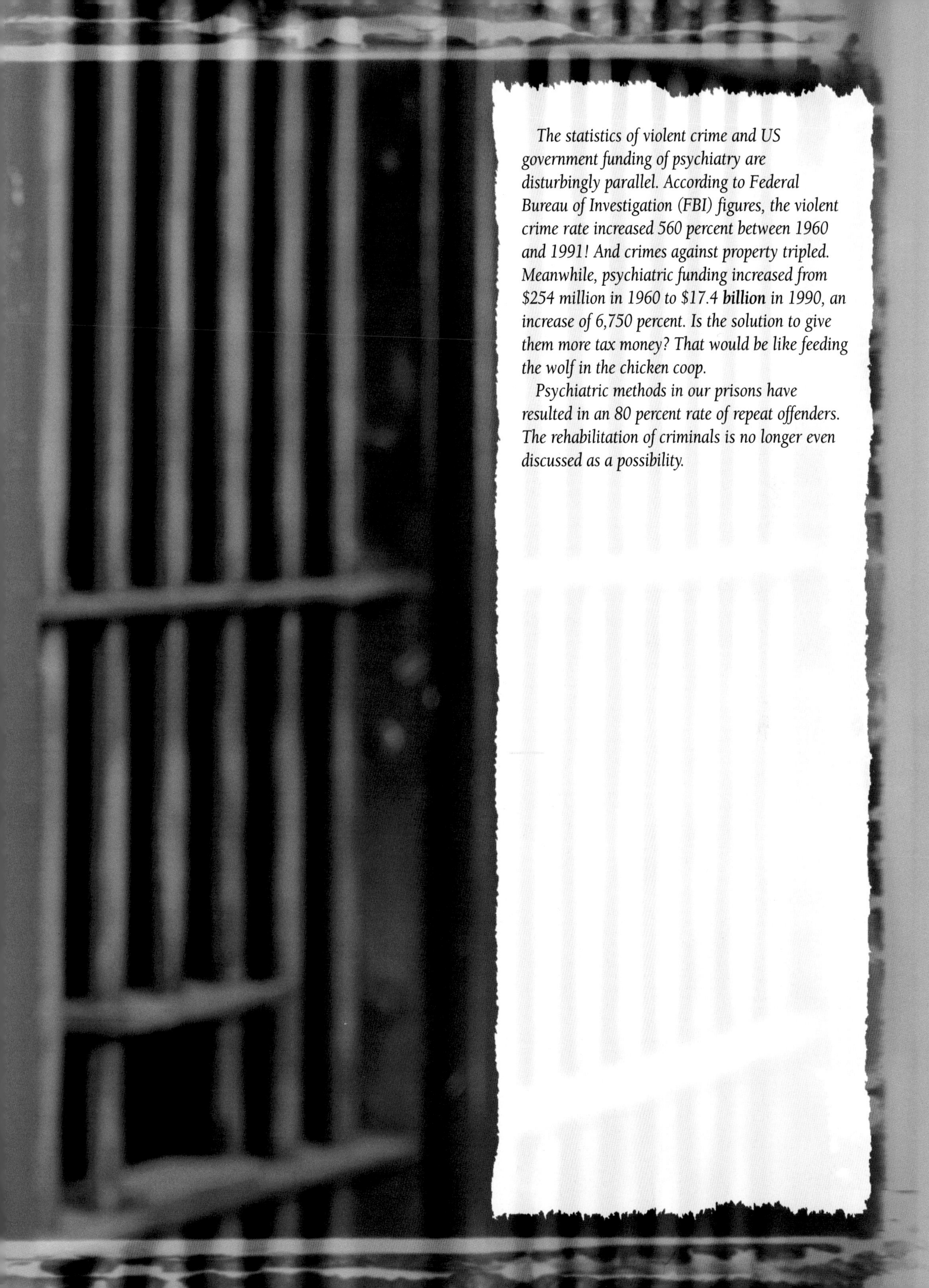

The statistics of violent crime and US government funding of psychiatry are disturbingly parallel. According to Federal Bureau of Investigation (FBI) figures, the violent crime rate increased 560 percent between 1960 and 1991! And crimes against property tripled. Meanwhile, psychiatric funding increased from $254 million in 1960 to $17.4 **billion** *in 1990, an increase of 6,750 percent. Is the solution to give them more tax money? That would be like feeding the wolf in the chicken coop.*

Psychiatric methods in our prisons have resulted in an 80 percent rate of repeat offenders. The rehabilitation of criminals is no longer even discussed as a possibility.

And ever since psychiatry began to meddle in matters between men and women, counseling them, filling popular magazines with their "solutions," and influencing the messages put forth by our gullible philosophers and artists, interpersonal relationships have, to put it kindly, become more strained than at any earlier time. If divorce rates continue to increase during the next twenty-five years as much as they did in the last, divorces will outnumber marriages in the United States.

Morally, mankind has often skated on thin ice, but it could be argued that the ice has never been as thin as it is today. In virtually every arena of life—from business to politics to our young—morals are at a low ebb. This too can be traced to materialistic ideas. If everything is material, who can say what is moral or immoral? Who can truly pin responsibility anywhere? Psychiatry? No field in the humanities or sciences is more ethically bankrupt than psychiatry, which encourages licentiousness as therapy in many cases, avidly chases the dollar without providing any valuable product in return, and heavily attacks the entire concept of morality—right and wrong. Many aspects of society have suffered for it. Psychiatrists have the stated goal of redefining the concepts of right and wrong to suit the arrogant-beyond-belief attitude they are the ones best suited to shape mankind's values and his future. And this from people who have the highest suicide rate of any profession.

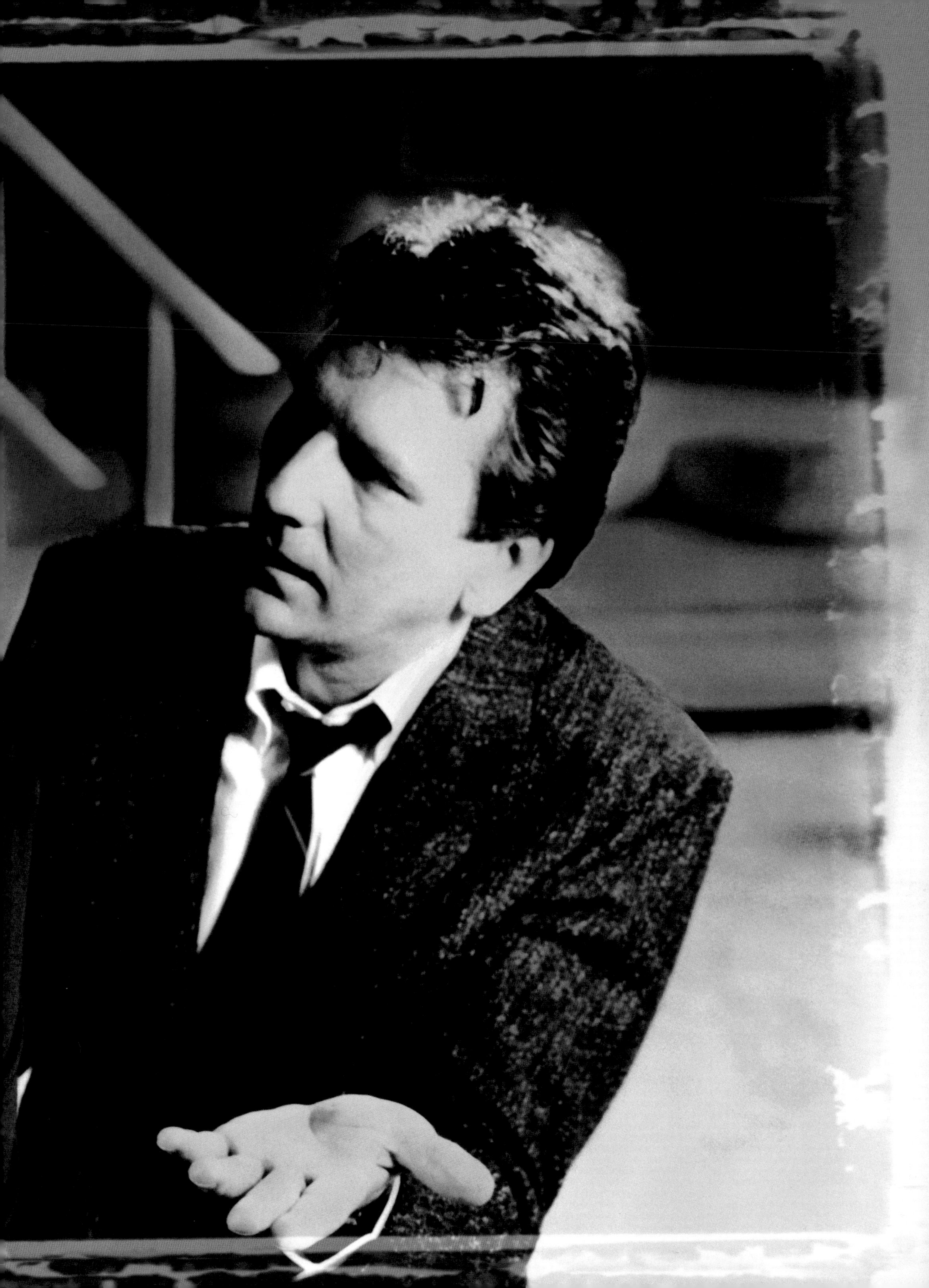

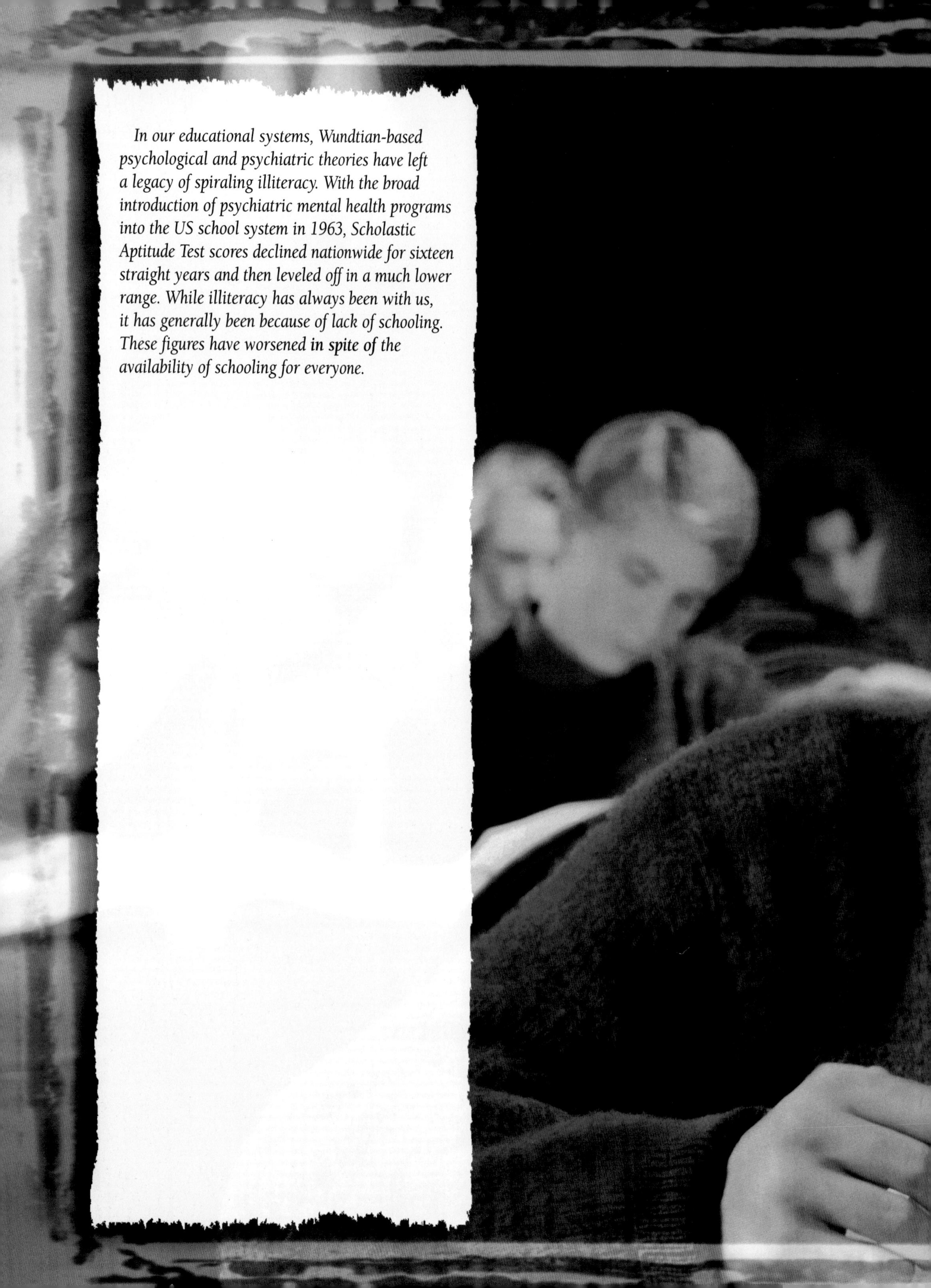

In our educational systems, Wundtian-based psychological and psychiatric theories have left a legacy of spiraling illiteracy. With the broad introduction of psychiatric mental health programs into the US school system in 1963, Scholastic Aptitude Test scores declined nationwide for sixteen straight years and then leveled off in a much lower range. While illiteracy has always been with us, it has generally been because of lack of schooling. These figures have worsened **in spite of** *the availability of schooling for everyone.*

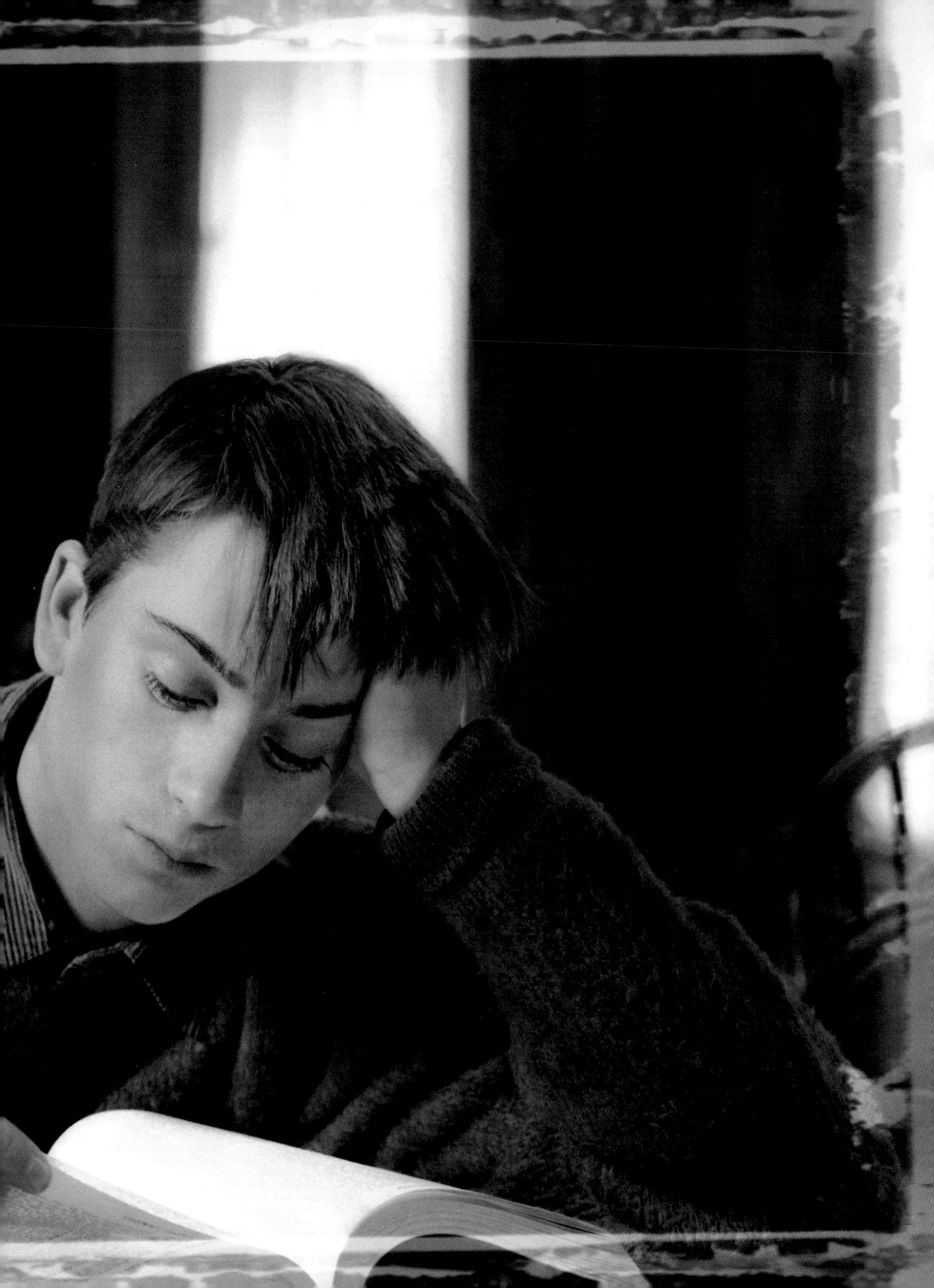

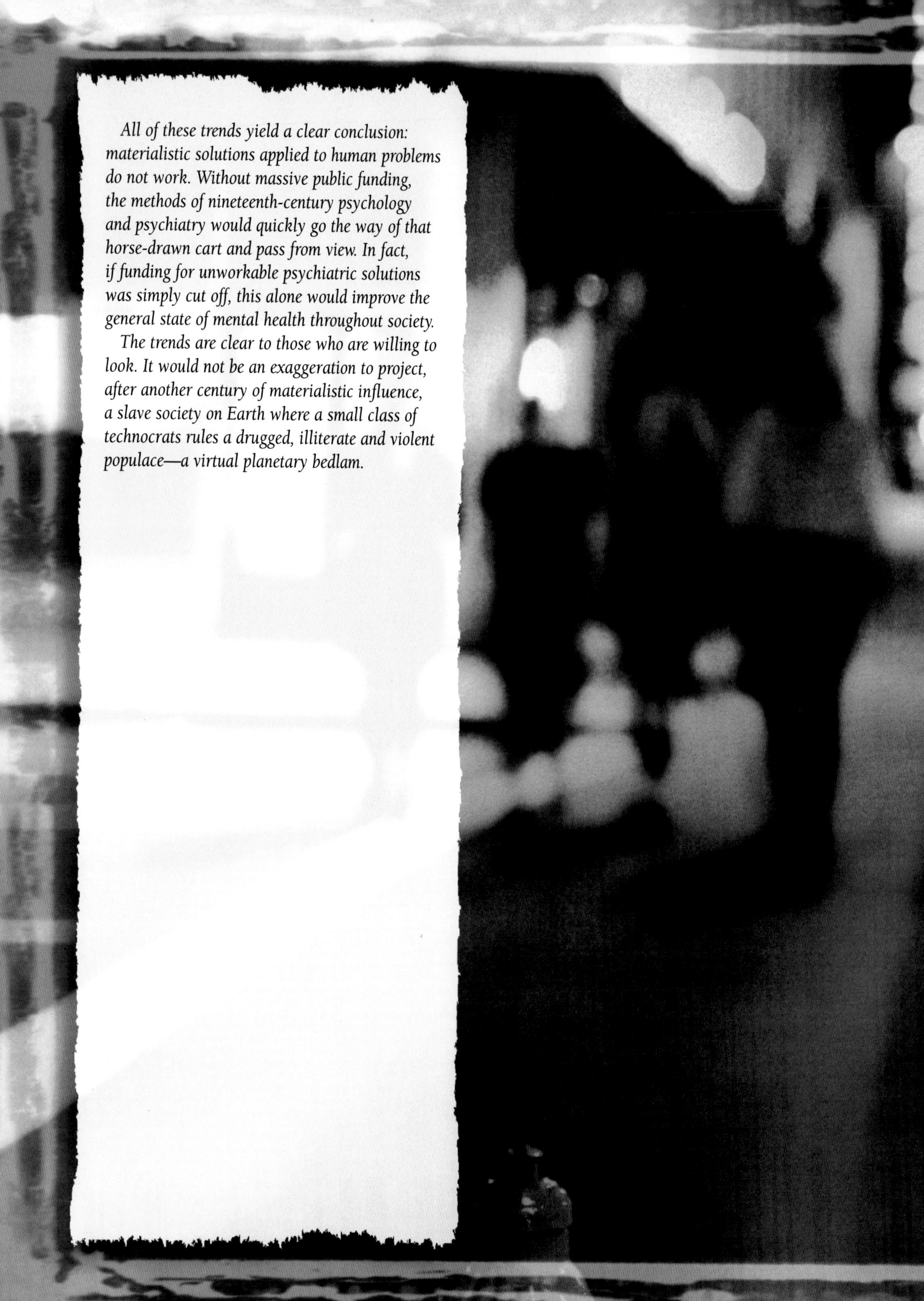

All of these trends yield a clear conclusion: materialistic solutions applied to human problems do not work. Without massive public funding, the methods of nineteenth-century psychology and psychiatry would quickly go the way of that horse-drawn cart and pass from view. In fact, if funding for unworkable psychiatric solutions was simply cut off, this alone would improve the general state of mental health throughout society.

The trends are clear to those who are willing to look. It would not be an exaggeration to project, after another century of materialistic influence, a slave society on Earth where a small class of technocrats rules a drugged, illiterate and violent populace—a virtual planetary bedlam.

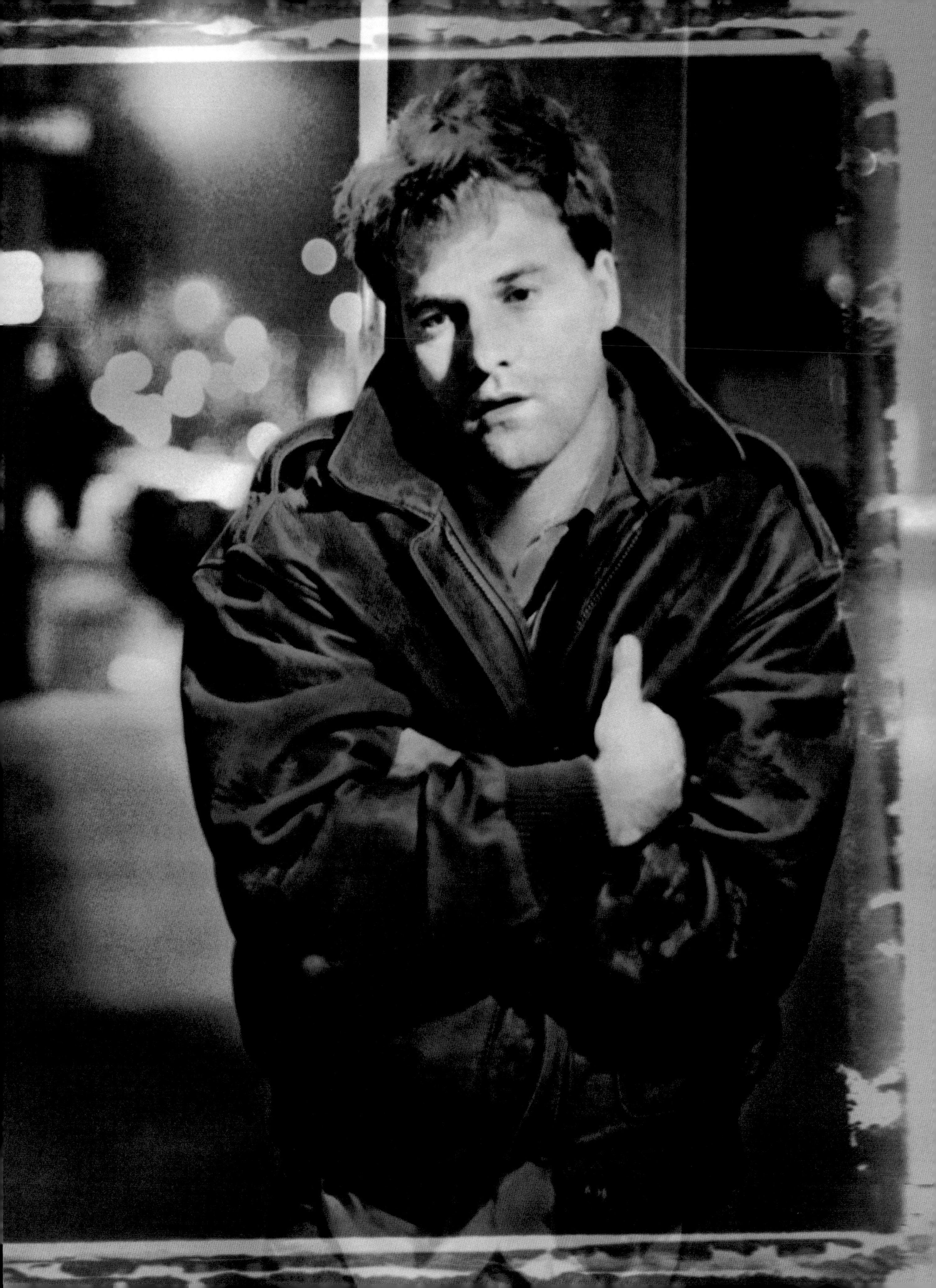

The Flaw in the Theory

No matter how many mechanical tricks the materialist can demonstrate through manipulation of matter, his basic assumption contained a serious flaw. Experimental psychology has never produced one convincing explanation for feelings, memories, expectations, desires, beliefs, thoughts, imaginings or intentions. Materialism cannot account for either the towering clouds of sound in a Beethoven symphony or the sense of delight in a child's laughter. By denying even the possibility that life itself was influenced by something other than mechanical factors, the materialist started off in a hole out of which he has never been able to dig himself.

And he ignored one of the most powerful forces in man.

If man is not an animal, as Wundt declared him to be, then what other view is there?

As Mr. Hubbard describes in his essay **Religious Influence in Society**, *it is no coincidence that the declining influence of religion in our society has seen a large increase in our problems.*

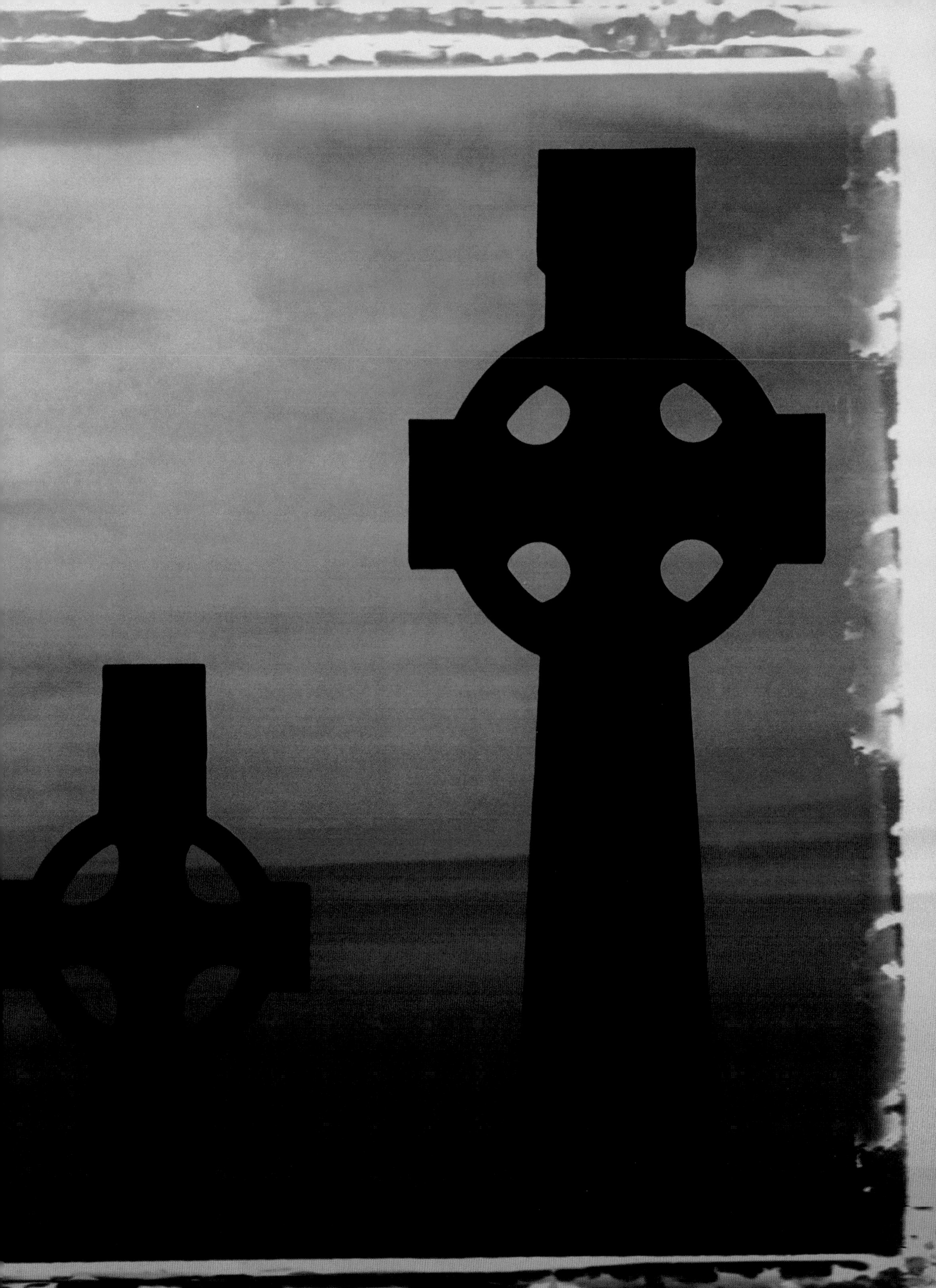

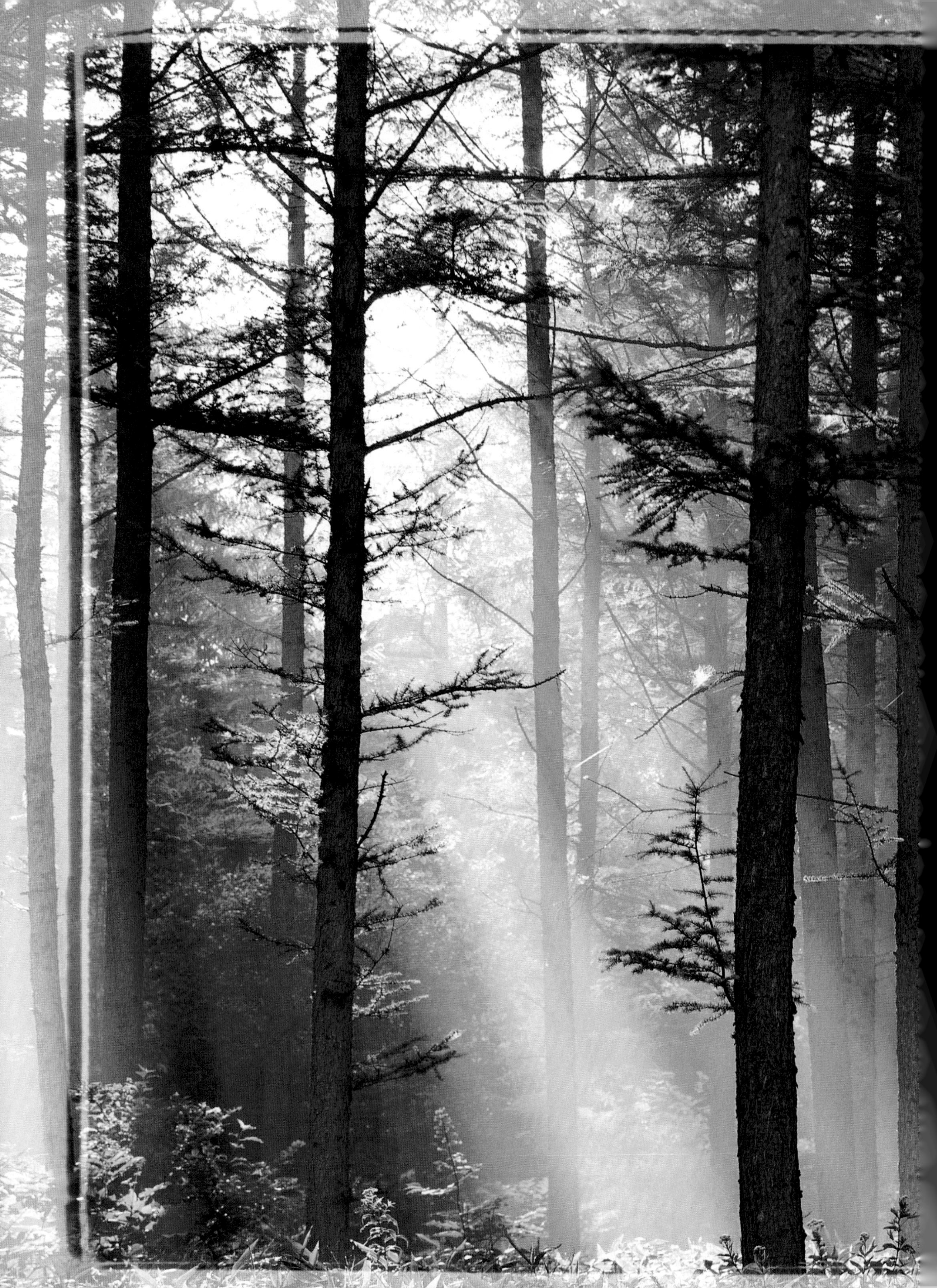

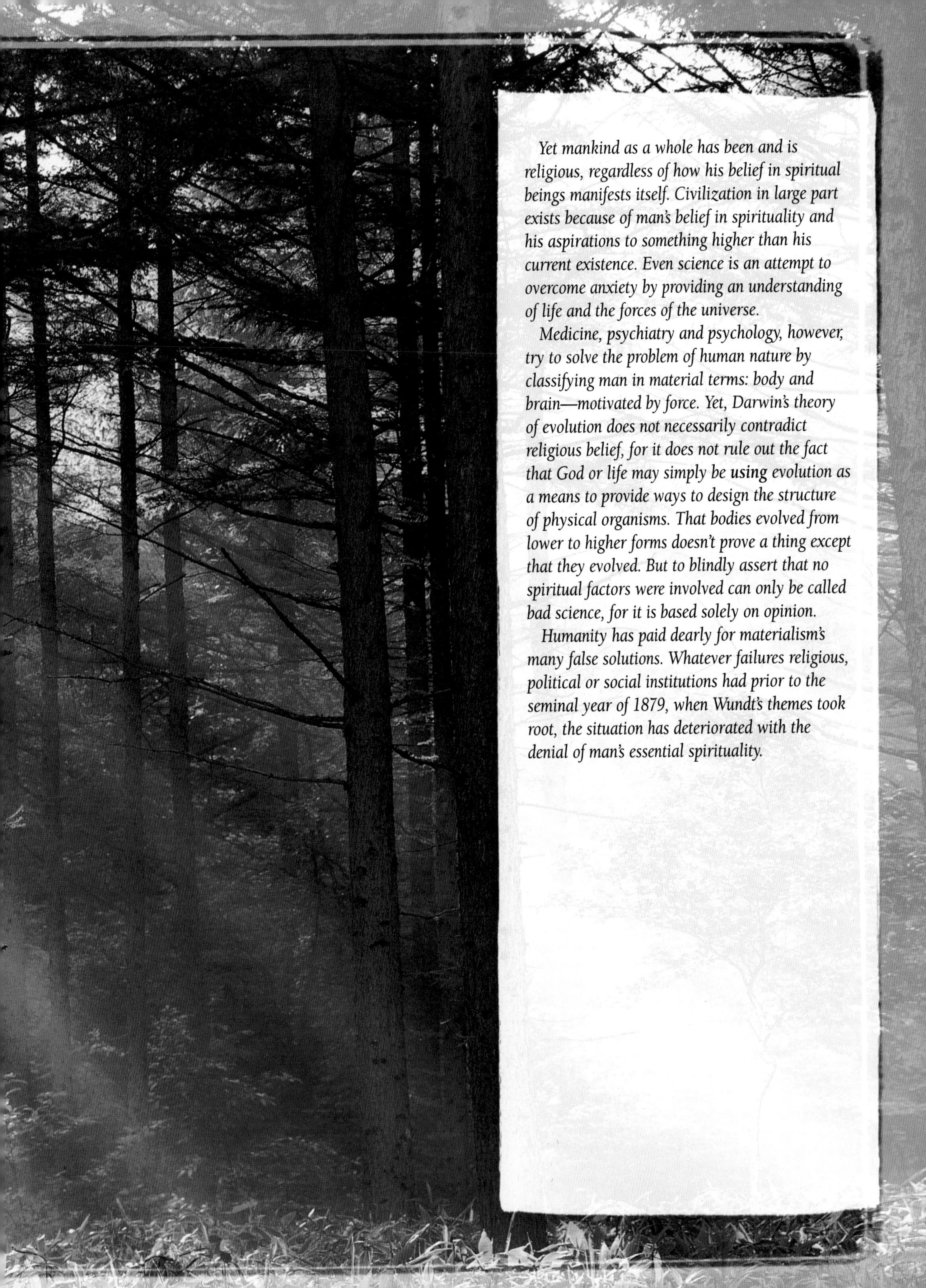

Yet mankind as a whole has been and is religious, regardless of how his belief in spiritual beings manifests itself. Civilization in large part exists because of man's belief in spirituality and his aspirations to something higher than his current existence. Even science is an attempt to overcome anxiety by providing an understanding of life and the forces of the universe.

Medicine, psychiatry and psychology, however, try to solve the problem of human nature by classifying man in material terms: body and brain—motivated by force. Yet, Darwin's theory of evolution does not necessarily contradict religious belief, for it does not rule out the fact that God or life may simply be using evolution as a means to provide ways to design the structure of physical organisms. That bodies evolved from lower to higher forms doesn't prove a thing except that they evolved. But to blindly assert that no spiritual factors were involved can only be called bad science, for it is based solely on opinion.

Humanity has paid dearly for materialism's many false solutions. Whatever failures religious, political or social institutions had prior to the seminal year of 1879, when Wundt's themes took root, the situation has deteriorated with the denial of man's essential spirituality.

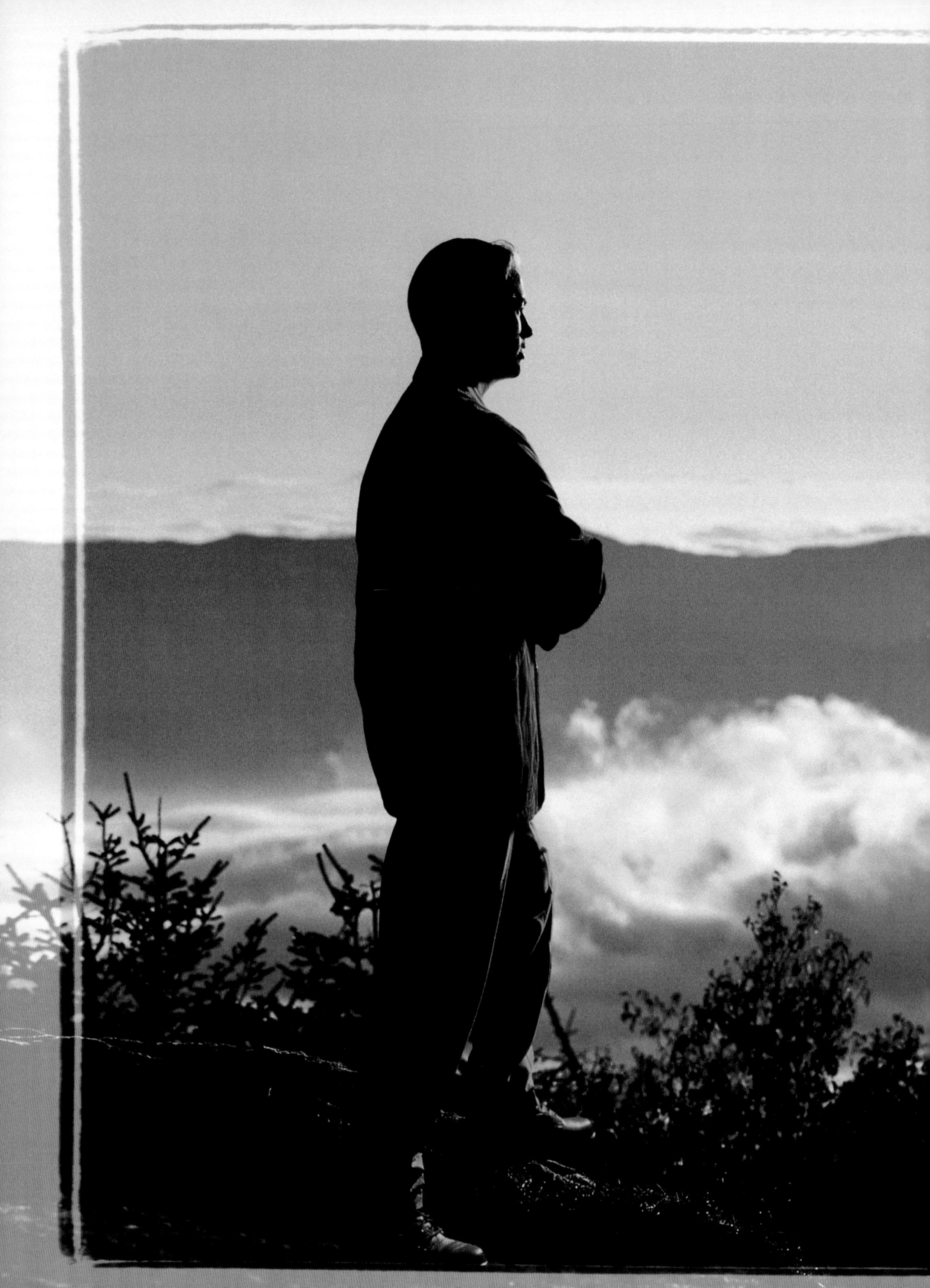

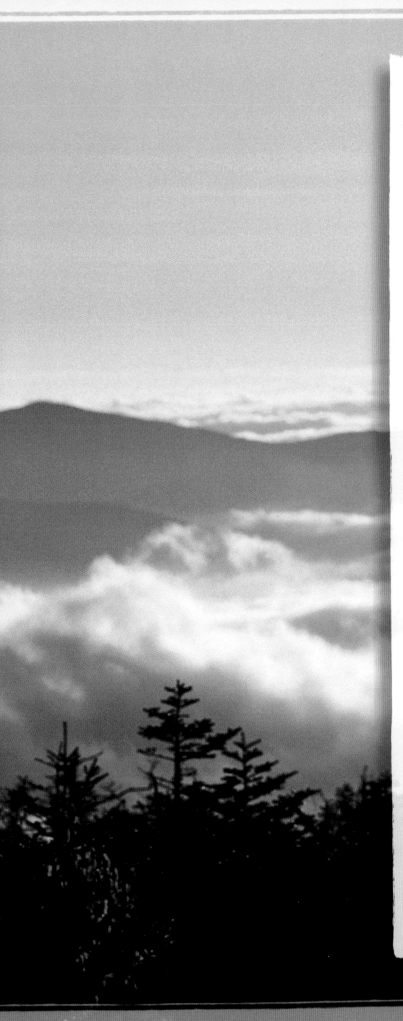

A New Hope for Man

In 1950, something new appeared. L. Ron Hubbard, who had traveled extensively in the Orient and been educated in Western science, broke through the barrier of ignorance that had stifled man's progress in the humanities. The result was an entirely new subject, Scientology, which means "knowing about knowing."

Scientology is an applied religious philosophy which contains workable answers to the problems people face in their lives. The subject matter of Scientology is **all** *life. It contains practical means through which predictable improvement can be obtained in any area to which it is applied.*

The philosophies of materialism and dualism can, and have been, endlessly argued, for they are opinions and not based on any hard evidence. Today, Scientology has the evidence to prove the existence of man's spiritual nature. It is based upon thousands of research hours and the results attained by millions of people.

Scientology recognizes that man is not just so many vials of chemicals fortuitously combined into a remarkable stimulus-response machine. Scientology views man as a spiritual being with native capabilities which can be improved far beyond what is generally believed possible. In fact, it has been demonstrated that man deteriorates to the degree that he denies his spiritual nature and ceases to live with moral values, such as trust, honesty, integrity and other sometimes intangible characteristics.

By seeing man as essentially spiritual, Scientology follows in the traditional view of man and his relationship to the universe. Scientology, however, is unique in that it contains practical means of enabling man to resolve his material concerns and so come to achieve his spiritual aspirations. In this regard Scientology is an improvement over any earlier practice in terms of what it can actually **do** *to help man.*

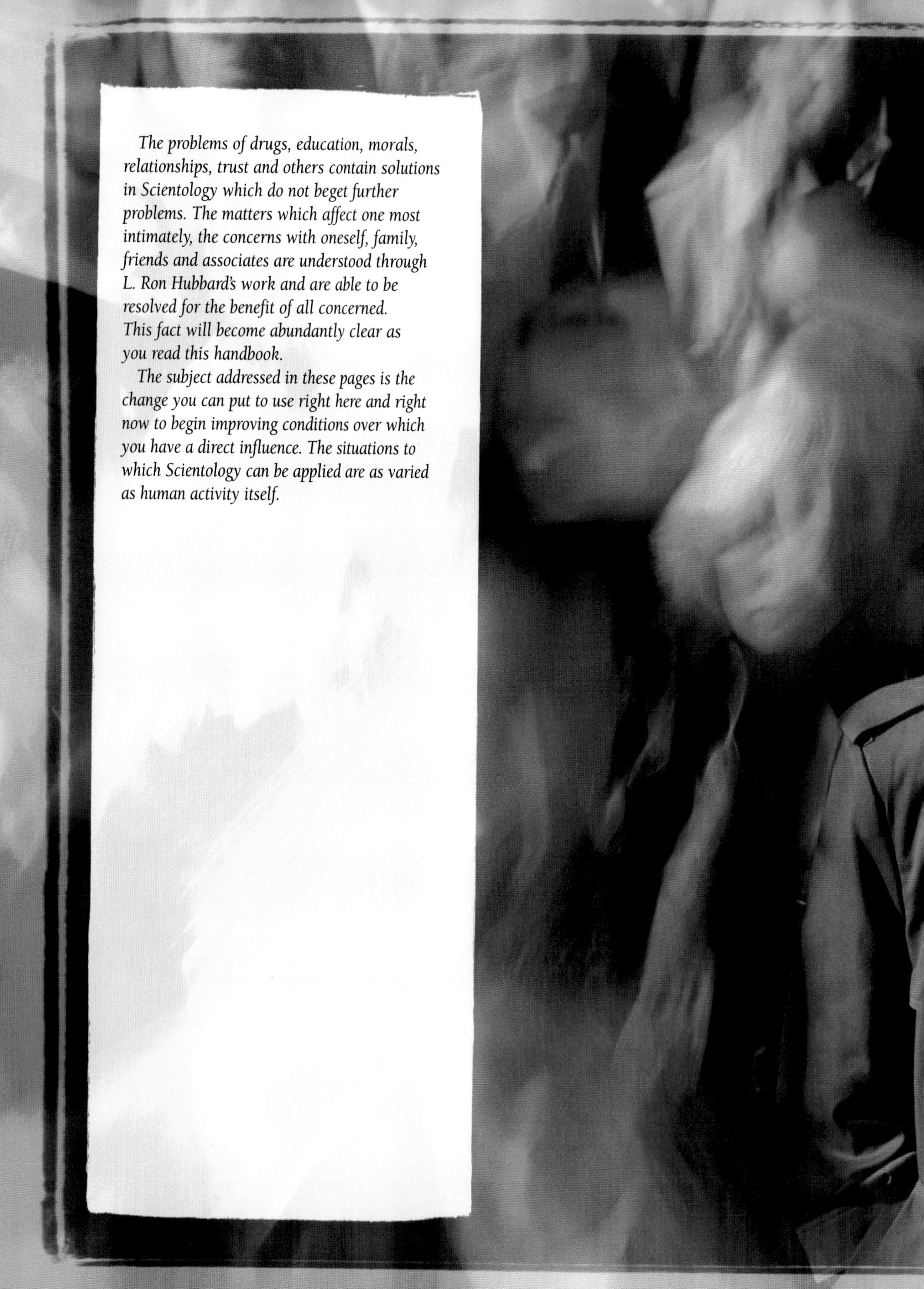

The problems of drugs, education, morals, relationships, trust and others contain solutions in Scientology which do not beget further problems. The matters which affect one most intimately, the concerns with oneself, family, friends and associates are understood through L. Ron Hubbard's work and are able to be resolved for the benefit of all concerned. This fact will become abundantly clear as you read this handbook.

The subject addressed in these pages is the change you can put to use right here and right now to begin improving conditions over which you have a direct influence. The situations to which Scientology can be applied are as varied as human activity itself.

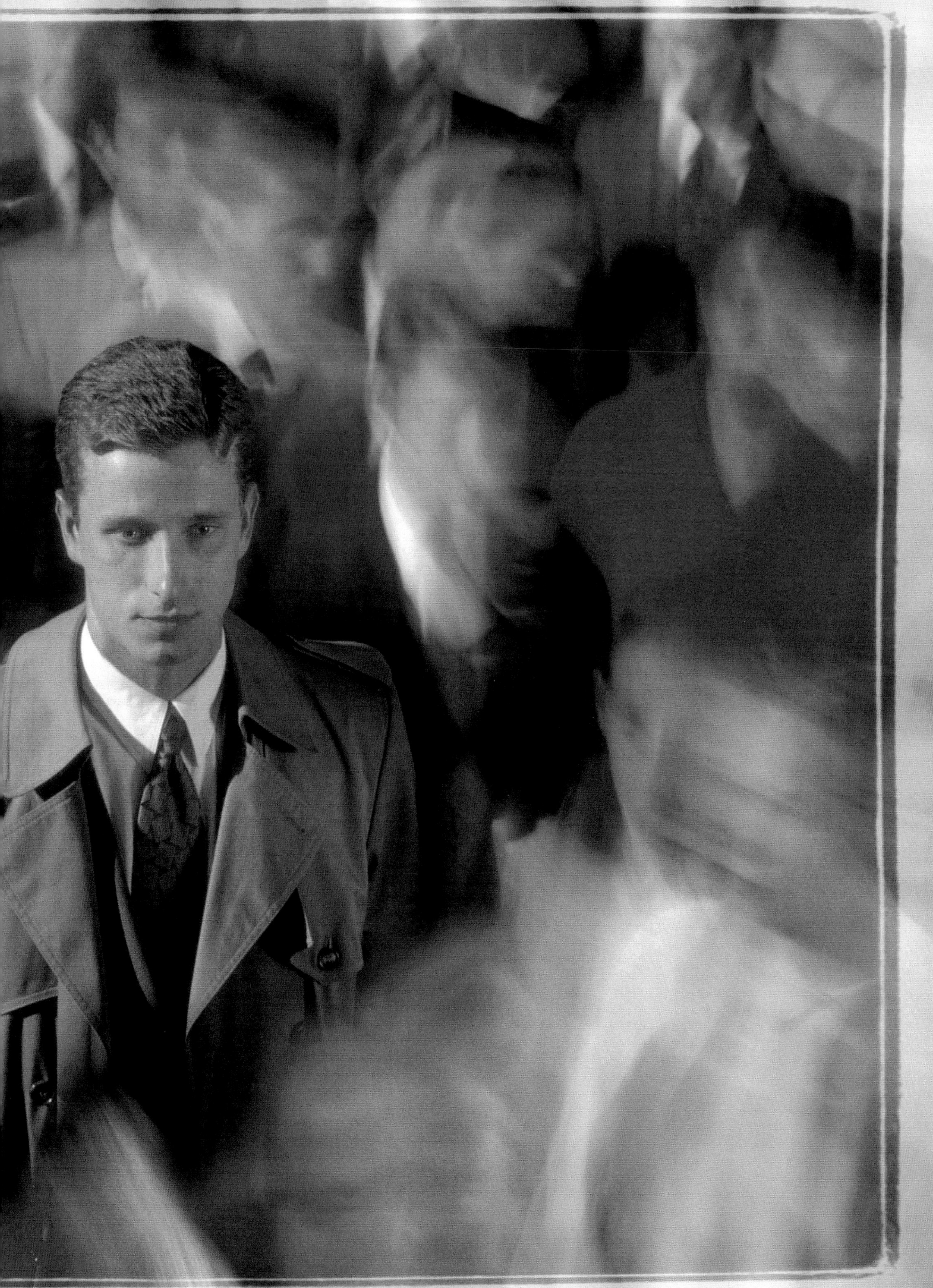

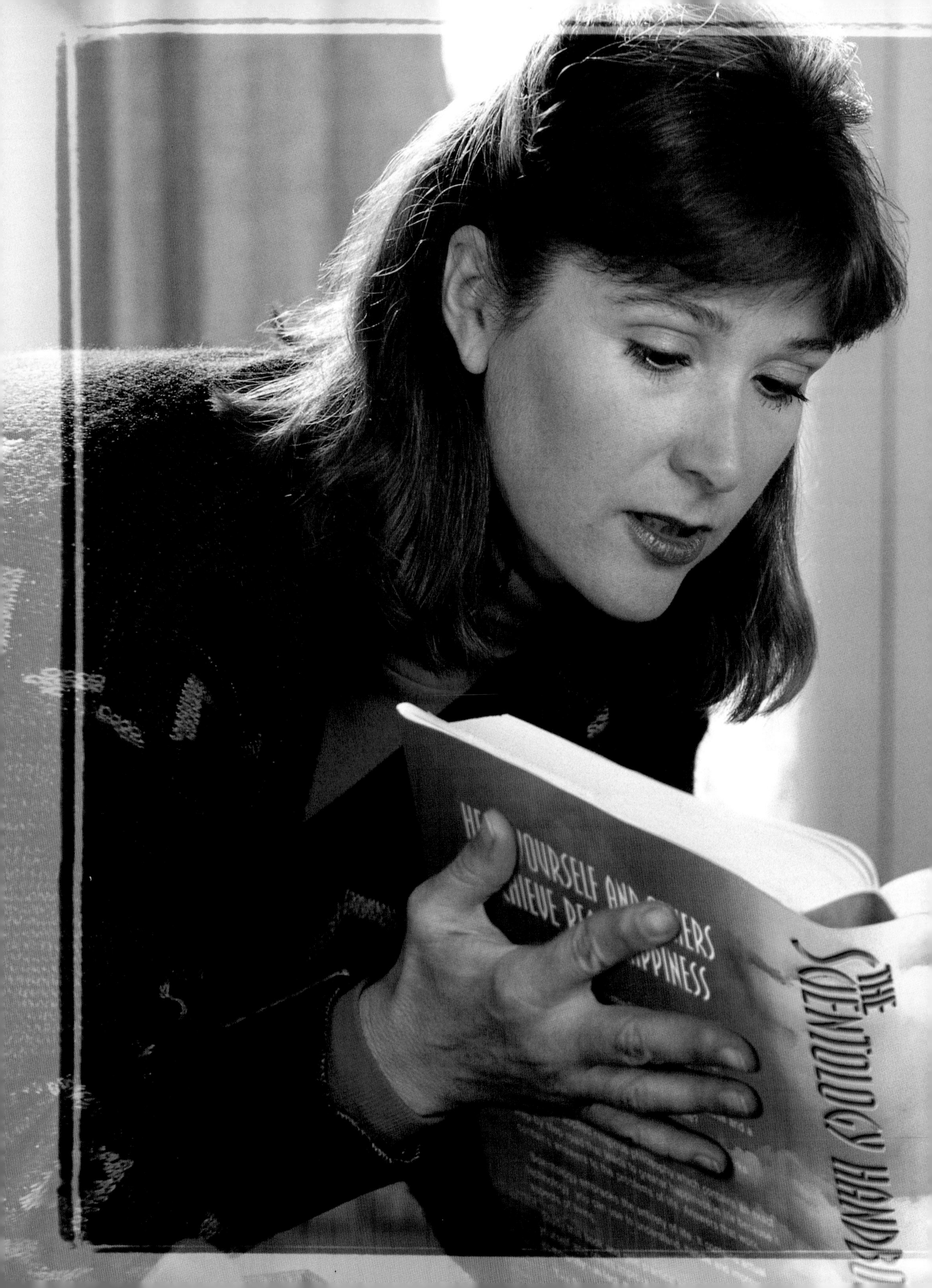
YOURSELF AND
THE

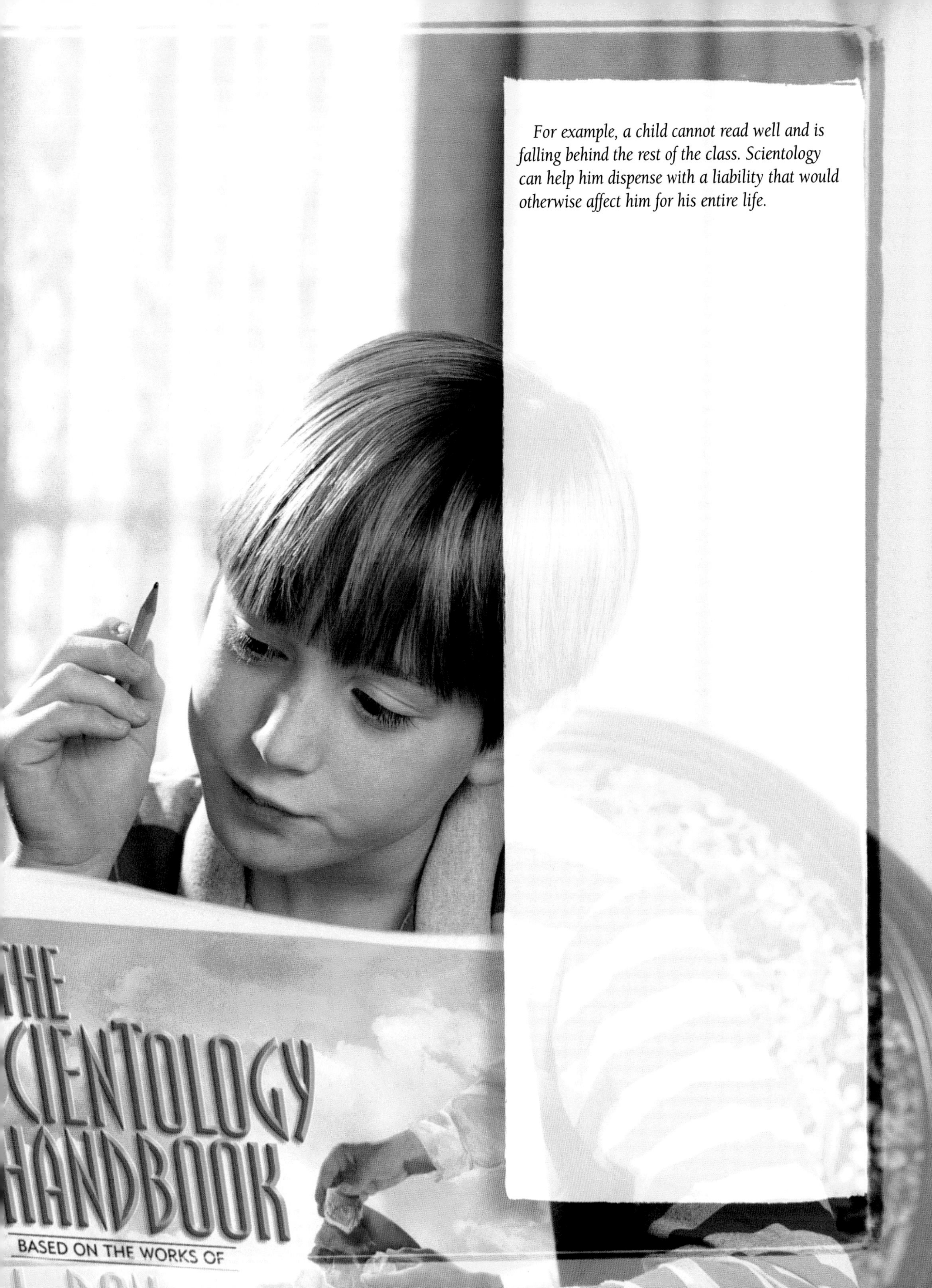

For example, a child cannot read well and is falling behind the rest of the class. Scientology can help him dispense with a liability that would otherwise affect him for his entire life.

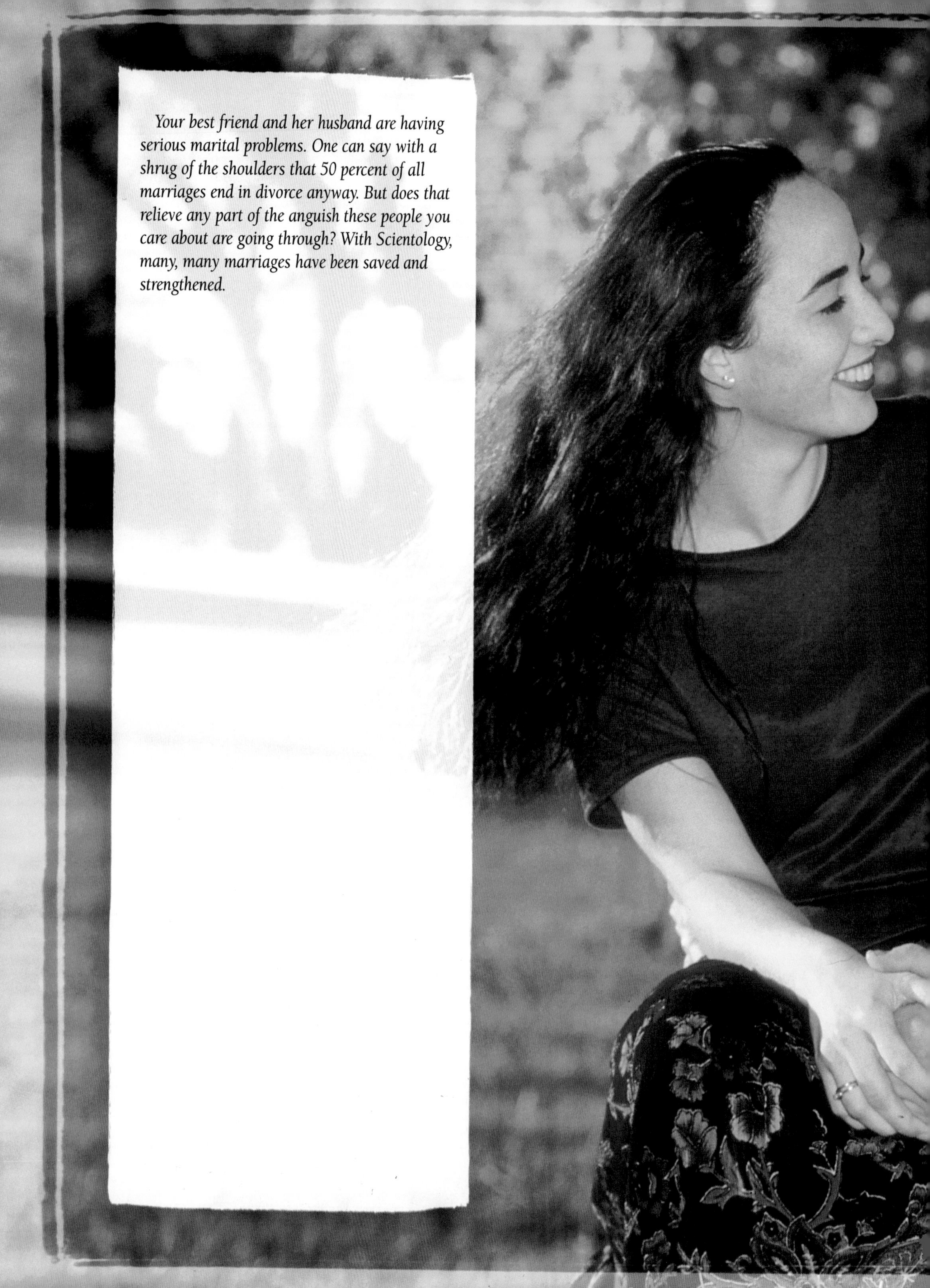

Your best friend and her husband are having serious marital problems. One can say with a shrug of the shoulders that 50 percent of all marriages end in divorce anyway. But does that relieve any part of the anguish these people you care about are going through? With Scientology, many, many marriages have been saved and strengthened.

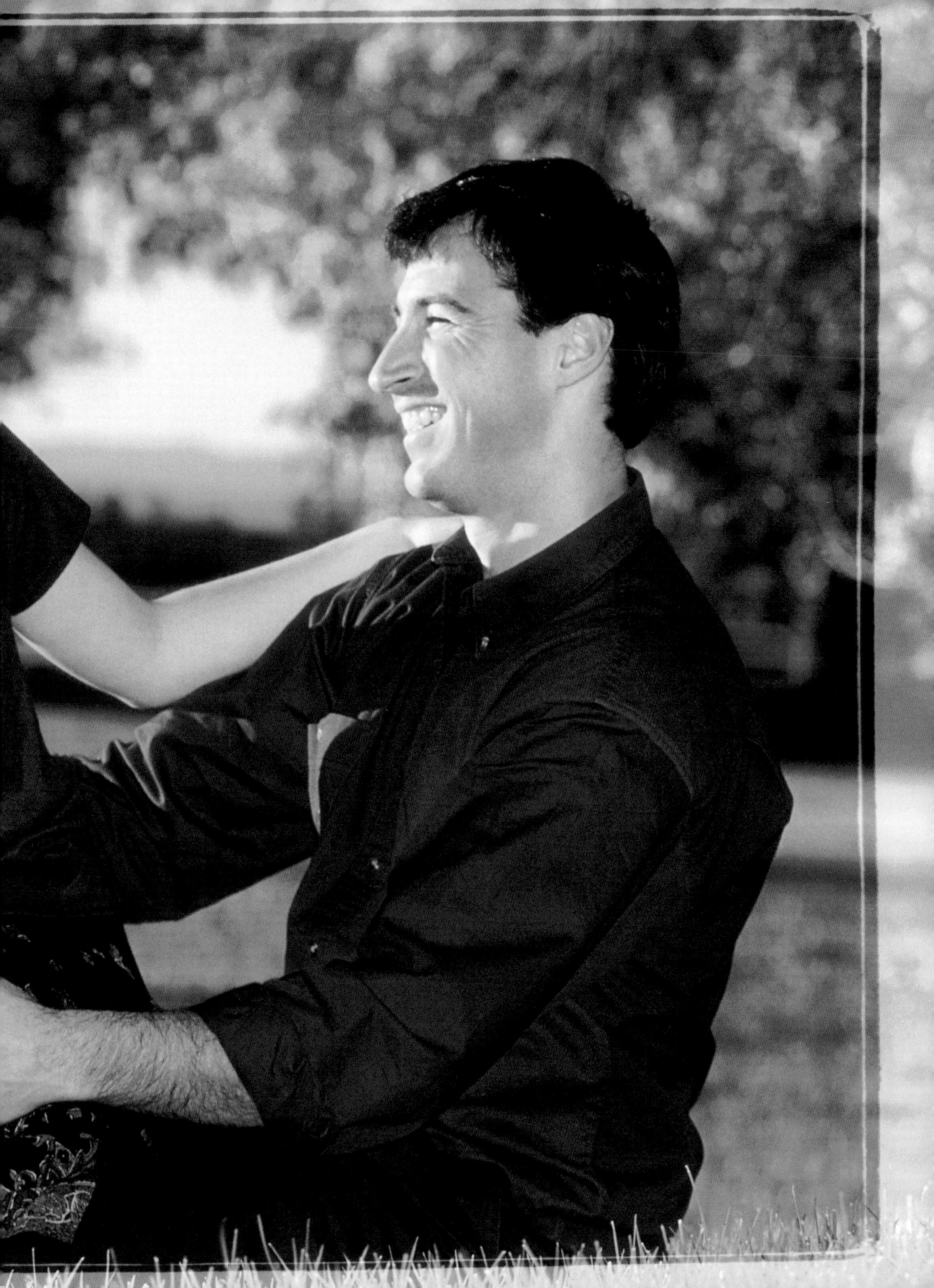

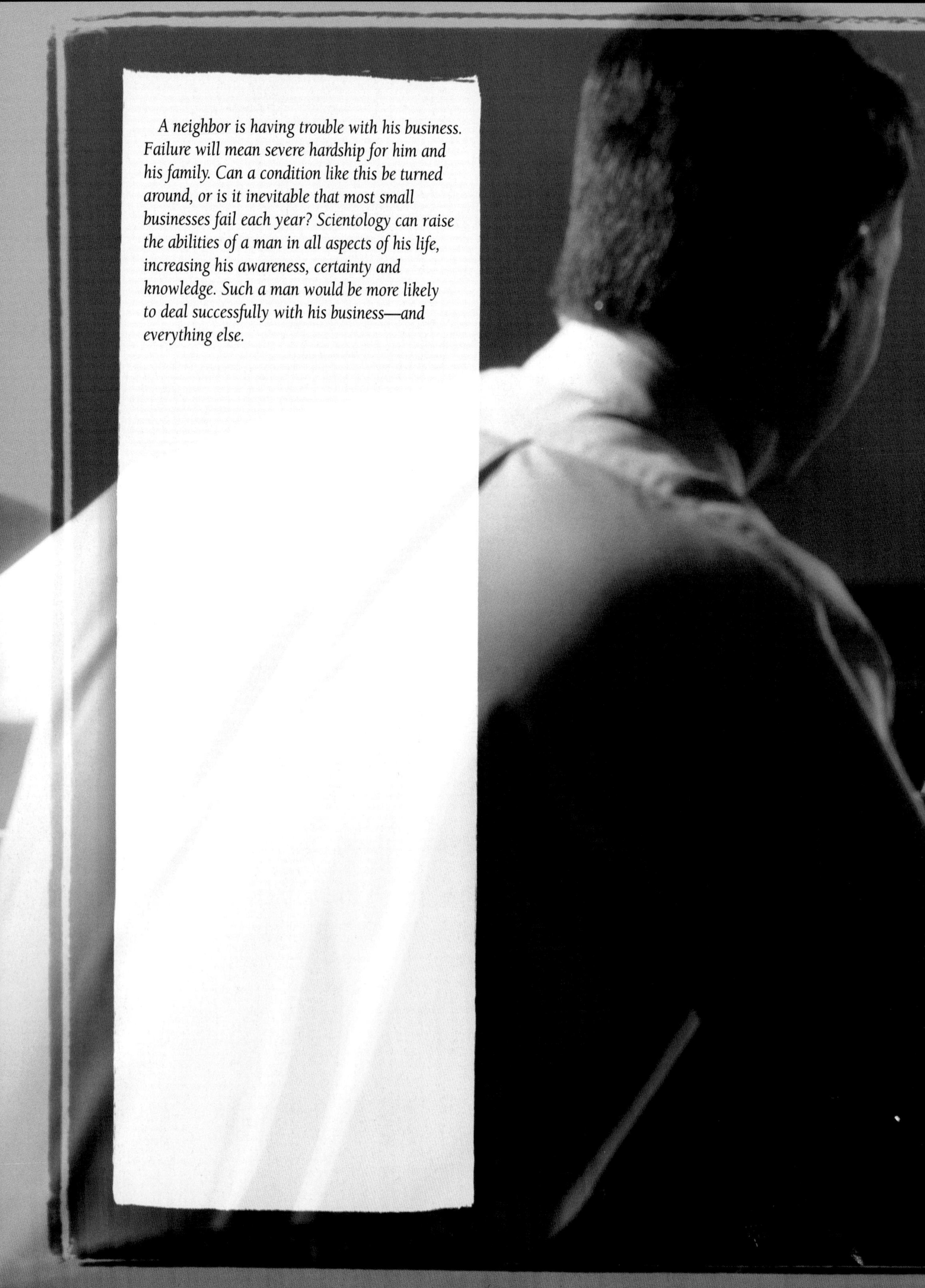

A neighbor is having trouble with his business. Failure will mean severe hardship for him and his family. Can a condition like this be turned around, or is it inevitable that most small businesses fail each year? Scientology can raise the abilities of a man in all aspects of his life, increasing his awareness, certainty and knowledge. Such a man would be more likely to deal successfully with his business—and everything else.

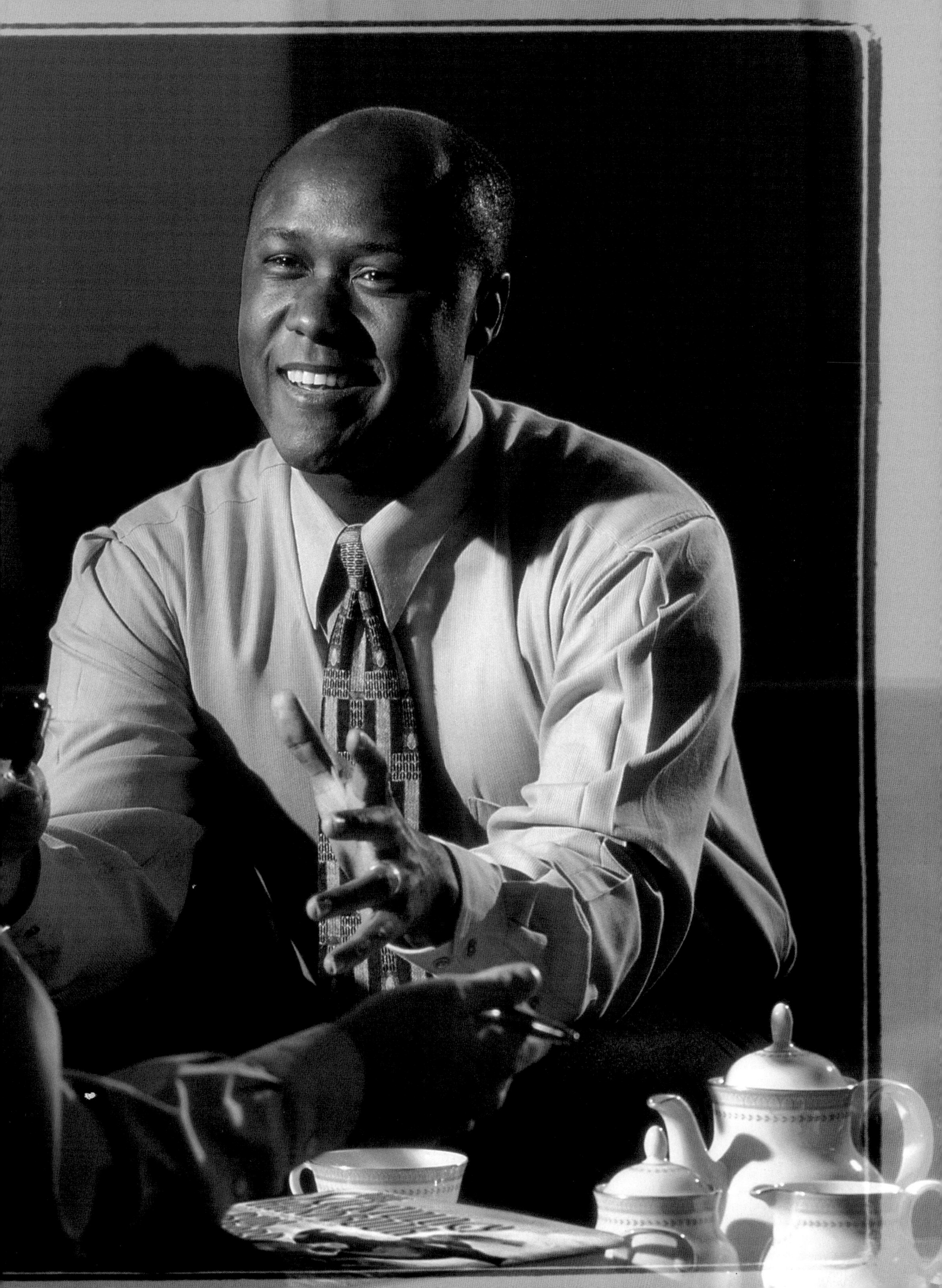

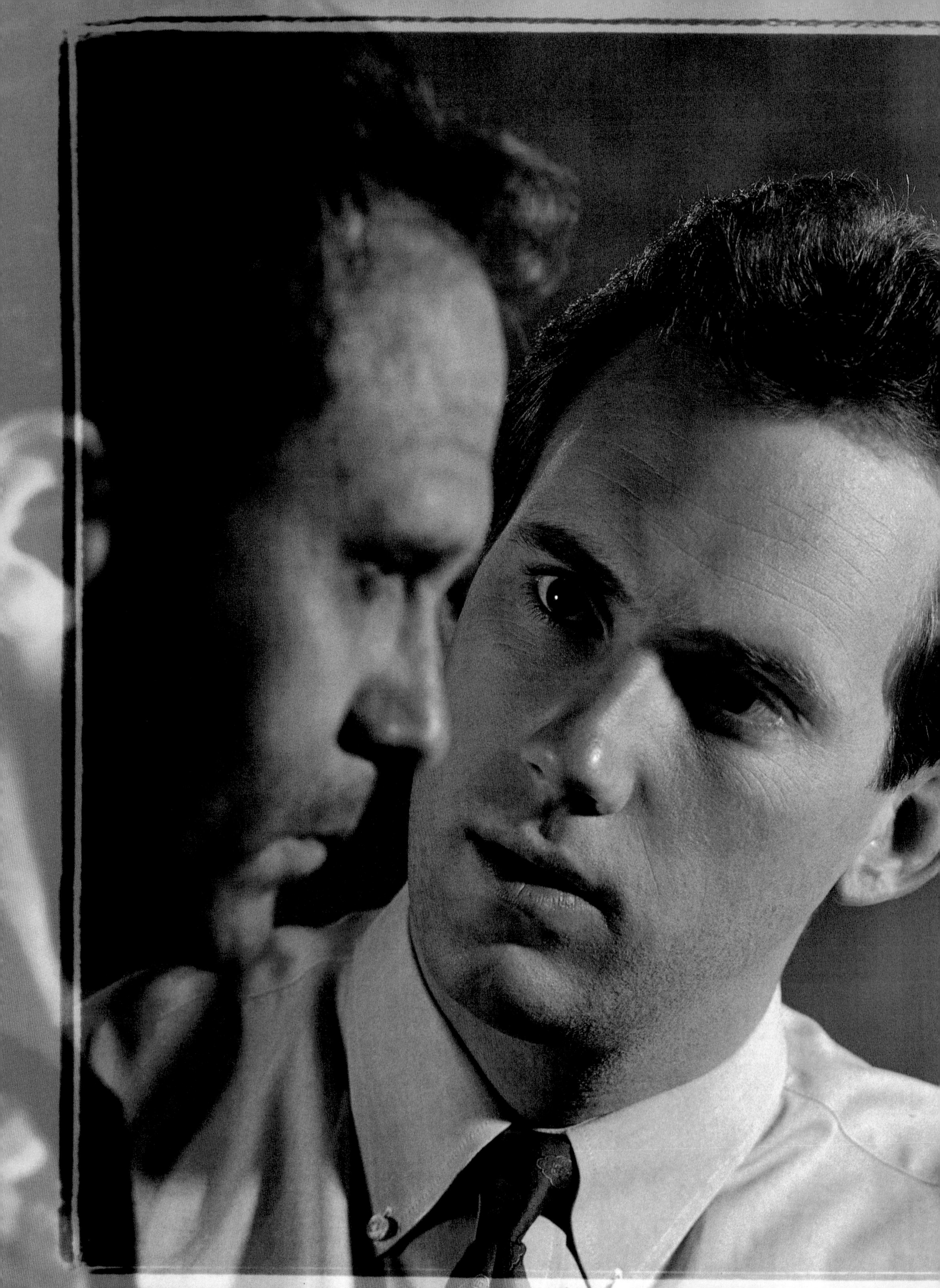

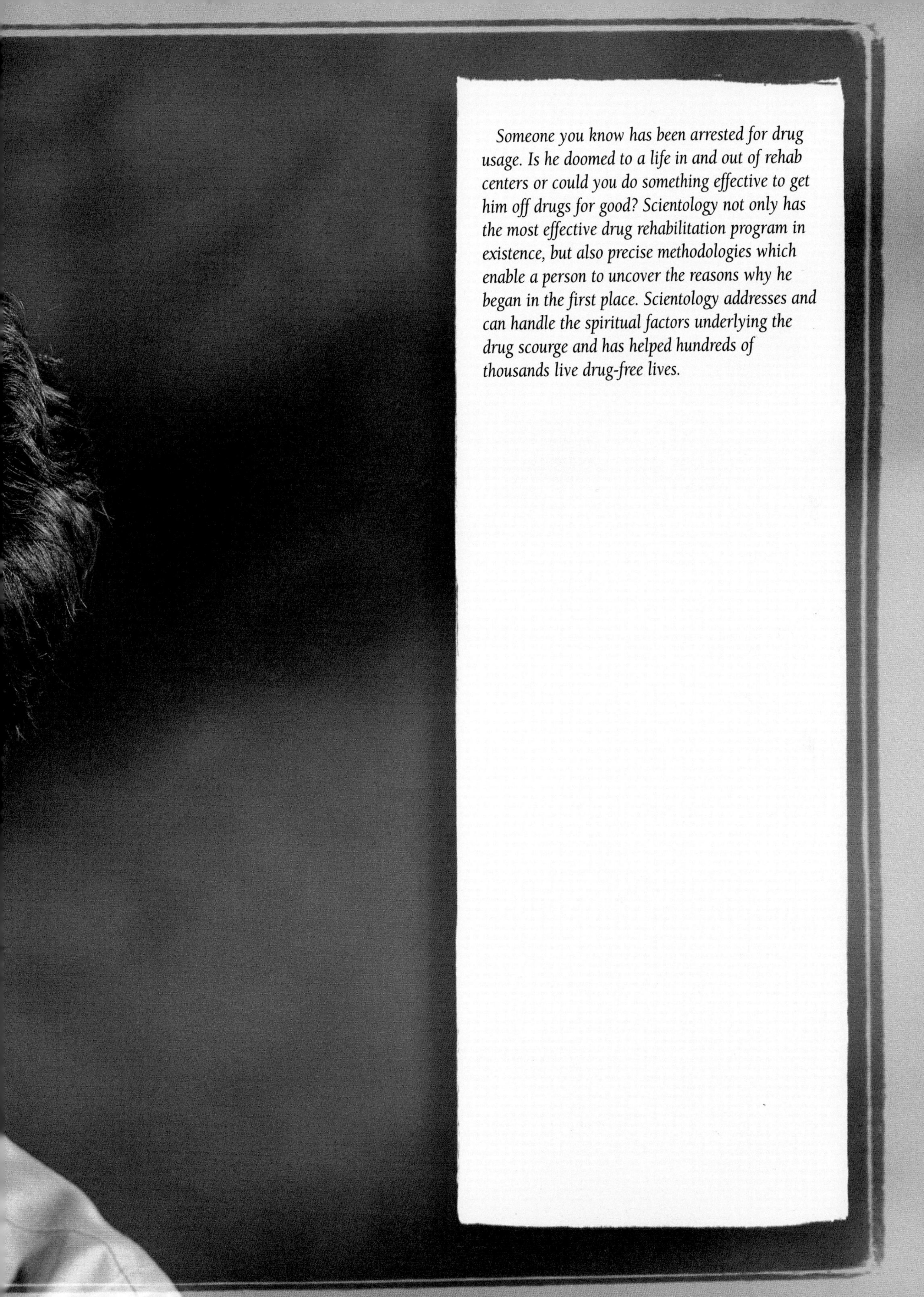

Someone you know has been arrested for drug usage. Is he doomed to a life in and out of rehab centers or could you do something effective to get him off drugs for good? Scientology not only has the most effective drug rehabilitation program in existence, but also precise methodologies which enable a person to uncover the reasons why he began in the first place. Scientology addresses and can handle the spiritual factors underlying the drug scourge and has helped hundreds of thousands live drug-free lives.

It is from the individual problems of men and women that the larger concerns of the world grow: drugs, crime, the environment, war, hatred, the economy and others. Each stems from individuals who dealt unsuccessfully, to a greater or lesser degree, with different aspects of living.

The emphasis in Scientology is on the **application** *of exact methodologies in order to bring about change in the conditions of an individual's life. Scientology's aim is to put a person into a condition where he can be more self-determined about living a happier, more fulfilling life. It is a firm conviction in Scientology that the way to a true resolution of a person's problems is to work toward putting him in a position where he is brighter and more able and where he can identify the factors of his life more easily. When this has been achieved, he has been put in a condition where he can understand the underlying sources of any situations he may face and so deal with life more successfully.*

The complete materials of Scientology contain more than forty million words in dozens of books, thousands of articles and thousands more recorded lectures. It is highly probable that this is the most extensive body of knowledge ever assembled on the subject of man, his mind, his capabilities and potentials and the different aspects of his existence.

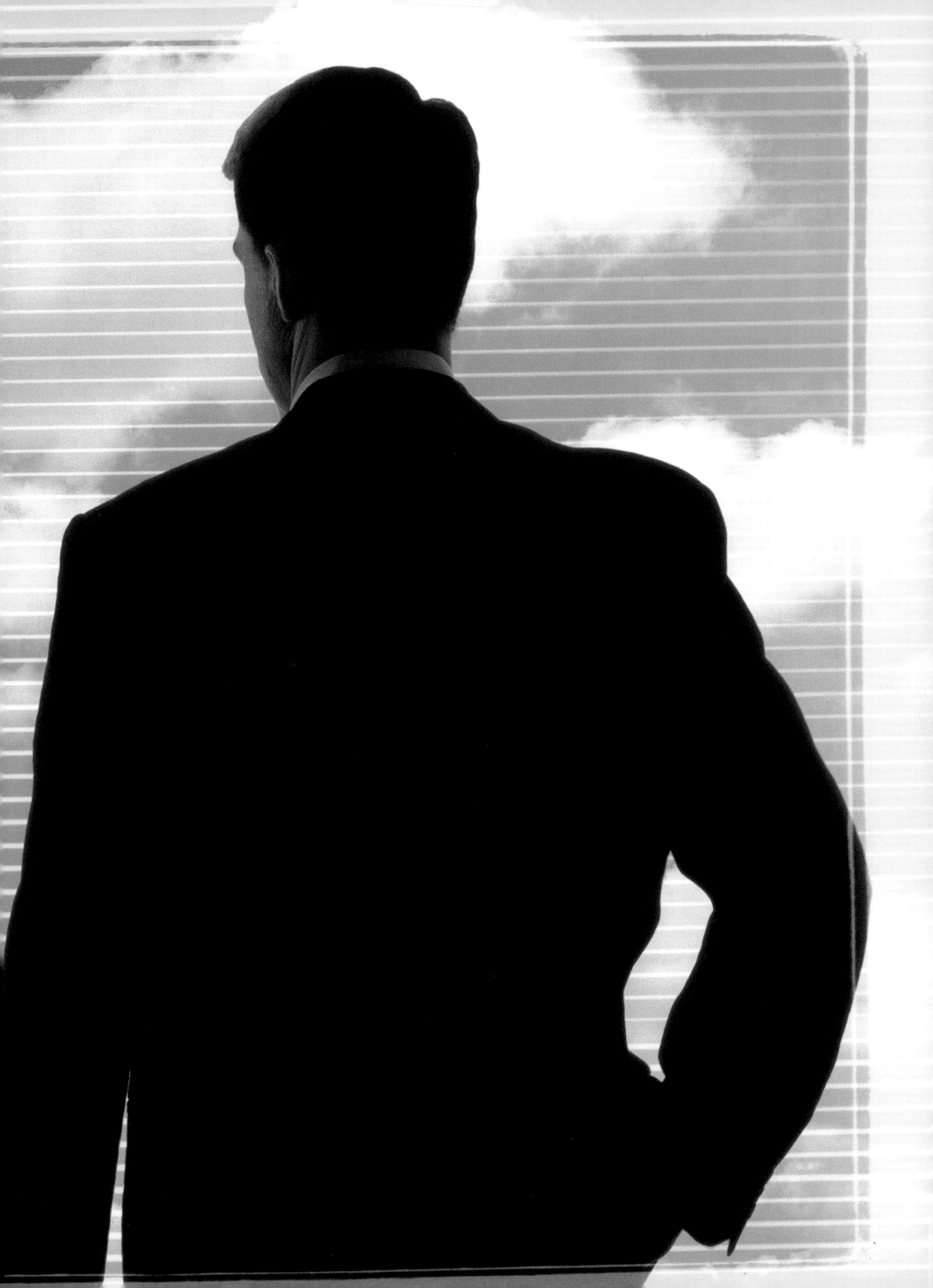

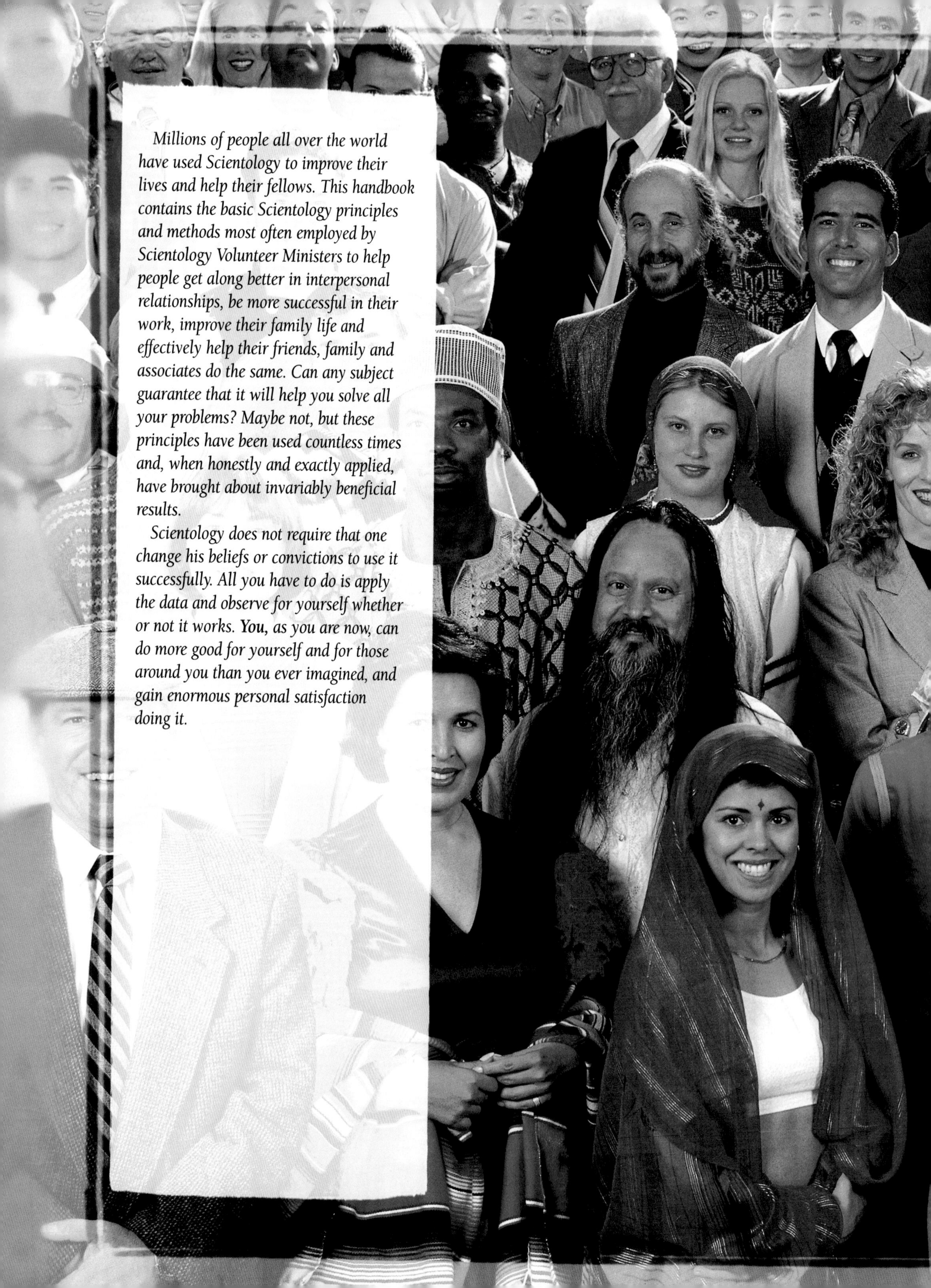

Millions of people all over the world have used Scientology to improve their lives and help their fellows. This handbook contains the basic Scientology principles and methods most often employed by Scientology Volunteer Ministers to help people get along better in interpersonal relationships, be more successful in their work, improve their family life and effectively help their friends, family and associates do the same. Can any subject guarantee that it will help you solve all your problems? Maybe not, but these principles have been used countless times and, when honestly and exactly applied, have brought about invariably beneficial results.

Scientology does not require that one change his beliefs or convictions to use it successfully. All you have to do is apply the data and observe for yourself whether or not it works. ***You,*** *as you are now, can do more good for yourself and for those around you than you ever imagined, and gain enormous personal satisfaction doing it.*

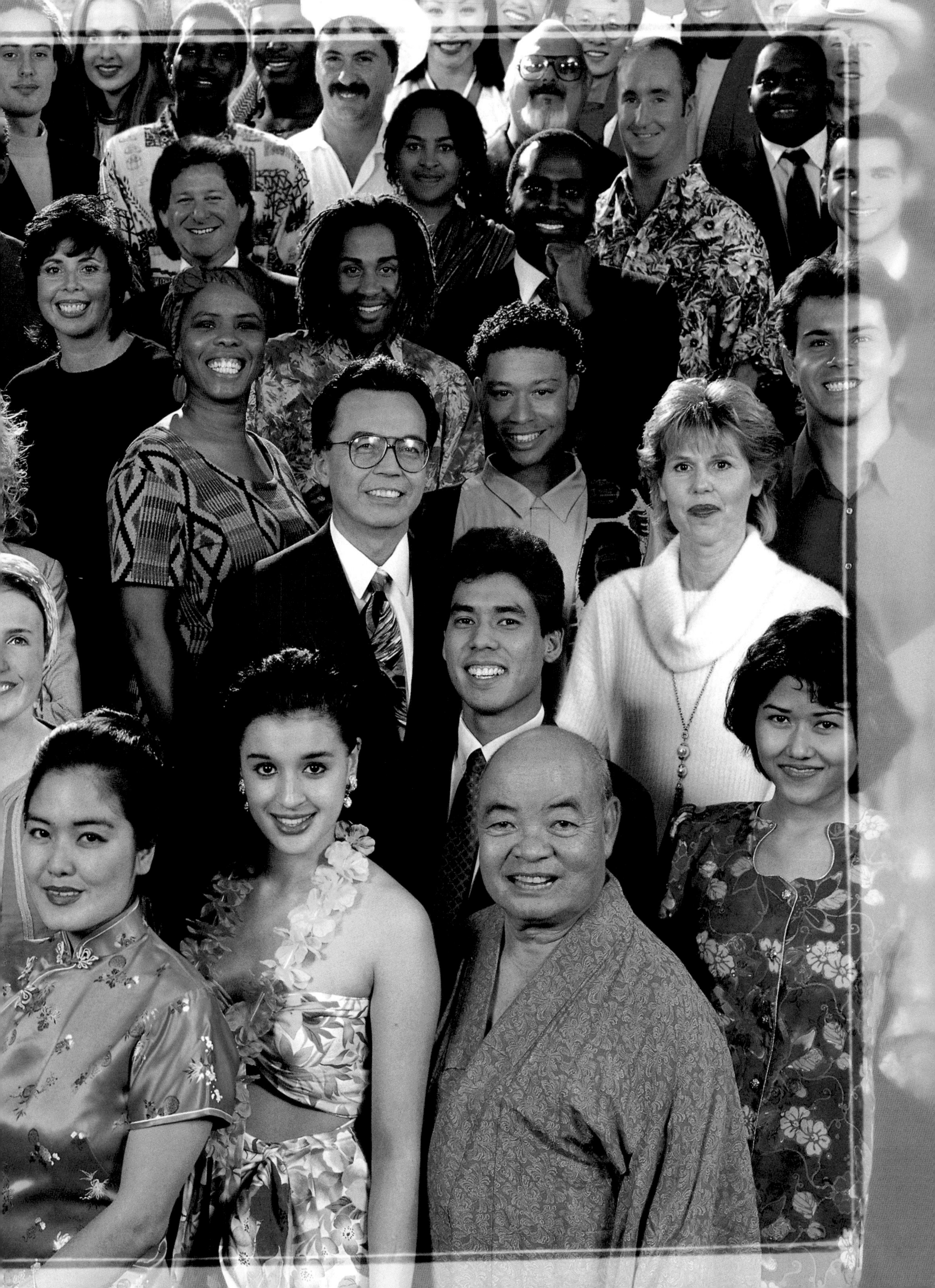

A sincere look at the conditions around you will reveal situations in the lives of people you know who would benefit from your help. Factually, there isn't a person you know who doesn't have something in his life he would improve if only he knew how. By reading this book, you'll gain these invaluable tools and be able to render real assistance wherever you find it is needed.

You only have to avail yourself of these tools. If enough people used the data in this book it would solve enough of the problems in their own spheres to elevate the entire society to a higher plateau. And ultimately, a civilization would form on Earth based on trust, decency, honesty and tolerance.

But knowing such tools exist and not using them would be like pouring water into the sand beside a man dying of thirst. It is an observable fact that nothing stays the same for long. Things either get better or else they worsen. Even if only by tiny increments, the conditions in a person's life, his environment and the society as a whole are always changing.

Man is at a crossroads in his history as man. He can begin to move upward towards a golden age or continue his descent into a new dark age of slavery to mechanistic principles where individuality and freedom are lost. With the data contained in this handbook, you can change conditions for the better. Such an opportunity never existed before Scientology. All man had was unreliable advice, superstition, unworkable remedies and the dim hope that somehow he would be saved.

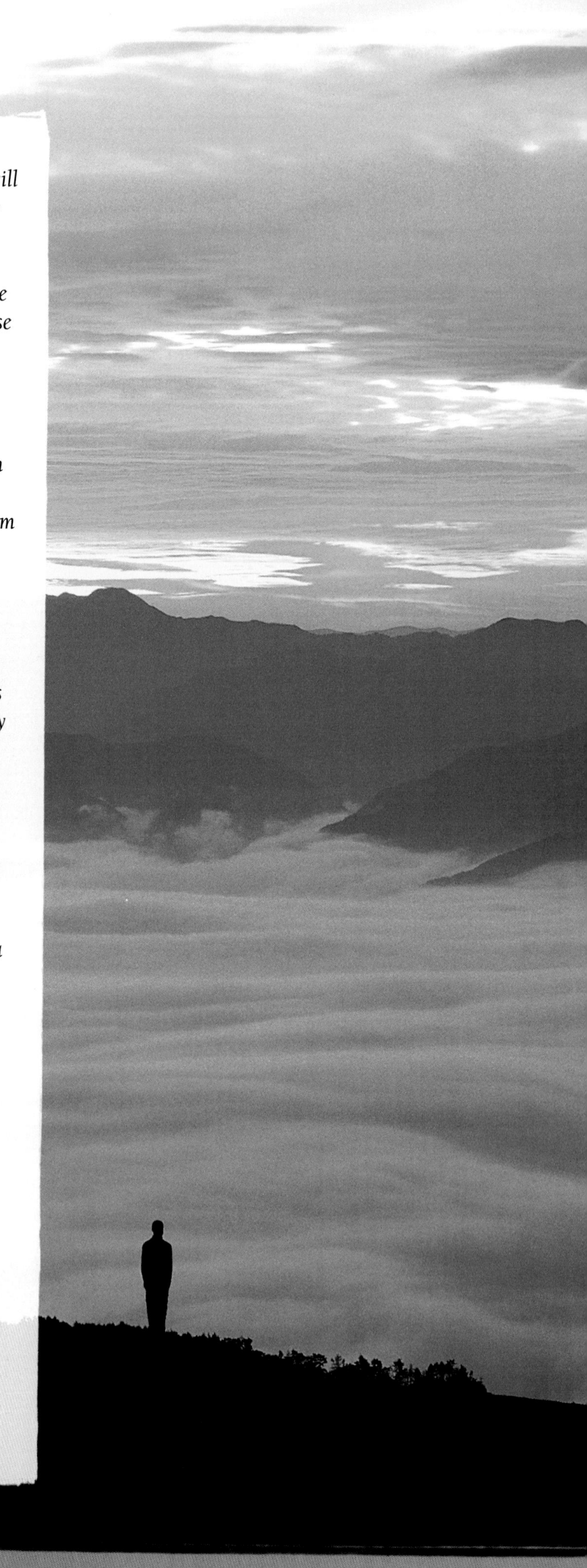

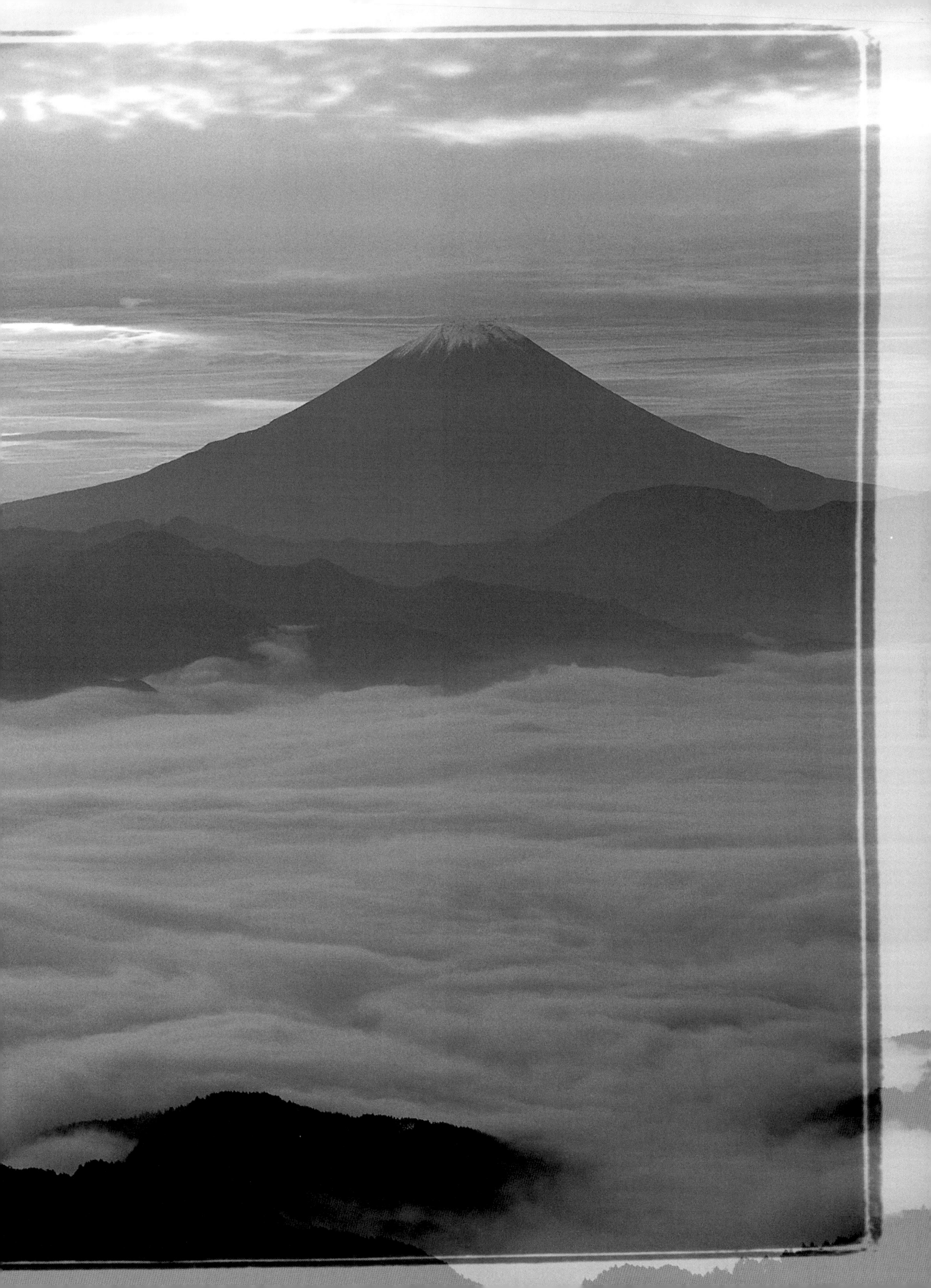

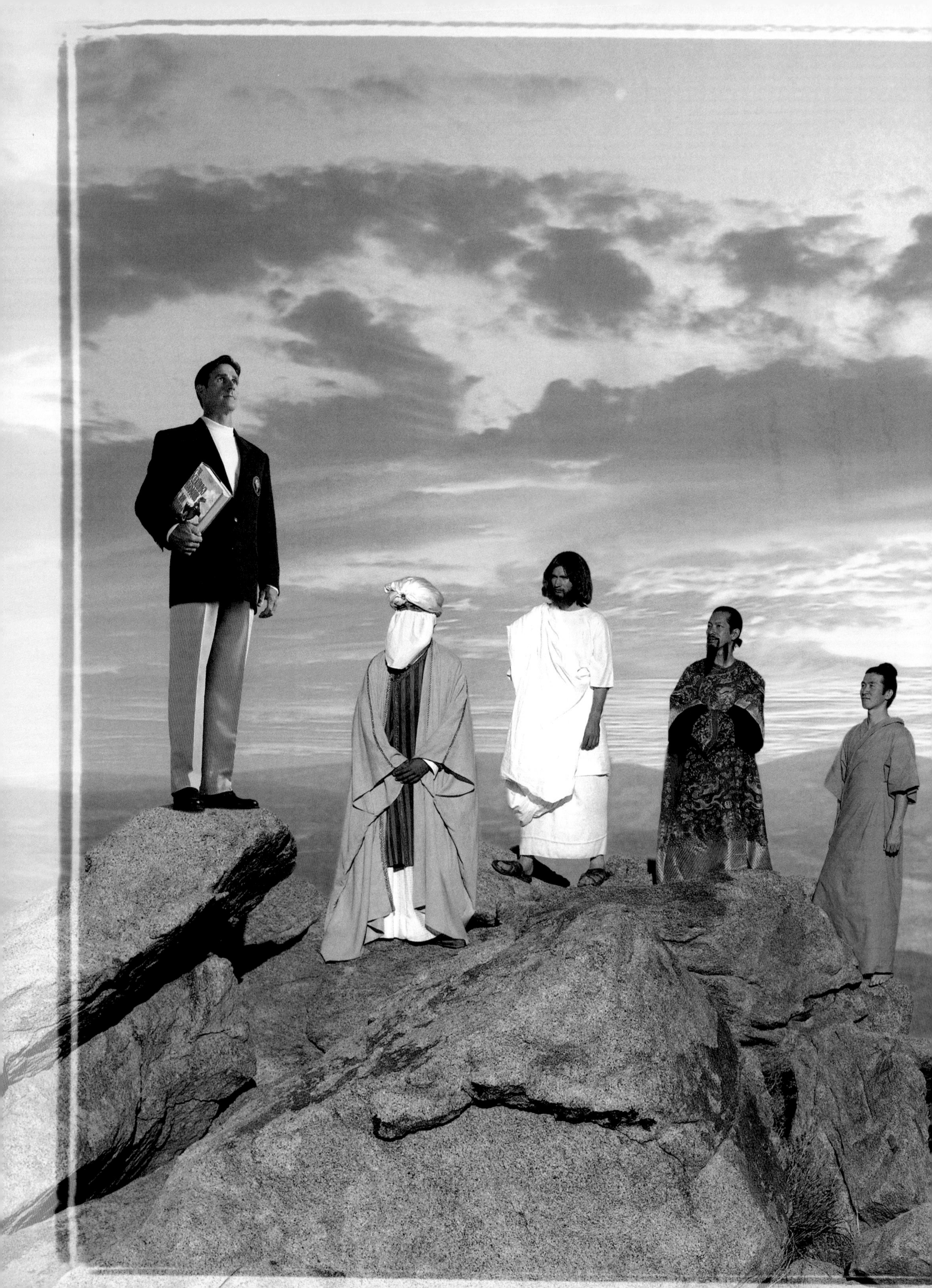

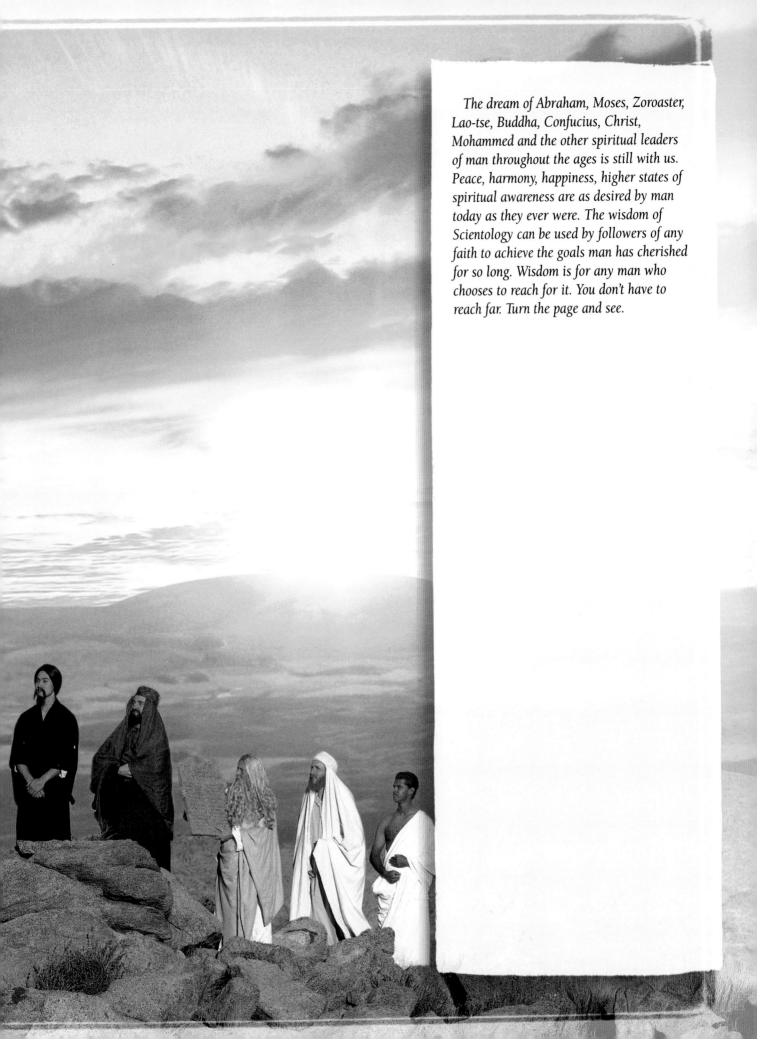

The dream of Abraham, Moses, Zoroaster, Lao-tse, Buddha, Confucius, Christ, Mohammed and the other spiritual leaders of man throughout the ages is still with us. Peace, harmony, happiness, higher states of spiritual awareness are as desired by man today as they ever were. The wisdom of Scientology can be used by followers of any faith to achieve the goals man has cherished for so long. Wisdom is for any man who chooses to reach for it. You don't have to reach far. Turn the page and see.

FUNDAMENTALS OF SCIENTOLOGY

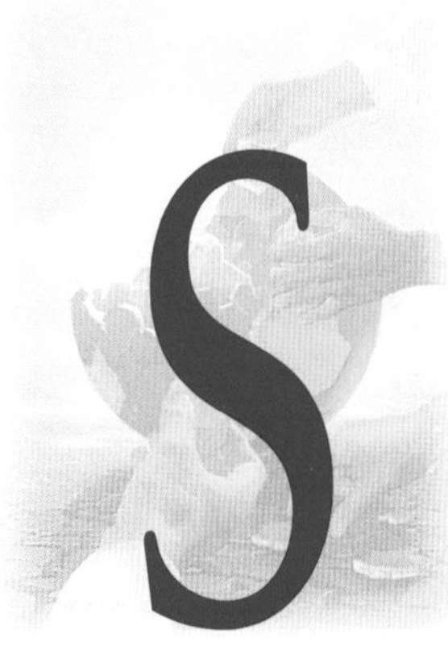

Scientology is a religious philosophy in its highest meaning, as it brings man to total freedom and truth.

The essential tenets of Scientology are these:

You are an immortal spiritual being.

Your experience extends well beyond a single lifetime. And your capabilities are unlimited, even if not presently realized.

Furthermore, man is basically good. He is seeking to survive. And his survival depends upon himself and his fellows and his attainment of brotherhood with the universe.

In Scientology, you are called a *thetan* (from the Greek letter *theta,* for thought or life or the spirit). This is to avoid confusion with previous conceptions of the soul.

The thetan *is* the spiritual being himself. It is the individual. It is *you.*

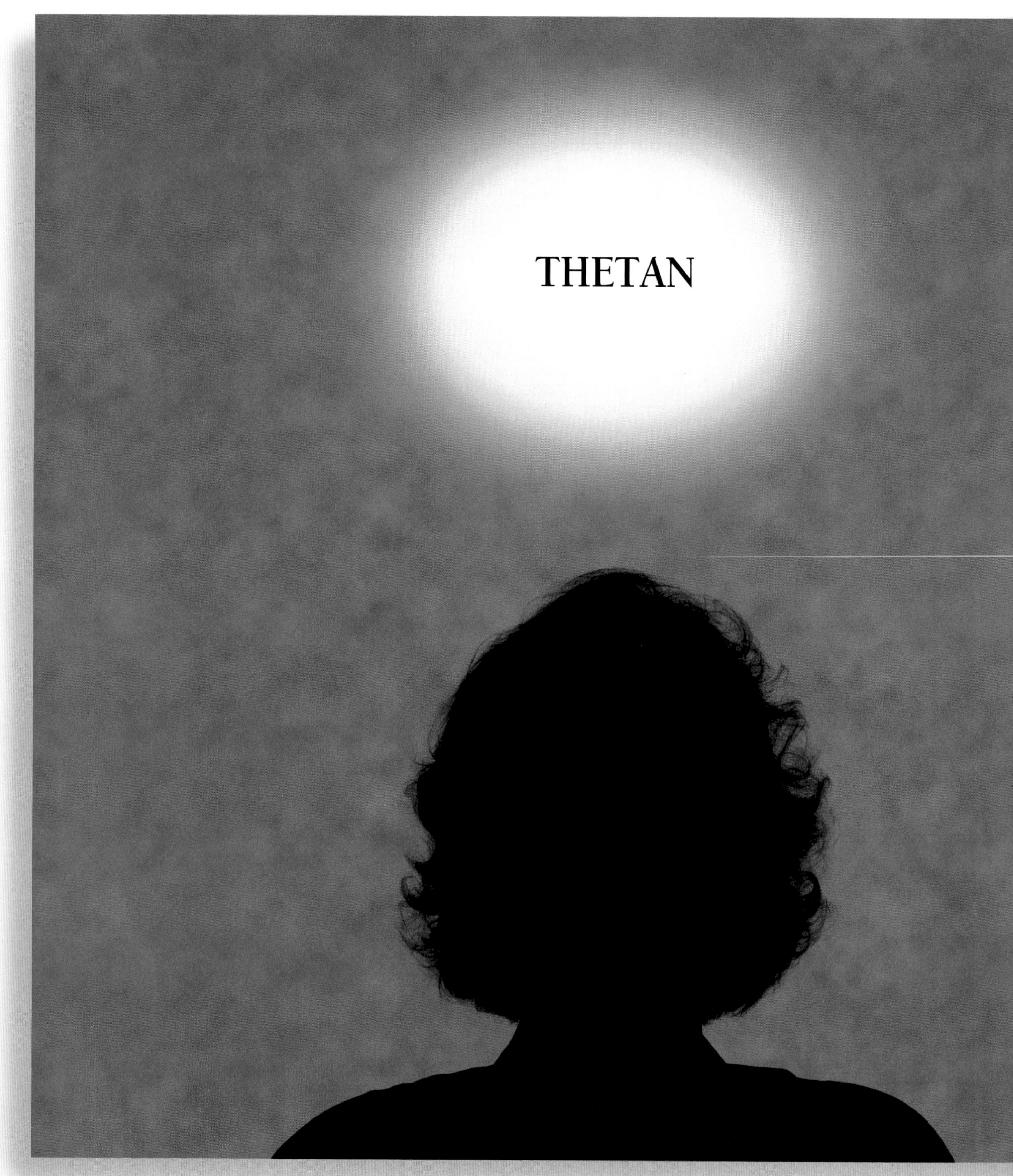
THETAN

You are a thetan, a spiritual being. Not your eyes, not your brain, but you. You do not *have* a thetan, something you keep apart from yourself; you *are* a thetan. You would not speak of *my* thetan; you would speak of *me*.

Although much of what Scientology holds true may be echoed in many great philosophic teachings, what it offers is entirely new: An exact route through which anyone can regain the truth and simplicity of his spiritual self.

Scientology, then, is a religious philosophy in the most profound sense of the word. It is concerned with nothing less than the full rehabilitation of the thetan, to increase his spiritual awareness, native capabilities, and certainty of his own immortality.

Scientology is organized along specific axioms that precisely define who we are, what we are capable of and, most importantly, how we might realize those abilities. The axioms further define the underlying causes and principles of reality as we know it, and thus unlock the very riddle of existence.

These axioms form the foundation of a vast area of observations in the humanities, a philosophic body that literally applies to the entirety of life. From this has been developed a great number of fundamental principles men can use to improve their lives. In fact, herein are found the methods and means of creating new ways of life.

The discoveries of Scientology are not only major philosophic breakthroughs, they are applicable principles; they explain the fundamental laws of life, why people behave the way they do, the impediments to survival and how best to overcome them. Indeed, Scientology offers nothing less than practical methods to better every aspect of our existence.

More than that, however, Scientology offers us the way to reclaim our spiritual heritage.

The spiritual being,
the thetan,
is who you are.

THE MIND

How is it that this potentially powerful spiritual being became but a puppet dancing on the end of unseen strings? How is it that he has become so burdened with the care and liability of a body, he has forgotten his own identity and believes he is a body? And that he now goes blindly from life to life, lacking memory, his self-awareness growing ever dimmer?

How is it that we cannot gain control of our lives, much less our destiny?

The answer is found in the nature of man's mind.

Just as you are not a body, neither are you a mind. While the nature of the mind has been argued endlessly in fields from philosophy to science, in Scientology it has been discovered that the mind is simply an accumulation of what are called mental image pictures. These mental image pictures are what we often think of as memory. They are three-dimensional color pictures with sound and smell and all other perceptions, plus the conclusions or speculations of the individual.

These pictures are actually composed of energy. They have mass, they exist in space and they follow some very, very definite routines of behavior, the most interesting of which is the fact that they appear when somebody thinks of something. For example, if you think of a cat, you will get a mental picture of a cat. This is what is called the *analytical mind.* This is the rational, conscious and aware mind which thinks, observes data, remembers it and resolves problems.

But there is more to the mind than this.

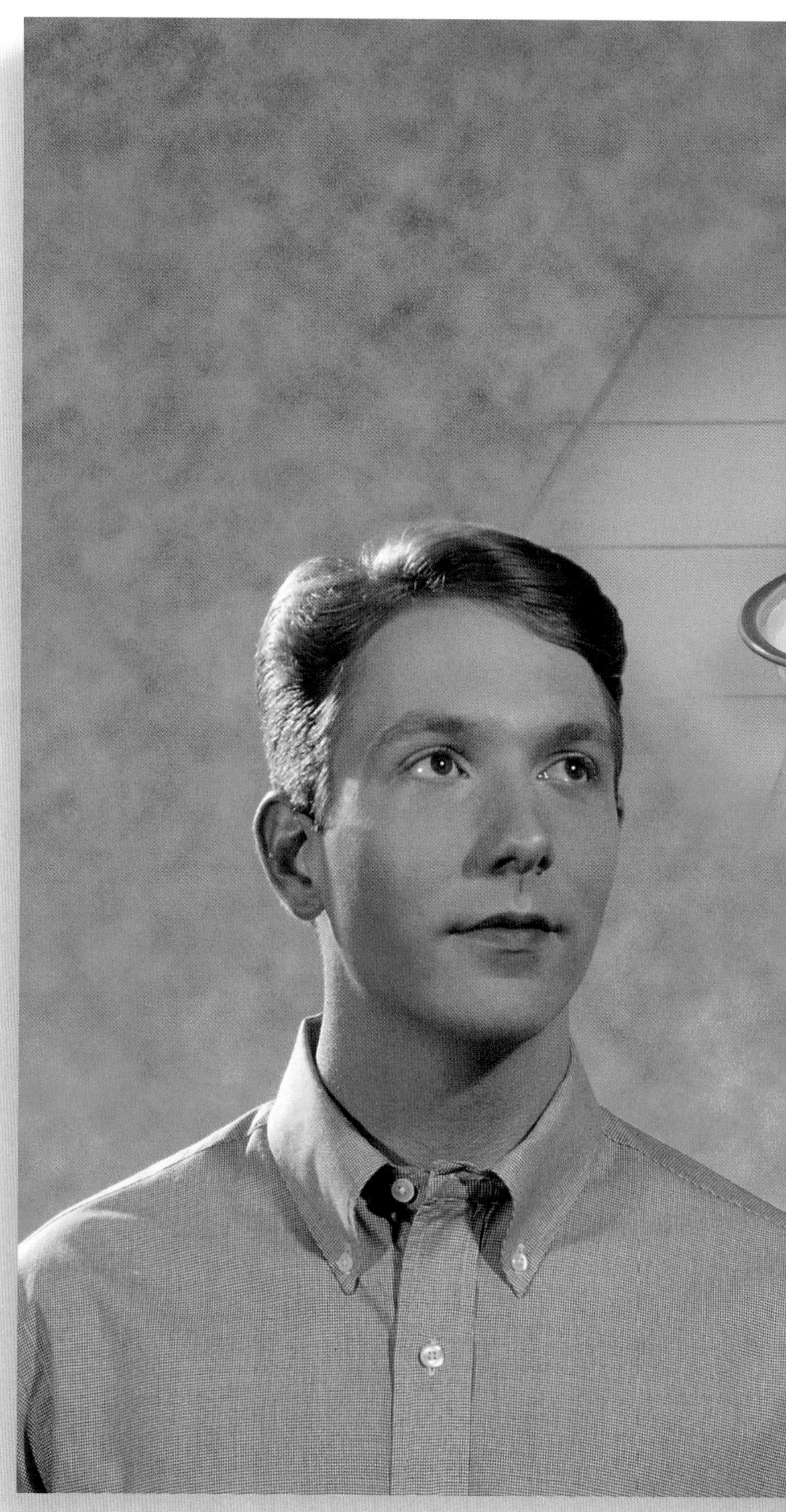

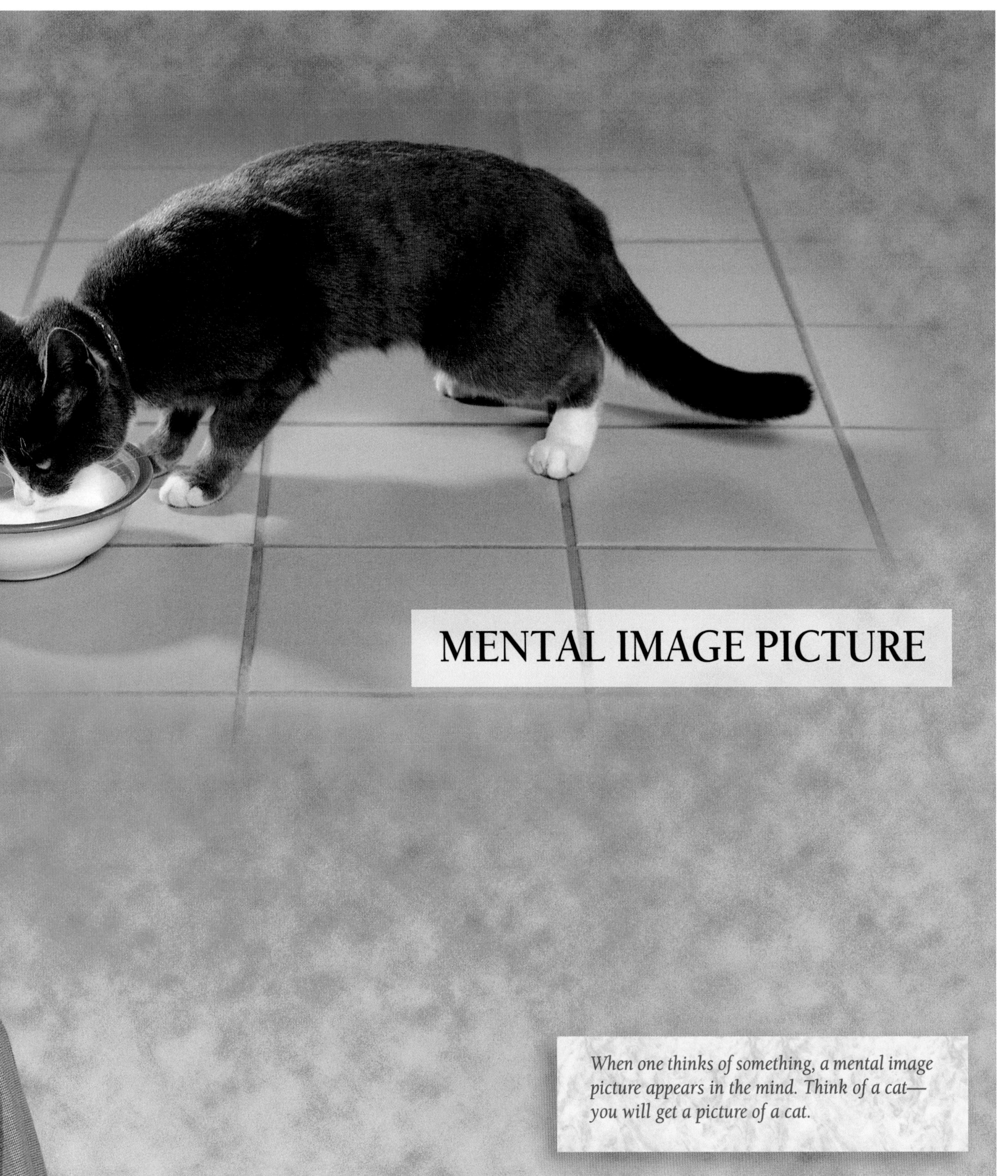
MENTAL IMAGE PICTURE
When one thinks of something, a mental image picture appears in the mind. Think of a cat—you will get a picture of a cat.

The accumulated record of all one's mental image pictures is called the *time track,* and it stretches very, very far back into the past.

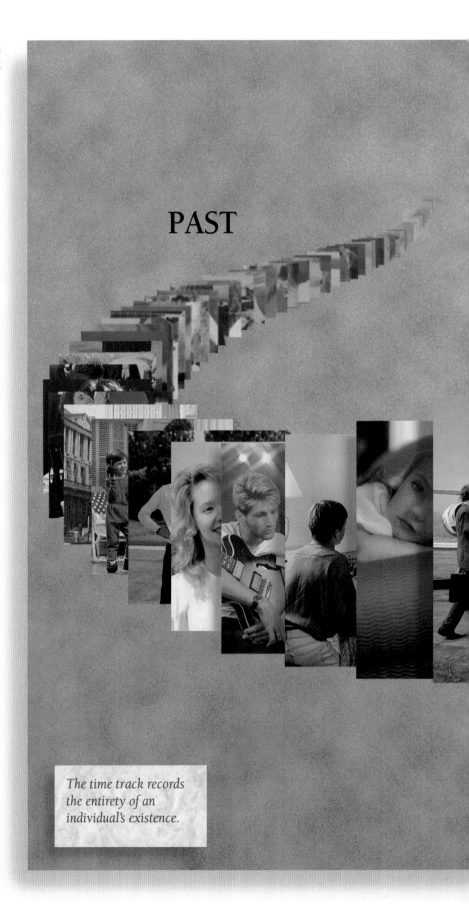

The time track records the entirety of an individual's existence.

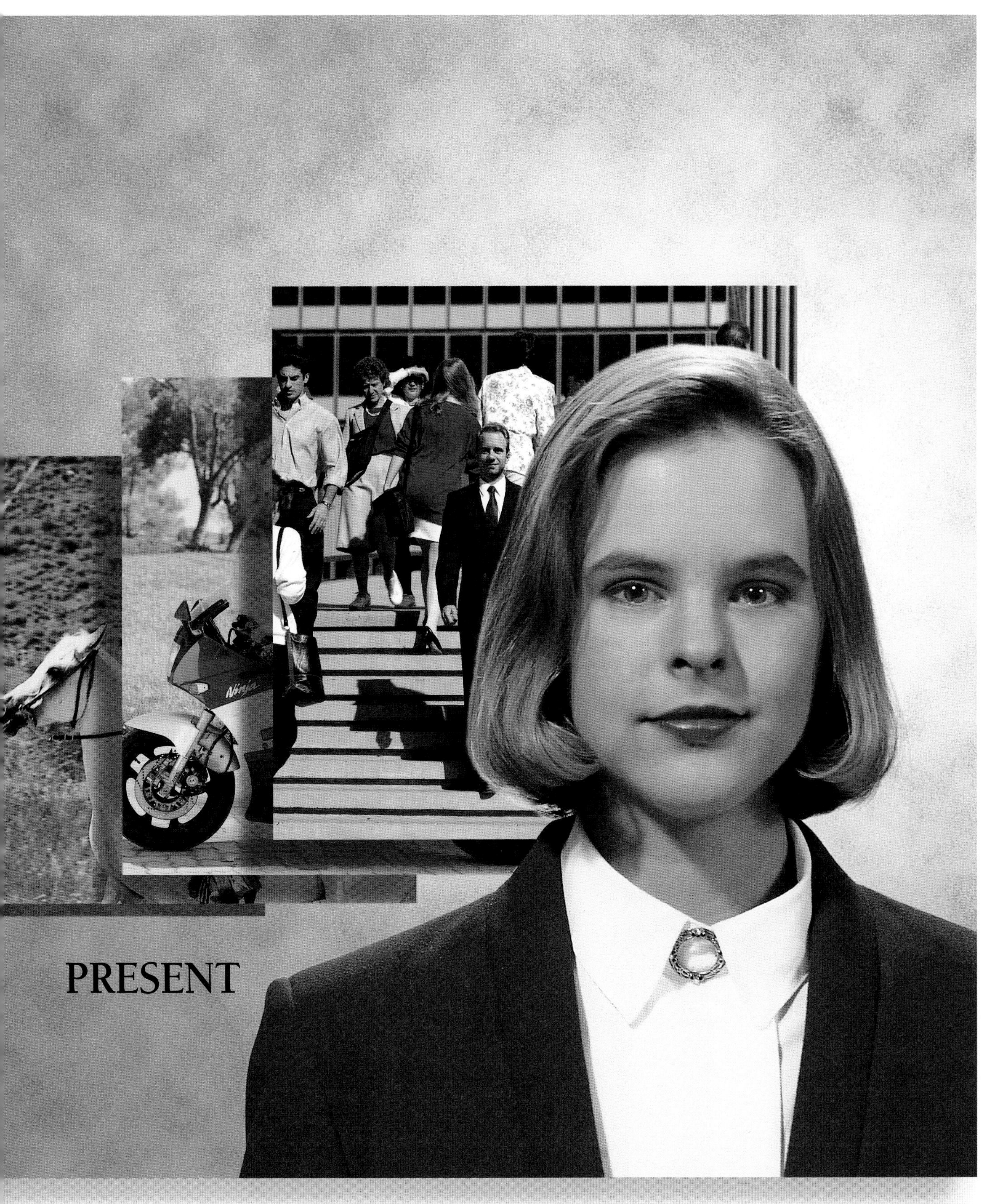
Ninja
PRESENT

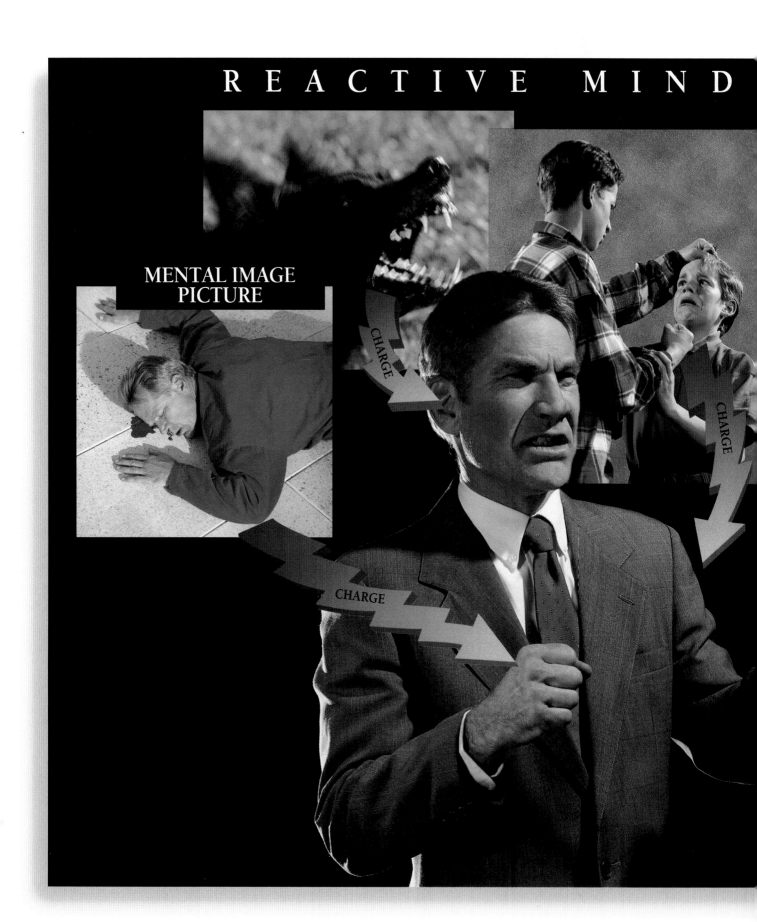
REACTIVE MIND
MENTAL IMAGE PICTURE
CHARGE
CHARGE
CHARGE

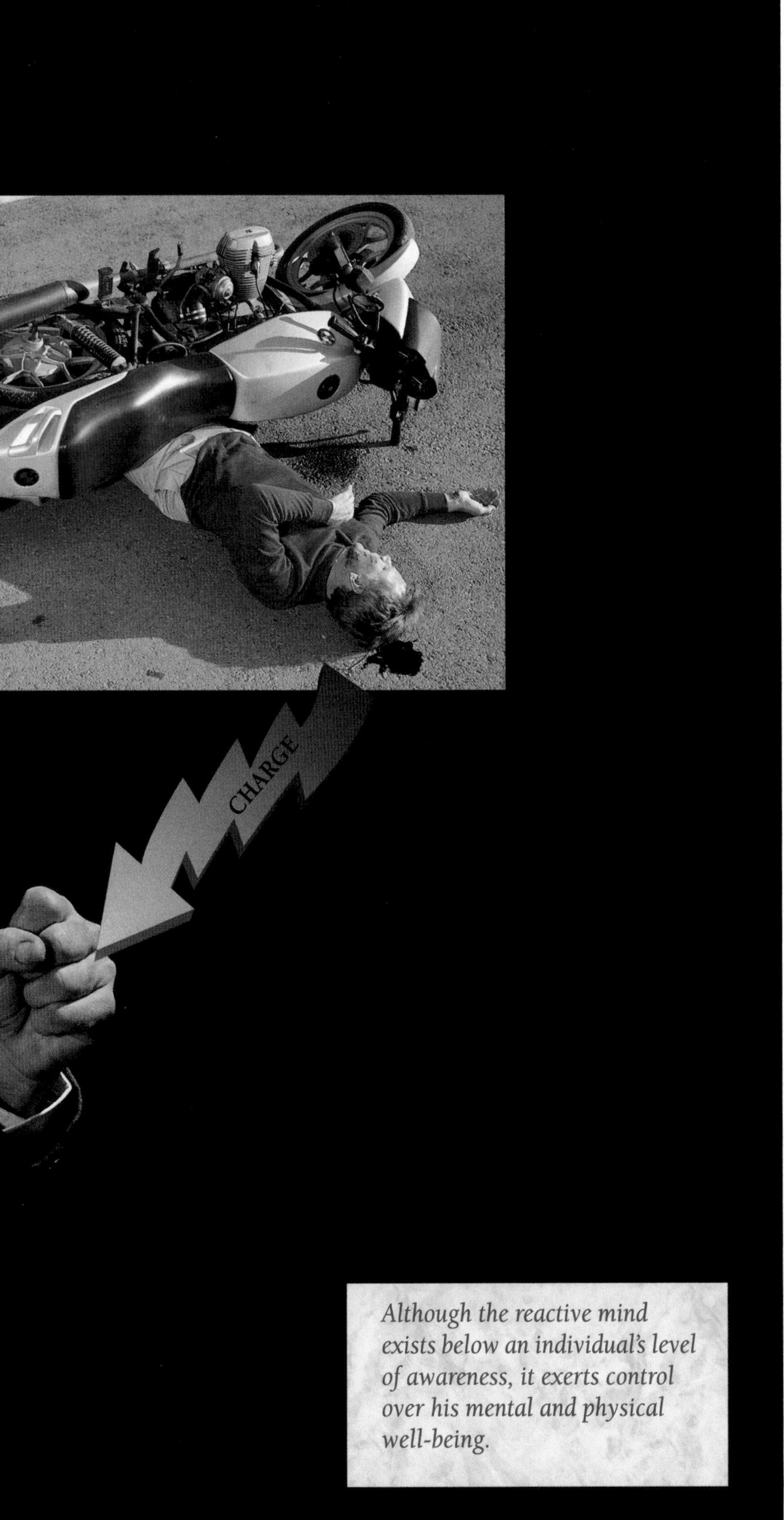

Although the reactive mind exists below an individual's level of awareness, it exerts control over his mental and physical well-being.

Although these experiences—good and bad—were long ago and long forgotten, the past trauma of *painful* moments is all too real in the here-and-now. In fact, that trauma is the source of much of what seems to trouble us today, including our problems, upsets, frustrations and the deeply rooted feeling that life is not what it should be.

Specifically, it is the mental energy within those pictures that impinges upon the individual. The energy and force in pictures of experiences painful or upsetting to a person can have a harmful effect upon him. This harmful energy or force is called *charge.*

The sum total of pictures that contain charge is called the *reactive mind.* All told, this reactive mind exacts a terrible toll. Although we are not conscious of it and it is not under our volitional control, this mind exerts force and the power of command over our awareness, purposes, thoughts, bodies and actions.

Until Mr. Hubbard's discovery of it, the reactive mind remained hidden, as did the key to unlock it. Nor was there any way to regain what it had taken from us, including the awareness, the goodness and remarkable abilities inherent in all spiritual beings.

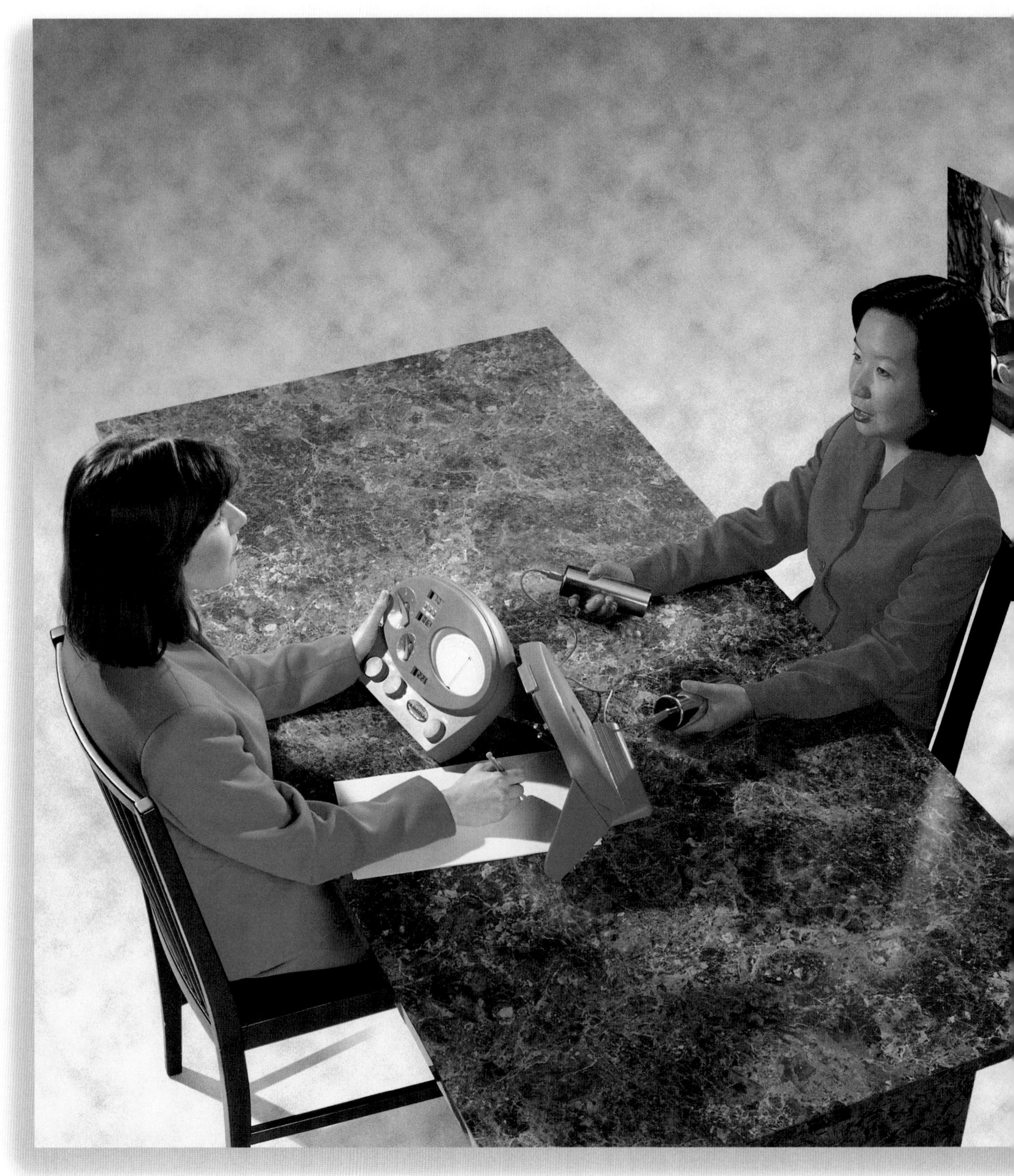

THE SOLUTION

The primary means by which Scientology's basic truths are applied to the rehabilitation of the human spirit is called *auditing*. It is the central practice of Scientology, and it is delivered by an *auditor,* from the Latin *audire,* "to listen." An auditor is "one who listens."

Auditing is not some vague form of mental exploration, and the auditor does not offer solutions, advice or evaluation. One of its essential principles rests upon the fact that only by allowing an individual to find his own answers to life's problems can improvements be made. This is accomplished by gradiently helping one examine his own existence and improve his ability to face what he is and where he is—peeling away the layers of experience that have weighed so heavily upon him. Thus, auditing is not something that is *done* to a person. Its benefits can only be achieved through active participation and good communication.

The specific techniques that have been developed to guide the person along auditing's road to self-discovery are called *processes*. A process is an exact set of questions asked or directions given by the auditor. There are many, many processes in Scientology, and all are aimed at improving one's perceptions and awareness, while removing unwanted impediments to spiritual growth.

The period of time during which auditing occurs is called an auditing *session.* Auditing requires a quiet, comfortable environment with the auditor and the individual receiving auditing seated across from one another.

ATTENTION

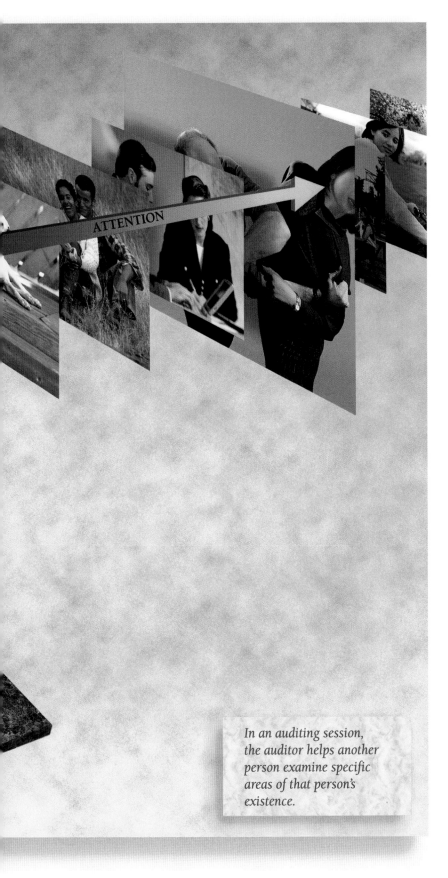

In an auditing session, the auditor helps another person examine specific areas of that person's existence.

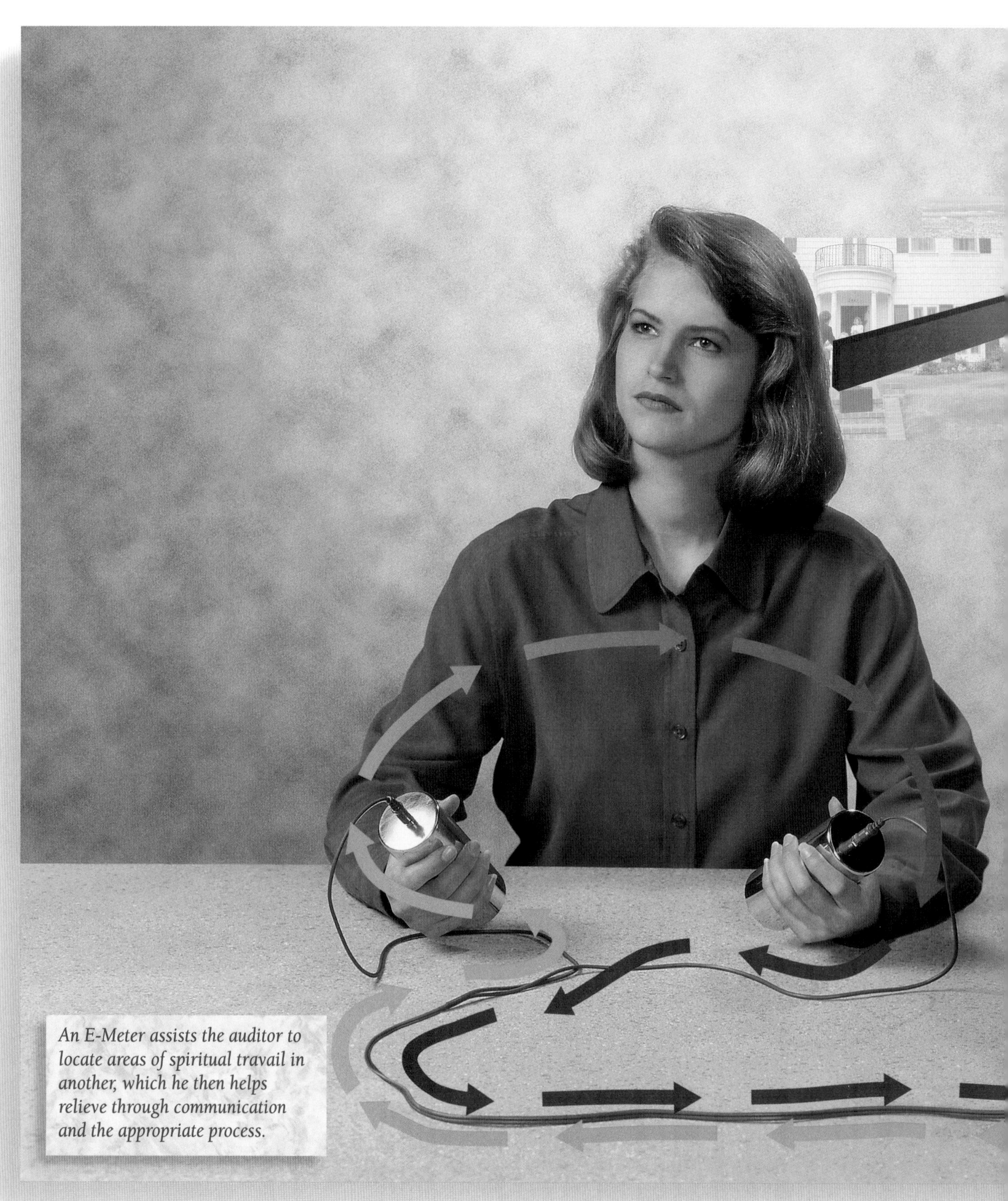

An E-Meter assists the auditor to locate areas of spiritual travail in another, which he then helps relieve through communication and the appropriate process.

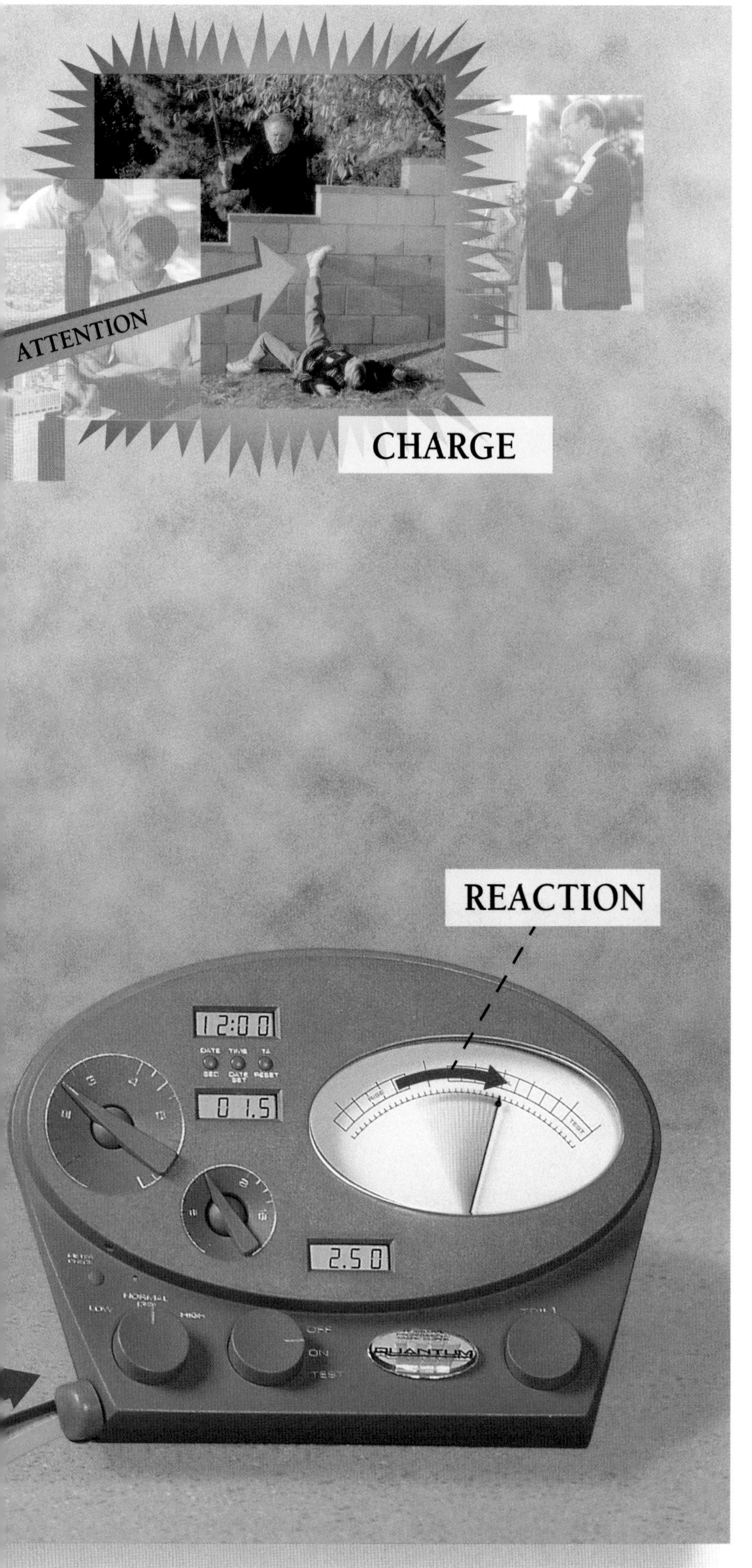

Given the precision of auditing and the fact it addresses long-hidden sources of travail, the auditor is assisted by a specially designed meter, called an electropsychometer or E-Meter for short. The E-Meter does not diagnose or cure anything. It simply measures the state or change of state of an individual.

When the meter is in operation and a person is holding its electrodes, a very tiny flow of electrical energy (about 1.5 volts—less than a flashlight battery) passes down the wires, through the person's body and back into the E-Meter. This flow of energy is so small there is no physical sensation when holding the electrodes. Nevertheless, when one thinks a thought, one is actually moving and changing mental energy and charge; and these changes are registered on the meter.

In the hands of an auditor, skilled at recognizing and interpreting the E-Meter's reactions, the E-Meter becomes the tool by which otherwise buried experience may be located and viewed.

The E-Meter does nothing by itself. Rather, it serves as a guide by registering charge and thereby indicating what should be addressed with auditing.

Factually, there are no parallels to auditing. There is nothing comparable to having one's attention directed to some long-buried source of emotional charge and then—simply by *viewing* it—causing its instant vanishment and relief from the distressing charge.

Nor is there any parallel to what auditing brings in the way of awareness, well-being and spiritual fulfillment.

And because there are no parallels, no verbal descriptions are enough; one must experience it.

With the advent of Dianetics in 1950, a new era of hope for mankind began. Dianetics, a substudy of Scientology, is most accurately defined as what the soul is doing to the body through the mind. With L. Ron Hubbard's discovery of Dianetics, man at last possessed the key to unlock the riddle of the mind.

Men have always known of what Dianetics calls the analytical mind. This is the rational, conscious and aware mind which thinks, observes data, remembers it and resolves problems. The reactive mind, of course, was another matter.

Mental image pictures are stored in the standard memory banks of the analytical mind. In moments of intense pain, however, the action of the analytical mind is suspended and the reactive mind takes over. These mental image pictures—ones containing pain and unconsciousness—are recorded by, and stored in, the reactive mind.

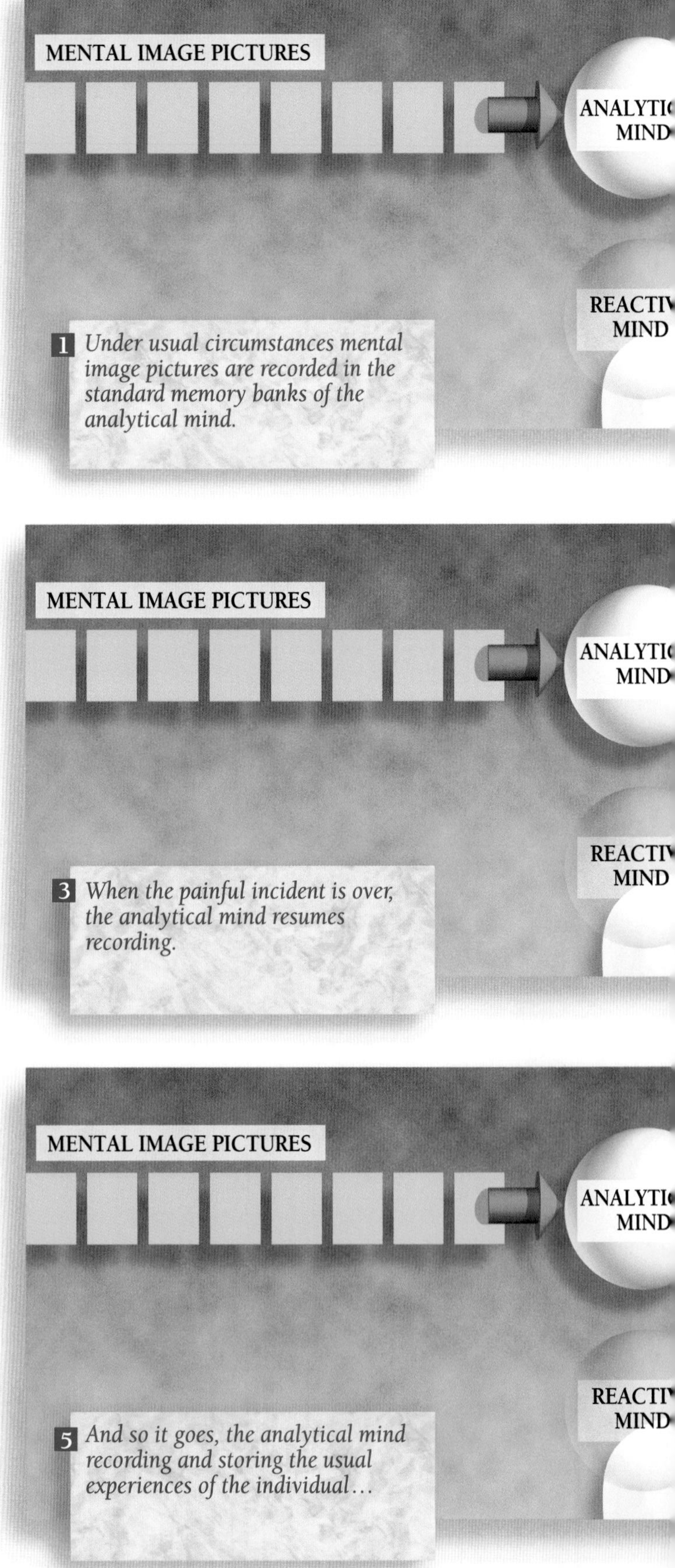
MENTAL IMAGE PICTURES
ANALYTIC
MIND
REACTIV
MIND
1 Under usual circumstances mental image pictures are recorded in the standard memory banks of the analytical mind.
MENTAL IMAGE PICTURES
ANALYTIC
MIND
REACTIV
MIND
3 When the painful incident is over, the analytical mind resumes recording.
MENTAL IMAGE PICTURES
ANALYTIC
MIND
REACTIV
MIND
5 And so it goes, the analytical mind recording and storing the usual experiences of the individual…

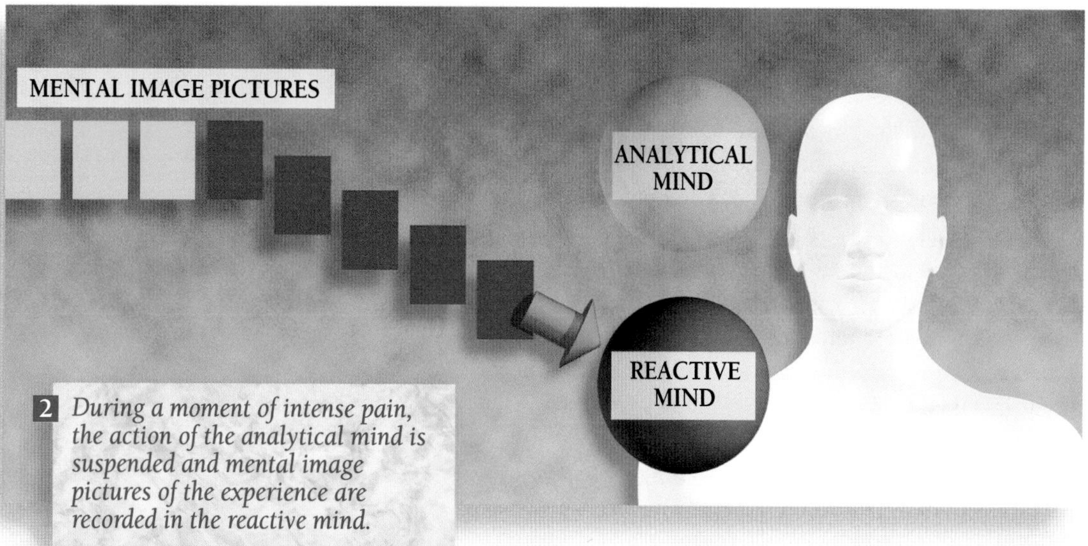

2 *During a moment of intense pain, the action of the analytical mind is suspended and mental image pictures of the experience are recorded in the reactive mind.*

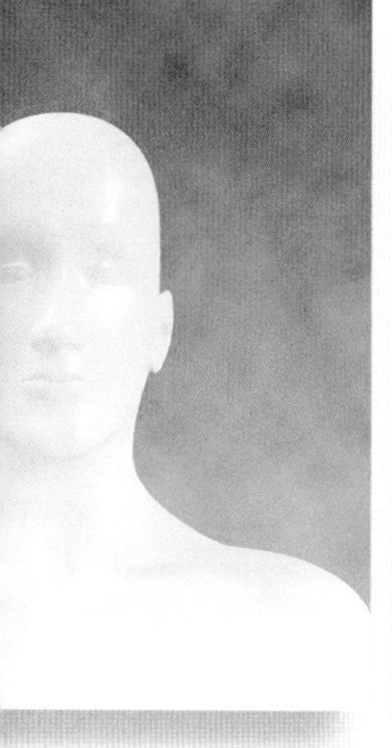

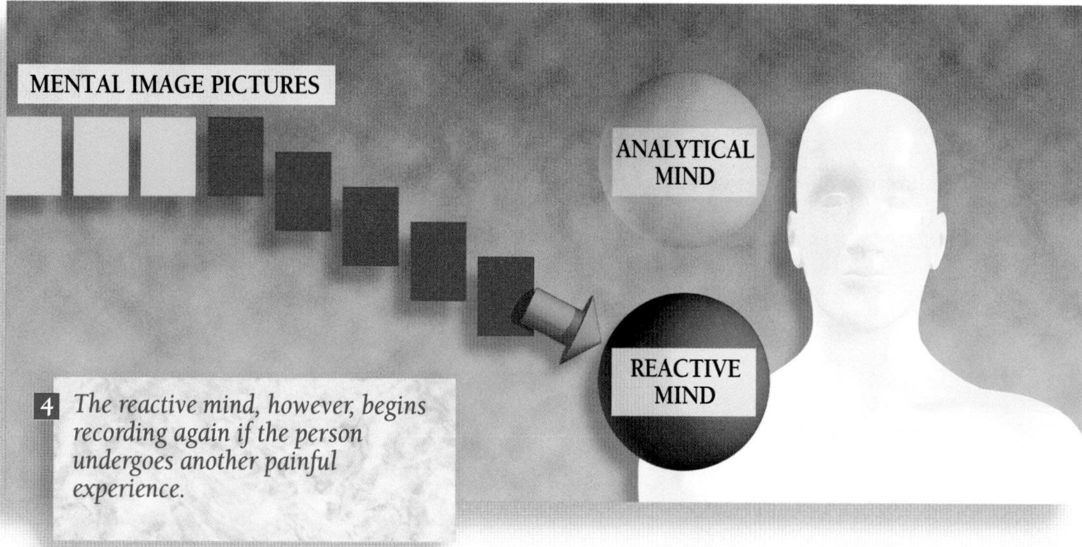

4 *The reactive mind, however, begins recording again if the person undergoes another painful experience.*

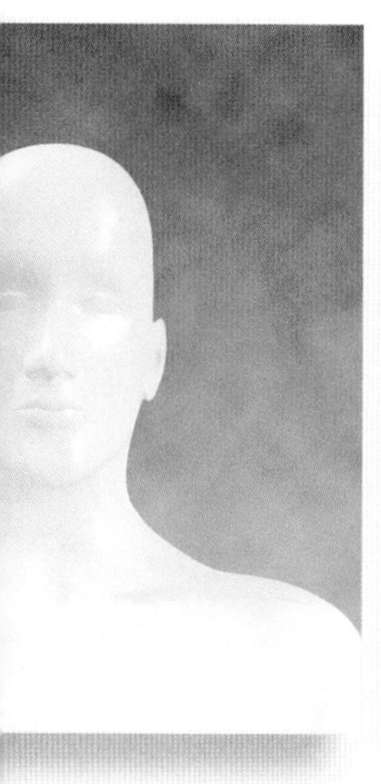

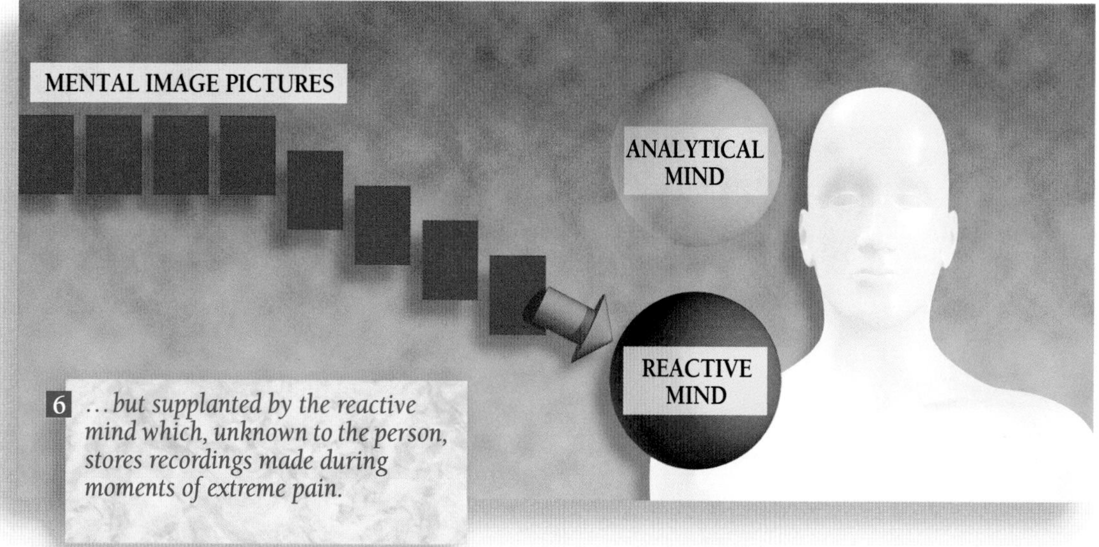

6 *…but supplanted by the reactive mind which, unknown to the person, stores recordings made during moments of extreme pain.*

No matter how "unconscious" the person may seem, when the analytical mind shuts down, the reactive mind continues to record. These incidents are not memories as such. Rather, they are called engrams, and they are a *complete* recording of every perception present in a moment of partial or full "unconsciousness."

All of the many human perceptions such as sight, taste, color, depth, smell, touch and sound are recorded in an engram. Of these stored perceptions the most insidious are spoken words, for they are taken literally and can later act upon the individual as commands. An engramic phrase such as "Don't talk" might produce a stammerer. The words "He can't feel a thing" spoken during a moment of pain and unconsciousness could lead to a shut-off of both emotions and physical perceptions. These phrases and thousands of variations spoken within the hearing of an "unconscious" person could later be enforced on him by the reactive mind as literal commands that must be obeyed.

The reactive mind is not at all selective. It faithfully records *everything* during a moment of pain and unconsciousness and is composed exclusively of these engrams.

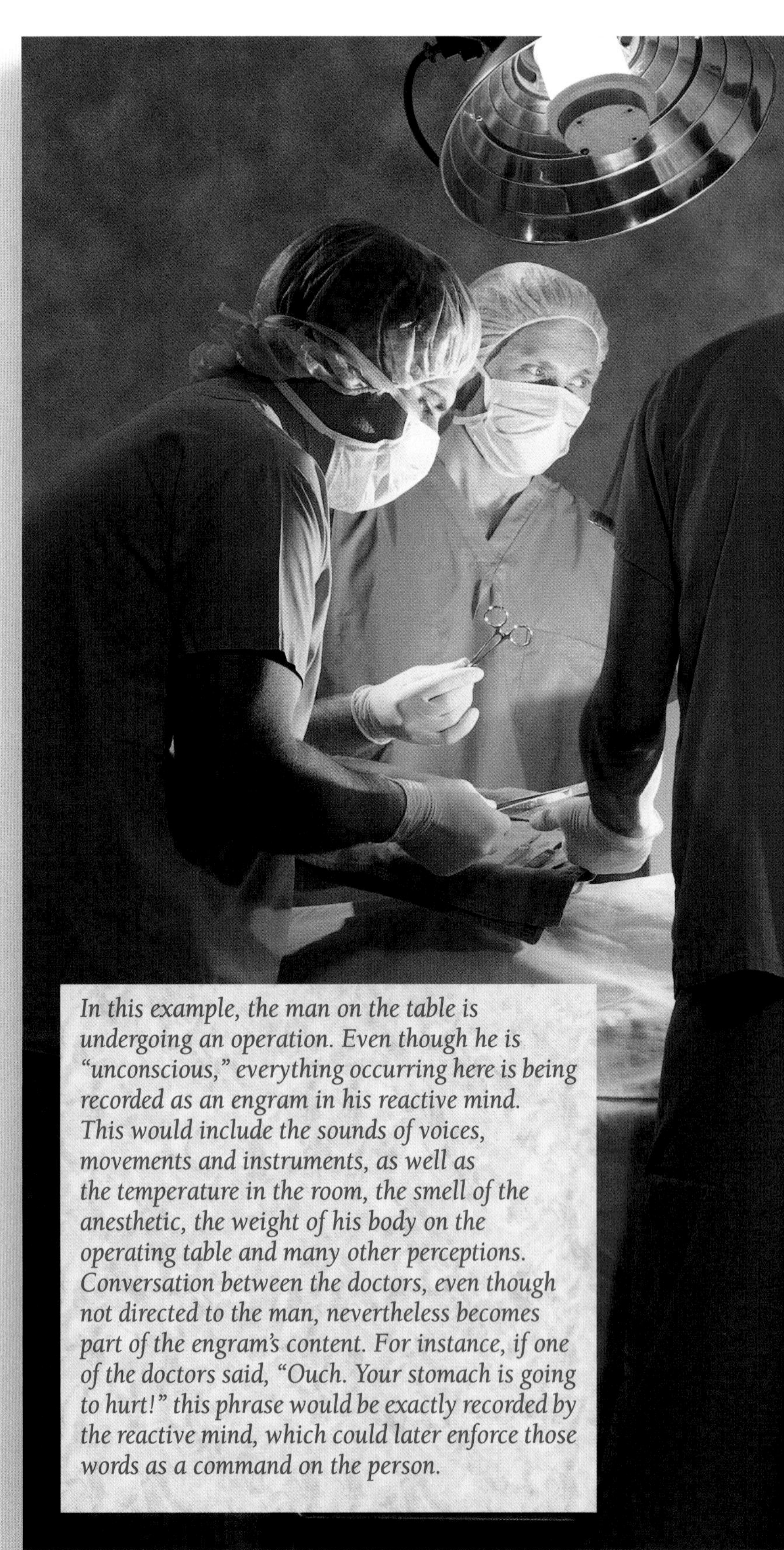

In this example, the man on the table is undergoing an operation. Even though he is "unconscious," everything occurring here is being recorded as an engram in his reactive mind. This would include the sounds of voices, movements and instruments, as well as the temperature in the room, the smell of the anesthetic, the weight of his body on the operating table and many other perceptions. Conversation between the doctors, even though not directed to the man, nevertheless becomes part of the engram's content. For instance, if one of the doctors said, "Ouch. Your stomach is going to hurt!" this phrase would be exactly recorded by the reactive mind, which could later enforce those words as a command on the person.

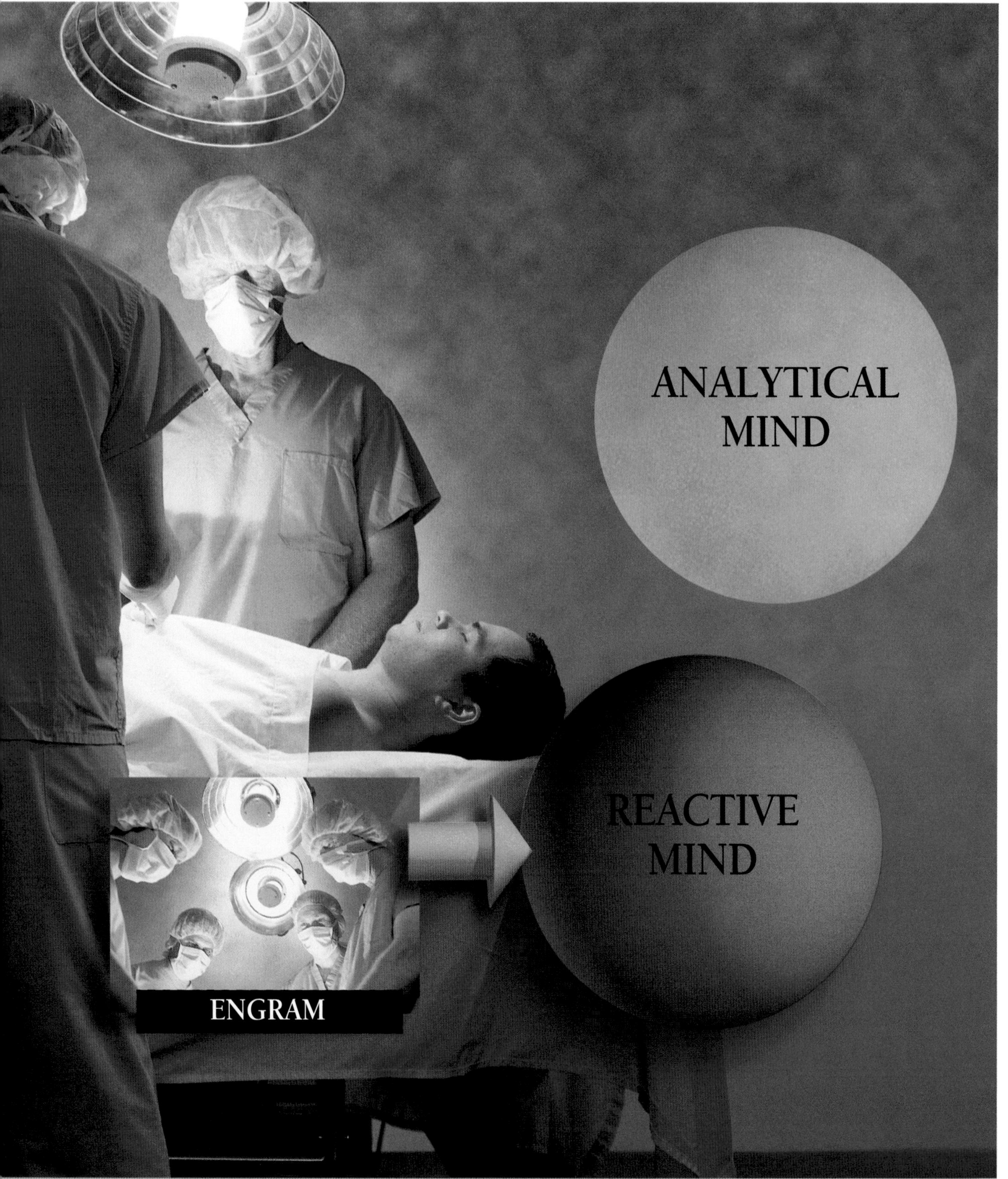
ANALYTICAL
MIND
REACTIVE
MIND
ENGRAM

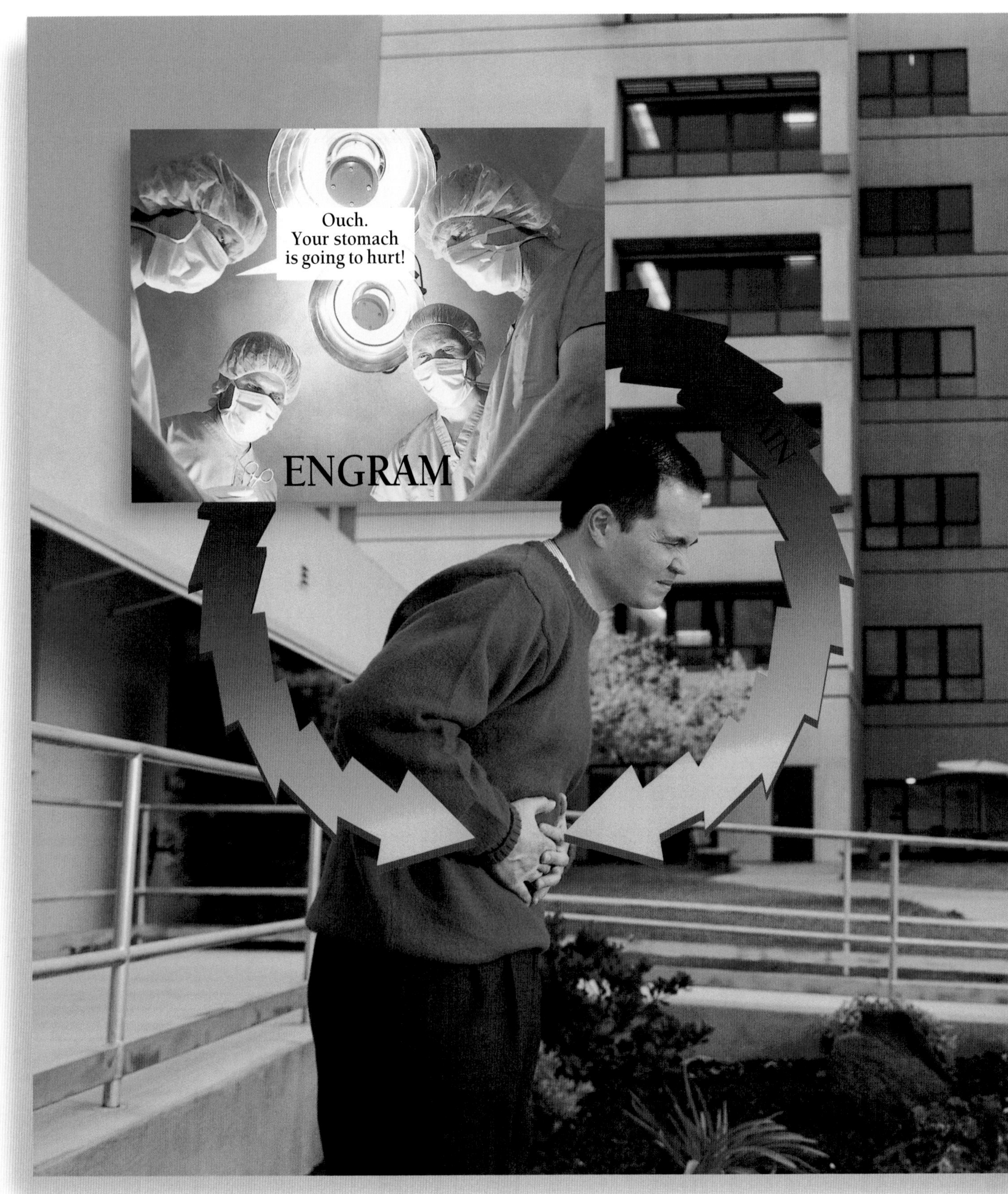
Ouch.
Your stomach
is going to hurt!
ENGRAM

In one sense, this reactive mind could be regarded as a survival mechanism. During moments of emergency or danger, it throws these pictures back at the individual so as to dictate his actions along lines which have been deemed "safe." This is called the "restimulation" of the engram.

Unfortunately, the reactive mind is not rational or logical. All it takes to restimulate an engram during moments of upset or illness or tiredness is something in the current environment that approximates the perceptions stored in the engram—words, sounds, smells, etc.

In such situations, the engram has the power of command over the individual's actions, body, thoughts, awareness and purposes. Thus we will find a person acting in a certain manner and not knowing why he is doing so. For remember, the reactive mind is hidden and below his level of conscious awareness.

So we have an obsessive strata of unknown, unseen, uninspected data which are forcing solutions, unknown and uninspected, on the individual.

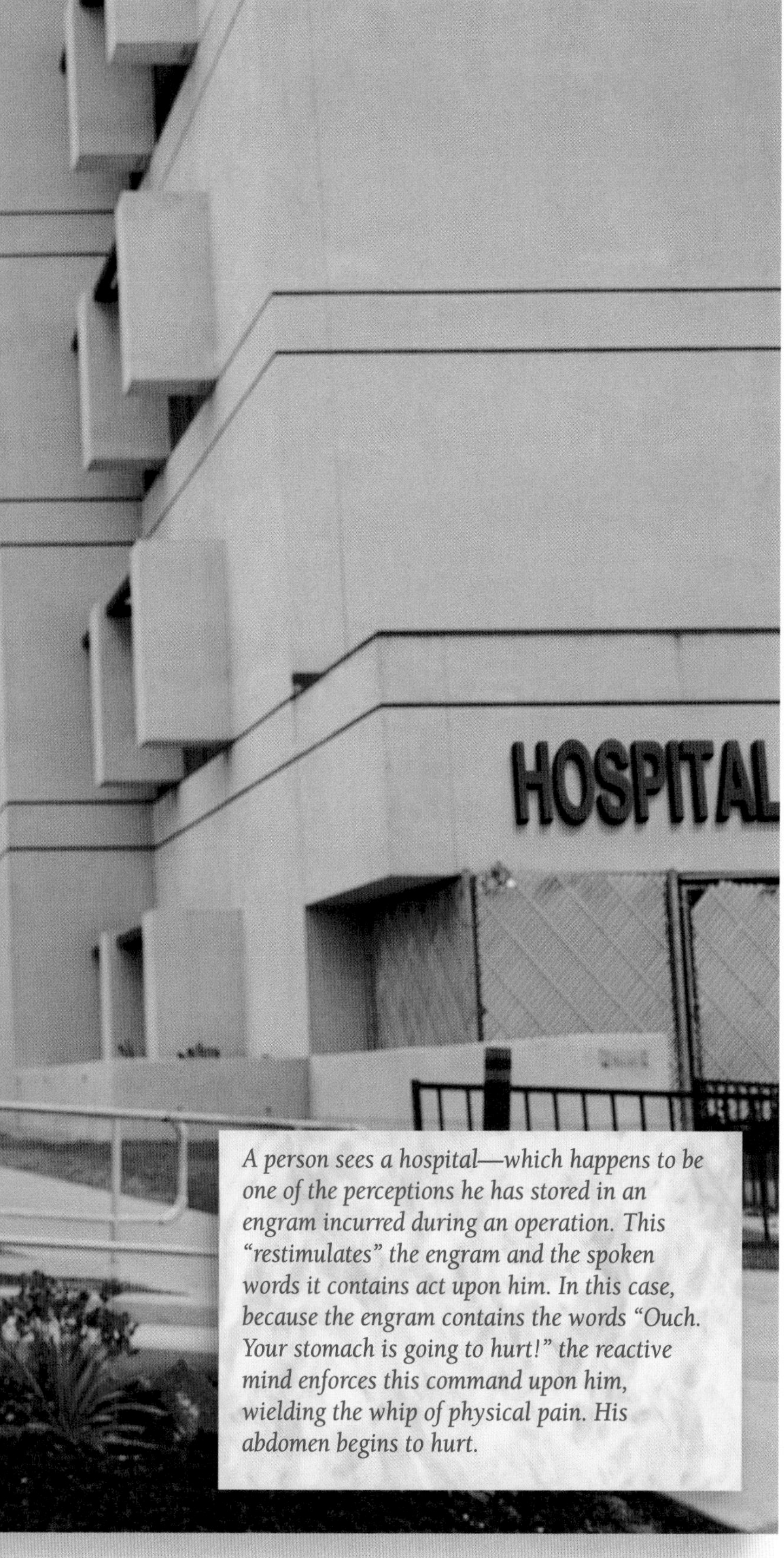

A person sees a hospital—which happens to be one of the perceptions he has stored in an engram incurred during an operation. This "restimulates" the engram and the spoken words it contains act upon him. In this case, because the engram contains the words "Ouch. Your stomach is going to hurt!" the reactive mind enforces this command upon him, wielding the whip of physical pain. His abdomen begins to hurt.

THE GOAL OF AUDITING

With Dianetics came the discovery of the source of man's irrationalities, psychosomatic illnesses, inappropriate emotions, neuroses and compulsions. And, through Dianetics auditing, a method for man to discover these engrams and eliminate their effects by erasing the charge connected to them. The experience is then refiled in the standard memory banks of the analytical mind.

The end result of Dianetics auditing is a new state for man—Clear. A Clear is very simply defined as a person who no longer has his own reactive mind. The spiritual ramifications of this breakthrough are profound.

The Clear has no engrams which, when restimulated, throw out the correctness of his computations by entering hidden and false data.

Becoming Clear strengthens a person's native individuality and creativity and does not in any way diminish these attributes. A Clear is free with his emotions. He can think for himself. He can experience life unencumbered by inhibitions reactively dictated by past engrams. Artistry, personal force and individual character are all residual in the basic personality of the person, not the reactive mind.

But with Dianetics came another vital question: *Who* exactly was looking at the pictures in the mind? The answer, of course, was the human spirit itself, the thetan.

And therein lay the answer to what constitutes the human being.

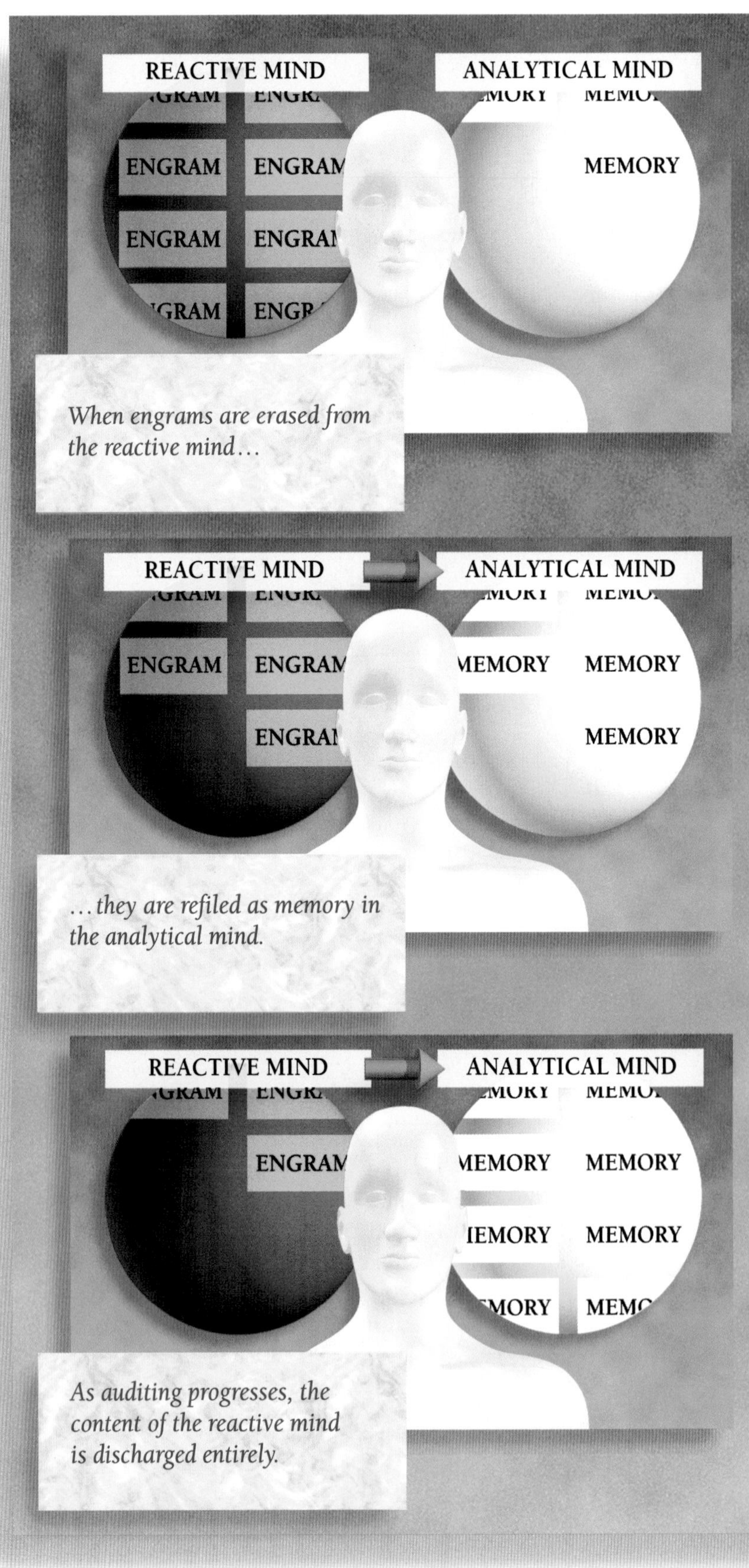

When engrams are erased from the reactive mind…

…they are refiled as memory in the analytical mind.

As auditing progresses, the content of the reactive mind is discharged entirely.

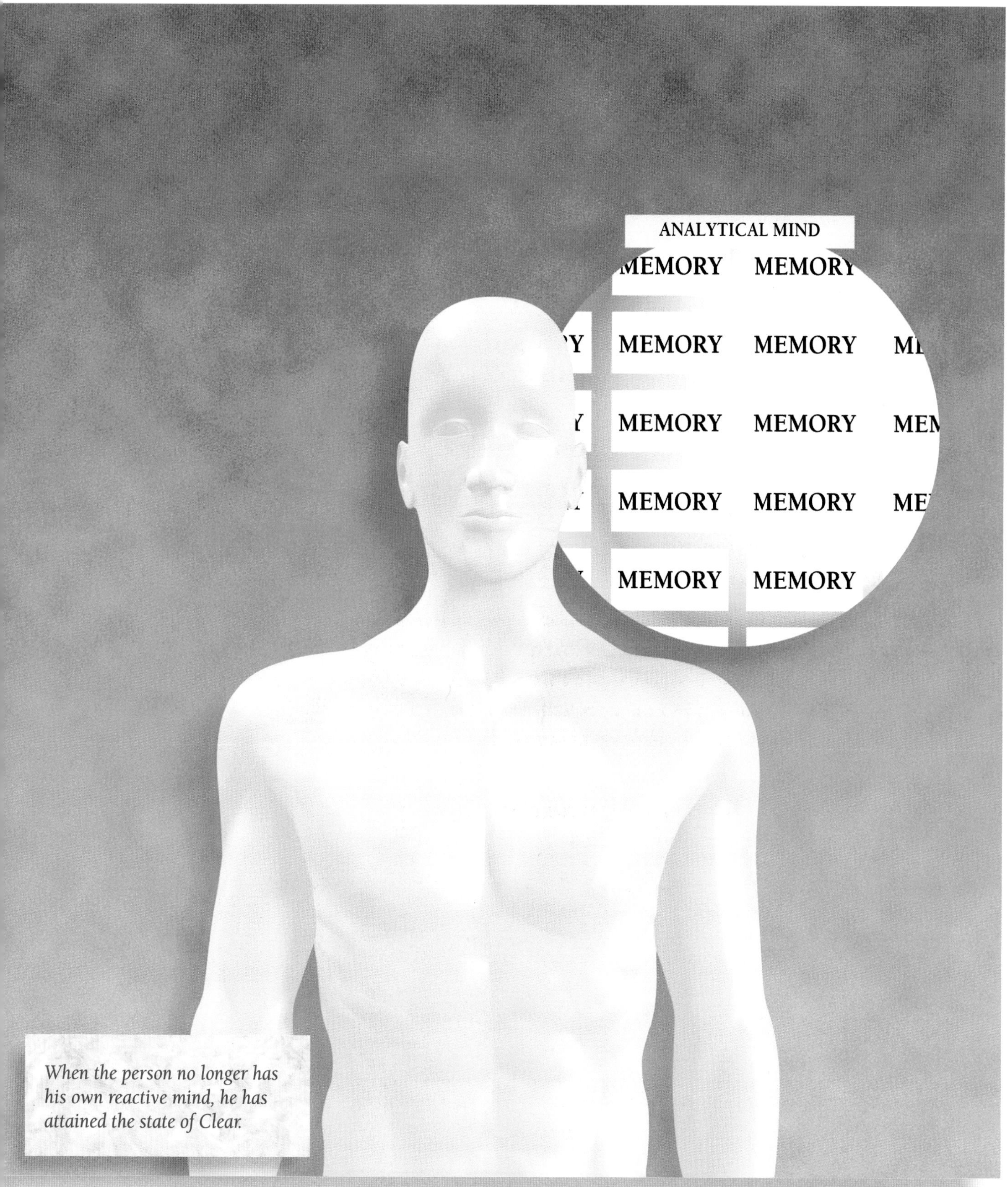

When the person no longer has his own reactive mind, he has attained the state of Clear.

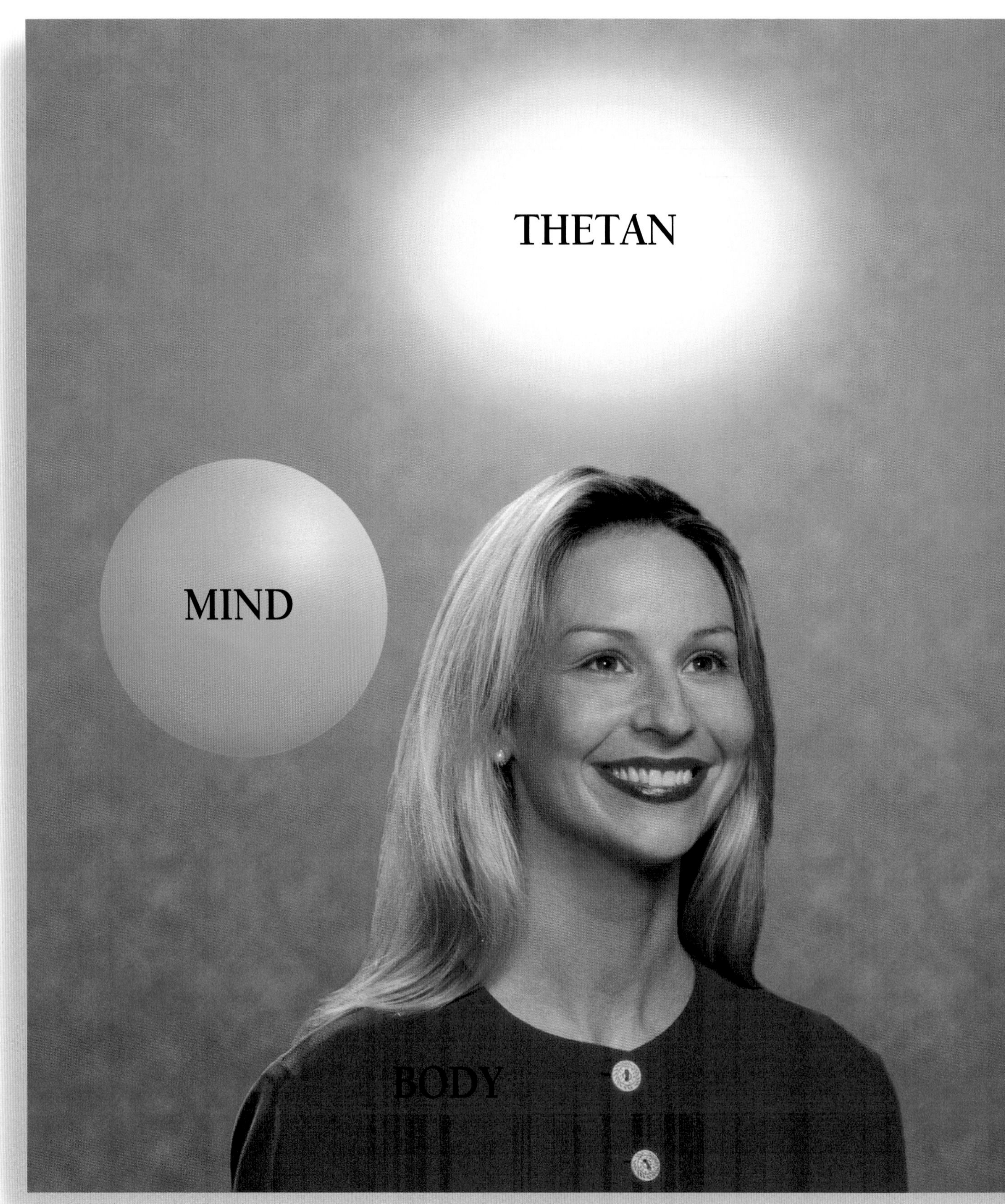
THETAN
MIND
BODY

Of the three parts to a human being, the thetan is senior.

Man consists of three parts: the body, little more than a machine; the mind, divided into the analytical and reactive, which computes and contains little more than a collection of pictures; and the thetan, life itself, the spirit which animates the body and uses the mind.

The point being, the thetan is senior to both body and mind. After all, it is none other than the thetan who actually erases engramic charge. In fact, as he gains control over his reactive mind through auditing, he likewise gains more control over the whole of life—regaining abilities and certainty of himself. But what are his limits? How high can he ultimately ascend?

From the search for these answers came the subject of Scientology, and the door opened to the full realization of spiritual potential.

That state is called Operating Thetan, and it is nothing short of what is delineated in this description of a spiritual being's native state: Although without mass, motion, wavelength or location in space or time, the thetan is nonetheless capable of accomplishing *anything*. Thus the Operating Thetan, or OT, may be defined as one who is at "knowing and willing cause over life, thought, matter, energy, space and time."

It is an ancient dream, this state of OT; and all great philosophic works either touch upon or echo it. Although it may seem remote to some in this postindustrial age, the thinking men of every major civilization up to this century not only would have grasped its meaning, but were themselves seeking on some level to attain it. For when one speaks of OT one is speaking of a transcendence over the travails of existence, and therein lies the ultimate dream of spiritual freedom.

It is not for nothing, then, that Scientology has been described as realizing man's most basic hope for spiritual freedom—by stripping away the accumulated impediments of the ages and returning to our native state, with all the abilities that are inherently ours.

Although the goal of OT is one every Scientologist has in common, one does not have to attain that state in order to realize he has embarked upon a journey the likes of which has never existed before. Every step, from the very first auditing session, is a landmark of realizations, increased awarenesses and regained abilities.

THE BRIDGE

Man has long envisioned a route across the chasm between his present state and higher levels of awareness. In Scientology that route is called the Bridge.

This bridge is gradiently laid out in an orderly progression so gains are incremental. It must be walked exactly, for each step represents attainable and known improvements—results that are readily apparent and predictable.

All steps on the Bridge are delineated on the Classification, Gradation and Awareness Chart of Levels and Certificates, an abridged version of which is shown here.

Classification, on the left side of the chart, refers to the study of the religious philosophy, its axioms, laws and procedures. This provides one with the wisdom and know-how to most effectively better conditions in life. Training is essential for a person to achieve complete spiritual freedom and fully half the gains available in Scientology come from this activity.

Gradation, on the right, refers to the ascending levels of auditing resulting in increased spiritual awareness and abilities for the thetan. The chart shows the proper step-by-step progression one takes to genuinely reach these levels.

In the center of the chart are the Awareness Characteristics from the lowest human states to the highest levels of spiritual awareness. Everyone is at one of these levels; it represents what he is personally aware of in his life, not what others may observe about his behavior. The Awareness Characteristics are part and parcel of the basics of the Scientology philosophy, as they relate not only to the level of an individual's own spiritual awareness and provide a means by which he can analyze his own life, but they also parallel his spiritual progress up the Bridge.

Like all else in Scientology, the Bridge is based upon traditional philosophy, and represents a dream of progressing to freedom that is as old as man himself.

The Grade Chart is a map anyone can follow to achieve higher awareness, greater ability and total freedom. An unabridged version of the chart is available upon request from the publisher at the address listed on page 824.

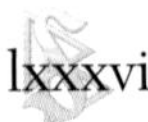

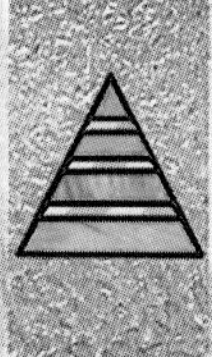

THE BRIDGE TO TOTAL FREEDOM

SCIENTOLOGY CLASSIFICATION GRADATION AND AWARENESS CHART OF LEVELS AND CERTIFICATES

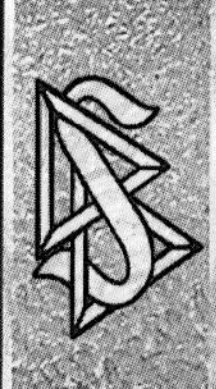

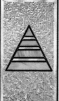

CLASSIFICATION
Training

Auditor's Class	Certificate
Class XII Auditor	Hubbard Class XII Auditor
Class XI Auditor	Hubbard Class XI Auditor
Class X Auditor	Hubbard Class X Auditor
Class IX Auditor	Hubbard Advanced Courses Specialist
Class VIII Auditor	Hubbard Specialist of Standard Tech
Class VII Auditor	Hubbard Graduate Auditor
Class VI Auditor	Hubbard Senior Scientologist
Class VA Graduate Auditor	Hubbard Expanded Dianetics Specialist
Class V Graduate Auditor	Hubbard Class V Graduate Auditor
Class V Auditor	Hubbard New Era Dianetics Auditor
Class IV Auditor	Hubbard Advanced Auditor
Class III Auditor	Hubbard Professional Auditor
Class II Auditor	Hubbard Certified Auditor
Class I Auditor	Hubbard Trained Scientologist
Class 0 Auditor	Hubbard Recognized Scientologist
Hubbard Professional Metering Course	Hubbard Professional Metering Course Graduate
Hubbard Professional Upper Indoctrination TR Course	Hubbard Professional Upper Indoctrination TR Course Graduate
New Hubbard Professional TR Course	New Hubbard Professional TR Course Graduate
The Student Hat	Hubbard Graduate of Study Technology

Total Freedom
Power on all 8 dynamics
21 Source
20 Existence
19 Conditions
18 Realization
17 Clearing
16 Purposes
15 Ability
14 Correction
13 Result
12 Production
11 Activity
10 Prediction
9 Body
8 Adjustment
7 Energy
6 Enlightenment
5 Understandings
4 Orientation
3 Perception
2 Communication
1 Recognition
–1 Help
–2 Hope
–3 Demand for Improvement
–4 Need of Change
–5 Fear of Worsening
–6 Effect
–7 Ruin
–8 Despair
–9 Suffering
–10 Numbness
–11 Introversion
–12 Disaster
–13 Inactuality
–14 Delusion
–15 Hysteria
–16 Shock
–17 Catatonia
–18 Oblivion
–19 Detachment
–20 Duality
–21 Secrecy
–22 Hallucination
–23 Sadism
–24 Masochism
–25 Elation
–26 Glee
–27 Fixidity
–28 Erosion
–29 Dispersal
–30 Disassociation
–31 Criminality
–32 Uncausing
–33 Disconnection
–34 Unexistence

GRADATION
Auditing

Pc Grade	Name of State
New OT XV	New Section XV OT
New OT XIV	New Section XIV OT
New OT XIII	New Section XIII OT
New OT XII	Future
New OT XI	Operating
New OT X	Character
New OT IX	Orders of Magnitude
New OT VIII	Truth Revealed
New OT VII	Solo New Era Dianetics for OTs
New OT VI	Solo New Era Dianetics for OTs Course
New OT V	Audited New Era Dianetics for OTs
New OT IV	New Section IV OT
OT III	Section III OT, "The Wall of Fire"
OT II	Section II OT
New OT I	New Section I OT
CLEAR	Clear. A being who no longer has his own reactive mind
Solo Auditor	New Hubbard Solo Auditor Course
New Era Dianetics	New Era Dianetics Case Completion
Grade IV Expanded	Ability Release
Grade III Expanded	Freedom Release
Grade II Expanded	Relief Release
Grade I Expanded	Problems Release
Grade 0 Expanded	Communications Release
ARC Straightwire Expanded	Recall Release
Happiness Rundown	Happiness Rundown Completion
TRs and Objectives	Objectives Completion
Purification Rundown	Purification Rundown Completion

Yet with the realization of this dream of greater freedom comes the realization of another philosophic tradition: ethics. The idea is as simple as it is intrinsic to Scientology. Because man is basically good—meaning his basic personality and basic intentions toward others are good—he naturally restrains himself from committing harmful acts. And when he finds himself committing too many evils, then, causatively, unconsciously or unwittingly, he employs an ethical solution by lessening his own abilities and causing his own downfall.

It is for this reason that one cannot hope to progress along the Scientology Bridge without honest participation, without a sincere desire for betterment and without the highest standards of integrity. Nor can one ever hope to hold his gains unless he maintains these standards.

Needless to say, ethics is a subject the Scientologist takes very seriously. As he moves up the Bridge and becomes more and more himself, he likewise grows more ethical, but he also views it as a matter of personal responsibility that extends well beyond this life. For unlike the materialist who believes death to be an end to life, conscience and accountability, the Scientologist sees it as a transition through which one carries his past—a past for which one continues to be accountable.

He also knows that the abilities he is regaining were, in part, lost because of transgressions and irresponsibilities. Thus, honesty, integrity, trust and concern for his fellows are more than just words. They are principles to live by.

THE ROAD TO TRUTH

Unquestionably man is a troubled being in very troubled times. Since the start of the twentieth century, an endless parade of convoluted ideas have been proposed to account for our lot: left-brain/right-brain theories, chemical imbalances, genetic flaws, pop-psychology pronouncements and New Age speculations.

Such theories left only questions: What is the real source of our problems? Why do past upsets continue to haunt us? Why is it difficult to understand others, and why do we end up regretting so much? Why are we so afraid of old age, illness and death, and why is our happiness so frail?

What is unique about Scientology is the way in which these matters are addressed—and the fact they are finally resolved only by recognizing man's essential nature. For if the human spirit is the source of all man's innate wisdom, capabilities, goodness and strength, it is also the source of his failings—and thus only by directly addressing it can one right what is wrong.

This, then, is what Scientology is all about. And why it is defined as the study and handling of the spirit in relationship to itself, universes and other life.

In such terms, Scientology may be seen as the culmination of a long and noble religious tradition, one that extends back at least ten thousand years through the Buddhist, Hindu and Vedic scriptures. One may draw further parallels to Celtic, Greek and early Christian teachings, which also saw man as an eternal spirit who accepted responsibility for future lives.

Of course, the technology of Scientology is wholly new, and the way in which it addresses the spirit is new. But the tradition is an ancient one. Indeed, it was only within the last hundred years that men began to lose all sight of themselves with the advent of materialistic theory.

Whereas society today has spent literally billions of dollars in fruitless pursuit of solutions to symptoms, only Scientology addresses the true source—the spiritual realm.

And therein lies the path to miracles.

Scientology is a vast subject, very probably the largest body of work on the mind and spirit ever produced. As its applications are as extensive as life itself, all of its tools cannot be mastered in a single day. But as you will see through the succeeding pages, there are benefits to be had from the very first step. ■

How to Use This Handbook

The Scientology Handbook is a companion work to the book *What Is Scientology?* which explains Scientology and describes its religious philosophy, practices, organizations and wide-ranging community and social betterment activities.

What Is Scientology? is an encyclopedic reference work which furnishes a comprehensive description of the Scientology religion and its impact on the world today. In it you will find a complete history of Scientology, a descriptive biographical view of L. Ron Hubbard's life, a full list of all the materials he developed, and an enlightening look at the application of Scientology by individuals in their lives and toward the betterment of society.

An in-depth view of the fastest growing religion on the face of the earth, *What Is Scientology?* contains a catechism which answers all the commonly asked questions about the Church. Additionally, it presents the Scientology Axioms which amount to nothing less than a remarkable and complete codification of the activities of life itself, an examination of the Church hierarchy and what happens in a church of Scientology, and a full account of Mr. Hubbard's numerous discoveries about man and life that are changing the face of the culture in which we live. It is a thorough examination of a vital religion and the unique scope of its technology.

The Scientology Handbook, on the other hand, provides basic Scientology techniques and principles so a person can *apply* them to life. It has been assembled for those involved in Scientology and those who have read *What Is Scientology?* But it has also been compiled to be a usable and valuable tool for someone who has no prior familiarity with the subject whatsoever. It is for *anyone* who sees the need for positive change in the world around him.

L. Ron Hubbard made many observations and breakthroughs regarding life. From these, the auditing techniques were developed that lead to entirely new states of spiritual freedom. But because these breakthroughs are fundamental to all of life, their application extends to every aspect of life. In fact, these principles stand alone as effective methods of betterment. And it is

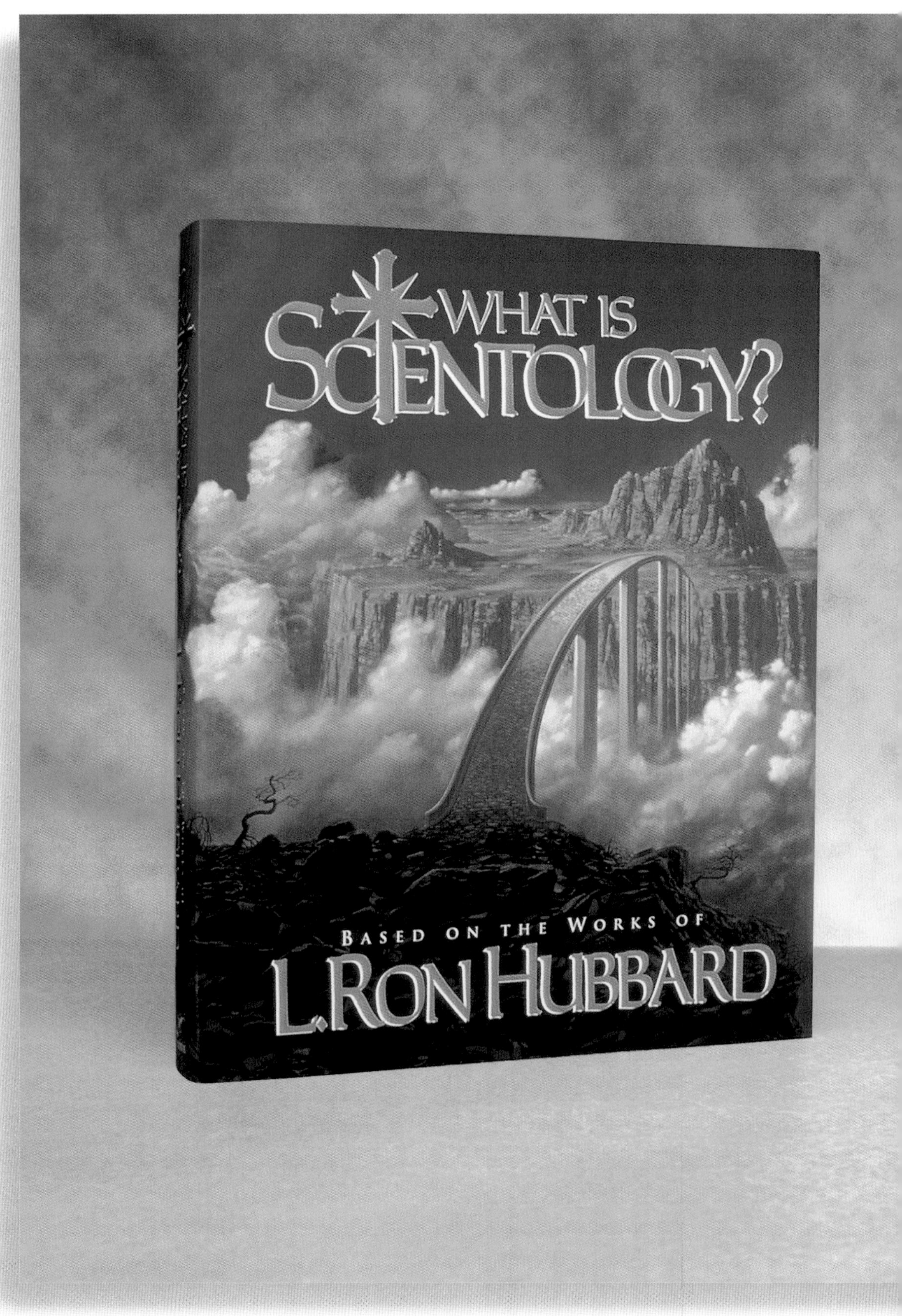
WHAT IS
SCIENTOLOGY?
BASED ON THE WORKS OF
L. RON HUBBARD

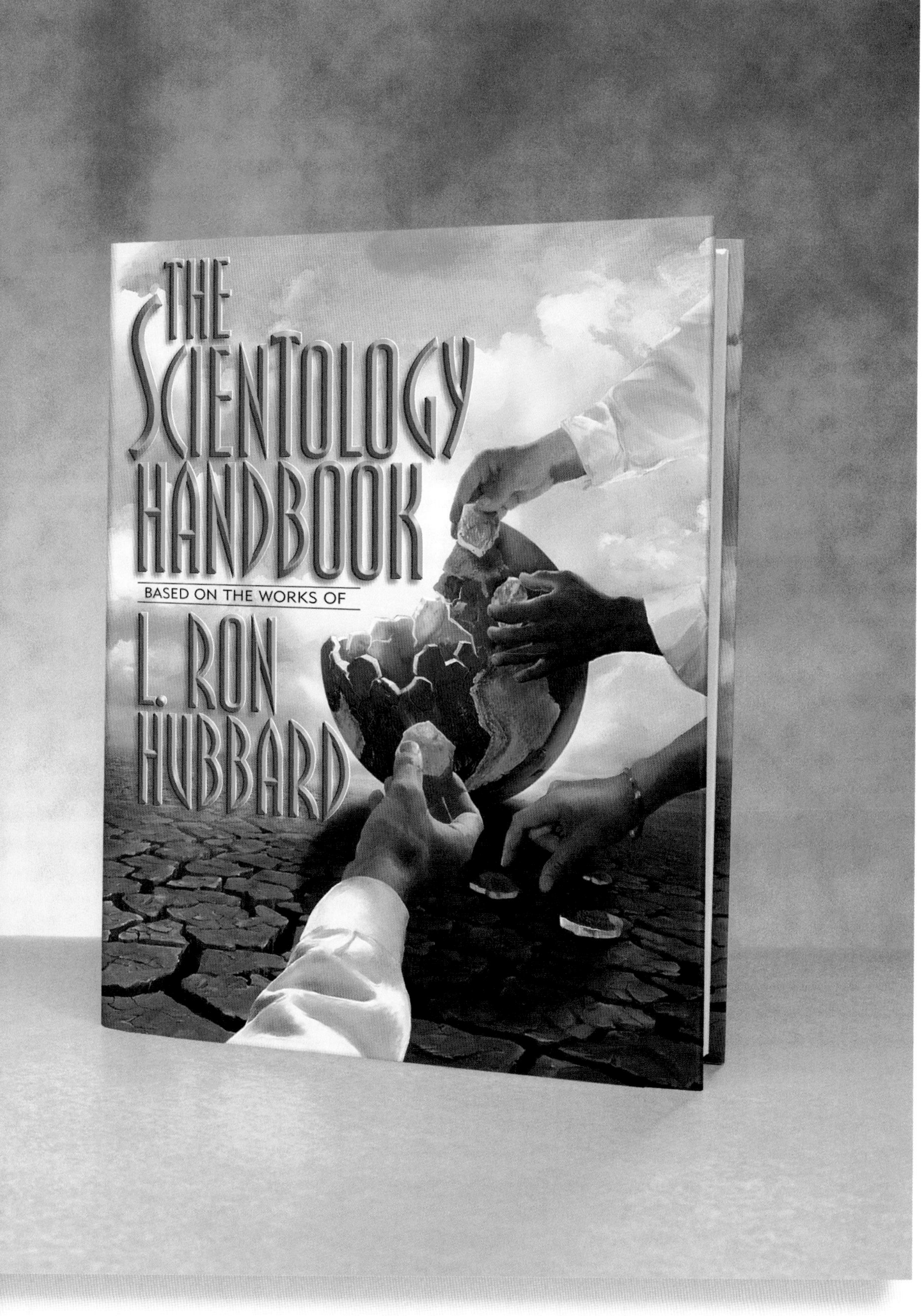

Together, **The Scientology Handbook** *and* **What Is Scientology?** *provide a thorough explanation of the philosophy and practical application of Scientology.*

this application of Scientology that forms the subject matter of this book. Even the employment of a single Scientology principle can dramatically change conditions.

For example, the knowledge that an engram contains all perceptions recorded during moments of pain and unconsciousness—including words—leads to a basic Scientology rule: Never speak in the vicinity of a person in such a condition. Silence is maintained around an injured or unconscious person so as not to add phrases to the contents of an engram, which can later be restimulated.

Scientology—all of it—is for use. It is a practical philosophy, something one does.

Thus *The Scientology Handbook* is a *practical* guide. In it are found many technologies of use in areas such as study, drug rehabilitation, interpersonal relationships, raising children and much more. These form the subject matter of this handbook. It places tools for solving the problems of life into the hands of those who read it.

Although this handbook contains only a small portion of the full technology of Scientology, it is intended to provide you with some of its most basic and practical aspects so you can improve your own life and the lives of others without extended study or practice. These are techniques and principles that have been successfully used countless times by millions of people in countries around the world.

What you will read here works when applied. And you will find actual stories of how people from all walks of life have used these tools to help themselves, their families and friends, co-workers and colleagues, even complete strangers.

This is a handbook for people who want to do something about the conditions they see in the world around them. It contains procedures which anybody can use to improve situations both in his own life and in the lives of others.

The Scientology Handbook is simple to use. You do not need to study the whole book to begin using the data which follow. Each chapter contains a body of material on a specific subject compiled from the writings of Mr. Hubbard. The editors have augmented these writings with a short introduction to the chapter's contents, a quiz of your understanding, practical exercises, examples of successful application and a list of materials available for further study for those who wish to gain a broader understanding of the entire subject.

You can find the chapter covering a particular situation in the table of contents or in the index. The index cross-references material from other chapters which augments data in the one you are reading. Using this index will broaden your knowledge of the procedures and how they can be applied to specific circumstances.

Each chapter can stand independent of subjects covered in other chapters. You could, for instance, learn to help an upset child by turning straight to Chapter 14 and reading it. In minutes, you could learn a technique to assist a co-worker recover from an on-the-job injury by reading Chapter 6. You could begin at once to discover the reason for a conflict in a relationship with someone and start to repair it by studying only Chapter 8.

Naturally, reading the entire handbook will show the relationships which exist among the various subjects and increase your understanding of how to use them.

Many new phenomena about man and life are described in Scientology, and so you may encounter terms in these pages you are not familiar with. These are described the first time they appear in a chapter. If you come to a term which is new to you, turn to the glossary at the back of the book. All Scientology terms which may be unfamiliar have been included there for your reference.

The tools which follow are for immediate use. But unlike a carpenter's saw that eventually dulls and needs sharpening, the more these procedures are used, the sharper they get. As one becomes more skilled in their application, the more benefit people receive.

One final note: there are many subjects in life that are taught from an authoritarian stance. One is force-fed the data and expected to swallow it. Such is not the case with this handbook. You are invited to inspect the data for yourself, apply it exactly as it is presented, and then decide for yourself whether or not it is true and whether it works. There is a very important datum in Scientology: "What is true for you is what you have observed yourself." Nothing in Scientology is true for you unless you have observed it and it is true according to your observation.

Millions have found that Scientology does indeed work. The object of *The Scientology Handbook* is to put this workable knowledge of life into the hands of every person on earth. Life *can* be improved. There is too much unhappiness, misery and distrust in the world. Too much attention is wasted on the negative side of life. Something can be done about it and this book tells you how. ■

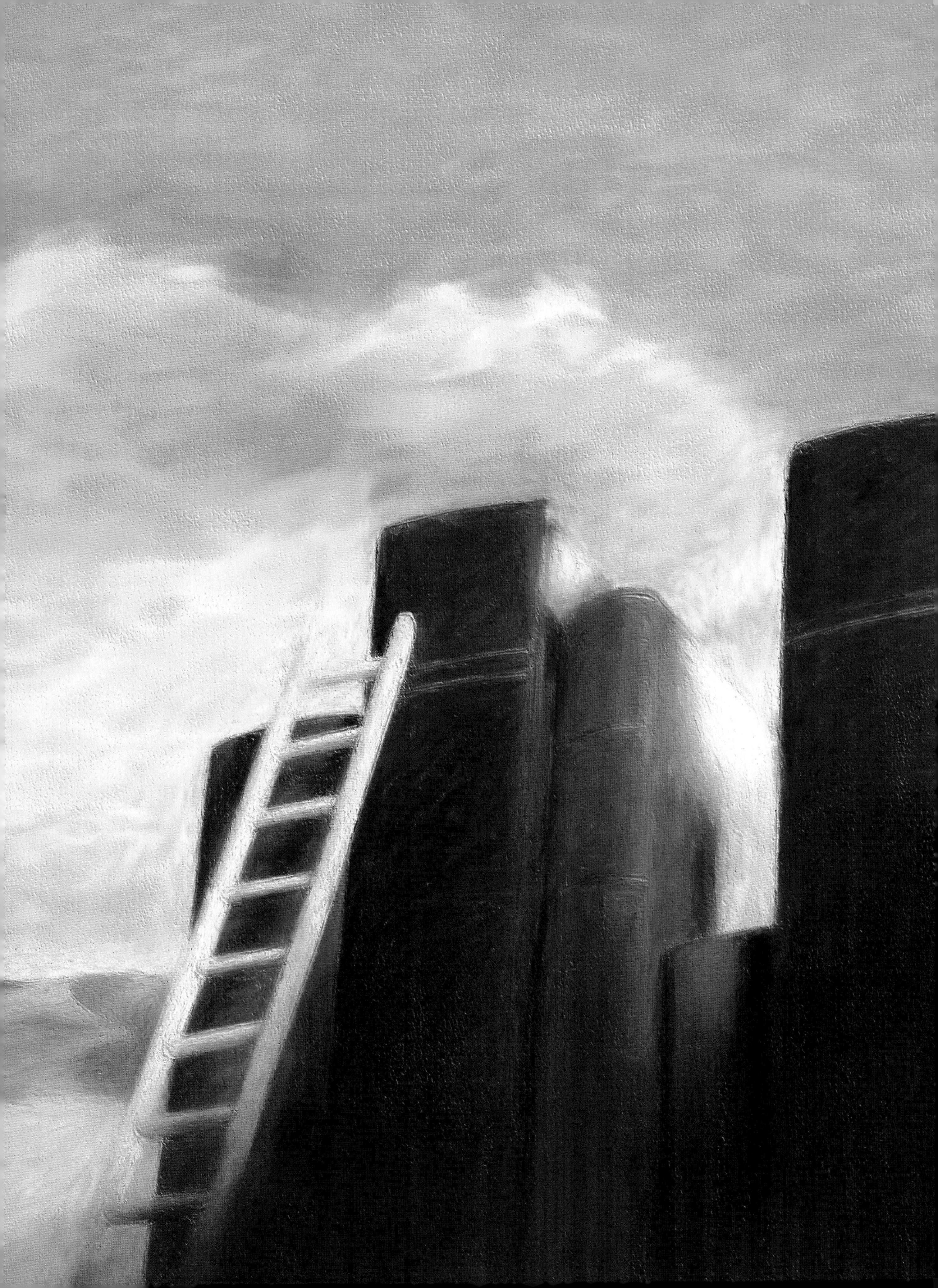

Chapter 1

THE TECHNOLOGY OF STUDY

Consider this for a moment: In all your schooling, did anyone ever teach you **how** *to study something?*

Today, people are graduating school unable to read or write at a level adequate to hold a job or deal with life. It is a huge problem. It is not that subjects cannot be learned; what isn't taught is **how** *to learn. It is the missing step in all education.*

L. Ron Hubbard filled this gaping hole by supplying the first and only technology of how to study. He discovered the laws on which learning is based and developed workable methods for anyone to apply. He called this subject "Study Technology."

This technology provides an understanding of the basics of learning and supplies exact ways to overcome all the pitfalls one can encounter during study.

Study Technology is not speed-reading or memory tricks. These have not been proven to raise one's ability to comprehend what was studied or to raise literacy. Study Technology shows **how** *one studies in order to comprehend a subject so one can* **apply** *it.*

Contained herein is only a small portion of the entire body of Study Technology developed by Mr. Hubbard. Regardless, this brief overview contains fundamentals which you can use to study more effectively. With this technology, **any** *subject can be learned by* **anyone***.*

Why Study?

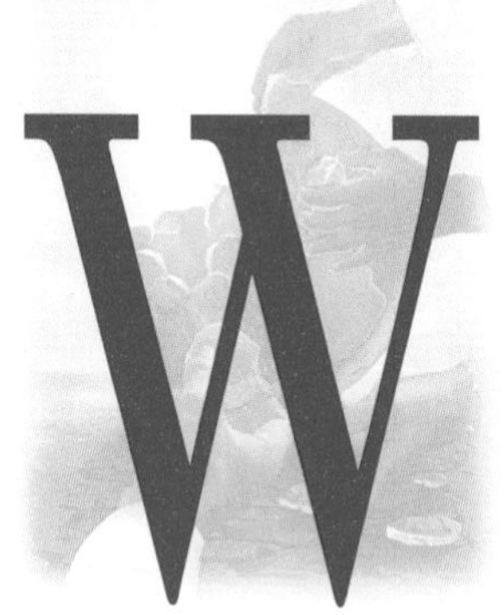

With all the emphasis placed on education in our society it is remarkable to realize that there has never been an actual technology of study or a technology of education. That sounds very far-fetched but it is true. There was a *school* technology, but it didn't have too much to do with *education*. It consisted of the technology of how you go to school, how you get taught and how you get examined, but there was no actual technology of education or *study*. Lacking such a technology, people find it difficult to achieve their goals. Knowing how to study is vitally important to *anyone*.

The first little gate that has to be opened to embark upon study is the willingness to know. If that gate remains closed, then one is liable to get into such things as a total memorized, word-for-word system of education, which will not result in the gain of any knowledge. Such a system only produces graduates who can possibly parrot back facts, but without any real understanding or ability to do anything with what they have been taught.

For what purpose, then, does one study? Until you clarify that, you cannot make an intelligent activity of it.

Some students study for the examination. The student is thinking to himself, "How will I repeat this back when I am asked a certain question?" or "How will I pass the examination?" That is complete folly, but unfortunately is what many students have done in a university.

Take the man who has been building houses for a long time, who one day gets an assistant who has just been trained in the university to build houses. He goes mad! The *academically* trained man has been studying it for years, yet knows nothing about it. And the *practical* man doesn't know why this is.

The reason why is that the man who just went through the university studied all of his materials so that he could be examined on them; he didn't study them to build houses. The man who has been out there on a practical line is not necessarily superior in the long run, but he certainly is able to get houses built, because all of *his* study is on the basis of "How do I apply this to house building?" Every time he picks up an ad or literature or anything else, he is asking the question throughout the entirety of his reading, "How can I apply this to what I'm doing?"

That is the basic and important difference between *practical* study and *academic* study.

This is why some people fail in practice after they graduate.

Instead of looking at data and thinking, "Is this going to be on the exam?" one would do much better to ask oneself, "How can I apply this material?" or "How can I really use this?"

By doing this a person will get much more out of what he studies and will be able to put what he studies to actual use.

The Student Who Knows All About It

On the subject of learning itself, the first datum to learn and the primary obstacle to overcome is: *You cannot study a subject if you think you know all about it to begin with.*

A student who thinks he knows all there is to know about a subject will not be able to learn anything in it.

A person might already be familiar with a subject from previous experience and, having had success in that field, now has the idea that he knows all about it. If such a person then took a course in that subject, he would be studying *through* a screen of "I know all about this."

With that obstacle in the way, one can become completely bogged down in his studies and not make forward progress.

This is true for a student of any subject.

If one can decide that he does not already know everything about a subject and can say to himself, "Here is something to study, let's study it," he can overcome this obstacle and be able to learn.

This is a very, very important datum for any student. If he understands this and applies it, the gateway to knowledge is wide open to him.

Barriers to Study

Being a successful student requires more than just a willingness to learn, however. Pitfalls do exist and students must know *how* to effectively learn in order to overcome them.

It has been discovered that there are three definite barriers which can block a person's ability to study and thus his ability to be educated. These barriers actually produce different sets of physical and mental reactions.

If one knows and understands what these barriers are and how to handle them, his ability to study and learn will be greatly increased.

The First Barrier: Absence of Mass

In Study Technology, we refer to the *mass* and the *significance* of a subject. By *mass* we mean the actual physical objects, the things of life. The *significance* of a subject is the meaning or ideas or theory of it.

Education attempted in the absence of the *mass* in which the technology will be involved is hard on a student.

If you were studying about tractors, the mass would be a tractor. You could study a textbook all about tractors, how to operate the controls, the different types of attachments that can be used—in other words, all the significance—but can you imagine how little you would understand if you had never actually seen a tractor?

Such an absence of mass can actually make a student feel squashed. It can make him feel bent, sort of dizzy, sort of dead, bored and exasperated.

Photographs or motion pictures can be helpful because they represent a promise or hope of the mass. But if one is studying about tractors, the printed page and the spoken word are not a substitute for an actual tractor!

Not having the mass of what one is studying about can make a student feel bent, dizzy, dead, bored and exasperated. The printed page is not a substitute for the actual mass.

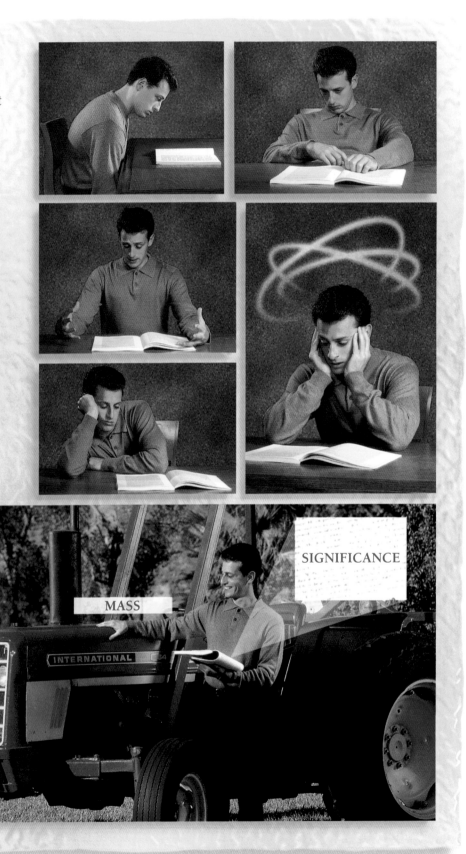

Educating a person in a mass that he does not have and which is not available can produce some uncomfortable and distracting physical reactions.

If you were trying to teach someone all about tractors but you did not show him any tractors or let him experience the mass of a tractor, he would wind up with a face that felt squashed, with headaches and with his stomach feeling funny. He would feel dizzy from time to time and often his eyes would hurt.

Students of any age can run into this barrier. Let us say that little Johnny is having an awful time at school with his arithmetic. You find out that he had an arithmetic problem that involved apples, but he never had any apples on his desk to count. Get him some apples and give each one of them a number. Now he has a number of apples in front of him—there is no longer a theoretical number of apples.

The point is that you could trace Johnny's problem back to an absence of mass and remedy it by supplying the mass; or you could supply an object or a reasonable substitute.

This barrier to study—the studying of something without its mass ever being around—produces these distinctly recognizable reactions.

Remedying an Absence of Mass

As not everyone studying has the actual mass available, useful tools to remedy a lack of mass have been developed. These come under the subject of demonstration.

Demonstration comes from the Latin *demonstrare:* "to point out, show, prove."

The *Chambers 20th Century Dictionary* includes the following definition of *demonstrate:* "to teach, expound or exhibit by practical means."

In order to supply mass, one would *do* a demonstration. One way of accomplishing this is with a "demonstration kit." A "demo kit," as it is called, is composed of various small objects such as corks, caps, paper clips, pen tops, rubber bands, etc. A student can use a demo kit to represent the things he is studying and help him to understand concepts.

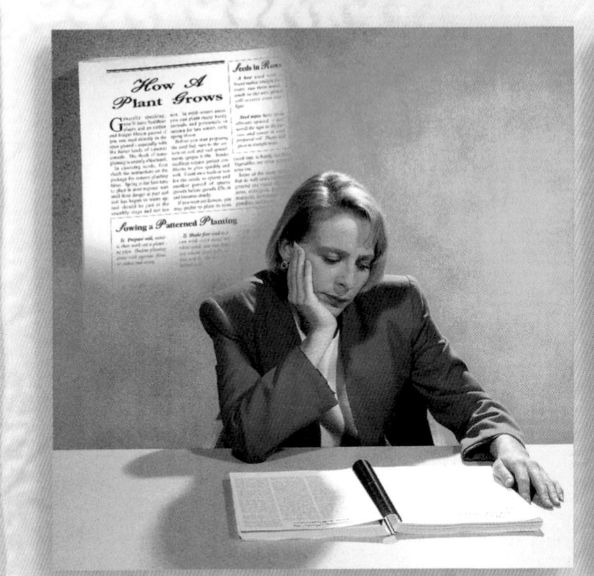

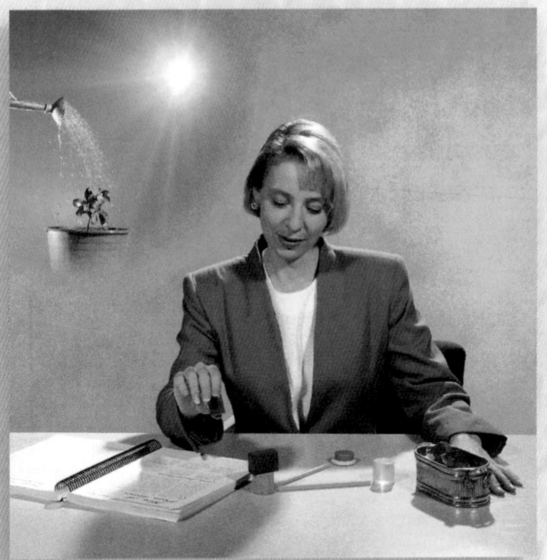

Demonstrating a concept with various small objects adds mass to what a person is studying. This increases understanding.

If a student ran into something he couldn't quite figure out, demonstrating the idea with a demo kit would assist him to understand it.

Anything can be demonstrated with a demo kit: ideas, objects, interrelationships or how something works. One simply uses these small objects to represent the various parts of something he is studying about. The objects can be moved about in relation to each other to show the mechanics and actions of a given concept.

Another means of demonstrating something is by sketching.

Someone sitting at his office desk trying to work something out can take a pencil and paper and, by sketching out or drawing graphs of what he was working with, get a grip on it.

There is a rule which goes *if you cannot demonstrate something in two dimensions, you have it wrong.* It is an arbitrary rule—based on judgment or discretion—but is very workable.

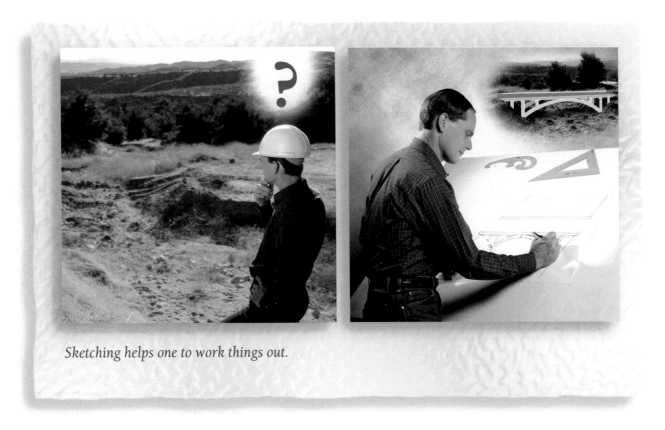

Sketching helps one to work things out.

This rule is used in engineering and architecture. If it cannot be worked out simply and clearly in two dimensions, there is something wrong and it couldn't be built.

Sketching and two-dimensional representation is all part of demonstration and of working something out.

A third means of supplying mass to clarify principles is through the use of modeling clay to make a *clay demonstration,* or "clay demo," of a principle or concept.

The purpose of clay demonstration is:

1. to make the materials being studied real to the student,

2. to give a proper balance of mass and significance,

3. to teach the student to *apply*.

The whole theory of clay demonstrations is that they add mass.

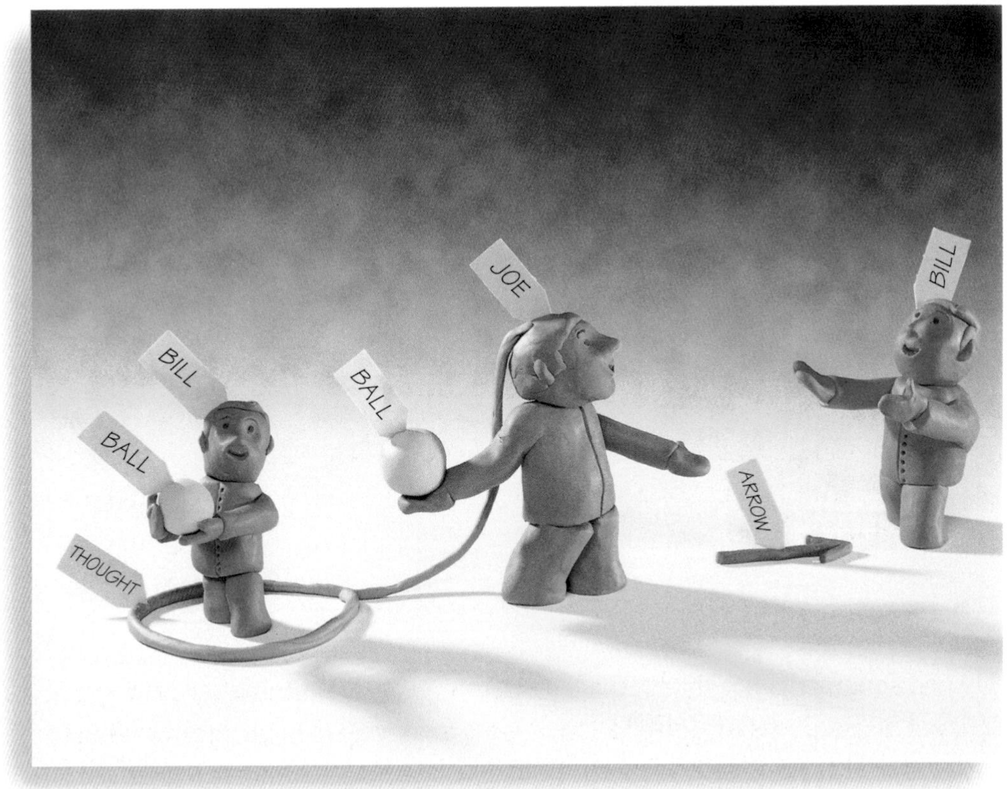

Objects, actions, thoughts, ideas, relationships or anything else can be demonstrated in clay.

A student needs mass in order to understand something. Without it, he only has thoughts or mental concepts. Given mass, he can sort it out because he has mass and space in which to then envision the concept he is studying.

Demo kit demonstrations work on this principle too, only a clay demonstration more closely represents the thing being demonstrated and provides more mass.

Any student can use clay to demonstrate an action, definition, object or principle. He sits at a table set up with different colors of modeling clay for his use. He demonstrates the object or principle in clay, labeling each part. The clay *shows* the thing. It is *not* just a blob of clay with a label on it. Small strips of paper are used for labels.

For example, say a student wants to demonstrate a pencil. He makes a thin roll of clay which is surrounded by another layer of clay—the thin roll sticking slightly out of one end. On the other end goes a small cylinder of clay. The roll is labeled "lead." The outer layer is labeled "wood." The small cylinder is labeled "rubber."

Simplicity is the keynote.

Anything can be demonstrated in clay if one works at it. And just by working on *how* to demonstrate it or make it into clay and labels brings about renewed understanding.

In the phrase "How do I represent it in clay?" is contained the secret of the teaching. If one can represent it in clay, one understands it. If one can't, one really doesn't understand what it is. So clay and labels work only if the term or things are truly understood. And working them out in clay brings about an understanding of them.

Art is no object in doing clay demo work. The forms are crude.

Each separate thing made in a clay demo is labeled, no matter how crude the label is. Students usually do labels on scraps of paper or light cardboard written on with a ballpoint. When making a label, a point is put on one end, making it easy to stick the label into the clay.

The procedure should go: student makes one object, labels it, makes another object, labels it, makes a third object and puts a label on it and so on in sequence. This comes from the datum that optimum learning requires an equal balance of mass and significance and that too much of one without the other can make the student feel bad. If a student makes all the masses of his demonstration at once, without labeling them, he is sitting there with all those significances stacking up in his mind instead of putting down each one (in the form of a label) as he goes. The correct procedure is to label each mass as one goes along.

Any object or principle or action can be represented by a piece of clay and a label. The mass parts are done by clay, the significance or thought parts by label.

Directions of motion or travel are usually indicated with little arrows. The arrow can be made out of clay or it can be made as another type of label. This can become important. Lack of clarity in the demo about which way what is going or which way what is flowing can make the demo unrecognizable.

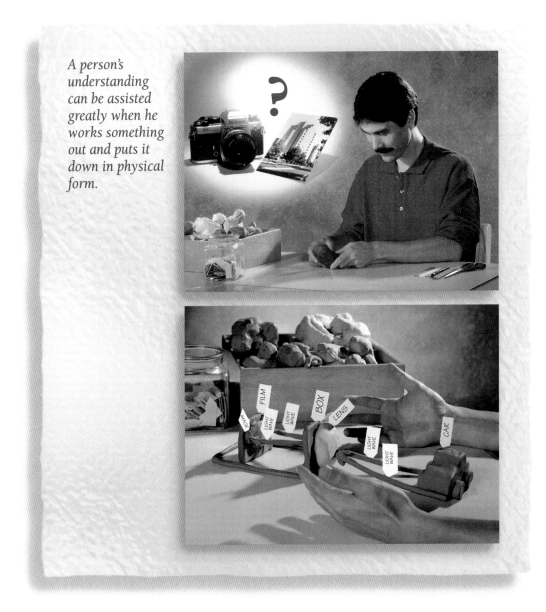

A person's understanding can be assisted greatly when he works something out and puts it down in physical form.

Clay demos must be large. One of the purposes of clay demonstrations is to make the materials being studied *real* to the student. If a student's clay demo is small (less mass), it may not be sufficiently real to the person. *Big* clay demos are more successful in terms of increasing student understanding.

A well-done clay demo, which actually does demonstrate, will produce a marvelous change in the student. And he will retain the data.

Each of these three methods of remedying an absence of mass—using a demo kit, sketching and clay demonstrations—should be used liberally in any educational activity. They can make a big difference in how well a student learns and can apply what he has studied.

The Second Barrier: Too Steep a Gradient

A *gradient* is a gradual approach to something taken step by step, level by level, each step or level being, of itself, easily attainable—so that finally, complicated and difficult activities can be achieved with relative ease. The term *gradient* also applies to each of the steps taken in such an approach.

When one hits too steep a gradient in studying a subject, a sort of confusion or reelingness (a state of mental swaying or unsteadiness) results. This is the second barrier to study.

The remedy for too steep a gradient is to cut back the gradient. Find out when the person was not confused about what he was studying and then find out what *new* action he undertook. Find out what he felt he understood well just *before* he got all confused.

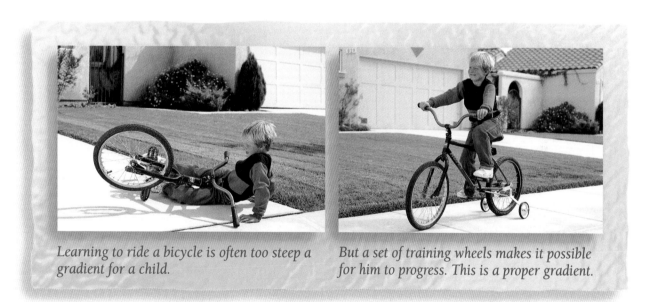

Learning to ride a bicycle is often too steep a gradient for a child.

But a set of training wheels makes it possible for him to progress. This is a proper gradient.

You will discover that there is something in this area—the part he'd felt he understood well—which he did not really understand.

When this is cleared up, the student will be able to progress again.

When a person is found to be terribly confused on the second action he was supposed to know or do, it is safe to assume that he never really understood the *first* action.

This barrier is most recognizable and most applicable when engaged in *doingness*—performing some action or activity—as opposed to just academic or intellectual study.

The Third–and Most Important–Barrier: The Misunderstood Word

The third and most important barrier to study is the misunderstood word. A misunderstood word is a word which is *not* understood or *wrongly* understood.

An entirely different set of physical reactions can occur when one reads past words he does not understand. Going on past a word that was not understood gives one a distinctly blank feeling or a washed-out feeling.

A "not-there" feeling and a sort of nervous hysteria (excessive anxiety) can follow that.

The confusion or inability to grasp or learn comes *after* a word that the person did not have defined and understood.

The misunderstood word is much more important than the other two barriers. The misunderstood word establishes aptitude and lack of aptitude; this is what psychologists have been trying to test for years without recognizing what it was.

This is all that many study difficulties go back to. Studying past misunderstood words produces such a vast range of mental effects that it itself is the prime factor involved with stupidity and many other unwanted conditions.

If a person didn't have misunderstood words, his *talent* might or might not be present, but his *doingness* in that subject would be present.

There are two specific phenomena which stem from misunderstood words.

First Phenomenon

When a student misses understanding a word, the section right after that word is a blank in his memory.

You can always trace back to the word just before the blank, get it understood and find miraculously that the former blank area is not now blank in the material you are studying.

It is pure magic.

When a person is reading down a page...

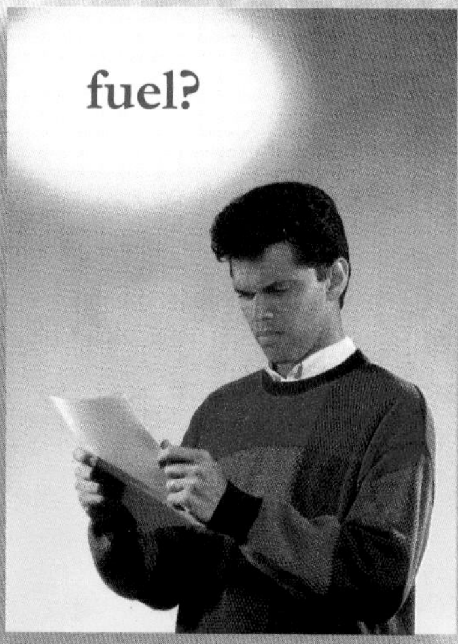

...and goes past a word for which he has no definition...

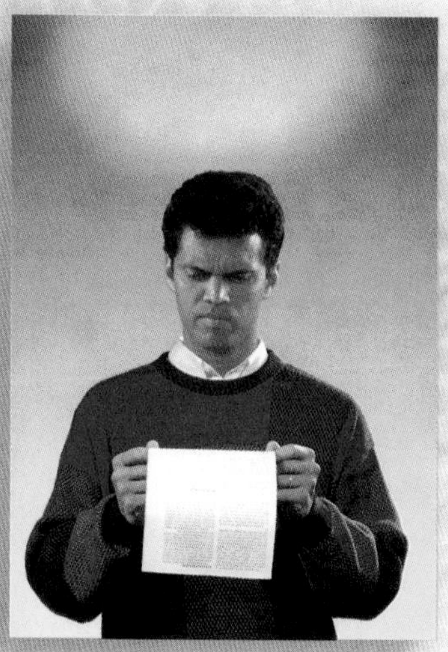

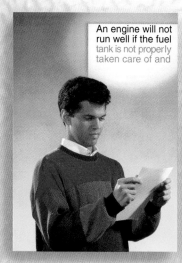

...the section after the misunderstood word will be blank in his memory. The misunderstood word is the most important barrier to successful study.

Have you ever had the experience of coming to the end of a page and realizing you didn't know what you had read? Somewhere earlier on that page you went past a word that you had no definition for or an incorrect definition for.

Here is an example: "It was found that when the crepuscule arrived the children were quieter and when it was not present, they were much livelier." What happens is you think you do not understand the whole idea, but the inability to understand comes entirely from the one word you could not define, *crepuscule*, which means twilight or darkness.

Second Phenomenon

A misunderstood definition or a not-comprehended definition or an undefined word can even cause a person to give up studying a subject and leave a course or class. Leaving in this way is called a *blow*.

We have all known people who enthusiastically started on a course of study only to find out some time later that the person dropped the study because it was "boring" or "it wasn't what they thought it would be." They were going to learn a skill or go to night school and get their degree but never followed through. No matter how reasonable their excuses, the fact is they dropped the subject or left the course. This is a blow. A person blows for only one primary reason—the misunderstood word.

A person does not necessarily blow because of the other barriers to study—lack of mass or too steep a gradient. These simply produce physical phenomena. But the misunderstood word can cause a student to blow.

There is a definite sequence of actions following a misunderstood word:

When a word is not grasped, the student then goes into a noncomprehension (blankness) of things immediately after. This is followed by the student's solution for the blank condition which is to *individuate* from it—meaning to separate himself from it and withdraw from involvement with it.

Now that the student is separated from the area he was studying, he does not really care what he does with regard to the subject or related things or activities. This is the attitude—being separate or different from—which precedes doing something harmful to something or someone.

For example, a student in school who has gone past misunderstood words in a course will not care about what happens in class, will probably bad-mouth the subject to his friends and may even damage class equipment or lose his textbook.

However, people are basically good. When an individual commits a harmful act, he then makes an effort to restrain himself from committing more harmful acts. This is followed by his finding ways he has been "wronged" by others, in order to justify his actions, and by complaints, faultfinding and a "look-what-you-did-to-me" attitude. These factors justify, in the student's mind, a departure or blow.

But most educational systems, frowning on blows as they do, cause the student to really withdraw himself from the study subject (whatever he was studying) and set up in its place mental machinery which can receive and give back sentences and phrases. A person can set up mental machinery when he becomes disinterested in what he is doing but feels he has to continue doing it.

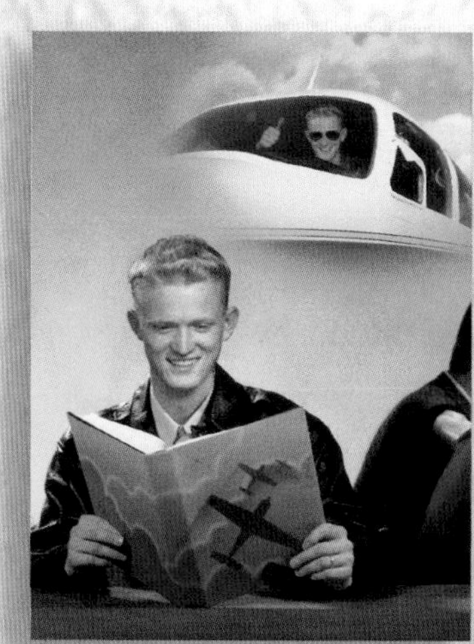

A person often starts study of a new subject with great eagerness.

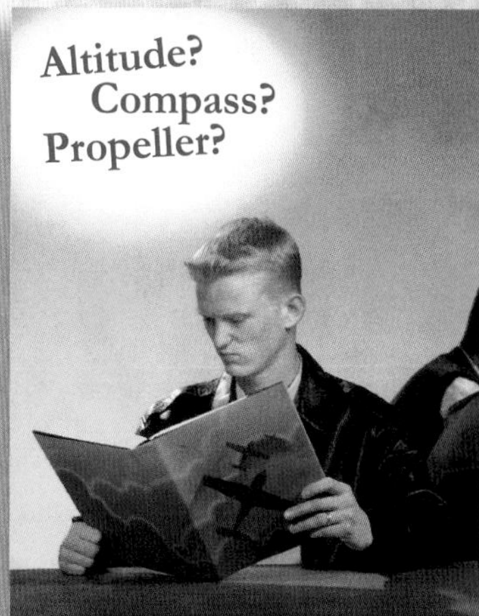

However, if he accumulates misunderstood words, his interest wanes.

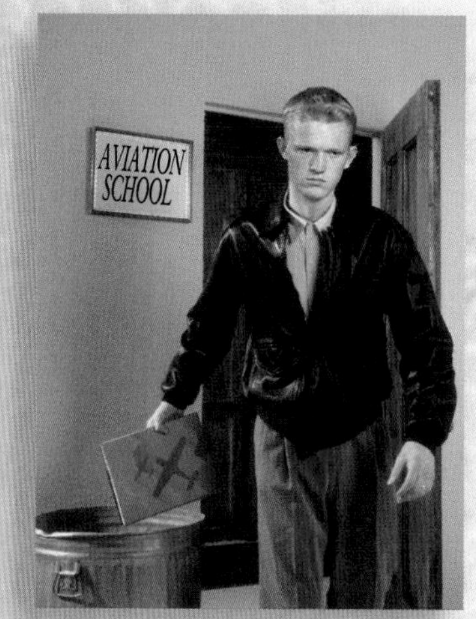

If he does not find these and get them defined, he will lose interest entirely and abandon the subject. This is called a blow.

We now have "the quick student who somehow never applies what he learns," also called a *glib student*.

The specific phenomenon then is that a student can study some words and give them back and yet be no participant to the action. The student gets A+ on exams but can't apply the data.

The thoroughly dull (stupid) student is just stuck in the noncomprehend blankness following some misunderstood word. He won't be able to demonstrate his materials with a demo kit or in clay, and such difficulties are a sure sign that a misunderstood word exists.

The "very bright" student who yet can't use the data is *not there* at all. He has long since ceased to confront (face without flinching or avoiding) the subject matter or the subject.

The cure for either of these conditions of "bright noncomprehension" or "dull" is to find the missing word.

This discovery of the importance of the misunderstood word actually opens the door to education. And although this barrier to study has been given last, it is the most important one.

CLEARING WORDS

A misunderstood word will remain misunderstood until one *clears* the meaning of the word. Once the word is fully understood by the person, it is said to be *cleared.*

The procedures used to locate and clear up words the student has misunderstood in his studies are called *Word Clearing.* The first thing to learn is the exact procedure to clear any word or symbol one comes across in reading or studying that he does not understand. All Word Clearing technology uses this procedure.

Steps to Clear a Word

1. Have a dictionary to hand while reading so that you can clear any misunderstood word or symbol you come across. A simple but good dictionary can be found that does not itself contain large words within the definitions of the words which themselves have to be cleared.

2. When you come across a word or symbol that you do not understand, look it up in a dictionary and look rapidly over the definitions to find the one which applies to the context in which the word was misunderstood. Read that definition and make up sentences using the word with that meaning until you have a clear concept of that meaning of the word. This could require ten or more sentences.

3. Then clear each of the other definitions of that word, using each one in sentences until you clearly understand each definition.

When a word has several different definitions, you cannot limit your understanding of the word to one definition only and call the word "understood." You must be able to understand the word when, at a later date, it is used in a different way.

Don't, however, clear the technical or specialized definitions (math, biology, etc.) or obsolete (no longer used) or archaic (ancient and no longer in general use) definitions unless the word is being used that way in the context where it was misunderstood. Doing so may lead off into many other words contained in those definitions and greatly slow one's study progress.

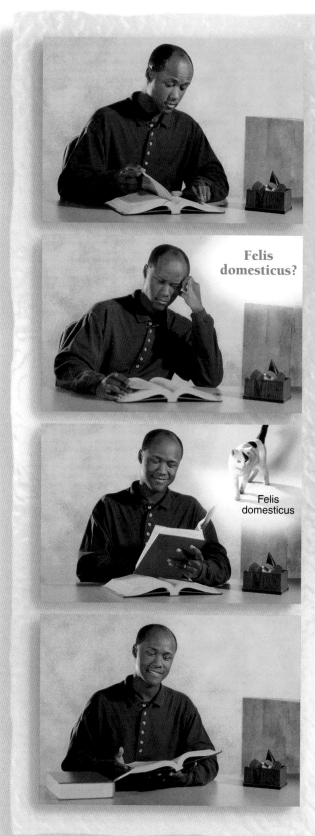

If a person encounters difficulty with what he is reading…

…there will be a misunderstood word earlier in his text. He must go back and locate the word.

When he looks up the word in a dictionary and defines it…

…the difficulty vanishes and he can progress.

Example of Clearing a Word

> I know that he has
> jobs. He used to clean chimneys for
> a living. It is actually quite
> extraordinary for a man his age.

■ *Let's say that you are reading the sentence, "He used to clean chimneys for a living," and you're not sure what "chimneys" means.*

> unreal, imaginary
> **chimney** 1. A flue for the smoke or
> gases from a fire. 2. A glass tube
> around the flame of a lamp. 3. A vent

■ *You find it in the dictionary and look through the definitions for the one that applies. It says "a flue for the smoke or gases from a fire."*

> fluctuation **n**
> **flue** (floo) **n** 1. a channel or passage
> for smoke, air or gases. 2. Any duct
> or passage for air, gas or the like. 3. A

■ *You're not sure what "flue" means so you look that up. It says "a channel or passage for smoke, air or gases." That fits and makes sense, so you use it in some sentences until you have a clear concept of it.*

> for smoke, air or gases.
> 2. Any duct or passage for air,
> gas or the like. 3. A tube, especially a
> large one. [OFr. *fluie*, a flowing]

■ *"Flue" in this dictionary has other definitions, each of which you would clear and use in sentences.*

> passage for air, gas or the like.
> tube, especially a large one. [OFr. *fluie*,
> a flowing]
> an organ pipe

■ *Next, read the derivation the dictionary gives for the word "flue." Now go back to "chimney." The definition, "a flue for the smoke or gases from a fire," now makes sense, so you use it in sentences until you have a concept of it.*

> **chimney**
> gases from a fire. 2. A glass
> tube around the flame of a lamp.
> 3. A vent as in a cliff or volcano
> fireplace

■ *You then clear the other definitions. If the dictionary you are using has specialized or obsolete definitions, you would skip them as they aren't in common usage.*

> 3. A vent as in a cliff or volcano
> [OFr. LL *caminata*, fireplace L.
> *caminus* Gr. *kaminos*, furnace]
> **corner** corner or side of a

■ *Now clear up the derivation of the word. You find that "chimney" originally came from the Greek word "kaminos," which means "furnace." If the word had any notes about its use, synonyms or idioms, they would all be cleared too. That would be the end of clearing "chimney."*

The above is the way any word should be cleared. When words are understood, communication can take place, and with communication any given subject can be understood.

4. The next thing to do is to clear the derivation, which is the explanation of where the word came from originally. This will help you gain a basic understanding of the word.

5. Most dictionaries give the idioms of a word. An idiom is a phrase or expression whose meaning cannot be understood from the ordinary meanings of the words. For example, "give in" is an English idiom meaning "yield." Quite a few words in English have idiomatic uses and these are usually given in a dictionary after the definitions of the word itself. If there are idioms for the word that you are clearing, they are cleared as well.

6. Clear any other information given about the word, such as notes on its usage, synonyms, etc., so as to have a full understanding of the word. (A synonym is a word which has a similar but not the same meaning to another word, for example, "thin" and "lean.")

7. If you encounter a misunderstood word or symbol in the definition of a word being cleared, you must clear it right away using this same procedure and then return to the definition you were clearing. (Dictionary symbols and abbreviations are usually given in the front of the dictionary.) However, if you find yourself spending a lot of time clearing words within definitions of words, you should get a simpler dictionary. A good dictionary will enable you to clear a word without having to look up a lot of other ones in the process.

Simple Words

You might suppose at once that it is the *big* words or the technical words which are most misunderstood.

This is *not* the case.

Words like *a, the, exist, such* and other words that "everybody knows" are found with great frequency as misunderstood words when doing Word Clearing.

It takes a *big* dictionary to define these simple words fully. This is another oddity. The small dictionaries also suppose "everybody knows what that word means."

It is almost incredible to see that a university graduate has gone through years and years of study of complex subjects and yet does not know what "or" or "by" or "an" means. It has to be seen to be believed. Yet when cleaned up, his whole education turns from a solid mass of question marks to a clean useful view.

A test of schoolchildren in Johannesburg, South Africa, once showed that intelligence *decreased* with each new year of school!

The answer to the puzzle was simply that each year they added a few dozen more crushing misunderstood words onto an already confused vocabulary that no one ever got them to look up.

Stupidity *is* the effect of misunderstood words.

In those areas which give man the most trouble, you will find the most alteration of fact, the most confused and conflicting ideas and of course the greatest number of misunderstood words.

THE EARLIEST MISUNDERSTOOD WORD IN A SUBJECT IS A KEY TO LATER MISUNDERSTOOD WORDS IN THAT SUBJECT.

In studying a foreign language it is often found that the grammar words of one's *own* language that tell about the grammar in the foreign language are basic to not being able to learn the foreign language.

It is important that these words be cleared.

Methods of Word Clearing

Nine different methods for clearing the meanings of words have been developed in Scientology.

They cover various ways to locate the misunderstood words underlying a person's difficulties. These range from finding misunderstood words in the text one is studying, to clearing the key words relating to one's job, to even tracing down the words that were misunderstood in subjects studied years earlier!

Three of these Word Clearing methods that are very applicable in everyday life are given here.

Basic Word Clearing

Basic Word Clearing is the method of finding a misunderstood word by looking earlier in the text for a misunderstood word than where one is having trouble. This is the most basic method of Word Clearing used in Scientology.

A student must know how to keep himself tearing along successfully in his studies. He should be able to handle anything that slows or interferes with his progress. He applies the Study Technology to assist himself.

A student who uses Study Technology will look up each word he comes to that he doesn't understand and will never leave a word behind him that he doesn't know the meaning of.

If he runs into trouble, the student himself, his study partner or his instructor (in Scientology called a Supervisor) uses Basic Word Clearing to handle anything that slowed or interfered with his progress.

Waiting to become groggy or to "dope off" (feel tired, sleepy or foggy as though doped or drugged) as the only detection of misunderstood words before handling is waiting too long. If you have ever seen a student falling asleep over his book, then you have seen dope-off. Long before that point, someone should have made the student look for a misunderstood word. The time to look for the misunderstood word is as soon as the student slows down or isn't quite as "bright" as he was fifteen minutes before. It is not a misunderstood phrase or idea or concept but a misunderstood WORD. This always occurs before the subject itself is not understood.

Basic Word Clearing is done as follows:

1. The student is not flying along and is not so "bright" as he was or he may exhibit just plain lack of enthusiasm or be taking too long on the course or be yawning or disinterested or doodling or daydreaming, etc.

2. The student must then look earlier in the text for a misunderstood word. There is one always; there are no exceptions. It may be that the misunderstood word is two pages or more back, but it is always earlier in the text than where the student is now.

3. The word is found. The student recognizes it in looking back for it. Or, if the student can't find it, one can take words from the text that could be the misunderstood word and ask, "What does _____ mean?" to see if the student gives the correct definition.

4. The student looks up the word found in a dictionary and clears it per the steps of clearing a misunderstood word described above. He uses it verbally several times in sentences of his own composition until he has obviously demonstrated he understands the word by the composition of his sentences.

5. The student now reads the text that contained the misunderstood word. If he is not now "bright," eager to get on with it, feeling happier, etc., then there is another misunderstood word earlier in the text. This is found by repeating steps 2–5.

6. When the student is bright and feeling happier, he comes forward, studying the text from where the misunderstood word was to the area of the subject he did not understand (where step 1 began).

The student will now be enthusiastic about his study of the subject, and that is the end result of Basic Word Clearing. (The result won't be achieved if a misunderstood word was missed or if there is an earlier misunderstood word in the text. If so, repeat steps 2–5.) If the student is now enthusiastic, have him continue studying.

Good Word Clearing is a system of backtracking. You have to look earlier than the point where the student became dull or confused and you'll find that there's a word that he doesn't understand somewhere before the trouble started. If he doesn't brighten up when the word is found and cleared, there will be a misunderstood word even before that one.

This will be very clear to you if you understand that *if it is not resolving, the thing the student is apparently having trouble with is not the thing the student is having trouble with.* Otherwise, it would resolve, wouldn't it? If he knew what he didn't understand, he could resolve it himself. So to talk to him about what he thinks he doesn't understand just gets nowhere. The trouble is *earlier.*

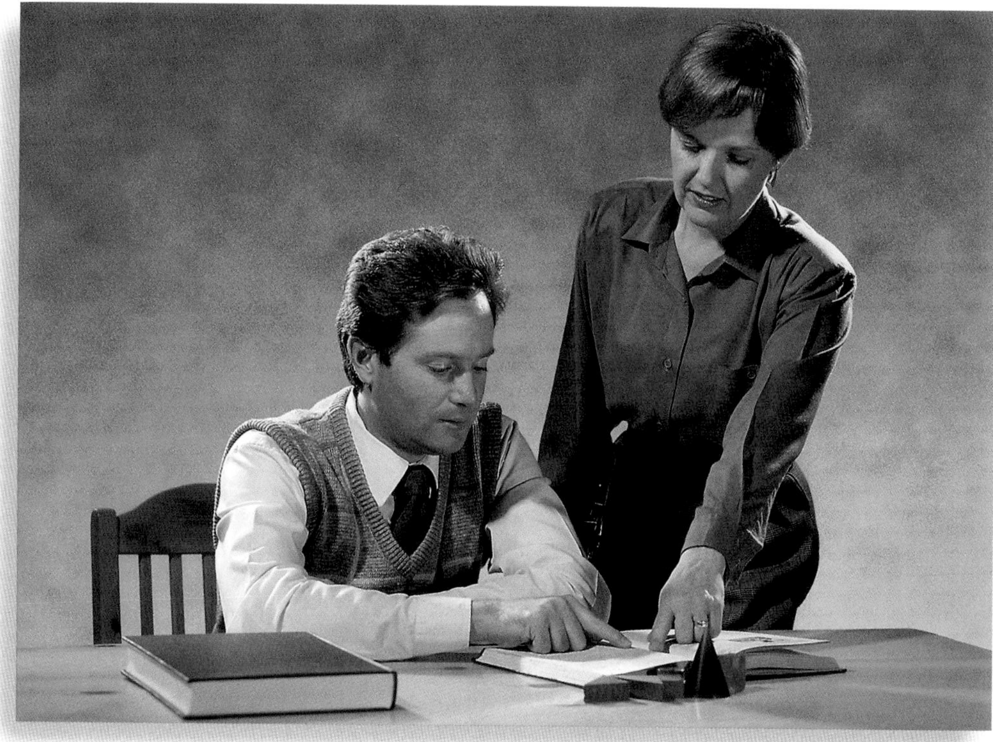

In Basic Word Clearing, the student must look earlier in the text for a misunderstood word. It is always earlier in the text than where the student is now.

Zeroing In on the Word

The formula is to find out where the student wasn't having any trouble and find out where the student is now having trouble and the misunderstood word will be in between. It will be at the tag end—the last part—of where he wasn't having trouble.

Basic Word Clearing is tremendously effective when done as described here.

Reading Aloud Word Clearing

A highly effective method of finding the words a person doesn't understand in a book or other written material is called Reading Aloud Word Clearing.

A student, when reading by himself, often does not know he has gone past misunderstood words. But whenever he does go by misunderstood words, he will have trouble with what he is reading.

In Reading Aloud Word Clearing, one has the person read the material aloud. The person he reads to helps him find and clear any misunderstood words and is called, appropriately, a *word clearer.*

Reading Aloud Word Clearing is commonly done by two persons on a turnabout basis: one student is the word clearer and word clears the other student, and then they switch around and the student who was just word cleared becomes the word clearer and word clears his partner.

A word can be misunderstood in many different ways. It is important that these different types of misunderstood words are known to the person doing Reading Aloud Word Clearing. A word can be misunderstood because of:

1. A *false* (totally wrong) definition—The person reads or hears the word "cat" and thinks "cat" means "box." You can't get more wrong.

2. An *invented* definition—When young, the person was always called "a girl" by his pals when he refused to do anything daring. He invents the definition of "girl" to be "a cowardly person."

3. An *incorrect* definition—A person reads or hears the word "computer" and thinks it is a "typewriter." This is an incorrect meaning for "computer" even though a typewriter and a computer are both types of machines.

4. An *incomplete* definition—The person reads the word "office" and thinks it means "room." The definition of the word "office" is "the building, room or series of rooms in which the affairs of a business, professional person, branch of government, etc., are carried on." The person's definition of "office" is incomplete.

5. An *unsuitable* definition—The person sees a dash (–) in the sentence "I finished numbers 3–7 today." He thinks a dash is a minus sign, realizes you cannot subtract 7 from 3 and so cannot understand it.

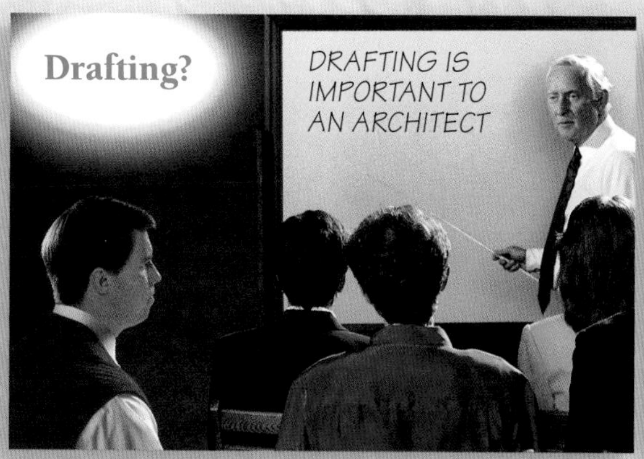

A misunderstood word can prevent the person's understanding of something.

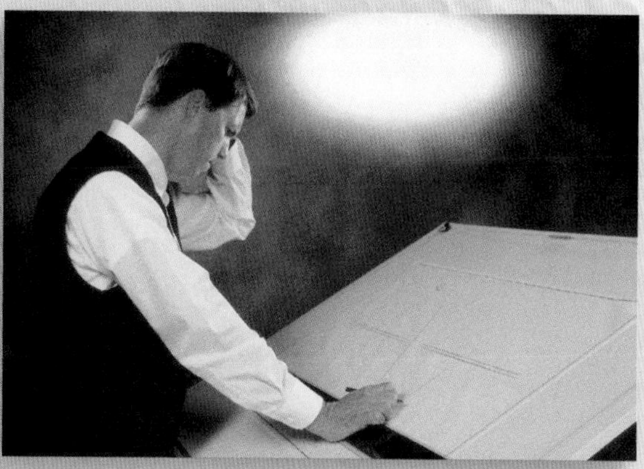

As a result, he can appear to have no aptitude for doing certain things, much to his frustration and unhappiness.

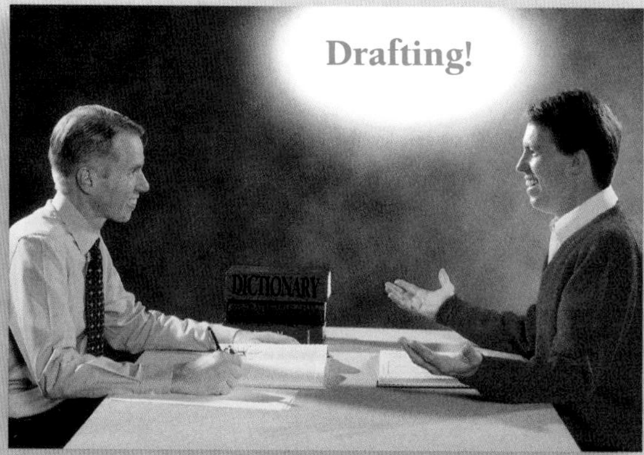

But, locating and fully clearing misunderstood words on a subject restores the ability to do in the area.

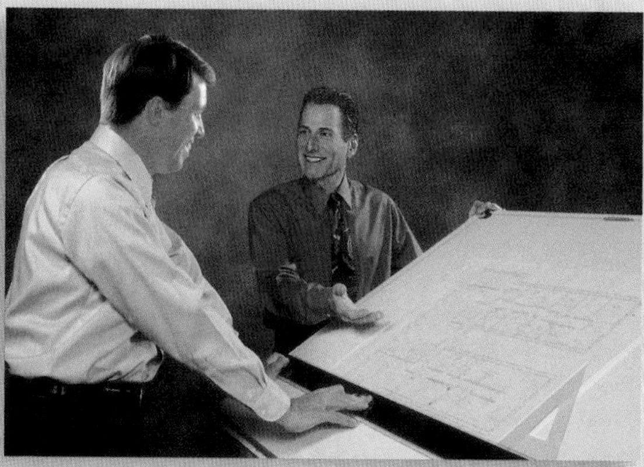

Clearing up misunderstood words is the key to resolve any difficulties in any subject the person is studying.

6. A *homonymic* (one sound or symbol which has two or more distinctly separate meanings) definition—The person hears the word "period" in the sentence "It was a disorderly period in history" and knowing that "period" comes at the end of a sentence and means stop, supposes that the world ended at that point.

7. A *substitute* (synonym) definition—The person reads the word "portly" and thinks the definition of the word is "fat." "Fat" is a synonym for the word "portly." The person has a misunderstood because the word "portly" means "large and heavy in a dignified and stately way."

8. An *omitted* (missing) definition—The person hears the line "The food here is too rich." This person knows two definitions for the word "rich." He knows that "rich" means "having much money, land, goods, etc." and "wealthy people." Neither of these definitions make much sense to him in the sentence he has just heard. He cannot understand how food could have anything to do with having a lot of money. He does not know that "rich" in this sense means, "containing plenty of butter, eggs, flavoring, etc."

9. A *no*-definition—A no-definition is a "not-understood" word or symbol. The person reads the sentence "The business produced no lucre." No understanding occurs, as he has no definition for "lucre." The word means "riches; money: chiefly a scornful word, as in *filthy lucre.*"

10. A *rejected* definition—The person refuses to look up the definition of asterisk (*). On discussion, it turns out that every time he sees an asterisk on the page he knows the material will be "very hard to read" and is "literary," "difficult" and "very intellectual."

If a person has habitually gone past many, many misunderstood words in his reading or his education (which most everybody in this present culture has), not only will his ability to read be lowered but also his intelligence. What he himself writes and says won't be understood, what he reads and hears he won't understand, and he will be out of communication. The probability is that the world will look like a very peculiar place to him, he will feel that he is "not understood" (How true!) and life will look a bit miserable to him. He can even appear to others to be criminal. At best he will become a sort of robot or zombie. So you see, it is very important to clear misunderstood words.

Why Reading Aloud Word Clearing Works

A student who understands all the words on the page he is reading will be able to read the page aloud perfectly. He will feel bright and alert and will fully understand what he reads. But when a student passes a word or symbol he doesn't understand, the misunderstood causes an interruption of his voice or physical beingness (his physical state). His voice may change, or he may stumble on a word or make a face or squint his eyes or react in some other way.

This is easy to understand if you remember that a person can go blank after he passes a word or symbol he doesn't understand. He may make a mistake in his reading right there at the point of the misunderstood, or he may

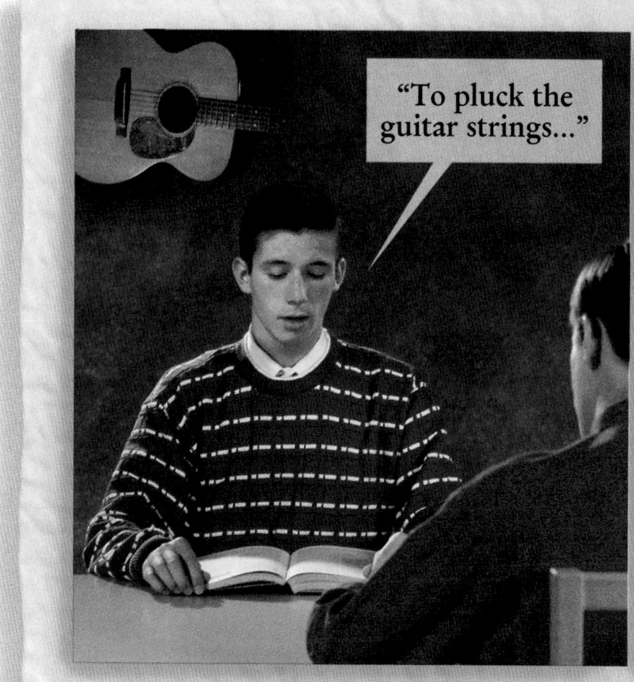

Reading Aloud Word Clearing is a thorough method of locating misunderstood words.

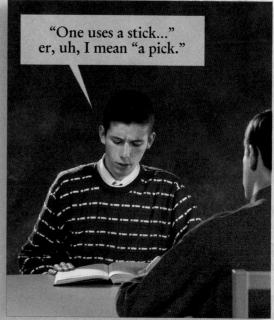

These become apparent through stumbles, alterations or in other ways as the student reads.

continue reading past the misunderstood and make a mistake on a later word or symbol. He will feel duller and he will try to make up for the dull feeling by reading with more effort. This will always be expressed by a nonoptimum action of some kind which must be noted and handled at once by the word clearer.

A *nonoptimum* reaction is anything the student does besides read the page easily, naturally and perfectly. Examples of *some* of the nonoptimum reactions that may show up are:

1. Student adding a word or leaving out a word or changing a word in the sentence he is reading.

2. Student stumbling on a word or saying it incorrectly.

3. Student pausing or reading more slowly.

4. Student frowning or looking uncertain.

5. Student going stiff or tensing a body part, such as squinting his eyes or tightening the grip of his hands, or biting his lip or some other physical reaction.

6. Student reading with effort.

7. Student reading with a glib, robotic attitude (which is how he gets after he has been forced to read "correctly" by someone who doesn't know anything about misunderstood words).

Other manifestations can occur.

The above is not a complete list of reactions but is intended to give an idea of what to look for. In all fairness, one can stumble when reading if he is trying to read in a dim light or he is having eye trouble or the print or handwriting or penciled corrections in the text are very hard to make out. Thus, it is necessary to do Reading Aloud Word Clearing only in bright light, and if the fellow is supposed to be wearing glasses, he should be wearing glasses, and the material being word cleared must not contain smudges and deletions itself. All possible reasons why he cannot *see* the text and unclear text must be removed. Otherwise, the student will simply say he couldn't see it or the light was bad or some other wrong Why (reason or cause).

Any time the person makes an error in his reading or reacts in some nonoptimum way, a misunderstood word will *always* be found *before* that point or sometimes *at* that point itself.

Example: The student is reading the page aloud. He reads, "Raymond walked home slowly and thoughtfully," then he frowns. The word clearer signals a halt by saying, "That's it," and then asks, "Is there some word or symbol there that you didn't understand?" (*If* the student wonders why he was stopped, the word clearer tells him what reaction he noticed.)

The student looks over what he has read. He feels uncertain about the word "slowly." He tells this to the word clearer and the word "slowly" is looked up in the dictionary and used in sentences until the student fully understands it.

When the word that was misunderstood is located and cleared, the student will brighten up and will begin reading clearly and correctly once again.

How to Do It

1. *Student and Word Clearer Sit Across from Each Other.*

The student and the word clearer sit across from each other at a table or desk. Each person has his own copy of the text to be word cleared. The word clearer must be able to see the student *and* the page in front of him at the same time.

2. *Dictionaries Are Available.*

A good, simple dictionary and any other dictionaries the student may need are available. (Above all things, do not use what is called a "dinky dictionary." This is different than a simple well-expressed dictionary. A dinky dictionary is what you commonly get off the paperback racks in drugstores. It quite often defines word A as word B and then defines word B as word A. It also omits all the alternative definitions and all the technical definitions.)

3. *Student Recognition of Misunderstood Words.*

Before the student starts reading, he should be told that if he reads anything he doesn't fully understand he should tell the word clearer, or if he sees a word he doesn't know the meaning of, he should stop and look the word up and clear it instead of going on past it. The student should be encouraged to find and clear misunderstood words himself. The word clearer on this method would never prevent the student from clearing a word that the student recognizes as misunderstood. Reading Aloud Word Clearing brings about the ability to do this, so that the student will find and clear his own misunderstood words in the future.

4. *Student Reads the Text Aloud to the Word Clearer.*

The student reads the text aloud to the word clearer. While the student reads, the word clearer follows his own copy of the same text, watches the student and listens to him.

The word clearer must be very alert and see or hear any nonoptimum reactions of the student while he is reading.

5. *Nonoptimum Reaction Equals Misunderstood Word.*

A nonoptimum reaction by the student to what he is reading is the clue to the word clearer that the student has encountered a misunderstood word. The word clearer and student must now locate the exact misunderstood word or symbol. It will be found *before* or sometimes *at* the point the nonoptimum reaction occurred.

6. *Find the Misunderstood.*

If it is not obvious to the student that he has reacted and he just continues reading, the word clearer says, "That's it. Is there some word or symbol there that you didn't understand?" It is the duty of the word clearer to steer the student to the misunderstood. It is either at the point of the nonoptimum reaction or before it. The point is that the student must be steered onto it. And it then is looked up.

The student may be able to spot his misunderstood word right away and tell the word clearer what it is. Or he may have difficulty finding it and the word clearer will have to help him find it.

The word clearer helps the student by getting him to look earlier and earlier in the text from the point where he reacted until the misunderstood word is found. The word clearer can also spot-check the student. Spot-checking means choosing words from the text the student has already read and checking with him to see if he knows the definitions of those words. The word clearer would choose an earlier word and simply ask, "What is the definition of _________?"

If the student is uncertain about any word or gives a wrong definition, then that word is taken up and cleared in the dictionary.

7. *Clear the Word.*

Once the misunderstood is found it must be fully cleared in the dictionary. Use the procedure in "Steps to Clear a Word" covered on page 18.

8. *Read the Sentence Again.*

The word clearer then asks the student to read once again the sentence in the text in which the misunderstood word or symbol was found. The student does so, and if he reads it correctly with understanding, he continues reading the text. Any further nonoptimum reactions are handled by finding the next misunderstood word and clearing it, as above.

9. *Reading Aloud Is Continued Until the Text Has Been Completed.*

Reading Aloud Word Clearing is continued until the text to be word cleared is completed.

At this point, where two students are doing Reading Aloud Word Clearing on each other, they switch around and the student who just completed being word cleared becomes the word clearer.

The student goes through the same section of text and then goes on to the next fresh passage.

They take it in turns like this, word clearing it section by section until they have both finished the whole text.

Cautions and Tips

It occasionally happens that the students doing the Word Clearing get into a quarrel or upset. If this happens, you know that one of two things has happened. Either:

1. "Misunderstood words" that were really understood were forced off on the student, or

2. Actual misunderstood words were not detected and were passed by.

You can clean up any falsely looked-up words by asking the student if he was made to look up words he understood. If this is the case, he will brighten up and tell you the word or words he was wrongly made to clear. This done, the Word Clearing can be resumed.

If the above doesn't handle it, then one knows that misunderstood words have been missed. Have the word clearer take the student back to when he was last doing well and then come forward in the text, following Reading Aloud Word Clearing procedure, picking up the missed misunderstood words. It will usually be found that several misunderstood words have been missed, not just one.

The end result of well-done Reading Aloud Word Clearing is a student who is certain he has no misunderstood words on that material so that he can easily study the material and apply it.

Reading Aloud Word Clearing is a great civilization saver.

It is vital that Reading Aloud Word Clearing is done correctly, exactly by the book. Otherwise, people will be denied the enormous wins that can be attained with it.

Special Reading Aloud Word Clearing

Whenever one is working with children or foreign-language persons or people who are semiliterate, Special Reading Aloud Word Clearing is used.

As in the Reading Aloud method, the person is made to read *aloud* to find out what he is doing.

It is a very simple method.

Another copy of the same text must also be followed by the word clearer as the person reads.

Startling things can be observed.

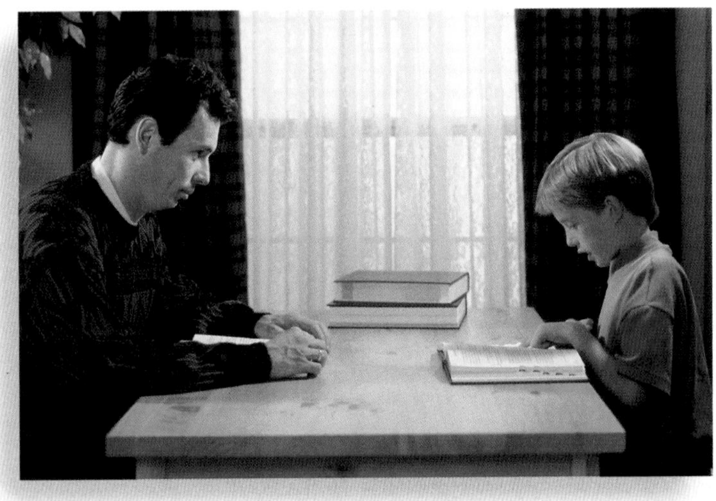

In Special Reading Aloud Word Clearing, the person reads aloud and each time he hesitates, has a physical reaction or alters a word, the word clearer helps him find and define the misunderstood word.

The person may omit the word "is" whenever it occurs. The person doesn't read it. He may have some strange meaning for it like "Israel" (actual occurrence).

He may omit "didn't" each time it occurs and the reason may trace to not knowing what the apostrophe is (actual occurrence).

He may call one word quite another word such as "stop" for "happen" or "green" for "mean."

He may hesitate over certain words.

The procedure is:

1. Have him read aloud.

2. Note each omission or word change or hesitation or frown as he reads and take it up at once.

3. Correct it by looking it up for him or explaining it to him.

4. Have him go on reading, noting the next omission, word change or hesitation or frown.

5. Repeat steps 2–4.

By doing this a person can be brought up to literacy.

His next actions would be learning how to use a dictionary and look up words.

Then a simple grammar text.

A very backward student can be boosted up to literacy by this Word Clearing method.

APPLYING THE TECHNOLOGY OF STUDY

Study Technology is a bridge to an education that will serve a student long after he leaves the classroom.

The difference between the "bright" student and the "dull" one, the student who is very, very fast and the one who is very, very slow, is really only the difference between the *careful* student and the *careless* student.

The careful student applies the technology of study. He studies with an intention to learn something. He handles any of the barriers to study which appear as he is working with his materials. If he is reading down a paragraph and suddenly realizes that he doesn't have a clue what he is reading about, he goes back and finds out where he got tangled up. Just before that there is a word he didn't understand. If he is a careful student, he doesn't continue—not until he finds out what that word is and what it means.

That is a careful student, and his brightness on the subject is dependent upon the degree he applies this technology. It isn't dependent on any native talent or anything else. It is his command of the subject of study that makes the difference.

This chapter is far from all there is to Study Technology. It is a comprehensive subject. But with what you have read in these pages, you now have the tools to study anything more successfully and help others do the same. ■

Test Your Understanding

Answer the following questions about Study Technology. Refer back to the chapter to check your answers. If you need to, review the chapter. Going over the material several times will increase your certainty and help you obtain better success in applying the knowledge.

- ❑ *What is the primary obstacle to learning?*
- ❑ *What are the barriers to study? Describe the physical and mental reactions that accompany each one.*
- ❑ *What are the two phenomena of a misunderstood word?*
- ❑ *How do you clear a word?*
- ❑ *At what point should a student apply Basic Word Clearing when studying?*
- ❑ *What is Reading Aloud Word Clearing?*
- ❑ *What is the difference between a "bright" student and a "dull" student?*

Practical Exercises

Here are exercises you can do to increase your ability to apply Study Technology. These will help you become proficient in your own studies and in helping others with anything they are trying to learn.

1 Think of someone you have seen or known who felt he already knew all about some subject. How would this attitude affect the person's ability to actually learn something new about that subject?

2 How would you handle these situations?

a. A friend is learning about different types of trees but has no idea what they look like. There are no actual trees nearby that can be shown to him. How could you help him?

b. In learning how to swim, a friend just learned to float in the water and is now being taught to swim across the pool, but is having a great deal of trouble with this. What could you do to help him?

c. A friend has been taking a course on how to manage his money, but has now decided he does not want to continue or go back to class. What should you do to handle this?

3 Think of or find a word you know you do not understand or are unsure of and clear it, using a dictionary.

4 Go back through the section "Barriers to Study," looking for and clearing any words you do not fully understand and restudying the section as you go.

5 Do Basic Word Clearing on yourself.

6 Do Basic Word Clearing on another person.

7 Drill Reading Aloud Word Clearing. Find another student or a friend to do this drill with you. One of you will be Student A and the other will be Student B. Decide who is going to be Student A and who is going to be Student B.

a. Student A (as word clearer) word clears Student B on the following paragraph, using Reading Aloud. Use a simple dictionary.

The quick brown fox jumped over the lazy dog. The dog was supposed to be guarding the chickens but had gone to sleep. The fox sneaked into the chicken coop without anyone noticing.

b. Student B (as word clearer) word clears Student A on the following paragraphs, using Reading Aloud. Use a simple dictionary.

The quick brown fox jumped over the lazy dog. The dog was supposed to be guarding the chickens but had gone to sleep. The fox sneaked into the chicken coop without anyone noticing.

As soon as the chickens noticed him they all made a dreadful row. The fox had to move very quickly; he grabbed hold of the nearest chicken by her neck and slunk off out of the coop.

c. Student A (as word clearer) word clears Student B on the following paragraphs, using Reading Aloud. Use a simple dictionary.

As soon as the chickens noticed him they all made a dreadful row. The fox had to move very quickly; he grabbed hold of the nearest chicken by her neck and slunk off out of the coop.

The farmer's wife came running out of the house when she heard the din, wondering what could possibly be going on with her chickens. She saw the fox disappearing into the nearby woods with the chicken.

d. Student B (as word clearer) word clears Student A on the following paragraphs, using Reading Aloud. Use a simple dictionary.

The farmer's wife came running out of the house when she heard the din, wondering what could possibly be going on with her chickens. She saw the fox disappearing into the nearby woods with the chicken.

She shrieked loudly and looked around for the dog whose prime duty it was to prevent this sort of occurrence. The dog looked quite abashed. The farmer's wife spent the next few minutes violently upbraiding him for his apathetic behavior.

e. Student A (as word clearer) word clears Student B on the following paragraph, using Reading Aloud. Use a simple dictionary.

She shrieked loudly and looked around for the dog whose prime duty it was to prevent this sort of occurrence. The dog looked quite abashed. The farmer's wife spent the next few minutes violently upbraiding him for his apathetic behavior.

8 Find someone who could benefit from Reading Aloud Word Clearing and do this to a satisfactory end result.

Results from Application

Study Technology, widely used from American universities to South African township schools, routinely demonstrates its workability in program after program.

In rural Alabama, children ranging in age from eight to sixteen took part in a seven-week program utilizing Study Technology for the stated purpose of increasing reading vocabulary and comprehension. Pre- and post-program standardized tests revealed an average increase of eight months per student in vocabulary and comprehension. One fourteen-year-old boy improved from a second grade level to sixth grade level in five and a half weeks on the program. This level of increase is virtually unheard of.

In London, a group of pupils received a short course in Study Technology consisting of approximately nine hours of instruction over a twelve-day period, while a control group received no instruction in Study Technology. Both groups otherwise continued their routine studies and both were tested before and after. The experimental group became an astonishing average of 1.29 years higher in reading ability after twelve days of instruction. The control group showed virtually no difference (0.03 decrease) in the second test. These impressive results speak for themselves.

Improvement in Reading Level

A 40-hour tutorial program for Washington, DC students using Study Technology demonstrated dramatic increases in reading levels.

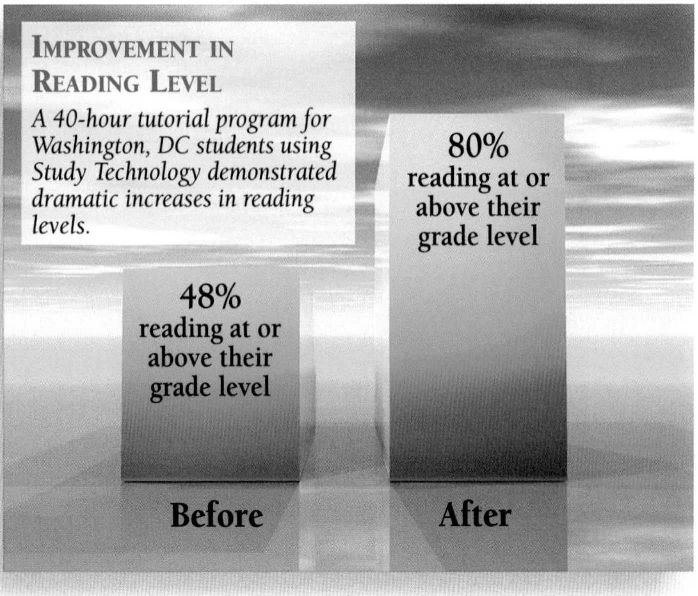

48%
reading at or above their grade level
Before

80%
reading at or above their grade level
After

The benefits of the Education Alive program in southern Africa have been validated by several studies in Bulawayo, Zimbabwe and the Transvaal, South Africa. One study demonstrated a 1.2 year improvement in reading ability over the course of a three-week program. Another program delivered over a four-week period yielded improvements averaging 1.8 years in reading ability. Another three-week program in the Transkei homeland in South Africa, showed a 2.3 year average improvement. A program run in an underprivileged high school resulted in a 91 percent pass rate on the country's Department of Education high-school examinations, compared to 27 percent in a control group. In South Africa, where 50 percent of the population is illiterate, this program brings about vitally needed improvement.

Compare these positive results to what is occurring elsewhere in school systems throughout the world: some inner city US high schools have drop-out rates approaching 50 percent; 42 percent of those surveyed in Great Britain could not add up the price of a hamburger, French fries, apple pie and coffee; and 700,000 students graduated from US high schools last year who were not literate enough to read their diplomas. Behind these figures lie many stories of personal frustration, broken dreams, low-quality workmanship, rising crime and bleak futures.

The stories of the people which follow are different. Luckily, these people from around the world found out about Study Technology and applied it and changed their lives and the lives of others for the better.

In Springfield, Virginia, a couple were distressed about their son's failures in school and problems at home. After being introduced to Study Technology and enrolling their son in a school which uses it, they wrote the following letter:

"Before Richard started at your school, and as a result of his inability to respond to the teaching methods of the Washington, DC public schools, he was a frustrated, unadjusted kid. Through the guidance and counseling provided, we were able to learn how to assist Richard in becoming a better person. More importantly, you sparked a renewed interest in him. He obtained the basic educational skills he had missed during the two years he spent in public schools. For the first time in two years, Richard wanted to go to school every day! He took the initiative to read books on his own. He became interested in various academic subjects, including science and geography. From the time his two cousins graduated from a prestigious high school, it had been Richard's dream to attend the same school. After learning Study Technology, he was accepted for enrollment in this school. We thank you from the bottom of our hearts for the big part you played in helping Richard to reach his goal."

Beside herself with worry, a London mother sought help for her ten-year-old son who was having great difficulty in school and could not concentrate. His teachers wanted to give him drugs. Instead, his mother found a tutorial program utilizing Study Technology. After the boy spent a short while on the program, his tutor wrote:

"During his first Saturday on the program, the boy spent three hours learning the basics of Study Technology. The boy's mother rang me during the next week as she noticed an immediate improvement and could not believe the change that had come over her son—the boy was doing his homework with no difficulties. The next Saturday, the boy returned to the program and learned more about how to study. A few days later the boy's mother told me that she received a call from his teachers wondering what had occurred with him. They had noticed such a change, they wanted to know

what was going on. The youngster's problems would not have been solved by drugs. It was simply that no one had ever taught him how to study."

A couple in Oregon were distraught about their eleven-year-old daughter who was barely reading at a second grade level and who had very low self-esteem. After her daughter started attending a school which uses Study Technology, the girl's mother wrote:

"My heart wrenched when my daughter came out of the room used for the entrance exam which she took on arriving at summer school. Tears streamed down her face and she asked for her green-tinted lenses which she thought she needed in order to read. She had scored very poorly, but in spite of reservations from all concerned she was given a chance to begin the summer program.

"At that moment the cumulative graph of her life which had been plummeting steeply took a sharp turn upward and it has been climbing ever since. She has now been at summer school for some months and the changes we have seen in her are nothing short of miraculous.

"She is reading now on her own, and even finds it hard to put her books down. She is back on track and has become a confident, happy kid, a great kid who will no doubt make an enormous contribution to the world—a contribution she could never have made if it were not for the study method of Mr. Hubbard and this incredible school you are creating! Thanks to every one of you for your efforts, your commitment and your vision."

A seven-year-old boy was having a hard time on his studies. He was studying and restudying the same materials for about six months. Fortunately, his mother knew Study Technology and realized that his teacher was not finding and correcting the real barriers and problems her son was running into.

"I have a very busy schedule with my own job and duties but I got him to bring home the materials he had been studying and I found what the real problem was. That was two months ago. The result is that he has become a model student in his class now. He no longer goofs off or gives others a hard time. He loves his studies and has been completing his assignments in record time. He came to me two nights ago and was spelling words which he had studied and properly cleared the definitions of. I know I could not even read when I was his age, let alone spell words like Antarctica, nurseries, patterns, penguin, polar bear, iceberg, etc. I realized that I had possibly salvaged his whole study future with what I had done earlier to resolve his study problems."

SUGGESTIONS FOR FURTHER STUDY

L. Ron Hubbard developed a considerable amount of material on the subject of learning and Study Technology which extends beyond the scope of this handbook. The materials shown here contain the *full* technology of study and give a complete understanding of the most basic factor of education: *how* to learn. Study Technology is available in its entirety in book and lecture form and in courses delivered in Scientology organizations as well as many educational groups all over the world. A list of these is in the back of this book. Millions of people have learned the basics of Study Technology and use them daily.

Learning How to Learn

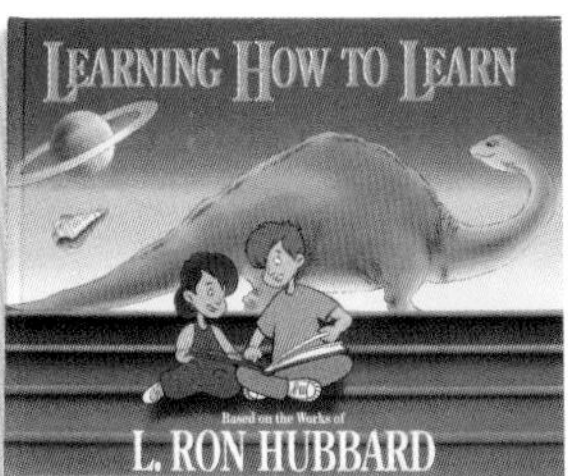

A beginning study book which teaches children how to study, using words and pictures. This provides a crucial foundation for any young student, for it covers the exact skills a child needs to begin successful schooling.

Study Skills for Life

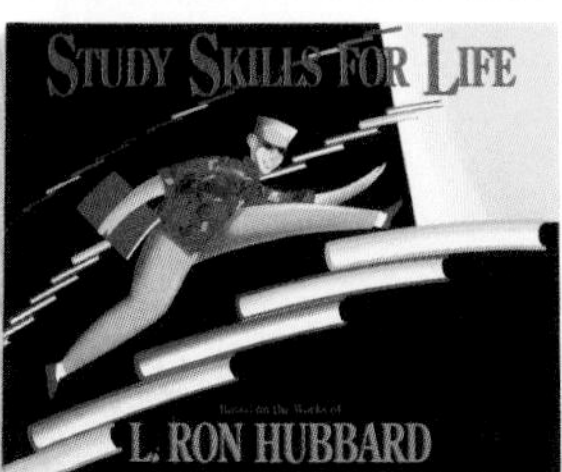

Covers many of the same study basics as *Learning How to Learn* but is written and illustrated for young teenagers. Success in life relies on one's competence; this book provides fundamentals for those approaching adulthood to acquire skill in a subject studied. All students, even those who have fallen prey to bad study habits, can benefit from this book.

How to Use a Dictionary Picture Book for Children

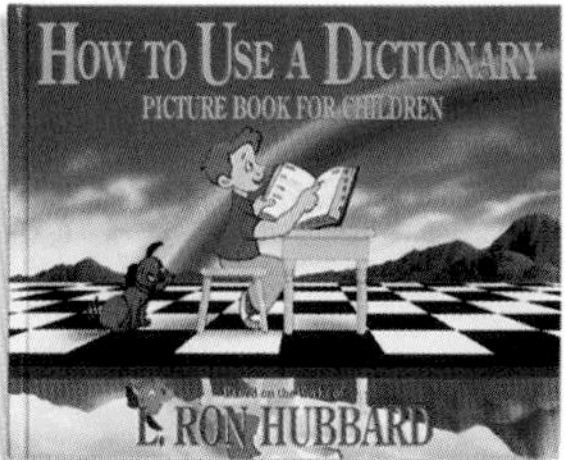

Teaches a child the vital skill of how to look up a word in a dictionary. This is a step that is often not taught to a child at all, yet can make the difference between success and failure in life.

Grammar and Communication for Children

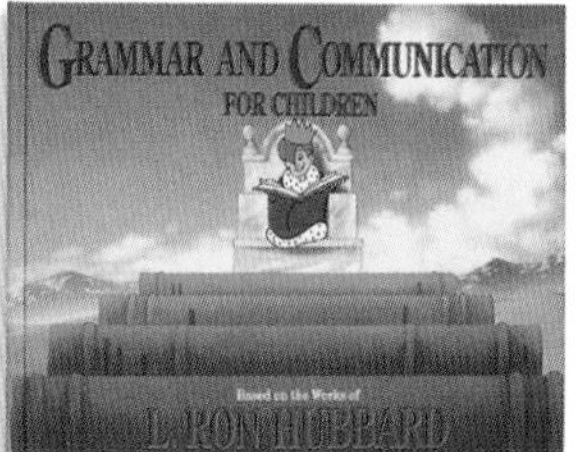

L. Ron Hubbard isolated grammar as a major factor in anyone's ability to study and communicate to others. He not only got rid of the complexities in the subject of grammar and developed a *new* grammar that is simple and easy to understand, but also made it possible for a child to learn it. This illustrated book contains the basics of the new grammar, a must for any child.

Basic Study Manual

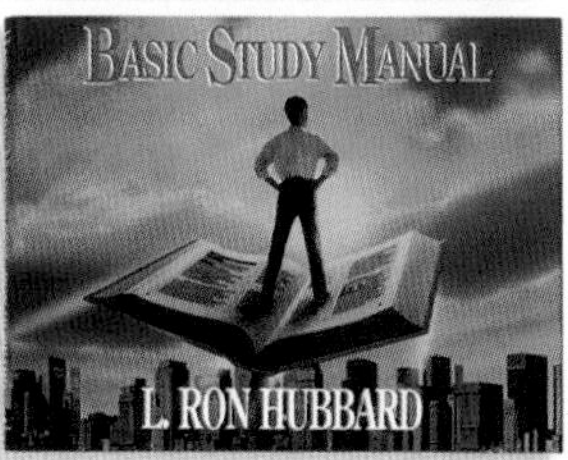

Describes each of the fundamentals of Study Technology for any age or academic level from teenagers to adult. With this basic data, an individual can grasp a subject and *apply* what he has learned to improve conditions in his life. Fully illustrated to increase understanding of concepts and procedures.

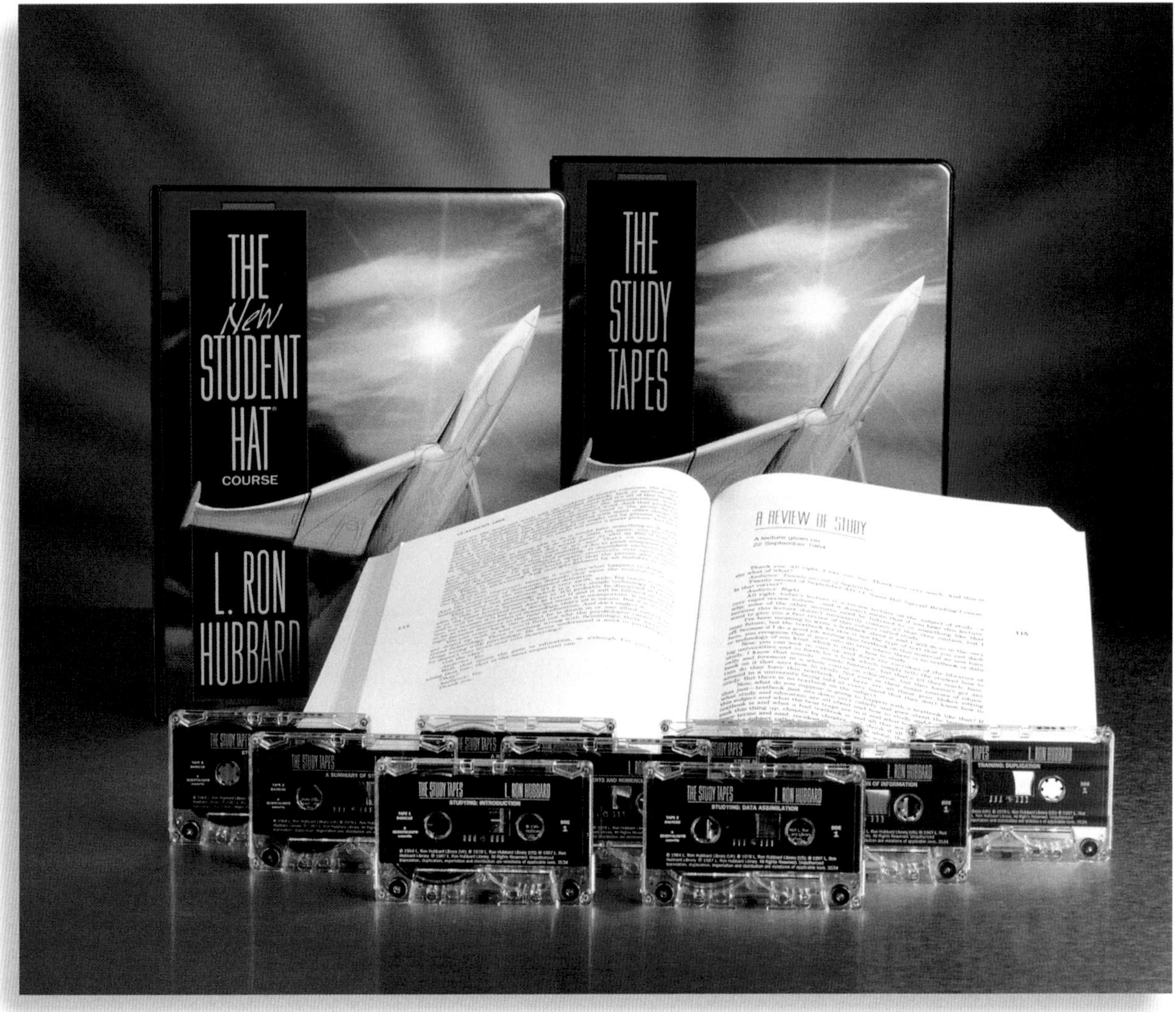

The Study Tapes

Here are the lectures in which L. Ron Hubbard gave the breakthroughs which were to revolutionize the field of study. In these nine recorded talks, a student will gain a full understanding of the barriers to study and how to apply this data in his own life. The material in these tapes contains the basics of study, essential for anyone who wants to improve his own study abilities or help others learn more effectively.

The Student Hat

A comprehensive course which contains *all* the technology on study. This is a required course for any person training to become a qualified Scientology practitioner. The Student Hat includes the nine Study Tapes described above as well as Mr. Hubbard's pertinent writings dealing with study and education. In two weeks' full-time study (eight hours a day, five days per week) one obtains a full grounding in skills that he can use in all endeavors in life. (Delivered in Scientology organizations throughout the world.)

How to Use a Dictionary Picture Book

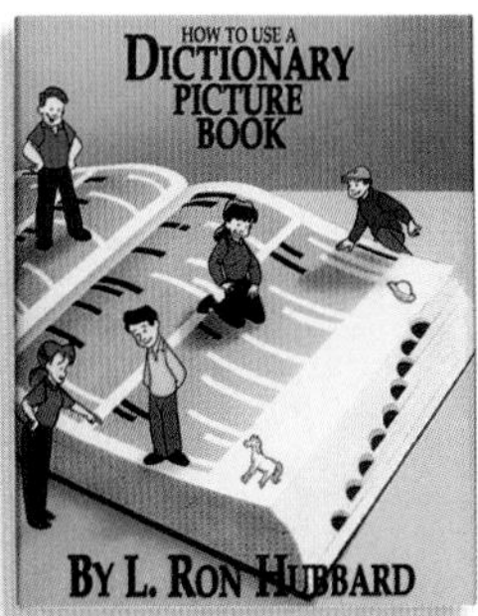

Using a dictionary is something people often take for granted. But few have ever been shown exactly how to gain all the benefits a dictionary can provide or how to use it efficiently. This illustrated and easy-to-understand text explains proper dictionary usage to both young students and adults, giving them this vitally needed skill. The book is part of the Hubbard Key to Life Course described below.

Small Common Words Defined

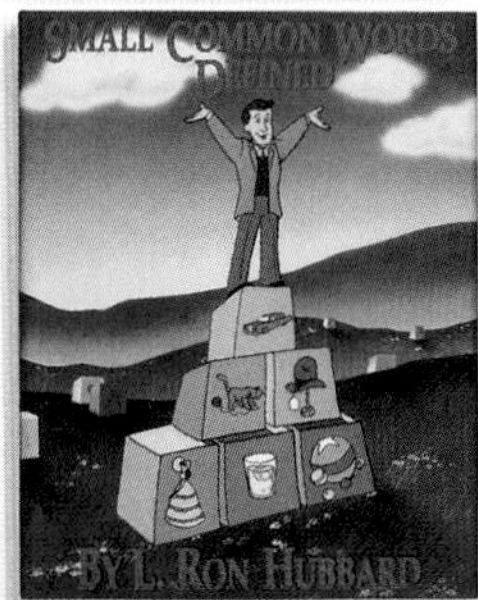

It is the small, common words that are most often misunderstood and form a major barrier to understanding. In this book, more than 3,000 illustrations clearly show each definition of the most common words in English. A unique method of providing a firm understanding of the basic building blocks of the language. Part of the Hubbard Key to Life Course.

The New Grammar

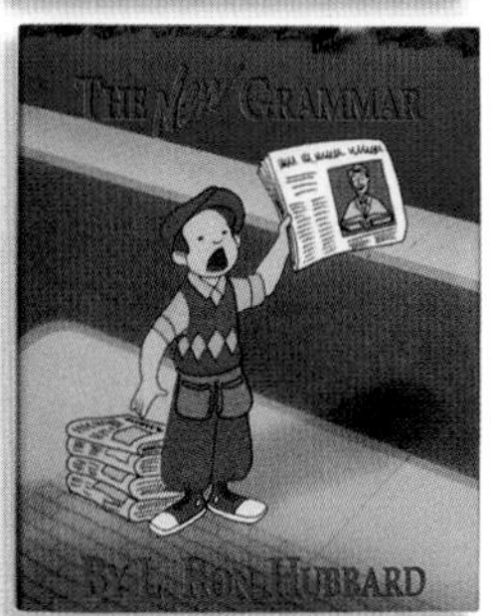

Mr. Hubbard researched the subject of grammar and isolated the exact basics to enable anyone to learn and effectively use this subject. Gone are the complexities and false data that have plagued grammar for many years. With *The New Grammar,* it is possible to greatly improve one's ability to communicate to others and understand others' communications to him. Part of the Hubbard Key to Life Course.

The Hubbard Key to Life Course

Communication is vital to all aspects of Scientology and its applications in life. Mr. Hubbard devised a unique method to increase the ability of *everyone* to comprehend and be comprehended, and thus be able to really communicate. The key to life *is* the ability to communicate, and this course elevates a person to a higher level of ability to do so. It also puts one in a position to gain a full conceptual understanding of all Scientology materials, whether basic or advanced. The Hubbard Key to Life Course contains much more than Study Technology; it puts a person into a much higher state where the potential for living is increased. (The course is delivered in Scientology organizations.)

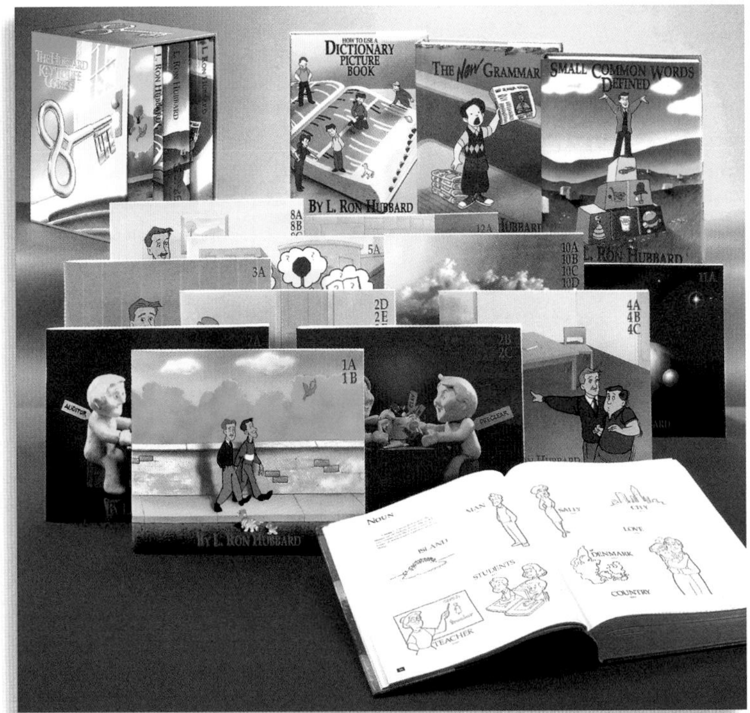

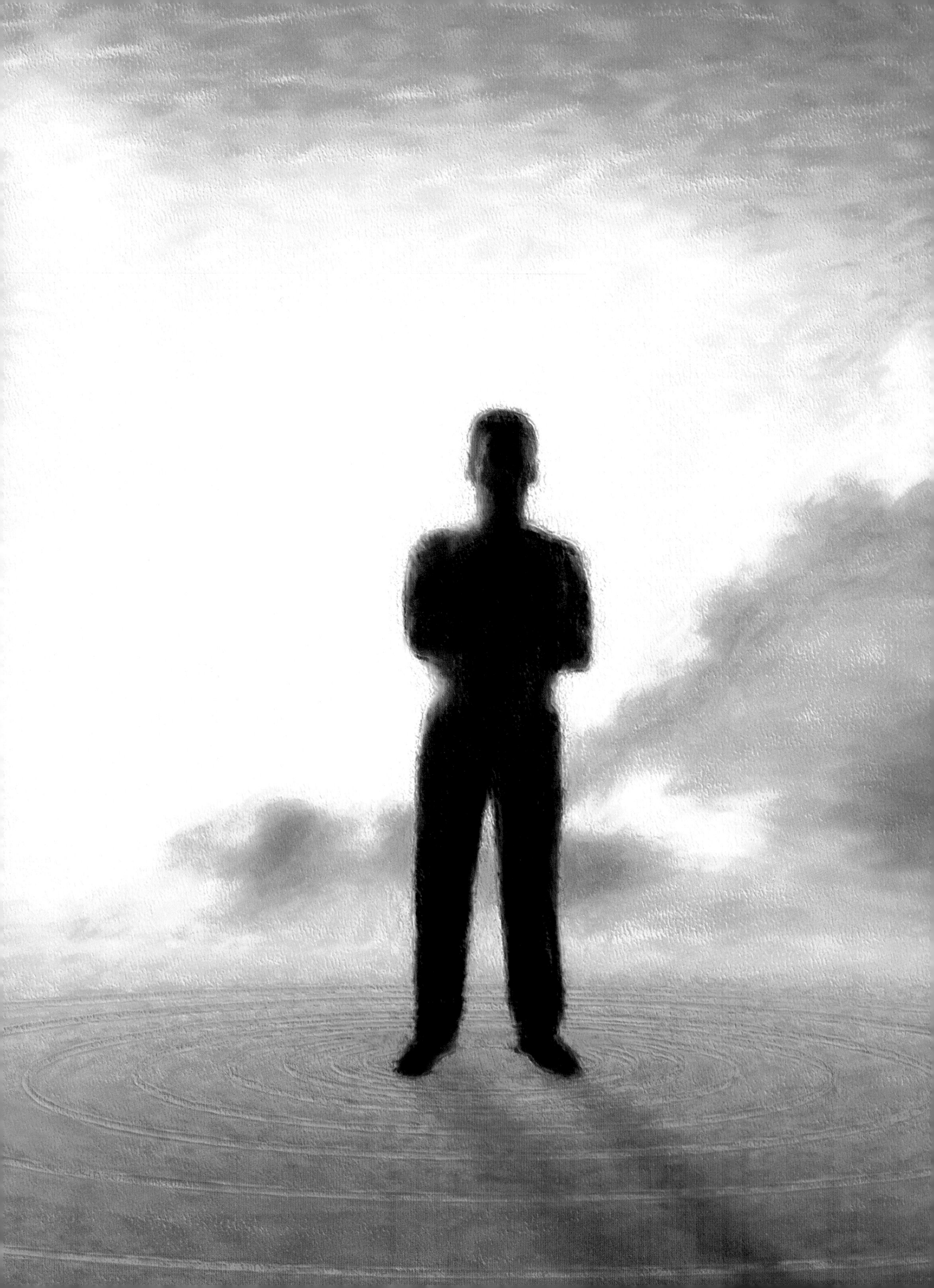

Chapter 2

THE DYNAMICS OF EXISTENCE

For millennia, man has attempted to assess his place in this material world. How should he relate to the rest of life, and to his fellows? What are his true responsibilities, and to whom?

Definitive answers were not forthcoming, not from the ancient Greeks, nor from the materialist thinkers of recent times.

And so it remained until L. Ron Hubbard realized his long sought-after goal: the discovery of a unifying principle that applied to all life, a common denominator by which all men and, indeed, all life, might be understood.

From this came a flood of discoveries that cast new light on the nature of man and life.

The principles in this chapter solve the ancient moral dilemma of right and wrong and bring about a new level of rationality. With them, one can now align the various factors of existence, invariably make the right decisions when faced with choices and achieve a new perspective on the directions available in his life.

Mr. Hubbard expanded upon these principles in numerous other writings and lectures. But what follows represents the essence of the subject and a practical approach to living successfully used by millions.

THE GOAL OF MAN

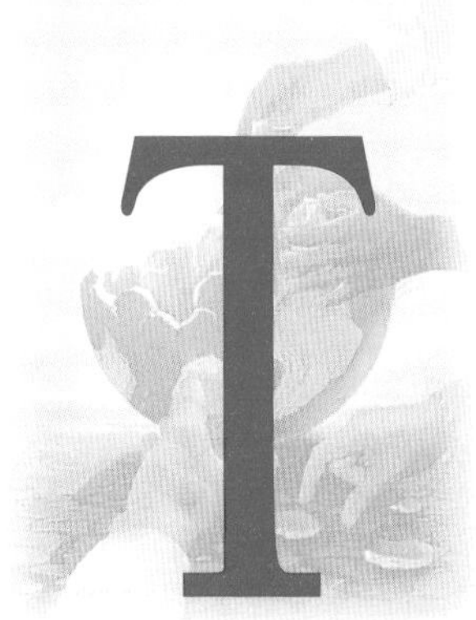

The goal of man, the lowest common denominator of all his activities, the dynamic principle of his existence, has long been sought. Should such an answer be discovered, it is inevitable that from it many answers would flow. It would explain all phenomena of behavior; it would lead toward a solution of man's major problems; and, most of all, it should be workable.

Such an answer has been discovered. It is:

The Dynamic Principle of Existence Is Survival.

The goal of life can be considered to be infinite survival. Man, as a life form, can be demonstrated to obey in all his actions and purposes the one command: "*Survive!*"

It is not a new thought that man is surviving. It is a new thought that man is motivated *only* by survival.

That his single goal is survival does not mean that he is the optimum survival mechanism which life has attained or will develop. The goal of the dinosaur was also survival and the dinosaur isn't extant anymore.

Obedience to this command, "*Survive!*" does not mean that every attempt to obey is uniformly successful. Changing environment, mutation (change in the form or nature of something) and many other things work against any one organism attaining infallible survival techniques or form.

What would be the optimum survival characteristics of various life forms? They would have to have various fundamental characteristics, differing from one species to the next just as one environment differs from the next.

This is important, since it has been but poorly considered in the past that a set of survival characteristics in one species would not be survival characteristics in another.

The methods of survival can be summed under the headings of food, protection (defensive and offensive) and procreation. There are no existing life forms which lack solutions to these problems. Every life form errs, one way or another, by holding a characteristic too long or developing characteristics which may lead to its extinction. But the developments which bring about successfulness of form are far more striking than their errors. The naturalist and biologist are continually resolving the characteristics of this or that life form by discovering that need rather than whim governs such developments. The hinges of the clam shell, the awesome "face" on the wings of the butterfly, have survival value.

The goals of man, then, stem from the single goal of survival through a conquest of the material universe. The success of his survival is measured in terms of the broad survival of all.

THE DYNAMICS

Every individual is made up of a central thrust through existence. This drive, this thrust through existence, is survival. It is the effort on the part of the organism to survive.

We call the urge toward survival a *dynamic*.

As this urge becomes enturbulated (put into a state of agitation or disturbance) or influenced by outside forces, it is either suppressed or it is diluted with other people's purposes. That is to say, other people force their purposes on the individual. In either way, the dynamic itself becomes to some slight degree enturbulated.

As the survival dynamic is cut back or as it is entered or acted upon by other influences—other people and the regular suppressors of life, such as the absence of food, clothing and shelter—this dynamic can become more and more enturbulated until it is headed toward death, or succumb, exactly in the opposite direction.

The dynamic goes toward succumb in the exact ratio that it is enturbulated. It goes toward survival in the exact ratio that it is clean and clear.

That is regarding it as just one dynamic. If we take a look at this dynamic through a magnifying glass, we find that in this one thrust there are actually eight thrusts, or *eight dynamics*.

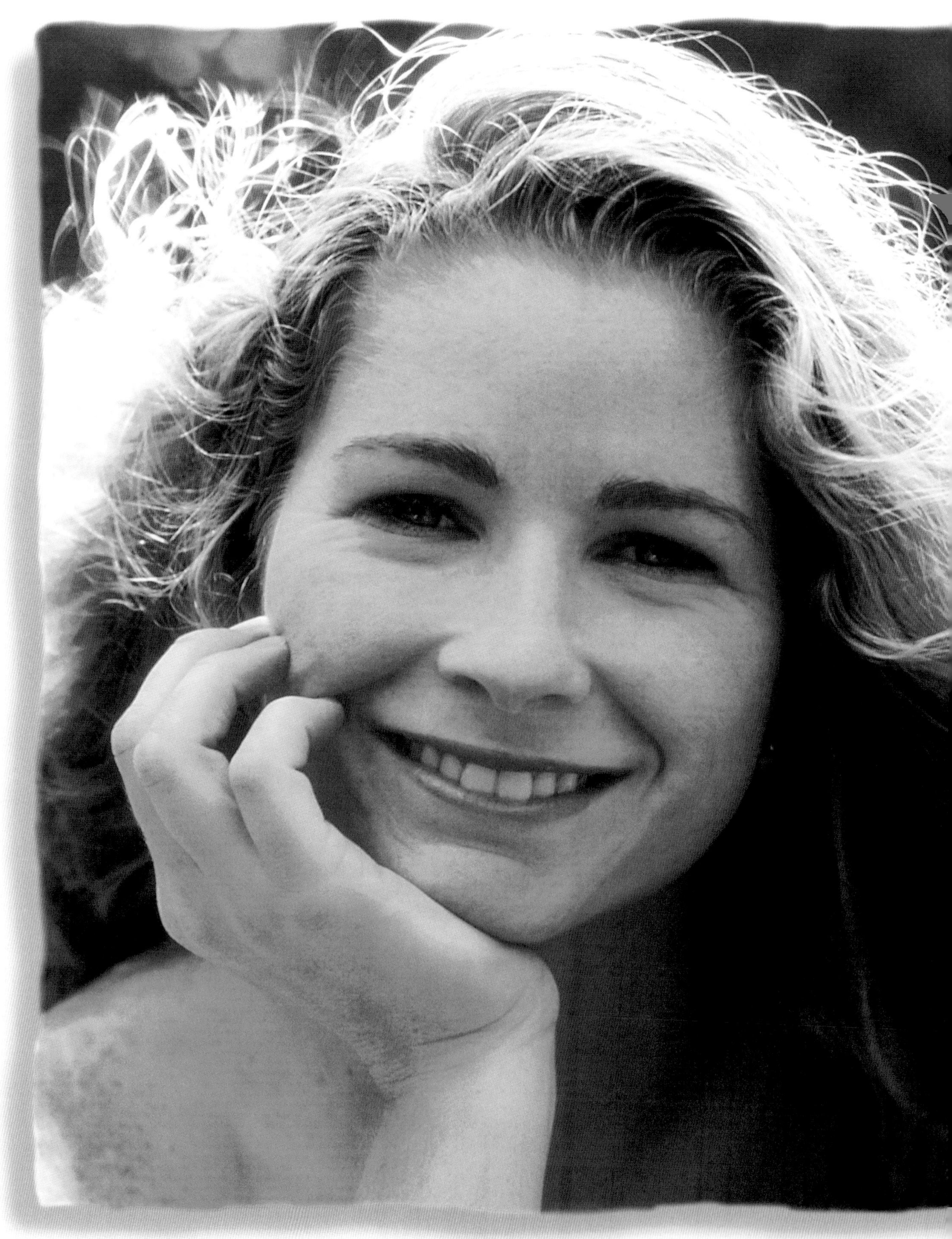

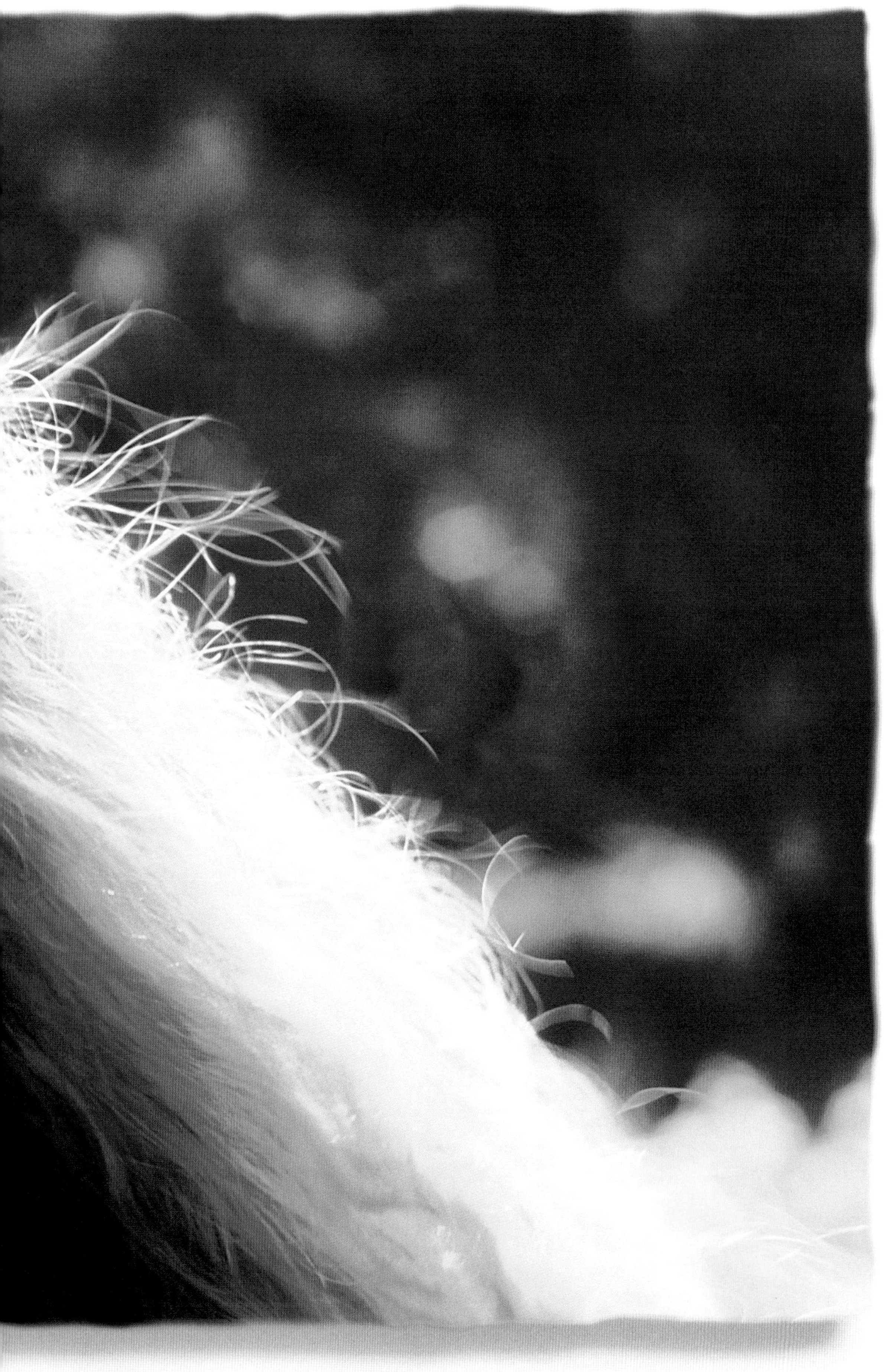

*The **first dynamic** is the urge toward existence as one's self. It is the effort to survive as an individual, to be an individual, to attain the highest level of survival for the longest possible time for self. Here we have individuality expressed fully.*

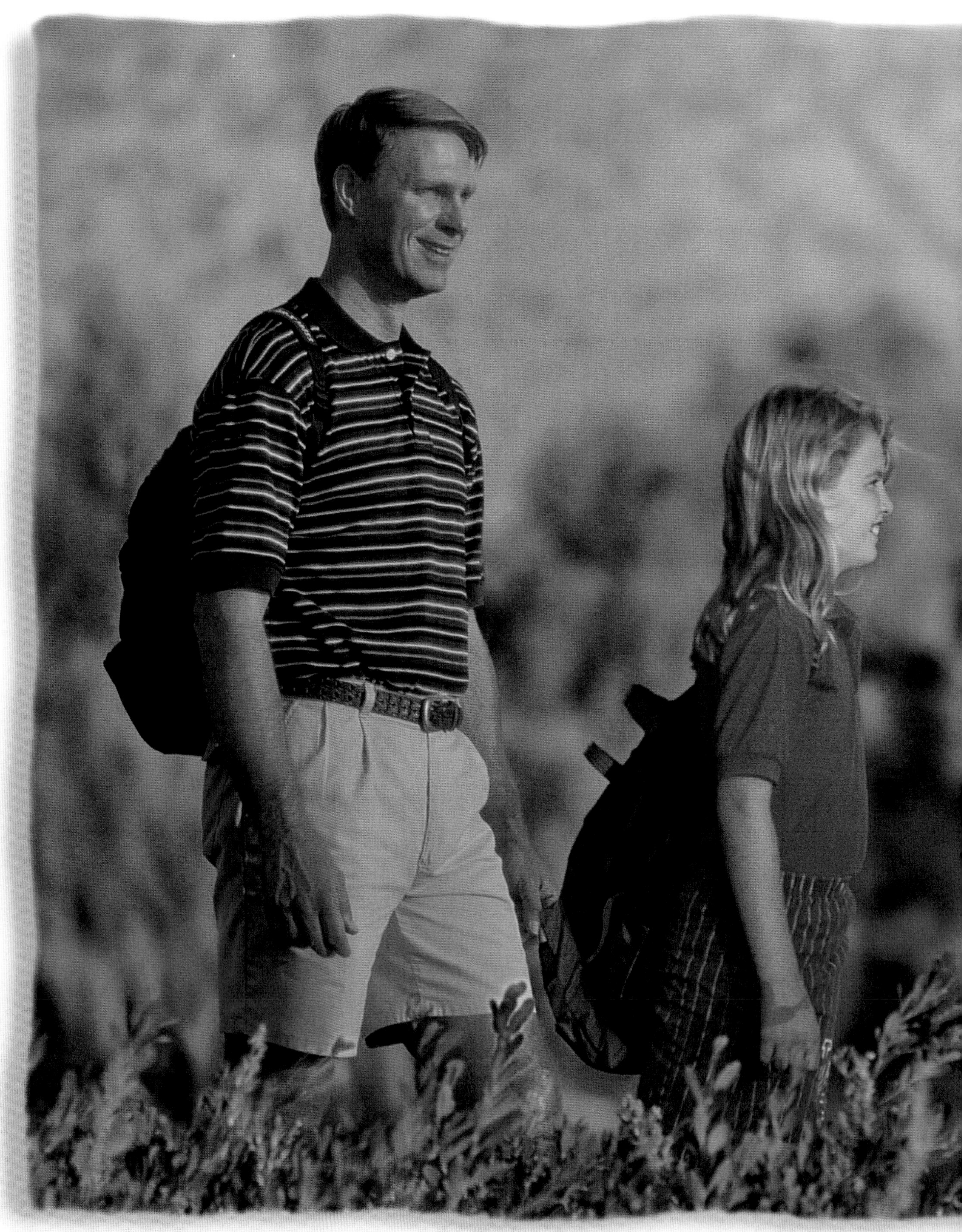

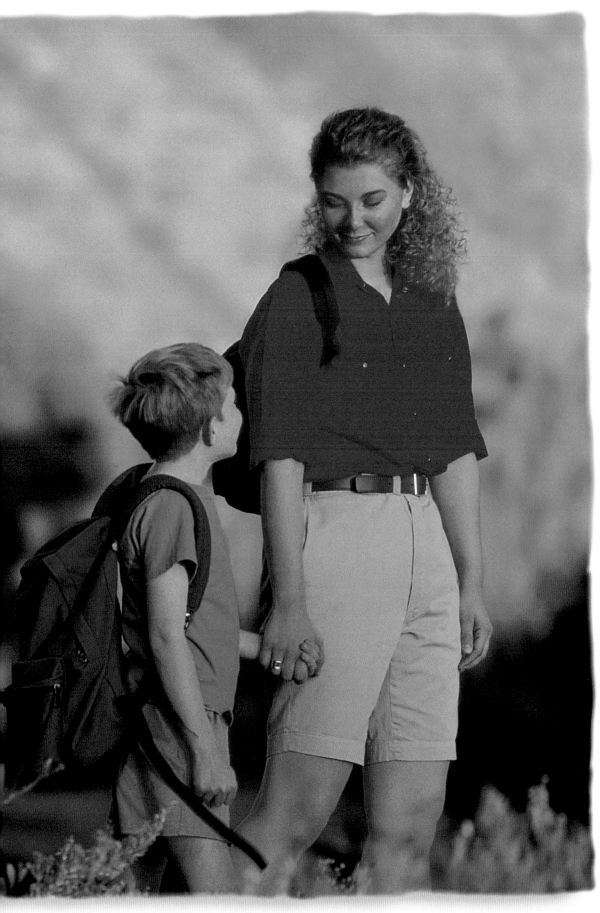

*The **second dynamic** is the urge toward existence as a future generation. It has two compartments: sex; and the family unit, including the rearing of children.*

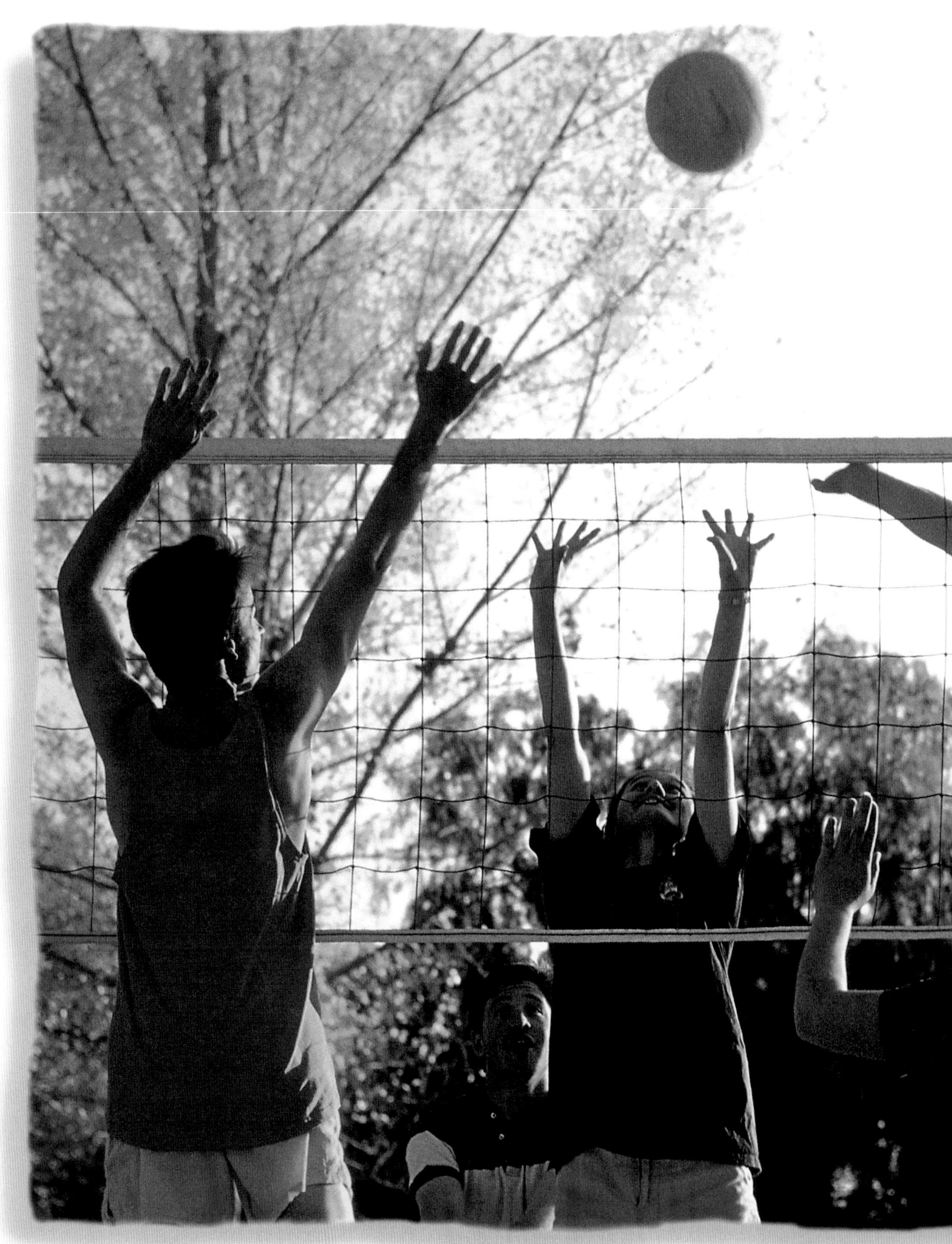

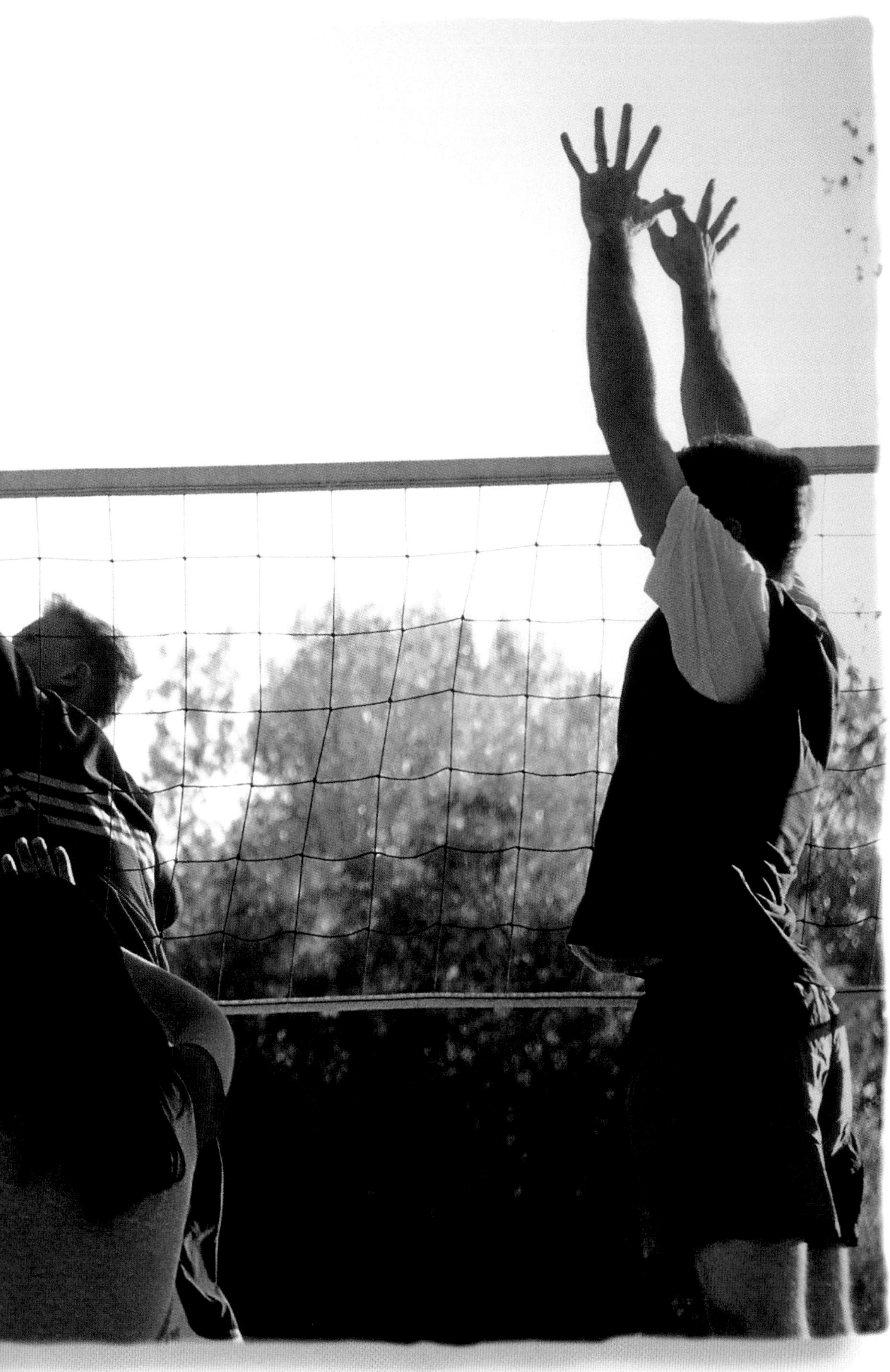

*The **third dynamic** is the urge to survive as part of a group, with the individual himself furnishing this motivation. Any group, temporary or permanent, political or social, is part of the third dynamic, and each one is a third dynamic.*

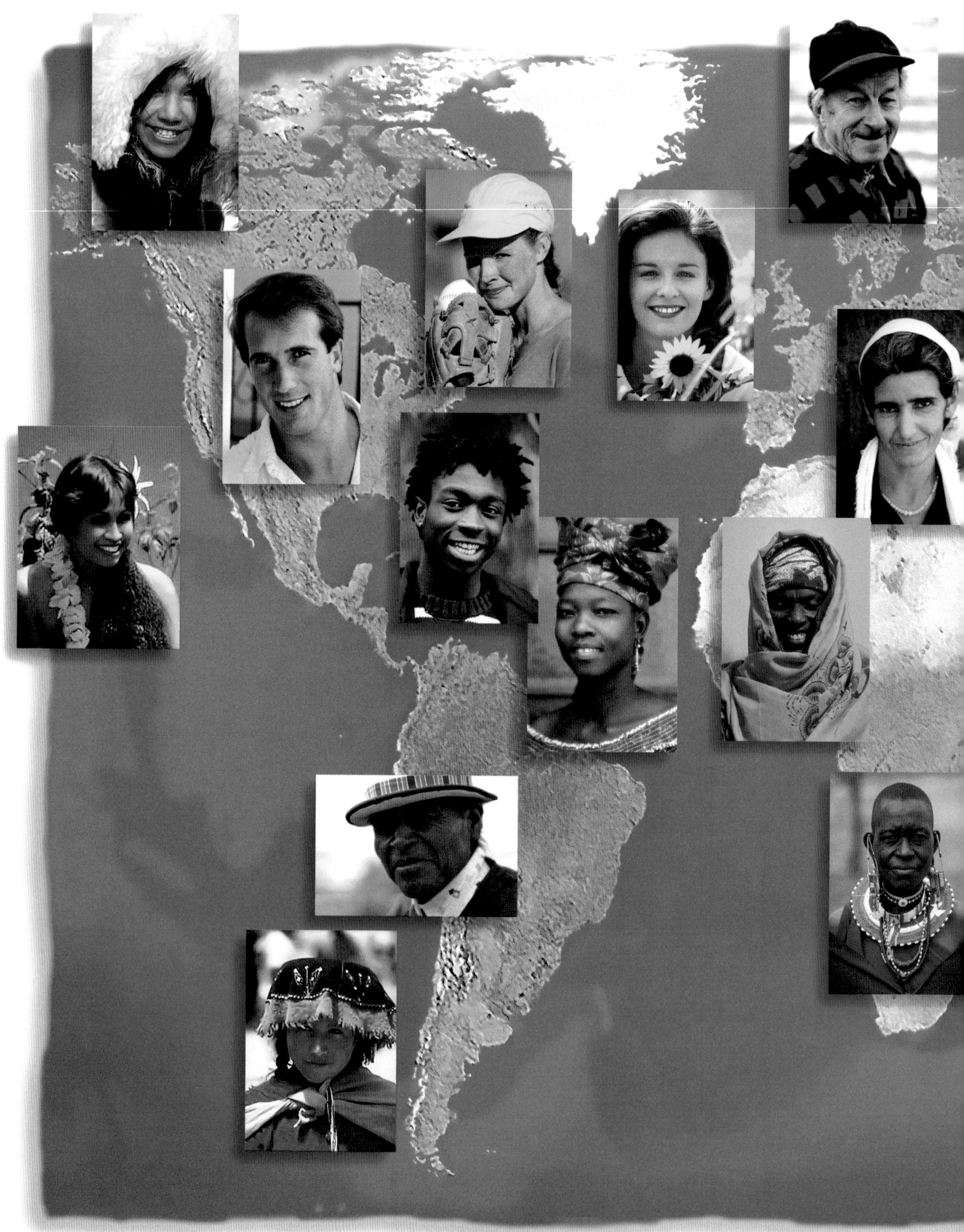

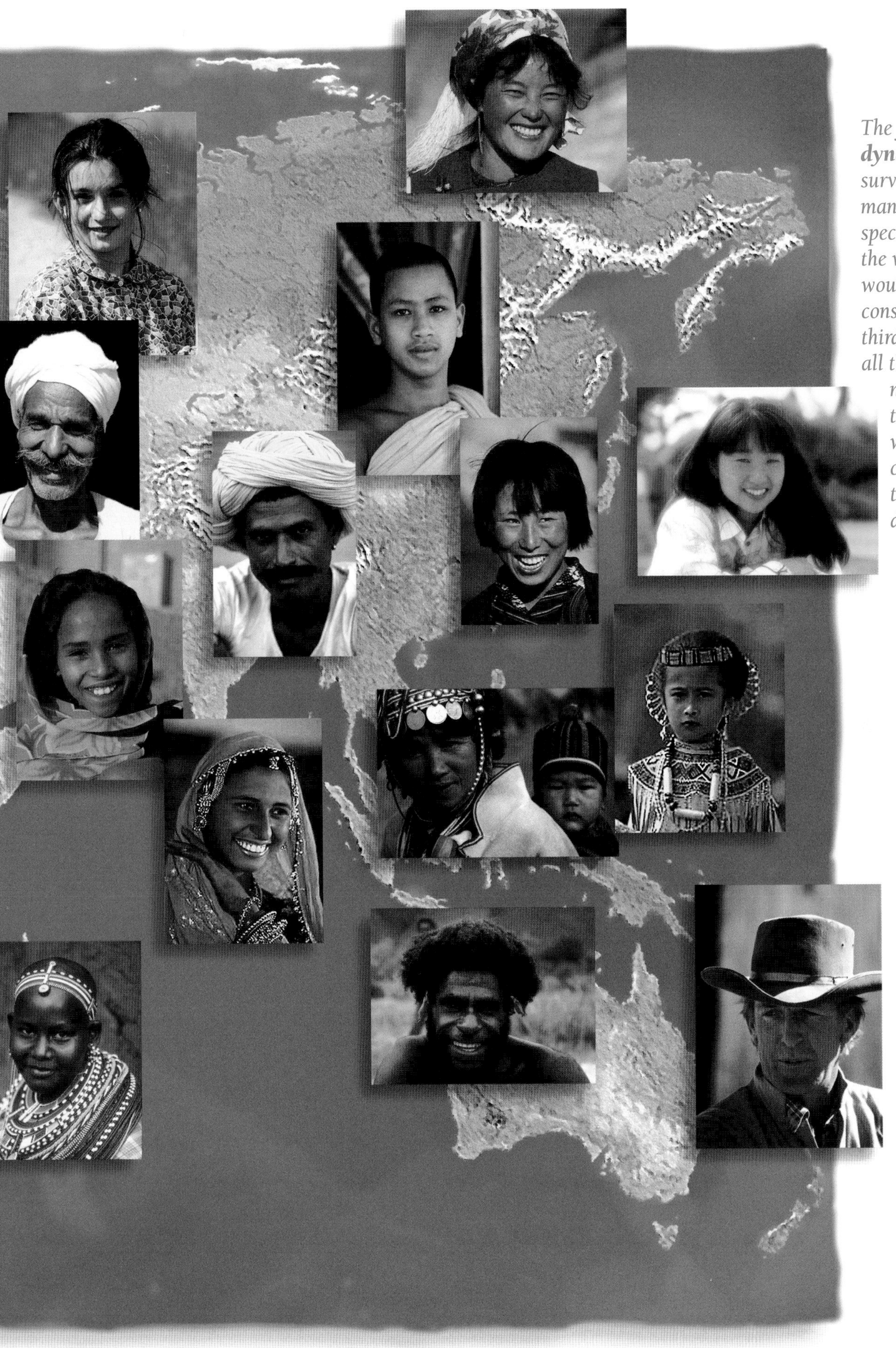

*The **fourth dynamic** is survival through man as a species. Whereas the white race would be considered a third dynamic, all the races of man together would be considered the fourth dynamic.*

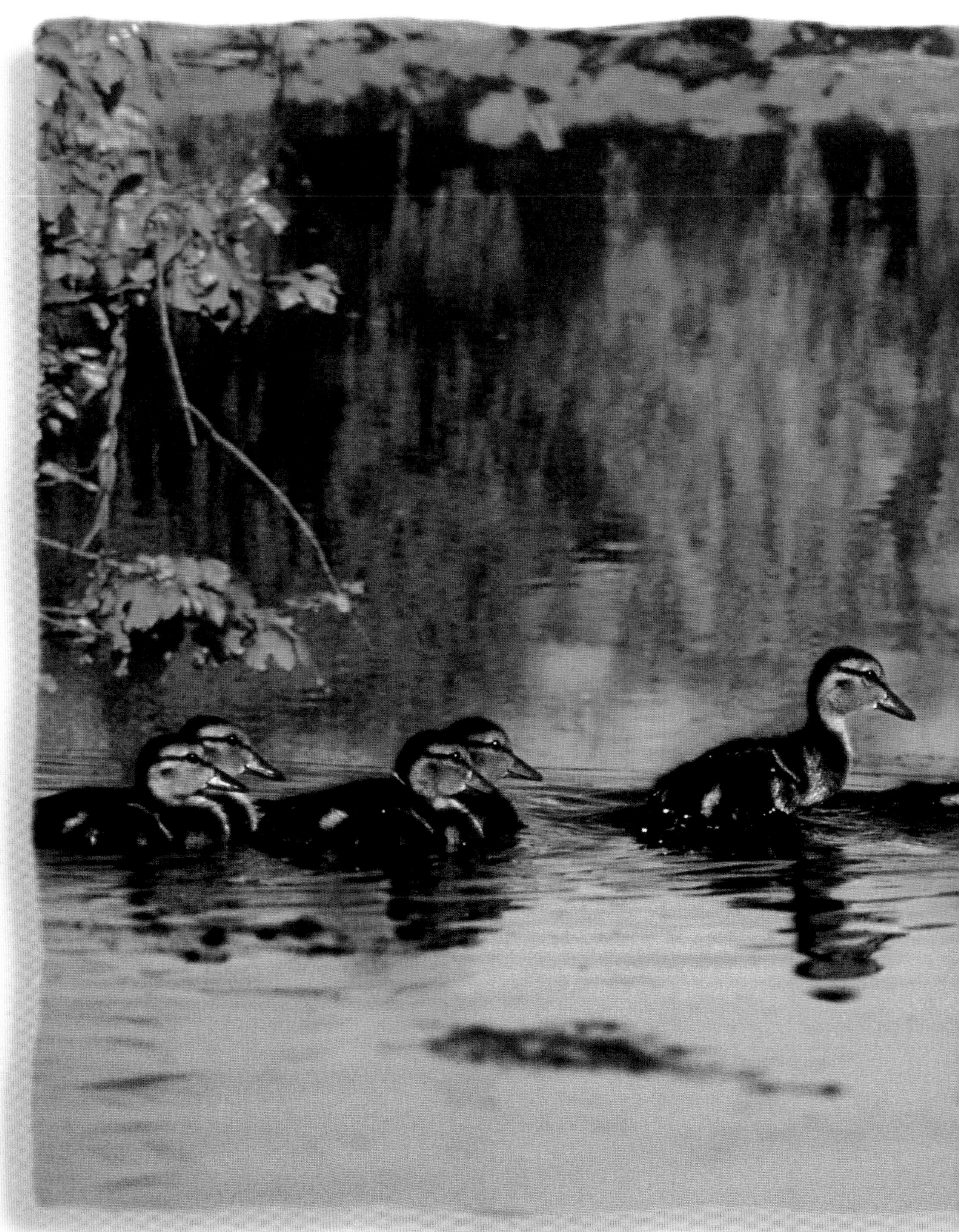

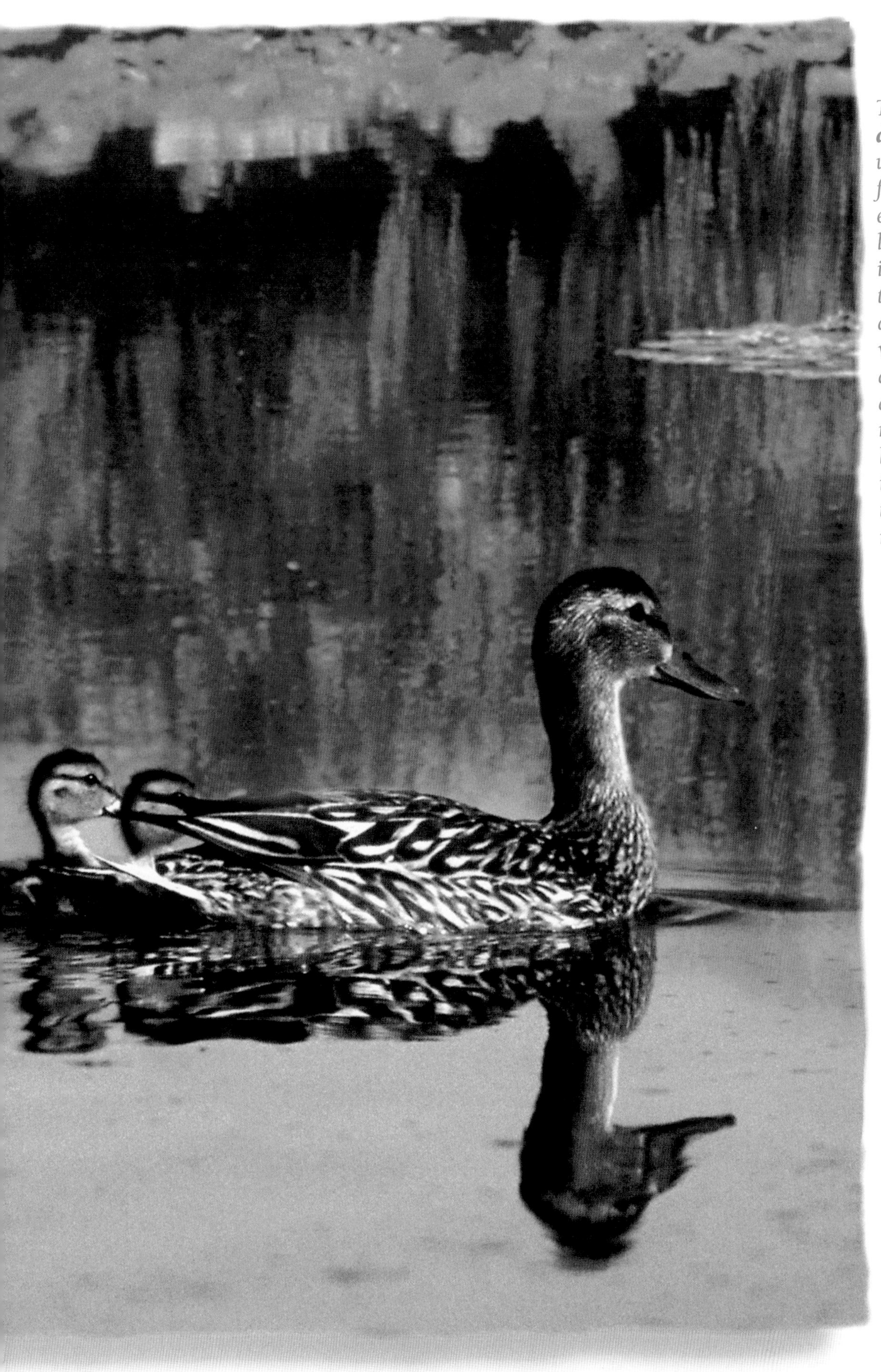

The ***fifth dynamic*** *is the urge to survive for any and every form of life. These would include all living things, whether animal or vegetable, anything directly and intimately motivated by life. It is the individual's effort to survive to make life survive.*

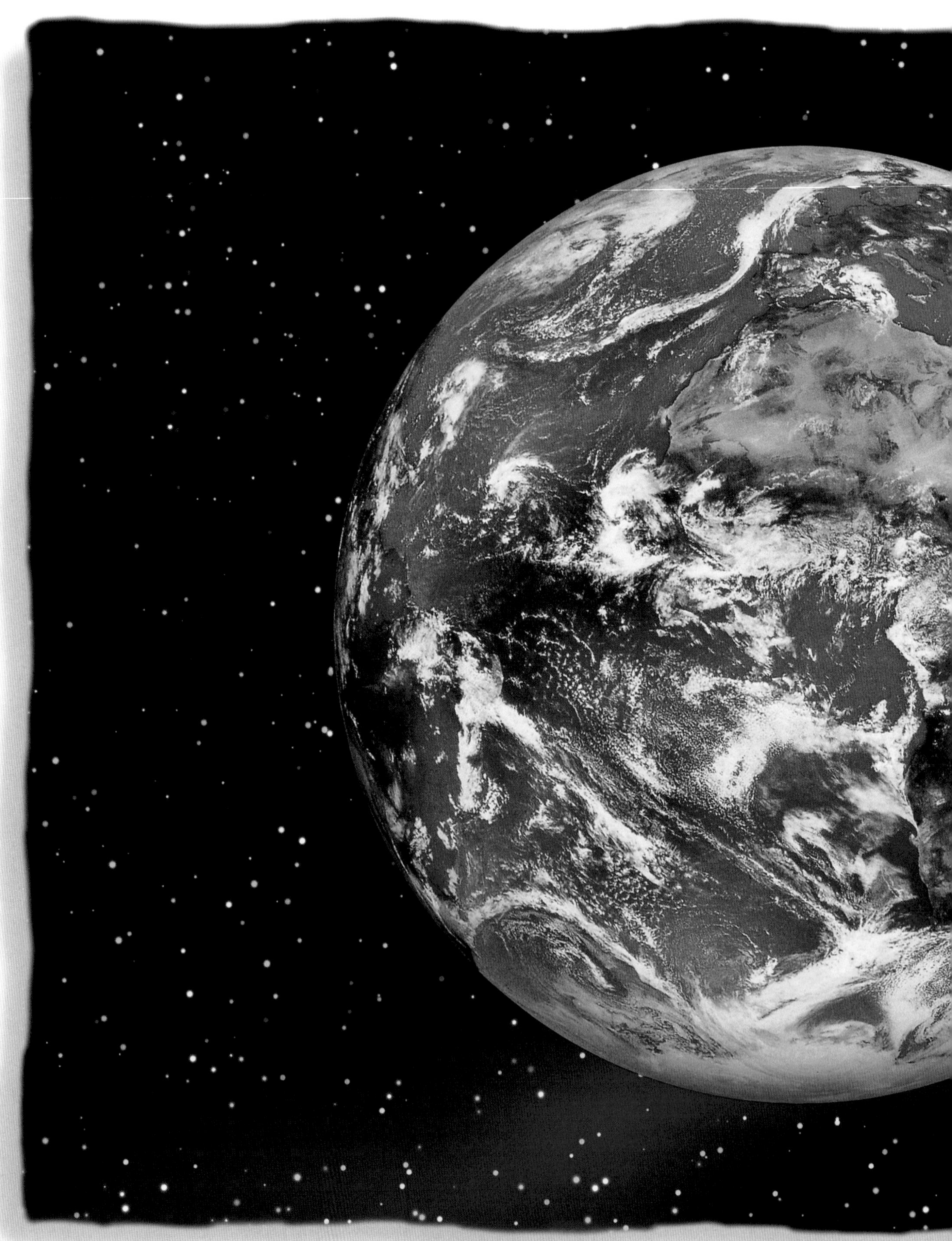

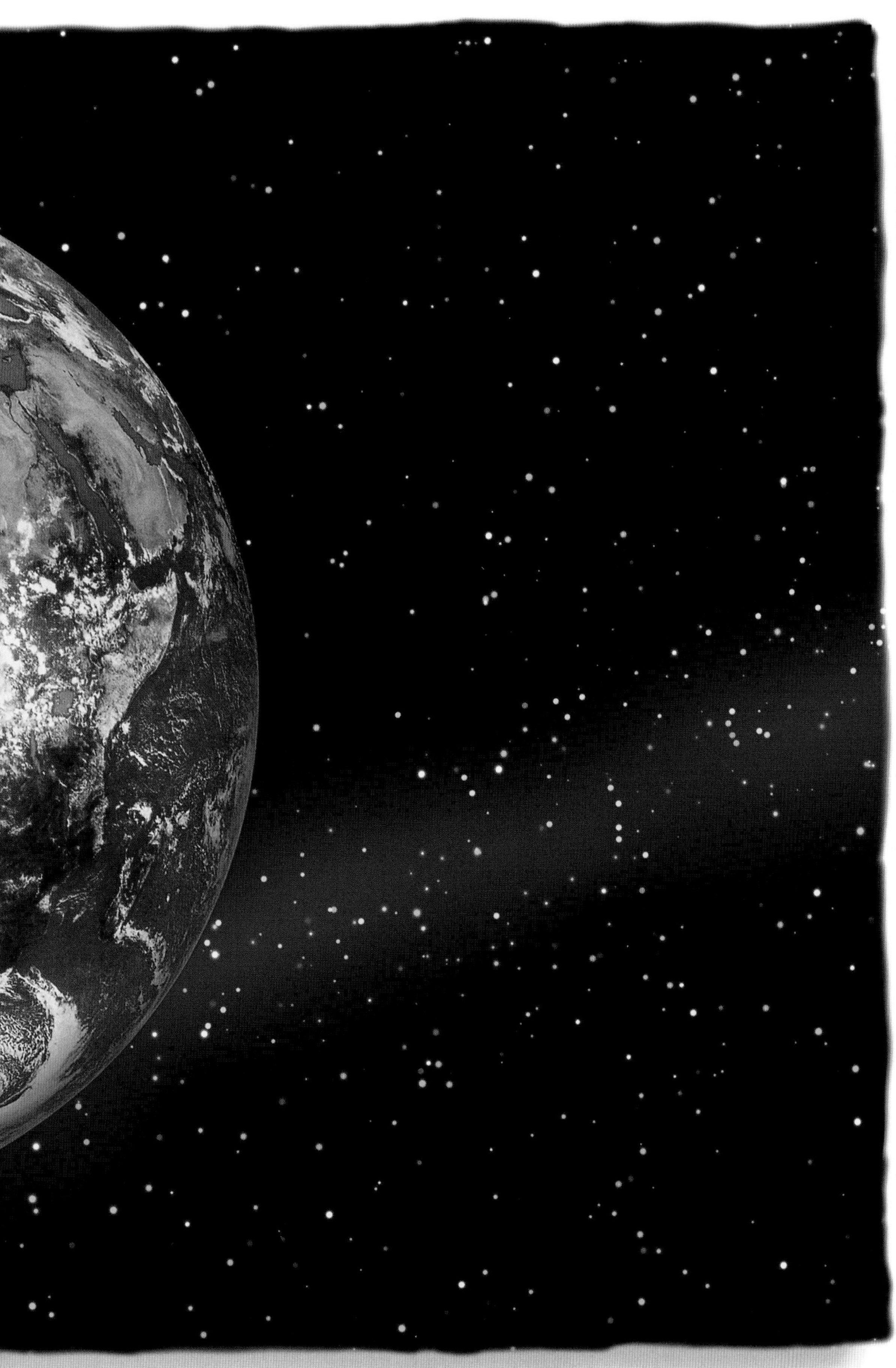

*The **sixth dynamic** is the urge toward existence as the physical universe. It is the drive of the individual to enhance the survival of all matter, energy, space and time—the component parts of the physical universe which we call **MEST**. The individual actually has a thrust for the survival of the material universe.*

*The **seventh dynamic** is the urge toward existence as or of spirits. Anything spiritual, with or without identity, would come under the heading of the seventh dynamic. This is separate from the physical universe and is the source of life itself. Thus there is an effort for the survival of life source.*

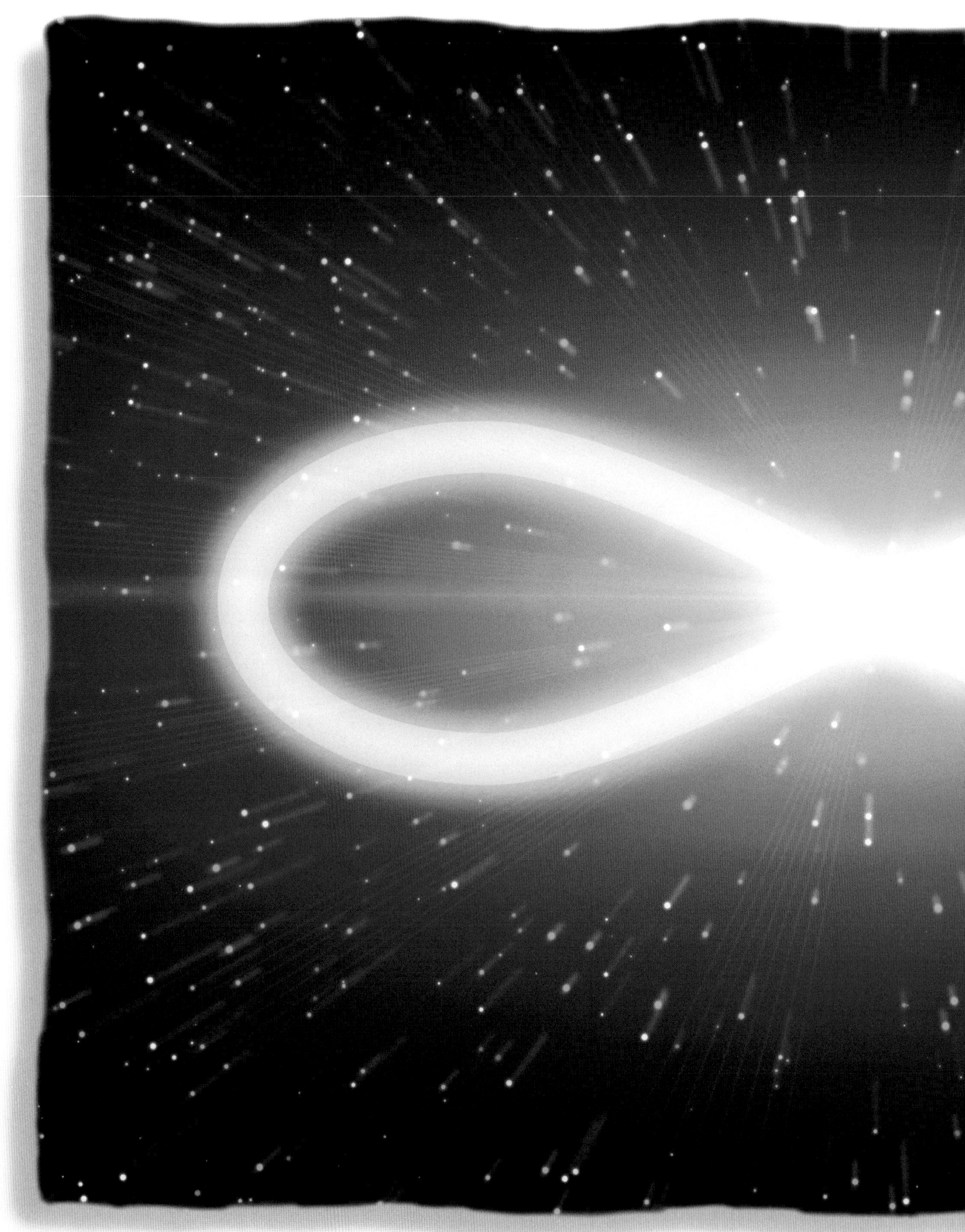

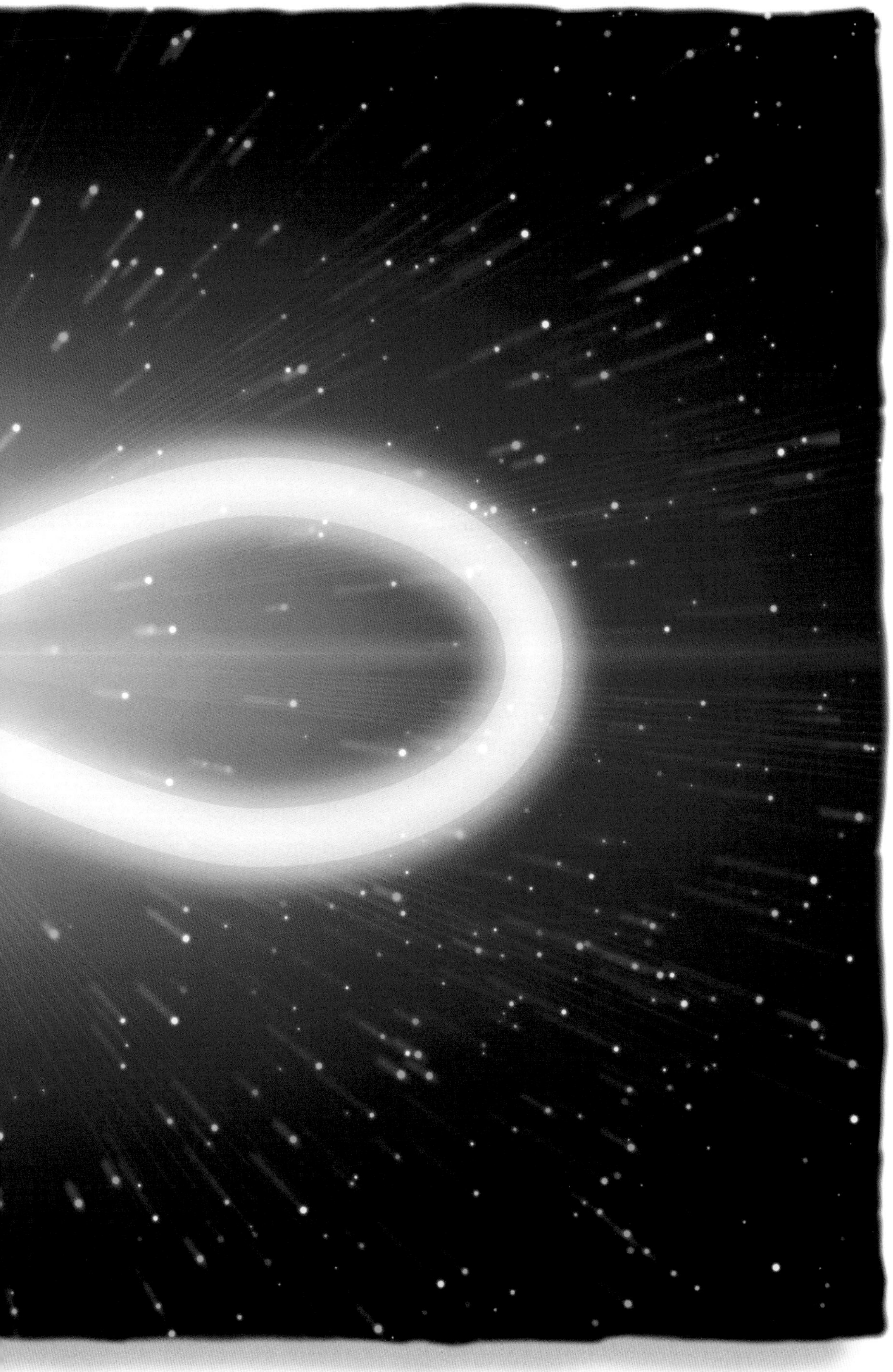

*The **eighth dynamic** is the urge toward existence as infinity. This is also identified as the Supreme Being. This can be called the infinity or God dynamic.*

The Individual and His Dynamics

By inspection of man himself, an individual seems to have a thrust in each one of these departments. In other words, an individual is interested in the survival of groups on a parity with his own survival.

As soon as you knock out one of these dynamics on a human being and you say "For this individual, this dynamic cannot possibly exist," you get trouble, because they *all* get knocked out. They come down on the same level. In other words, if you cut out half of one dynamic, you have cut out half of the rest of the dynamics. This package of dynamics is very vital to the survival of an individual.

Right now we have a whole society which is educated along the line of "man thinks for himself alone." People have to be forced, whipped, beaten and educated to have a third dynamic. They have to be jailed, they have to be sent to school, they have to be punished, fined, taxed, made to go to the polls and vote Democratic. All of these various things have to be done in order to make a person have a third dynamic.

In other words, in this society they are working like mad to build something which is already there. But take away all of these big structures which train the individual to adapt to society and you will find lying behind these structures a much prettier structure and a much stauncher one than any artificial structure being built.

It is the same way on the fourth dynamic. Have you ever known anyone who thought only cats were fit to associate with and that man was no good? There are such people. "Men are no good. Men are cruel, they're beasts, they do terrible things. And the human race is no good and man is no good. But cats and dogs and dear little dumb animals, these are what are nice." In other words, this person throws it all over on the fifth dynamic. She will be all right and she can go on living only until that concept fails on her, because it is an artificial concept.

Man can do almost anything he wants to these dynamics as long as he is consistent about it. The second he gets inconsistent along any line he is in bad shape.

There is no thought or statement here that any one of these eight dynamics is more important than the others. While they are categories of the broad game of life they are not necessarily equal to each other. It will be found among individuals that each person stresses one of the dynamics more than the others, or may stress a combination of dynamics as more important than other combinations.

The purpose in setting forth this division is to increase an understanding of life by placing it in compartments. Having subdivided existence in this fashion, each compartment can be inspected as itself and by itself in its relationship to the other compartments of life. In working a puzzle it is necessary to first take pieces of similar color or character and place them in groups. In studying a subject it is necessary to proceed in an orderly fashion. To promote this orderliness it is necessary to assume for our purposes these eight arbitrary compartments of life.

A further manifestation of these dynamics is that they could best be represented as a series of concentric circles wherein the first dynamic would be the center and each new dynamic would be successively a circle outside it. The idea of space adjoining enters into these dynamics.

The basic characteristic of the individual includes his ability to so expand into the other dynamics, but when the seventh dynamic is reached in its entirety one will only then discover the true eighth dynamic.

As an example of use of these dynamics, one discovers that a baby at birth is not perceptive beyond the first dynamic, but as the child grows and its interests extend it can be seen to embrace other dynamics. As a further example of use, a person who is incapable of operating on the third dynamic is incapable at once of being a part of a team and so might be said to be incapable of a social existence.

How does man act so as to operate successfully along the dynamics? With the state of the world around us, there is no evidence that an answer has been forthcoming. It may seem to be a gift of natural insight in a few individuals; however, this is far from the truth. Any person can acquire the knowledge he needs to determine the most favorable course of action for his survival.

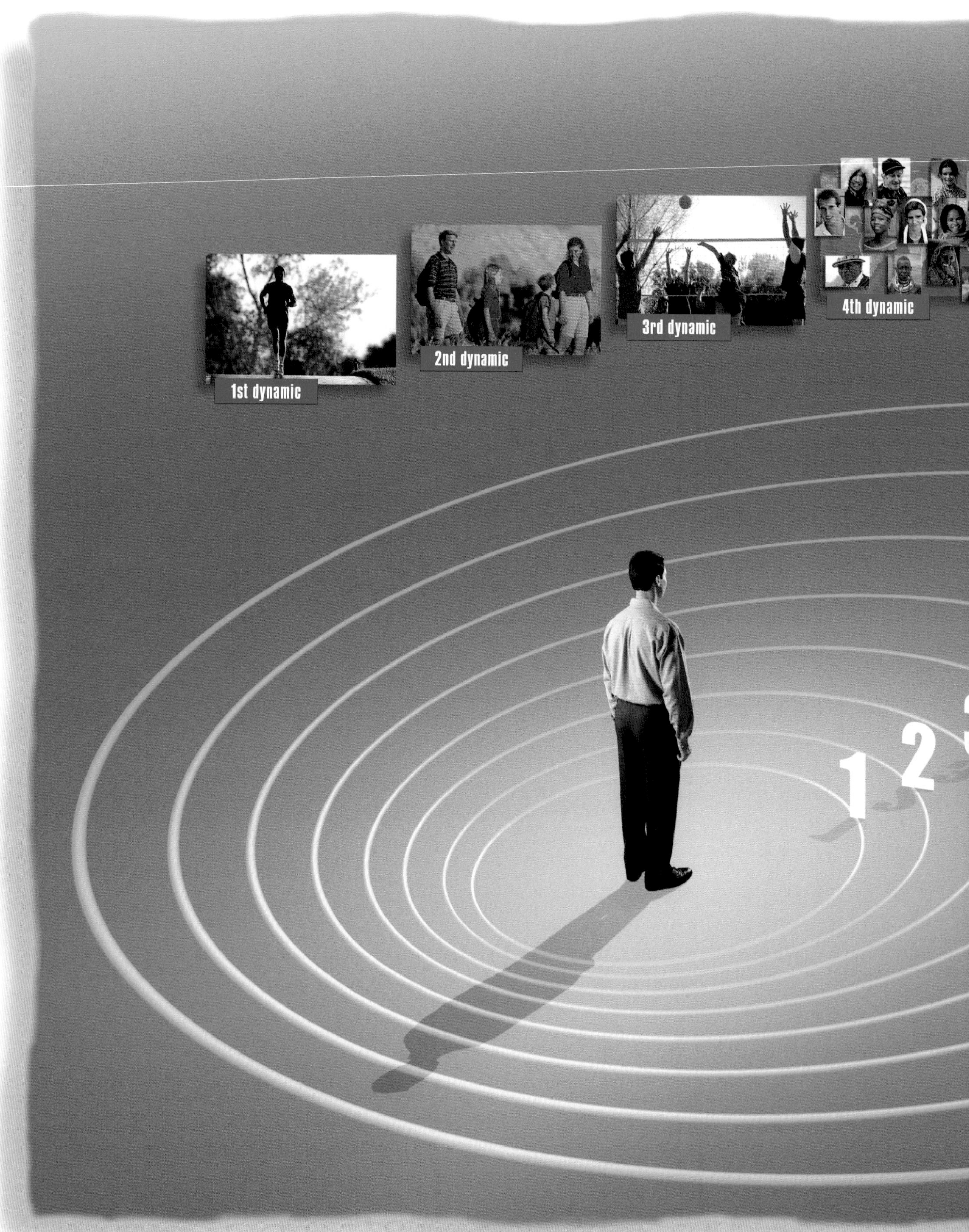

1st dynamic
2nd dynamic
3rd dynamic
4th dynamic
1
2

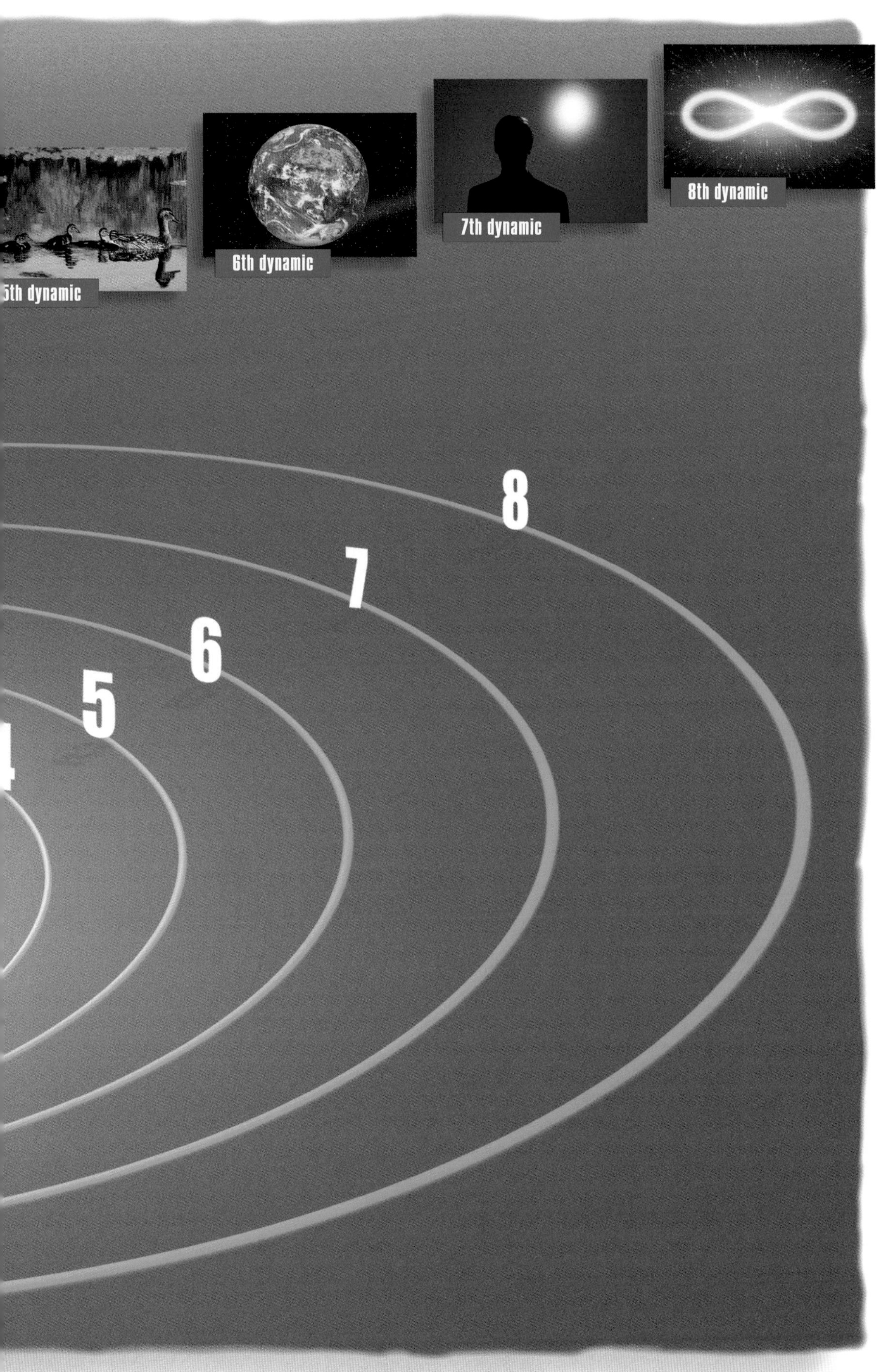

The dynamics can be represented as a series of concentric circles with the first dynamic at the center. The individual expands outwards as he embraces the other dynamics.

Determining Optimum Solutions

An optimum solution of life takes into account the maximum survival for everything concerned in the problem.

This does not mean that one cannot destroy. It so happens that if we didn't have destruction as one of the operating methods of existence, we would be in pretty bad shape. Do you realize that every fern tree that was growing back in the earliest ages would still be growing, and this would be in addition to every tree that had grown since? And we would have live, growing trees on the face of the earth until we would probably be walking about eight hundred feet above the soil. Death—destruction—has to come in there and clear the way for advances and improvements. And destruction, when used in that way, is very legitimate.

For instance, you can't build an apartment house without knocking down the tenement that stood there before. Somebody comes along and says, "Oh, that's very bad; you're destroying something. You're destroying an old landmark."

"We're trying to put up an apartment house here, lady."

"Yes, but that's a famous old landmark."

"Lady, that thing is about ready to fall into the street."

"Oh, it's very bad to destroy things."

That is pretty aberrated (not supported by reason, departing from rational thought or behavior), because you have to destroy something once in a while. Just think what would happen, for instance, if every piece of paper that had ever been given you in your lifetime was still in your possession and then you had to move, and it was very bad to destroy things so you had to keep on lugging all these things around with you. You can see how ridiculous it would get.

There is an actual equation involved in this: One must not destroy beyond the necessity required in construction.

If one starts to destroy beyond the necessity required in construction, one gets into pretty bad shape very hurriedly. One gets into the shape Nazi Germany was in. They destroyed everything; they said, "Now Austria, now Czechoslovakia, now let's knock apart Stalingrad!" So they did and Stalingrad was an awful mess. So was Germany.

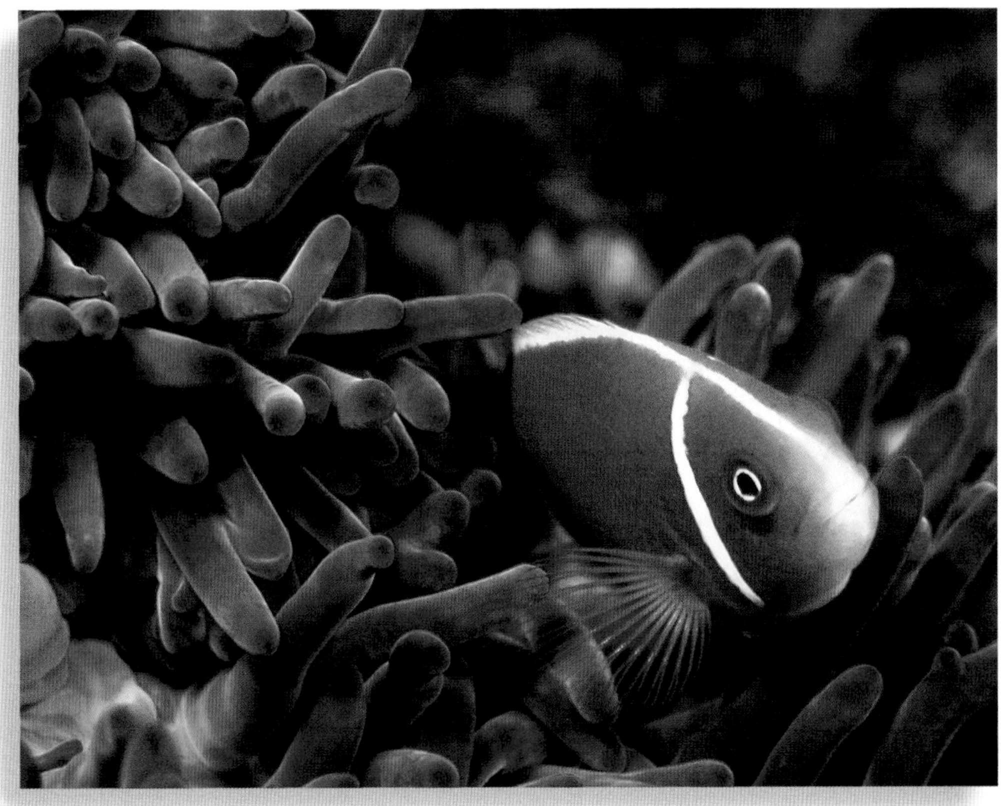

The solution to the problem that does not consider all the dynamics is not an optimum solution. Waste dumped into the sea may be expedient for some company's disposal problems but at huge expense to the fifth and sixth dynamics.

There is an old self-evident truth, "Never send to know for whom the bell tolls; it tolls for thee." Nothing is truer. People start looking at this and they get superstitions about it. They say, "Well, I don't dare harm anybody else because then I would be harmed someplace or other." This is not necessarily true. But on the overall equation of life and existence, the willful destruction of something can upset the survival of the other entities in its vicinity. It can upset and overbalance things to a point where, for example, we don't have any more passenger pigeons. People didn't stop and think, back there over a hundred years ago, that one of these fine days there wouldn't be any—obviously, there were all kinds of them all over the sky.

So man has had to go into a tremendous game-conservation program in order to restore the wildlife which his grandfathers wiped out. Man will do this quite instinctively.

The dynamics mean, simply, how many forms of survival are there? How does an individual survive? You can work this out that the individual survives solely because of himself and cooperates only because of selfishness. But you can also work it out that he survives only for future generations and prove it all very beautifully that way. You can work it out, as they did in Russia, that the individual survives solely for the state and is only part of an ant society, a collectivist, one who lives in a system where all property is owned or controlled by the state. And so it goes, one right after the other. You can take these ways he survives and you can make each one *it*. But when you put it to the test, you find out that you need all of the dynamics.

The number of dynamics merely add up to the number of fields or entities a man has to be in cooperation with in order to get along.

The optimum solution to any problem would be that solution which did the maximum construction or creation along the maximum number of dynamics pertinent to the problem.

Solutions which injure one dynamic for the benefit of another dynamic result in eventual chaos. However, optimum solutions are almost possible to attain and human thinking seeks at its highest level only to bring the greatest order and the least chaos.

When an individual is in a low emotional tone, he will stress one or two dynamics at the expense of the rest and so lives a very disorderly existence and is productive of much chaos for those around him.

The soldier, flinging away his life in battle, is operating on the third dynamic (his company, his nation) at the expense of his first dynamic, the fourth and all the rest. The religionist, someone devoted to religion, may live on the eighth, seventh, fifth and fourth at the expense of the first and sixth. The "selfish" person may be living only on the first dynamic, a very chaotic effort.

There is nothing particularly wrong with bad emphasis on these dynamics until such emphasis begins to endanger them broadly, as in the case of a Hitler or a Genghis Khan or the use of atomic fission for destruction. Then all man begins to turn on the destroyers.

The whole of *survival* is a dynamic, the only dynamic. But *survive* breaks down into these eight.

The abilities and shortcomings of individuals can be understood by viewing their participation in the various dynamics.

The equation of the optimum solution would be that a problem has been well resolved which portends (signifies or means) the maximum good for the maximum number of dynamics. That is to say that any solution, modified by the time available to put the solution into effect, should be creative or constructive for the greatest possible number of dynamics. The optimum solution for any problem would be a solution which achieved the maximum benefit in all the dynamics.

It is through application of these principles by oneself and by assisting others to understand and apply them that an individual can attain an increased level of survival for himself, those with whom he associates and, indeed, all life. ■

TEST YOUR UNDERSTANDING

Answer the following questions about the eight dynamics. Refer back to the chapter to check your answers. If you need to, review the chapter. Going over the material several times will increase your certainty and help you better apply it.

- ❑ *What is all life trying to do?*
- ❑ *What is a dynamic?*
- ❑ *What are the eight dynamics?*
- ❑ *What is the optimum solution to any problem?*

PRACTICAL EXERCISES

Here are exercises relating to the eight dynamics. Doing these exercises will help increase your understanding of the knowledge contained in this chapter.

1 Look around the environment and notice things that are surviving. How many things can you find that are surviving? Go around and spot examples of survival until you are certain that the goal of life is survival.

2 Look around your immediate environment and see how many of the eight dynamics you can find. Look out a window or take a walk outside and see how many examples you can find of the dynamics.

3 Select a situation or problem in your own life or in the life of someone you know. Using what you have learned about the eight dynamics, determine the optimum solution for it.

4 Now, help another person determine the optimum solution to a problem in his life.

Results from Application

Knowing the dynamics of life makes it possible for hitherto unresolvable problems to be resolved with ease. Any concept in Scientology is considered useful to the degree it can be applied. These pages contain examples of the application of these fundamentals.

In Adelaide, Australia, a woman who had studied about the eight dynamics noticed that an employee in the same company was always "in trouble" and was, in fact, being threatened with termination. As he seemed to be trying to do a good job, she sat down with him and proceeded to find out what was happening.

"After listening to him for some time, I realized that he had been neglecting himself totally. He wasn't sleeping well or eating enough, he didn't spend any time doing anything to improve himself—nothing—and he therefore was doing poorly at work. I showed him the definitions of the dynamics. It was as if it were an entirely new idea to him that he should look after himself. He had somehow imagined that he could do well at work while completely neglecting himself and he soon realized why he had been doing poorly at work. He immediately set about correcting the situation. While not neglecting the third dynamic, he slept an adequate amount, took better care of his appearance, spent time with his family, and took a course to improve himself and his job performance. As a result, his job performance improved, he was happier and his worth to the company was noticed by his superiors. He was no longer continuously 'in trouble' and, in fact, earned a promotion."

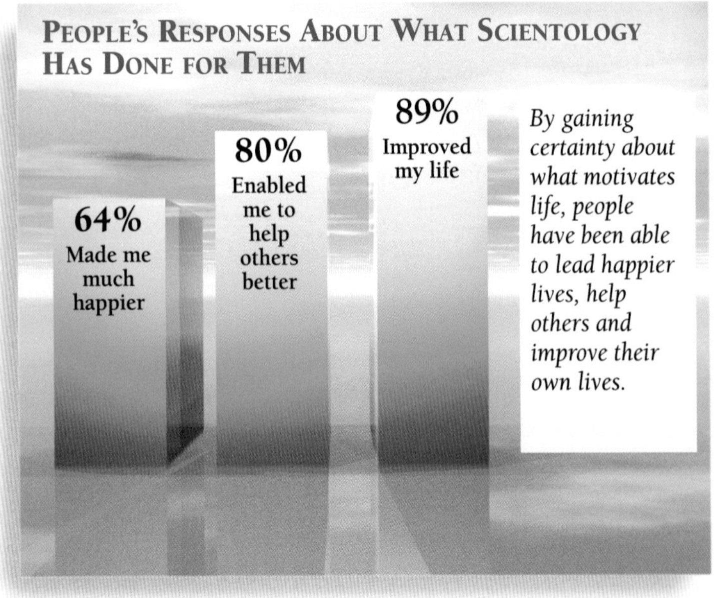

People's Responses About What Scientology Has Done for Them

64%	80%	89%
Made me much happier	Enabled me to help others better	Improved my life

By gaining certainty about what motivates life, people have been able to lead happier lives, help others and improve their own lives.

A young man from Milano, Italy, was leading an active life. He played soccer on a local team and had a girlfriend of whom he was very fond. Life was fun. Then some not-so-well-meaning acquaintances started him using drugs. As his use of drugs increased, his life began falling apart. He was fortunate enough to be shown data on the eight dynamics and halted the disastrous slide of his life. He said:

"Some time ago, I went against all the dynamics starting from the first one, and as

time went on, all the other dynamics went to pieces, one after the other. My girlfriend left me because I drugged myself. Then my soccer team threw me out because I couldn't play as well as I could before. All the rest of my dynamics went like this because I started to drug myself which was destroying my first dynamic. When I read the data on the eight dynamics, I understood what had happened in my life and I knew how to put my life back together, piece by piece. This knowledge gave me the strength and courage it took to get off drugs and now I devote all my time to getting other people off drugs. I am surviving on all my dynamics and I always insist that others around me have the data on the eight dynamics so that they can make the correct decisions about their lives. It makes me think that if everyone had this data, the world would be a happy place and the people in it would fare very well."

In Australia, a fifteen-year-old girl who knew the technology of the eight dynamics, started to spend time with a girl at her school and quickly discovered that her new friend was drinking, taking drugs, being sexually promiscuous, and fighting with her mother constantly. She had already been kicked out of her home once by her mother and had left home of her own accord a number of times, despite being only fifteen years old. The girl needed help with her life. Here is how her new friend provided it:

"I showed my friend some basic technology on the eight dynamics and got her to see how her own actions could be affecting the behavior of her mother toward her; that the upsets were not necessarily 'all her mother's fault.' I told her the solution was to get in **more** *communication, not less, and to be open with her mother rather than ignoring that part of her second dynamic. As a result of her own realizations about the dynamics, in a matter of a few weeks, she was* **really** *in communication with her mother and was stably living at home. She had stopped smoking dope and cut down on her drinking, so was doing much better on the first dynamic. She even got a steady boyfriend. She did better in school and started getting better grades. After a while she got a part-time job and started contributing financially to her parents. This was some real improvement in her life across all the dynamics."*

SUGGESTIONS FOR FURTHER STUDY

Only a small portion of the data L. Ron Hubbard amassed on man and the dynamics was able to be included in this chapter. However, it should be noted that his discovery of the common denominator "Survive!" led to all his further advancements. Therefore, anything in Scientology could classify as further study of these basics. However, here is a selection of additional *basic* references which expand and clarify these concepts.

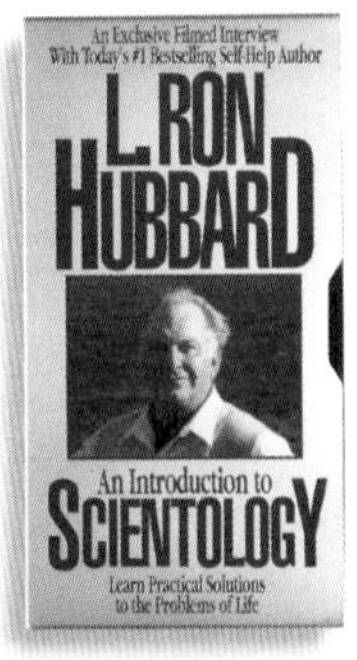

An Introduction to Scientology

This video presents a rare one-hour interview with L. Ron Hubbard, who provides candid answers to many commonly asked questions about Scientology. Mr. Hubbard relates his researches into life and the development of Scientology, its fundamentals, procedures and organizations.

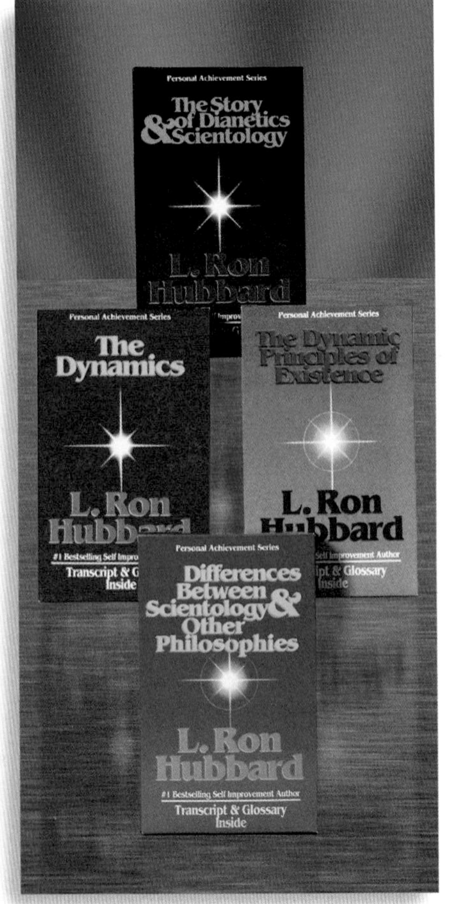

The Personal Achievement Series Lectures

There are nearly 3,000 lectures by Mr. Hubbard on the subjects of Dianetics and Scientology. Those which provide introductory Dianetics and Scientology materials form this series. Several of these taped hour-long lectures are suitable for additional study about the dynamics and are listed here.

The Story of Dianetics and Scientology

A compelling account of Mr. Hubbard's experiences while developing Dianetics and Scientology. Here he shares his earliest insights into human nature.

The Dynamics

Additional data on the eight dynamics including how man creates on his dynamics and the troubles which ensue when a person gets fixated on just one dynamic.

The Dynamic Principles of Existence

Some people seem more interested and involved in life than others, and generally have more fulfilling lives as a result. Discusses the importance of being a knowing part of and participant in any and all of the functions of life.

Differences Between Scientology and Other Philosophies

A look at the research approach taken to develop Scientology which resulted in advancements, where others' investigations into man and life yielded little of value. Covers the essential reasons which enable a person in Scientology to find his own answers, not authoritarian fixed ideas, which lead nowhere.

Scientology: The Fundamentals of Thought

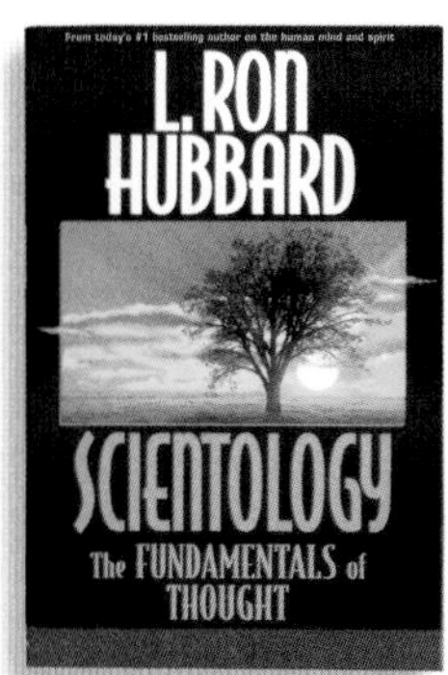

This book explains many basic principles of Scientology, greatly expanding on the materials in this chapter. Each of the subjects covered supplies a person with knowledge he can apply in his life to increase ability. Mr. Hubbard gives a broad summation of his research into life and the spirit, providing the first workable explanation of *how* life operates.

Scientology: A New Slant on Life

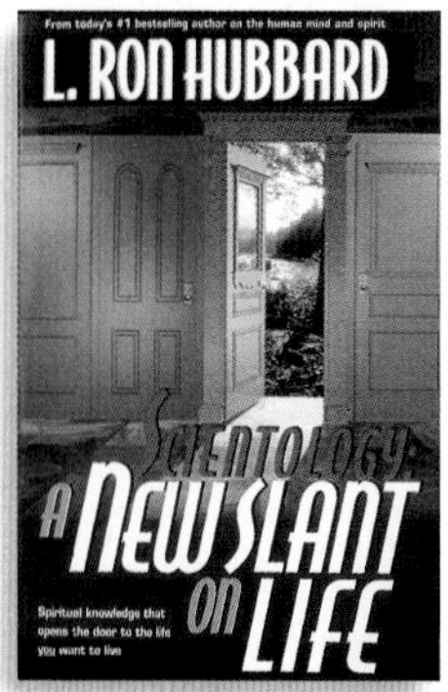

This new look at life helps you really know yourself, as you are and as you could be. Thirty of Mr. Hubbard's essays on a variety of subjects present many of the fundamental principles of Scientology, including additional data on the dynamics, and show how you can gain greater happiness and success in life.

The Dynamics of Life

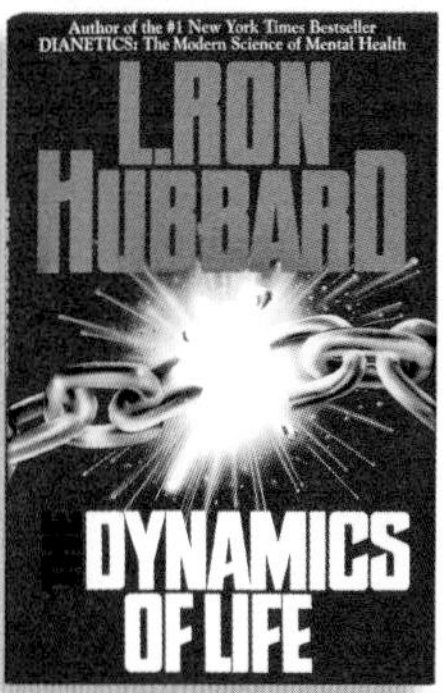

The first formal record of Mr. Hubbard's researches on the function of the human mind. Contains the original thesis on his work and explains the ideas which formed the basis of his research.

Dianetics: The Modern Science of Mental Health

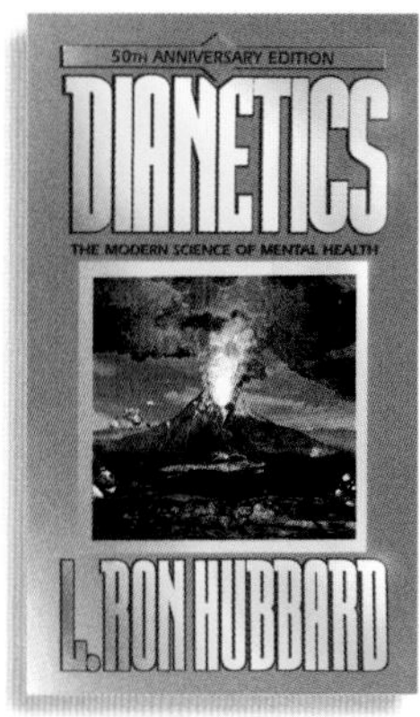

The bestselling self-help book of all time. This is the original manual of Dianetics techniques developed by L. Ron Hubbard. *Dianetics* became an overnight sensation after its release in 1950, and has remained a bestseller ever since. *Dianetics* provides the first accurate description of the human mind, what it consists of and how it operates, together with techniques that bring about new levels of happiness and rationality. This book marks a turning point in man's knowledge and understanding of himself. *Dianetics* laid the foundation for Mr. Hubbard's further researches which soon led into the realm of the human spirit, and from this developed Scientology. *Dianetics* has spread to nearly every country on earth. Daily, it reaches more and more people with the message that an understanding of the mind exists and that something effective can be done to improve it and thus, one's ability to handle life.

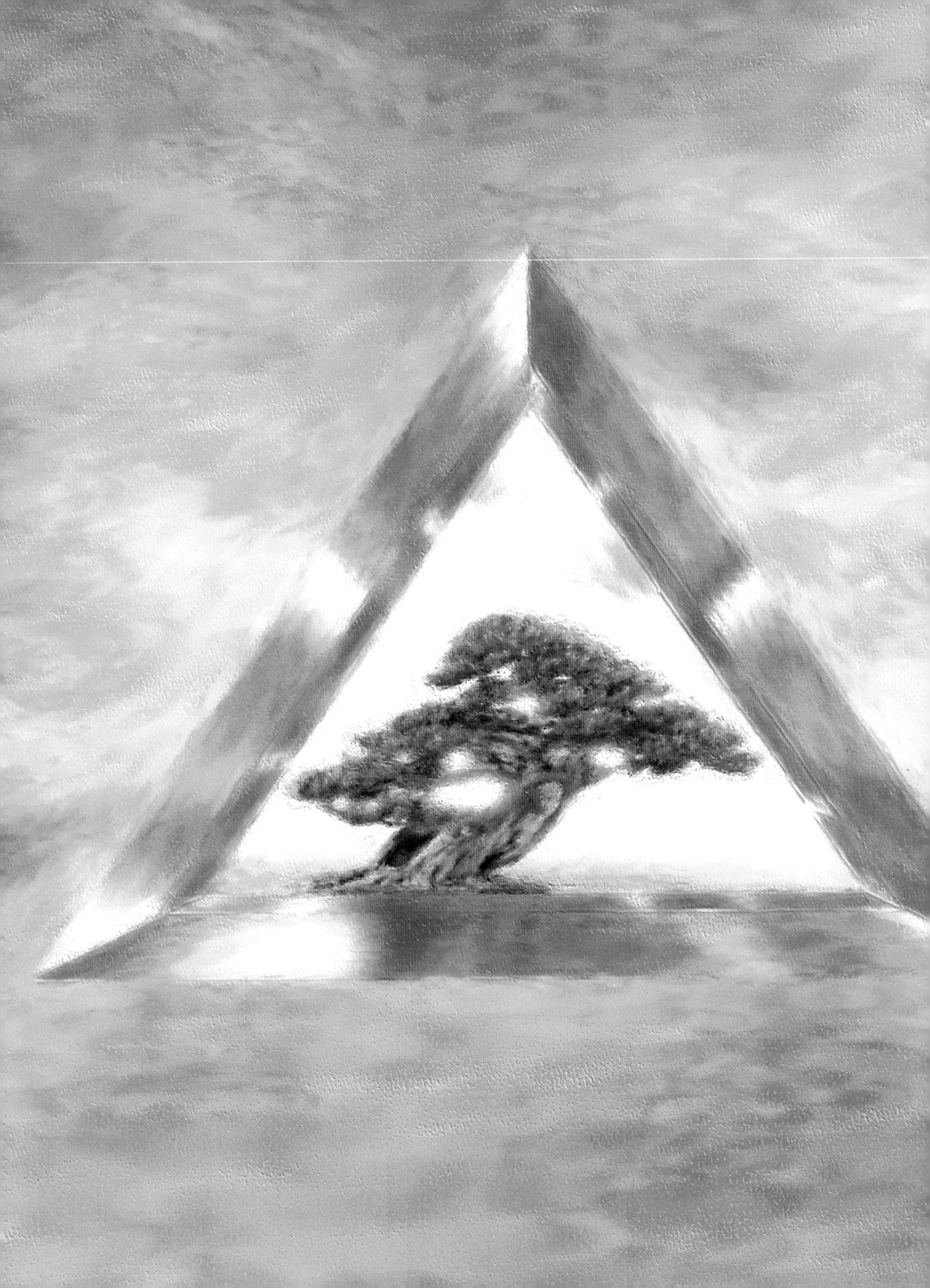

Chapter 3

The Components of Understanding

The self-improvement shelves of bookstores, the airwaves and self-help speakers who travel the lecture circuit all offer myriad solutions to the problems of understanding life. Yet the endless stream of man's difficulties still do not resolve.

In this chapter, L. Ron Hubbard goes beneath all these "solutions" to provide the basic knowledge of what actually constitutes understanding.

What can you do with this knowledge? By knowing what understanding really is, you have the tools to handle life itself. This means that you have the tools to increase your understanding of just about anything—including the people you know and come into contact with.

This knowledge will enable you to help others who are experiencing the travails caused by misunderstandings, differing viewpoints, broken relationships and other ills that make man's life a string of successive hardships. You will learn the components of understanding, how they interrelate and bring about understanding. With the skills one can acquire from a study of the fundamentals contained herein, you can help bring others back into understanding with their fellow man and the world around them.

Although only a portion of the full technology Mr. Hubbard developed on this subject is contained here, it is enough to change your approach to life. And its use will help you flourish in any aspect of human activity.

If lack of understanding is, indeed, a source of man's problems, imagine his potentials without this hindrance. Millions of people who apply this knowledge are reaching heights they once only dreamed of—and are successfully assisting others to do the same.

AFFINITY, REALITY AND COMMUNICATION

There are three factors in Scientology which are of the utmost importance in handling life. These three factors answer the questions: How should I talk to people? How can I give new ideas to people? How can I find what people are thinking about? How can I handle my work better?

These three factors in Scientology are called the ARC triangle. The abbreviation ARC (pronounced A-R-C rather than *arc*) is one of the most useful terms yet devised.

The ARC triangle is called a triangle because it has three related points. The first of these points is affinity. The second of these points is reality. The third of these points and the most important is communication.

These three factors are related. By affinity we mean emotional response. We mean the feeling of affection or lack of it, of emotion or misemotion (irrational or inappropriate emotion) connected with life. By reality we mean the solid objects, the *real* things of life. By communication we mean an interchange of ideas between two terminals (persons who can receive, relay or send a communication). Without affinity there is no reality or communication. Without reality there is no affinity or communication. Without communication there is neither affinity nor reality.

Application of the ARC triangle in the day-to-day circumstances one encounters in life requires an understanding of each of the triangle's components and their interrelationship.

Affinity is any emotional attitude which indicates the degree of liking for someone or something.

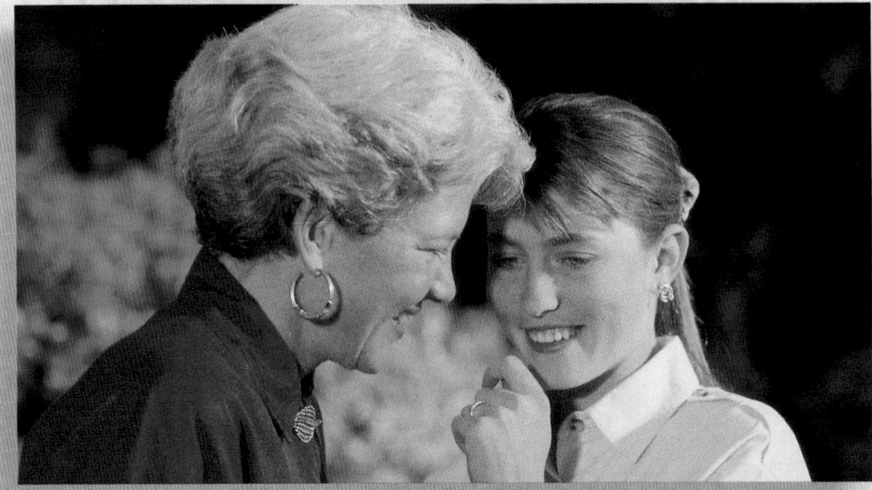

Reality is the degree of agreement reached by people. It also includes the solid objects, the real things of life.

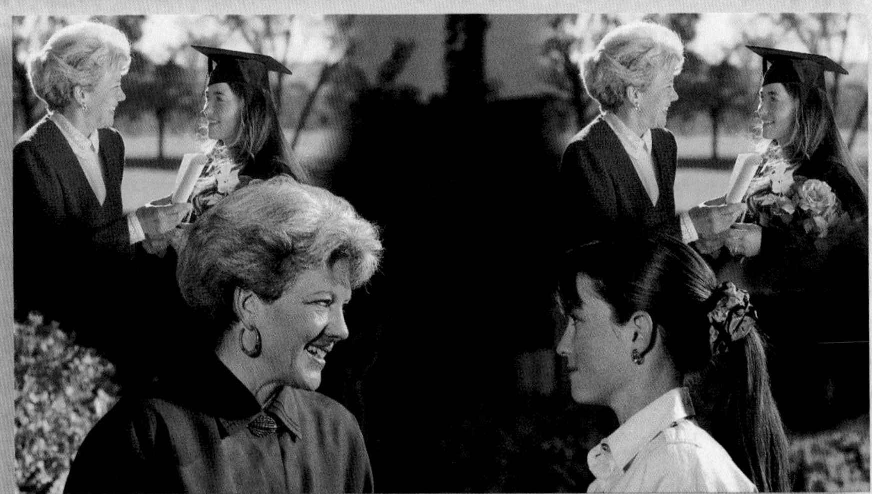

Communication is the interchange of ideas across space.

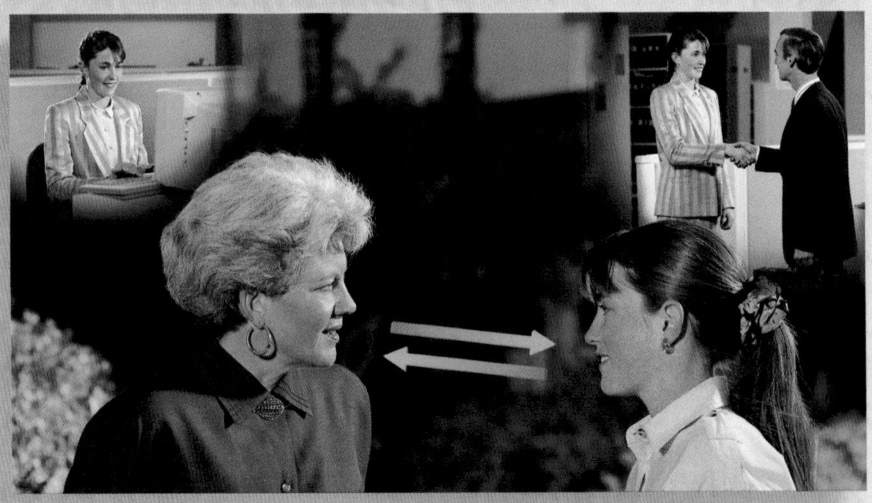

Affinity

The first corner of the triangle is affinity.

The basic definition of *affinity* is the consideration of distance, whether good or bad. The most basic function of complete affinity would be the ability to occupy the same space as something else.

The word *affinity* is here used to mean love, liking or any other emotional attitude. Affinity is conceived in Scientology to be something of many facets. Affinity is a variable quality. *Affinity* is here used as a word with the context "degree of liking."

Man would not be man without affinity. Every animal has affinity to some degree, but man is capable of feeling an especially large amount. Long before he organized into cities, he had organized into tribes and clans. Before the tribes and clans there were undoubtedly packs. Man's instinctive need for affinity with his fellow human beings has long been recognized, and his domestication of other animals shows that this affinity extends also to other species. One could have guessed that the race which first developed affinity to its highest degree would become the dominant race on any planet and this has been borne out.

A child is full of affinity. Not only does he have affinity for his father, mother, brothers and sisters and his playmates but for his dogs, his cats and stray dogs that happen to come around. But affinity goes even beyond this. You can have a feeling of affinity for objects: "I love the way the grain stands out in that wood." There is a feeling of oneness with the earth, blue skies, rain, millponds, cartwheels and bullfrogs which is affinity.

Affinity is never identification (becoming one with another in feeling or interest) nor does it go quite so far as empathy (the power or state of imagining oneself to be another person and even share *his* ideas or feelings). You remain very much yourself when you have affinity for something but you also feel the essence of the thing for which you have affinity. You remain yourself and yet you draw closer to the object for which you have affinity. It is not a binding quality. There are no strings attached when affinity is given. To the receiver it carries no duties and no responsibilities. It is pure, easy and natural and flows out from the individual as easily as sunlight flows from the sun.

Affinity begets affinity. A person who is filled with the quality will automatically find people anywhere near him also beginning to be filled with affinity. It is a calming, warming, heartening influence on all who are capable of receiving and giving it.

One can readily observe the level of affinity between individuals or groups. For instance, two men talking with each other either are in affinity with each other or they aren't. If they are not, they will argue. If they are in affinity with each other, two other things have to be there: they have to have agreed upon a reality and they have to be able to communicate that reality to each other.

This brings us to the next corner: reality.

Reality

Reality could be defined as "that which appears to be." Reality is fundamentally agreement. What we agree to be real is real.

Reality, physical-universe reality, is sensed through various channels; we see something with our eyes, we hear something with our ears, we smell something with our nose, we touch something with our hands, and we decide, then, that there is something. But the only way we know it is through our senses and those senses are artificial channels. We are not in direct contact with the physical universe. We are in contact through our sense channels with it.

Those sense channels can be blunted. For instance, a man loses his eyesight, and as far as he is concerned there is no light or shape or color or depth perception to the physical universe. It still has a reality to him, but it is not the same reality as another person's. In other words, he is unable to conceive a physical universe completely without sight. One can't conceive these things without senses. So the physical universe is seen through these senses.

Two men can take a look at a table and agree it is a table. It is made out of wood, it is brown. The men agree to that. Of course, one understands that when he says "brown" and the other hears "brown," brown actually to the first man may be purple but he has agreed that it is brown because all his life people have been pointing to this color vibration and saying "brown." It might really be red to the second man, but he recognizes it as brown. So both men

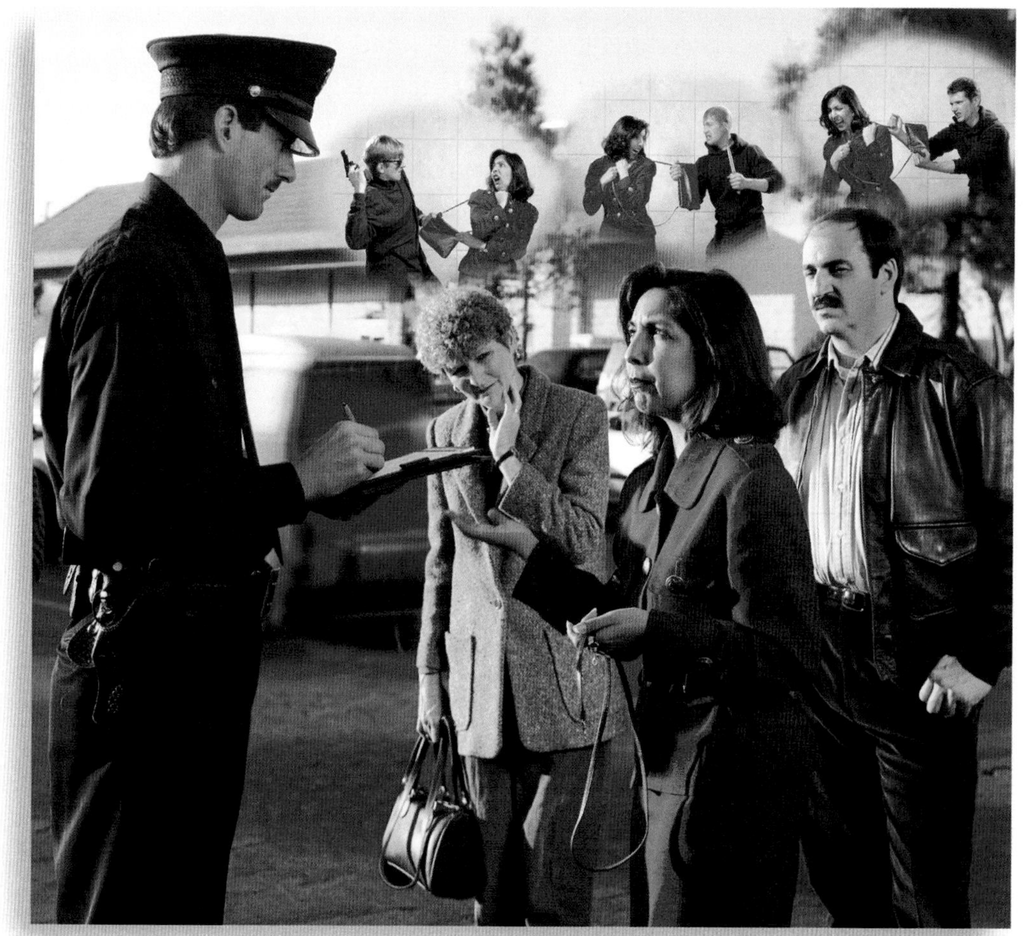

Eyewitnesses at the scene of an accident or crime often present differing accounts of what occurred. Each person here has a different reality of what happened to a woman who had her purse snatched.

are in agreement although they might be seeing something different. But they agree this is brown, this is wood, this is a table. Now a third fellow walks in the door, comes up and takes a look at this thing and says, "Huh! An elephant!"

One man says, "It's a table, see? Elephants are ..."

"No, it's an elephant," replies the third man.

So the other two men say the third one is crazy. He doesn't agree with them. Do they attempt further to communicate with him? No. He doesn't agree with them. He has not agreed upon this reality. Are they in affinity with him? No. They say, "This guy is crazy." They don't like him. They don't want to be around him.

Now let's say two individuals are arguing, and one says, "That table is made out of wood," and the other says, "No, it is not. It's made out of metal which is painted to look like wood." They start arguing about this; they are trying to reach a point of agreement and they can't reach this point of agreement. Another fellow comes up and takes a look at the table and says, "As a matter of fact, the legs are painted to look like wood, but the top is wood and it is brown and it is a table." The first two men then reach an agreement. They feel an affinity. All of a sudden they feel friendly and they feel friendly toward the third man. He solved the problem. The two individuals have reached an agreement and go into communication.

For an individual, reality can only consist of his interpretation of the sensory perceptions he receives. The comparative unreliability of this data is clearly shown by the varying reports always received in the description of, say, an automobile accident. People who have studied this phenomenon report that there is an amazing degree of difference in the description given of the same scene by different observers. In other words, the reality of this situation differed in details for each of the observers. As a matter of fact, there is a wide area of agreement, extremely wide, the common agreement of mankind. This is the earth. We are men. The automobiles are automobiles. They are propelled by the explosion of certain chemicals. The air is the air. The sun is in the sky. There is usually an agreement that a wreck happened. Beyond this basic area of agreement there are differing interpretations of reality.

For all practical purposes, reality consists of your perception of it, and your perception of reality consists, to a large extent, of what you can communicate with other people.

Communication

The third and most important corner of the ARC triangle is communication. In human relationships this is more important than the other two corners of the triangle in understanding the composition of human relations in this universe. Communication is the solvent for all things. It dissolves all things.

How do people go into communication with each other?

In order for there to be communication, there must be agreement and affinity. In order for there to be affinity, there must be agreement on reality and communication. In order for there to be reality and agreement, there must be affinity and communication—one, two, three. If you knock affinity out, communication and reality go. If you knock reality out, communication and affinity will go. If you knock communication out, they will all go.

There are several ways to block a communication line (the route along which a communication travels from one person to another). One is to cut it, another one is to make it so painful that the person receiving it will cut it, and another one is to put so much on it that it jams. Those are three very important things to know about a communication line. Also, that communication must be *good* communication: the necessary data sent in the necessary direction and received.

All that communication will be about, by the way, is reality and affinity concerning the physical universe. Discussions will be whether there is or is not affinity, or whether there is or is not agreement and where the agreement is particularly disagreed with on the physical universe.

Affinity can be built up in a number of ways. You can talk to people and build up an affinity with them. But remember this is communication, not just talk. There are many, many ways to communicate. Two people can sit and look at each other and be in communication. One of the ways to go into communication is by tactile, the sense of touch. You can pet a cat, and the cat all of a sudden starts to purr; you are in communication with the cat. You can reach out and shake a person's hand and you are in communication with him because tactile has taken place. The old-school boys with the tooth-and-claw idea that "everybody hates everybody really, and everybody is on the defensive and that is why we have to force everybody into being social animals" said that the reason men shake hands is to show there is no weapon in the hand. No, it is a communication. In France, Italy, Spain and so forth they throw their arms around each other; there is lots of contact and that contact is communication.

If a person is badly out of communication and you reach out and pat him on the shoulder and he dodges slightly (he considers all things painful) even though he doesn't go on, you will find he is also out of communication vocally. You try to say something to him. "You know, I think that's a pretty

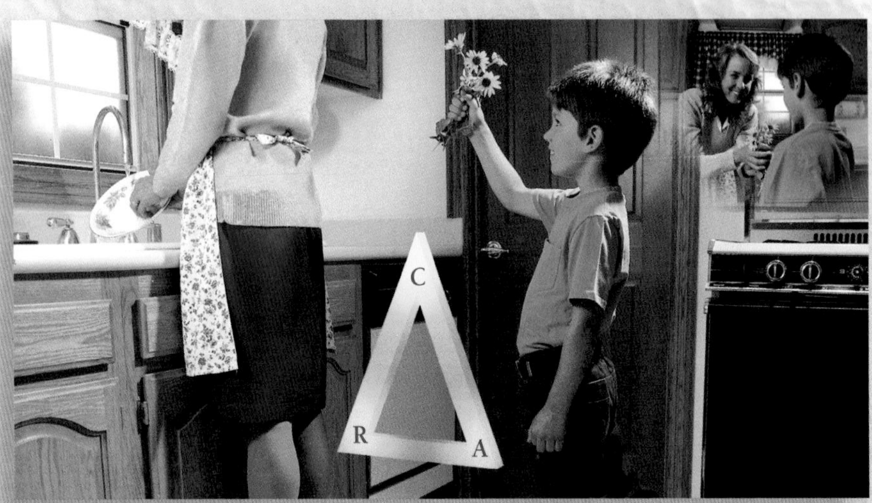

If one corner of the ARC triangle is knocked out the remaining corners also get knocked out. Here, a child cheerfully approaches his mother to give her flowers.

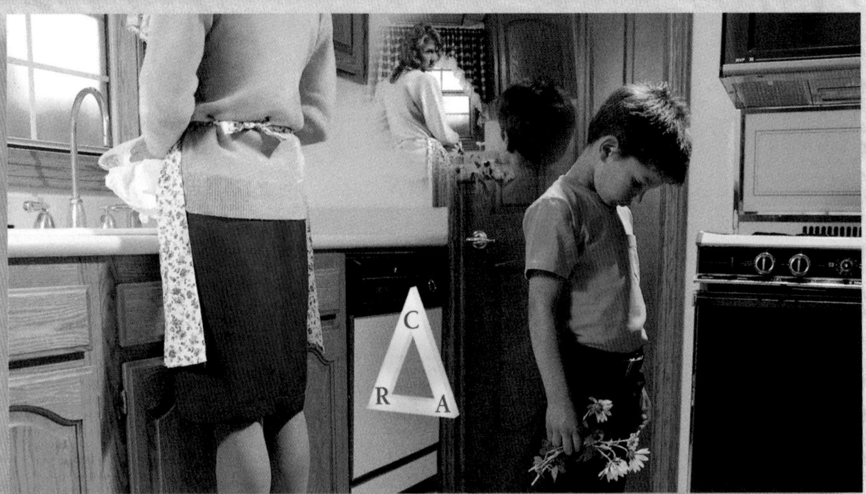

Preoccupied with housework, the mother ignores the child's communication, which becomes knocked out, followed soon after by less affinity and less reality.

good project, Project 342A, and I think we ought to go along with it." He will sit there and look at you and nod, and then he will go down and complete Project 36.

You say, "Project 36 has just been thrown out. We weren't going to go through with that at all," but he hardly knows you are talking to him. He dodges everything you say. Or he may talk to you so hard and so long you don't get a chance to tell him you want to do Project 342A. That is dodging you, too. In other words, he is out of communication with you. Therefore his affinity is low and he won't agree with you either. But if you can get him into agreement, communication will pick up and affinity will pick up.

This is about the most important data run across in the field of interpersonal relations.

You can take any group of men working on a project and take one look at the foreman and the men and tell whether or not these people are in communication with one another. If they aren't, they are not working as a coordinated team. They are not in communication, perhaps, because they are not agreed on what they are doing.

All you have to do is take the group, put them together and say, "What are you guys doing?" You don't ask the foreman, you ask the whole group and the foreman, "What are you guys doing?"

One fellow says, "I'm earning forty dollars a week. That's what I'm doing." Another one says, "Well, I'm glad to get out of the house every day. The old woman's pretty annoying." Another one says, "As a matter of fact, I occasionally get to drive the truck over there and I like to drive the truck, and I'll put up with the rest of this stuff. I drive the truck, and I've got to work anyhow." Another man might say, if he were being honest, "I'm staying on this job because I hate this dog that you've got here as a foreman. If I can devote my life to making him miserable, boy, that makes me happy."

All the time you thought that those men thought they were grading a road. Not one of them thought they were grading a road. You thought they were building a road. Not one of them was building a road; not one of them was even grading.

This crew may be unhappy and inefficient, but you get them together and you say, "Well, you know, some day a lot of cars will go over this road. Maybe they'll wreck themselves occasionally and so forth, but a lot of cars will go over this road. You boys are building a road. It's a pretty hard job, but somebody's got to do it. A lot of people will thank you boys for having built this road. I know you don't care anything about that, but that's really what we are doing around here. Now, I'd like a few suggestions from you people about how we could build this road a little bit better." All of a sudden the whole crew is building a road. Affinity, reality and communication go right up.

The ARC Triangle

Every point on the ARC triangle is dependent on the other two, and every two are dependent on one. One can't cut down one without cutting down the other two, and one can't rehabilitate one without rehabilitating the other two. On the positive side, one can rehabilitate any point on the triangle by rehabilitating any other point on it.

The interrelationship of the triangle becomes apparent at once when one asks, "Have you ever tried to talk to an angry man?" Without a high degree of liking and without some basis of agreement there is no communication. Without communication and some basis of emotional response there can be no reality. Without some basis for agreement and communication there can be no affinity. Thus we call these three things a triangle. Unless we have two corners of a triangle, there cannot be a third corner. Desiring any corner of the triangle, one must include the other two.

The triangle is not an equilateral triangle. Affinity and reality are very much less important than communication. It might be said that the triangle begins with communication, which brings into existence affinity and reality.

Since each of these three aspects of existence is dependent on the other two, anything which affects one of these will also similarly affect the others. It is very difficult to suffer a reversal of affinity without also suffering a blockage of communication and a consequent deterioration of reality.

Consider a lovers' quarrel: One of the pair offers affinity in a certain way to the other. This affinity is either reversed or not acknowledged. The first lover feels insulted and begins to break off communication. The second lover, not understanding this break-off, also feels insulted and makes the break in communication even wider. The area of agreement between the two inevitably diminishes and the reality of their relationship begins to go down. Since they no longer agree on reality, there is less possibility of affinity between them and the downward spiral goes on.

There are three ways of reversing this spiral. One is through raising of the necessity level of the individual. Another is by the intervention of some outside agency which will force the two lovers to agree or communicate. The third is by Scientology processing.

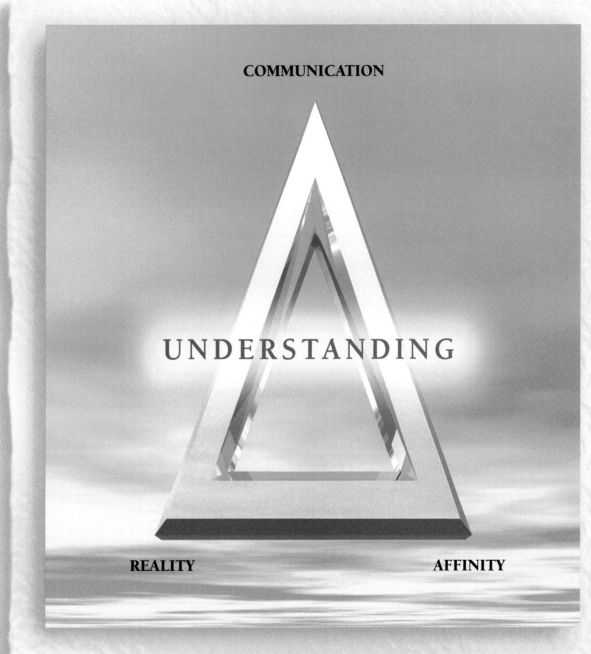

Affinity, reality and communication form the ARC triangle, with each point dependent upon the other two. These are the component parts of understanding.

Scientology processing is a precise, thoroughly codified activity with exact procedures. It is a very unique form of personal counseling which helps an individual look at his own existence and improves his ability to confront what he is and where he is.

Unless one of these three ways of reversing the spiral is utilized, eventually all of the reality of the relationship which had grown up between this pair of lovers would vanish and both of the people would be damaged in their total reality, their total ability to communicate, their total capacity for affinity.

Fortunately the spiral works both ways. Anything which will raise the level of affinity will also increase the ability to communicate and add to the perception of reality.

Falling in love is a good example of the raising of the ability to communicate and of a heightened sense of reality occasioned by a sudden increase in affinity. If it has happened to you, you will remember the wonderful smell of the air, the feeling of affection for the good solid ground, the way in which the stars seemed to shine brighter and the sudden new ability in expressing yourself.

If you have ever been alone, and in a dwindling spiral, only to have the telephone ring and the voice of a friend come across, you will have experienced the halting of a downward spiral through a lift in communication. This is particularly true if the friend happens to be a person with whom you converse easily and who seems to understand the communication which you try to give him. After such an experience, you are probably aware of a great deal more interest in the things around you (reality) and the increase of the feelings of affinity within you.

A troopship was slowly approaching the Golden Gate Bridge filled with troops who had been overseas for several months. As the ship slowly approached the bridge, all on board grew very quiet until at last no one was talking at all. Suddenly, as though by prearranged signal, just as the bow of the ship cleared the bridge, the men standing there broke into a tremendous cheer which carried on down the length of the ship as she went under the bridge. Suddenly everyone was talking to everyone excitedly. Men who scarcely knew each other were pounding each other on the back as though they were brothers. America regained some of its reality for these men and communication and affinity suddenly went up. Fast!

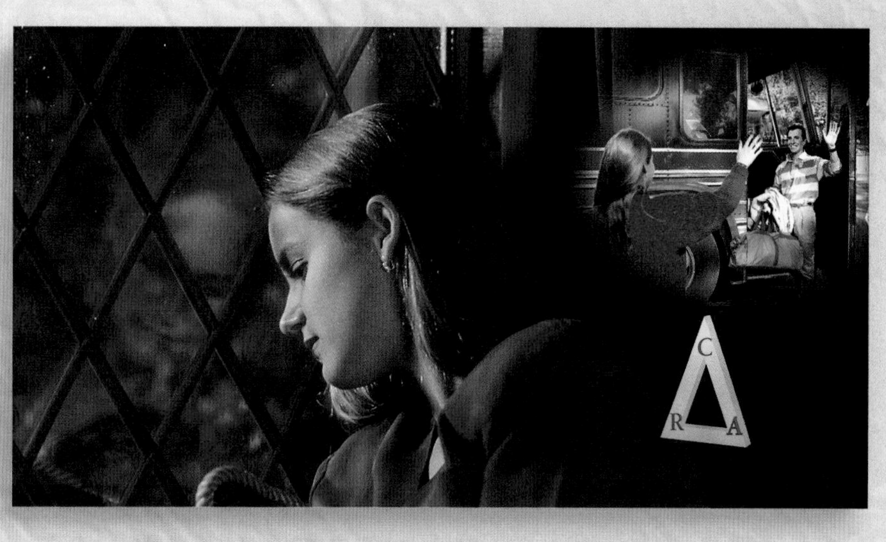

A person's ARC can be in a low state...

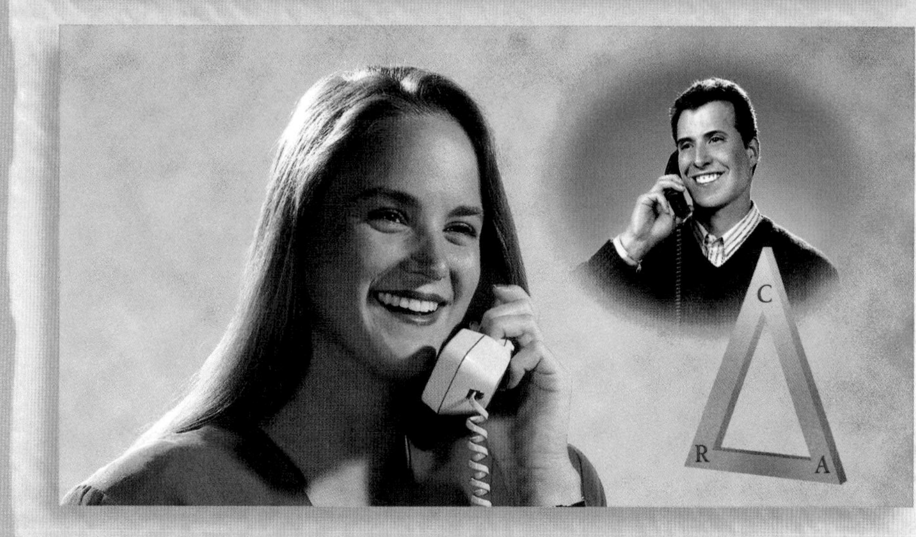

...but can be raised rapidly by communication from someone with whom ARC is high.

Affinity, reality and communication are part of everyday life—from a child going to school, through familial relations to governing a nation. And ignorance of their existence and application is equally as widespread; otherwise, one would not be continually swamped with the daily news of turmoil, strife and suffering due simply to lack of understanding.

However, knowledge of these components will only carry one so far. They must be applied. But how is that done?

How to Raise ARC

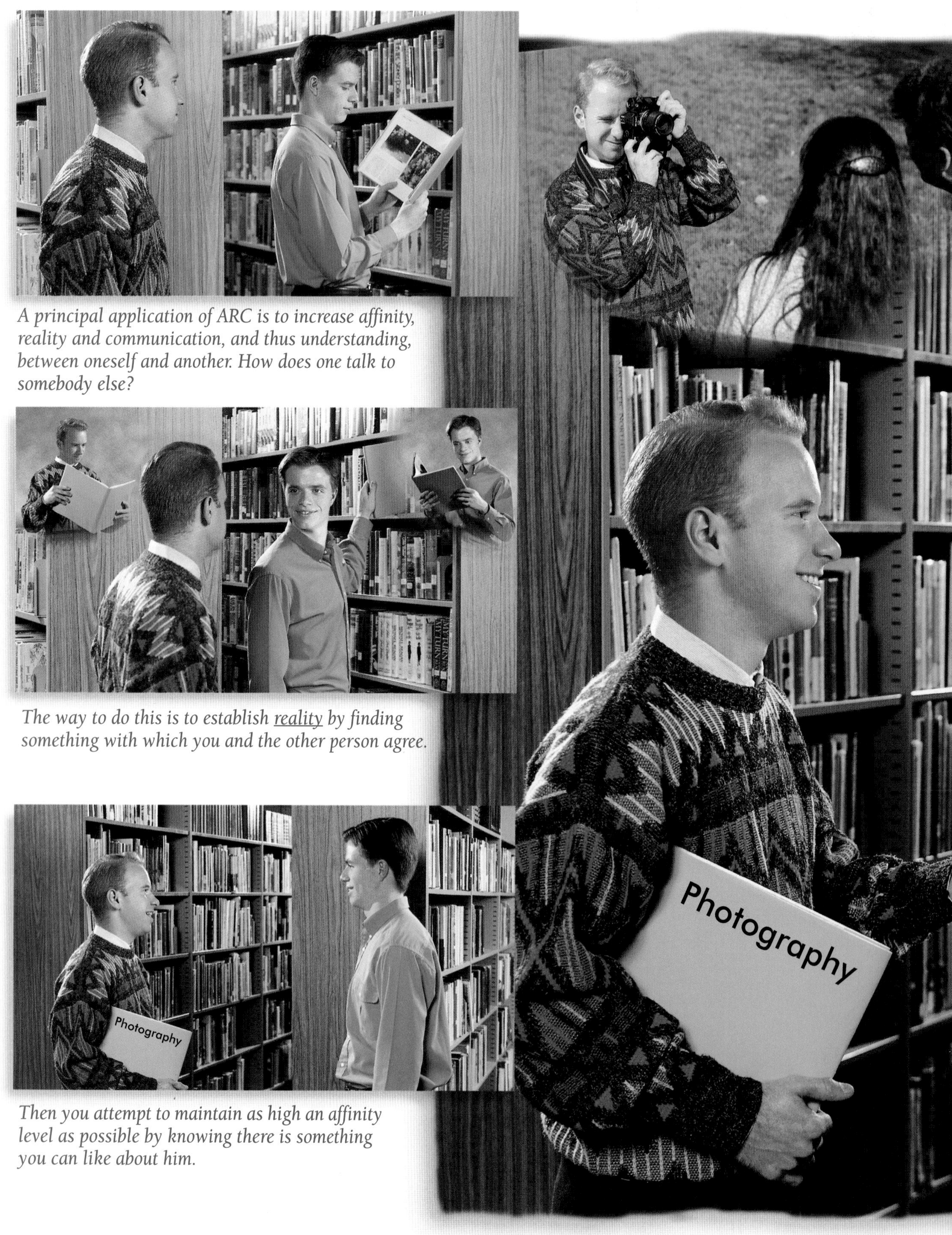

A principal application of ARC is to increase affinity, reality and communication, and thus understanding, between oneself and another. How does one talk to somebody else?

The way to do this is to establish reality by finding something with which you and the other person agree.

Then you attempt to maintain as high an affinity level as possible by knowing there is something you can like about him.

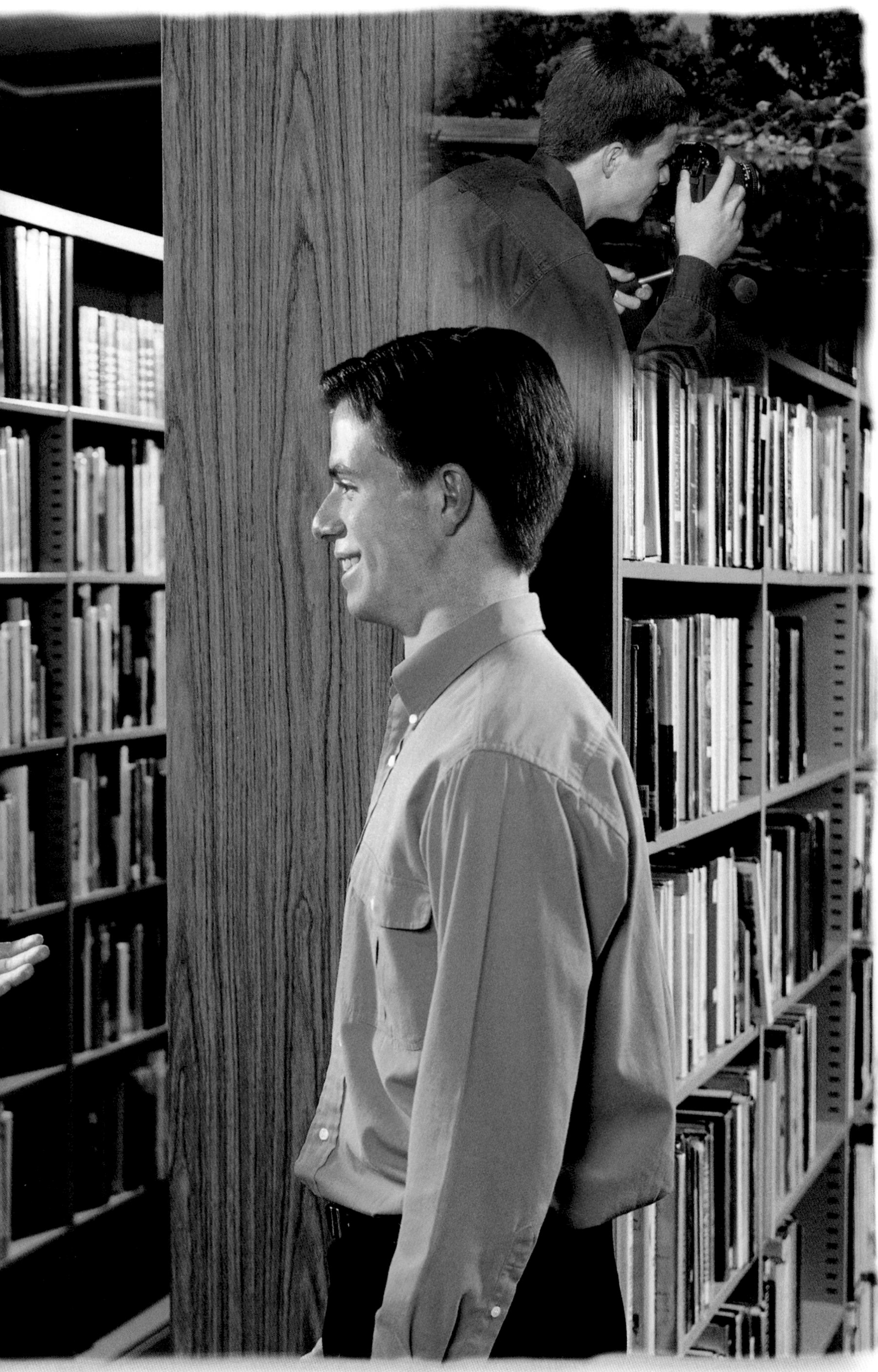

All three corners of the ARC triangle will have been established and you are then able to talk to him. Understanding will be possible because the three components of life—affinity, reality and communication—are present.

HOW TO USE THE ARC TRIANGLE

Given these principles of the ARC triangle and its components, how would you talk to a man?

You cannot talk adequately to a man if you are in a subapathy (a state of disinterest below apathy) condition. In fact, you would not talk to him at all. You would have to have a little higher affinity than that to discuss things with anyone. Your ability to talk to any given man has to do with your emotional response to any given man. Anyone has different emotional responses to different people around him. In view of the fact that two terminals, or, that is to say, two people, are always involved in communication, one could see that someone else would have to be somewhat real. If one does not care about other people at all, one will have a great deal of difficulty talking to them, that is certain. The way to talk to a man, then, would be to find something to like about him and to discuss something with which he can agree. This is the downfall of most new ideas: One does not discuss subjects with which the other person has any point of agreement at all. And we come to a final factor with regard to reality.

That with which we agree tends to be more real than that with which we do not agree. There is a definite coordination between agreement and reality. Those things are real which we agree are real. Those things are not real which we agree are not real. On those things upon which we disagree we have very little reality. An experiment based on this would be an even joking discussion between two men of a third man who is present. The two men agree on something with which the third man cannot agree. The third man will drop in emotional tone and will actually become less real to the two people who are discussing him.

How do you talk to a man then? You establish reality by finding something with which you both agree. Then you attempt to maintain as high an affinity level as possible by knowing there is something you can like about him. And you are then able to talk with him. If you do not have the first two conditions, it is fairly certain that the third condition will not be present, which is to say, you will not be able to talk to him easily.

Affinity, reality and communication are interdependent one upon the other, and when one drops the other two drop also. When one rises the other two rise also. It is only necessary to improve one corner of this very valuable triangle in Scientology in order to improve the remaining two corners. It is only necessary to improve two corners of the triangle to improve the third.

Understanding

Understanding is compounded of affinity, reality and communication. When an individual's understanding is great, his ARC is quite high, and when an individual's ability to understand is small, his ARC is accordingly small.

When we have raised these three parts we have raised somebody's understanding. It is use of the ARC triangle which accomplishes this.

This triangle is the keystone of living associations. It is the common denominator of all life activities. Its use means a greater understanding of life itself. ■

TEST YOUR UNDERSTANDING

Answer the following questions about the ARC triangle. Refer back to the chapter to check your answers. If you need to, review the chapter. Going over the material several times will increase your certainty and help you better apply the data.

- ❑ *What is affinity?*
- ❑ *What is reality?*
- ❑ *What is communication?*
- ❑ *How do affinity, reality and communication relate?*
- ❑ *Of affinity, reality and communication, which is most important and why?*
- ❑ *How do you raise ARC with a person?*

Practical Exercises

The following exercises will help you understand ARC better and increase your ability to apply it.

1 Look around the environment and spot ten instances where an individual is displaying affinity.

2 Look around the environment and spot ten examples where two or more individuals have reality on something.

3 Look around the environment and spot ten examples of communication.

4 Spot more examples of affinity, reality and communication, noticing how they interrelate. Continue to spot examples of affinity, reality and communication as above until you clearly see the relationship between these and are sure that each depends on the other two.

5 Using the data you have learned about the ARC triangle, raise the reality between yourself and another person. Establish reality by finding something with which you and the other person agree. Repeat this with different people as many times as needed until you can raise reality between yourself and another with ease.

6 Using the data you have learned about the ARC triangle, increase the affinity between yourself and another person. Find something you can like about the person, and note the difference in affinity you have for the person as a result. Repeat this with different people as many times as needed until you can raise affinity between yourself and another with ease.

7 Using the data you have learned about the ARC triangle, raise the communication level between yourself and another person. Repeat this with other people, over and over, until you are confident you can raise the communication level between yourself and others.

8 Using the data you have learned about the ARC triangle, raise the ARC between yourself and another person. Repeat this with other people, over and over, until you are confident you can raise ARC between yourself and others.

Results from Application

Those who know and use the components of understanding—affinity, reality and communication—gain control over situations that, without this knowledge, could leave them impotent to act. The mechanics of ARC are simple yet powerful when used to resolve aspects of life.

In dealing with others, whether it be creating new relationships, maintaining good relationships or repairing those that have gone awry, the use of the ARC triangle is *the* key that unlocks previously closed doors to harmony and understanding.

Lovers' spats, relatives who won't speak to one for years, angry bosses, "natural" antipathies, the generation gap, all dissolve under the soothing balm of ARC. Once learned, the use of the ARC triangle is never forgotten or left unused; it swiftly becomes a way of handling life. Those who use it say they couldn't imagine surviving without. That it is one of the "ABCs" of life is reflected in the examples that follow.

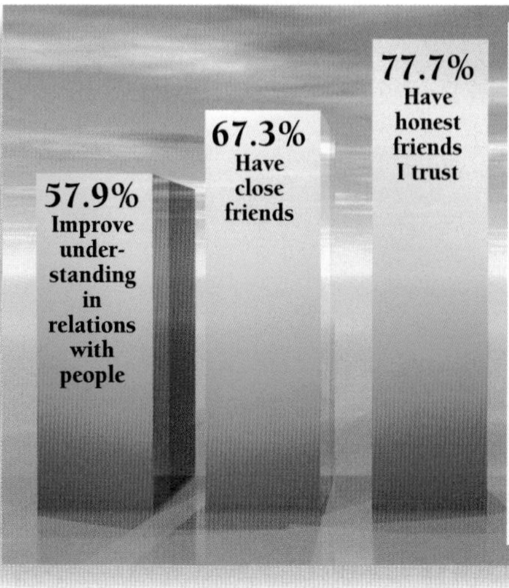

57.9% Improve understanding in relations with people

67.3% Have close friends

77.7% Have honest friends I trust

Relationships

A recent survey reflects how people consider it vital to improve understanding in their relations with others, have close friends and friends that one can trust. By applying the data in this chapter, numerous individuals have overcome the barriers that have kept them from achieving better relations.

A court reporter in Los Angeles was having tremendous difficulty getting along with her parents. She had upset them and, consequently, could no longer face them and had stopped communicating with them. Her father sent letters which expressed upset with her and which, in turn, upset her immensely since she loved and respected her parents. A friend came along about this time and showed her L. Ron Hubbard's materials on ARC to help her with this situation. Here is what came to pass:

"My parents and I had become more and more estranged. This data from Mr. Hubbard showed me exactly what was wrong and gave me a very easy-to-apply solution. I was able to communicate with my parents without upsetting them by establishing reality with them. After that, my dad wrote to me and for the first time ever in my life, said, 'I love you.' I could have died of happiness. Applying this data not only restored our relationship, it made it warmer than it had ever been."

The zing had gone out of the marriage of a couple with five children. A friend of theirs listened to the wife complaining that they no longer had anything in common and were drifting apart. She decided to do something to help both the children and the couple.

"To do something about this, I told my friend about the ARC triangle, and went over all the parts of it with her. She realized that she and her husband were not in communication and had no common reality anymore. She was involved with raising her

five children, while he was involved with work. It was quite different from when they courted as teenagers.

"So we worked out a solution. They went out, just the two of them. She used the tools of the ARC triangle to get in communication with her husband about points of common reality, which started with a movie that they had seen together. From that point, they got into further communication with one another and the marriage improved and continued to improve. It was really great to be able to use such a basic and simple tool to keep a family with five children together."

In Los Angeles, a young woman had a troubled relationship with her brother. Since childhood they had always picked on each other, clashing constantly. Her brother had become involved with hard drugs and grew more and more critical of others. The woman, after learning some of the fundamental principles about affinity, reality and communication in Scientology, decided to handle this relationship and his criticism of her and life in general. She applied her new skills and got into communication with him.

"I applied what I had learned about communication and found the exact thing ruining his life. He had been one of the most promising athletes in his high-school years, but had failed to follow through on his goals. He told me that he wanted to have things to strive for in life and that he wanted to achieve them. He realized when talking to me that the abandonment of his goals had probably led him into doing drugs in the first place. After that, my brother handled his drug problem and began to take even more positive actions to improve his life. He previously had gone from one relationship to another for years, but after that, he actually settled down and got married. Our relationship improved from that point and he now respects me for what I do."

By the end of high school, a young man had transformed from being an extroverted, happy teenager to an introverted and miserable one. Abilities he had enjoyed previously, such as the simple ability to help people just by listening to them, and a native ability to cheer people up and make them feel good about themselves—all of these seemed to have *vanished* by the time he graduated school. He was using drugs and was confused and losing.

"I thought I would never get those abilities back. Then I found Scientology, and things changed. I learned about a very simple but powerful principle known as the ARC triangle. Anyone can use this principle in day-to-day living. I found that with it, I could improve any part of my life. I learned exactly how to use communication with other people to increase affinity and reality and bring about understanding. It works. I can help people as never before, through my new understanding of communication and the ARC triangle. There is such a thing as real help, and real hope, as long as Scientology is in use by people like you and I. But don't listen to me—read L. Ron Hubbard's books and see for yourself!"

SUGGESTIONS FOR FURTHER STUDY

The principle of ARC underlies the application of all other Scientology data. Further study of these writings and lectures of L. Ron Hubbard is highly recommended for anyone wishing a fuller grasp and ability to apply Scientology to his life.

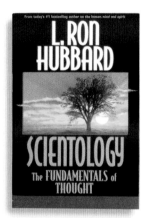

Scientology: The Fundamentals of Thought

Covers many essential principles, giving a complete description of Scientology's most fundamental ideas. Exact, succinct presentations of how life operates. Augments data from many chapters in this handbook by supplying a foundation for all further studies in Scientology.

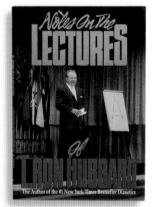

Notes on the Lectures of L. Ron Hubbard

Compiled from Mr. Hubbard's early lectures, this volume contains his first description of the ARC triangle and its relationship to helping another with Scientology. Understanding of and ability to apply ARC is a key to help an individual make gains in any therapeutic activity, a datum heavily stressed in Scientology. This book explains why.

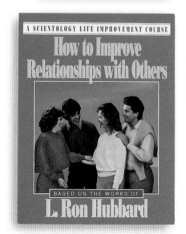

How to Improve Relationships with Others

A "how to" course delivered in Scientology organizations which can bring immediate improvement in a person's relationships. Teaches several important Scientology basics, fully illustrated with stress on application. Can be completed in a few evenings' study.

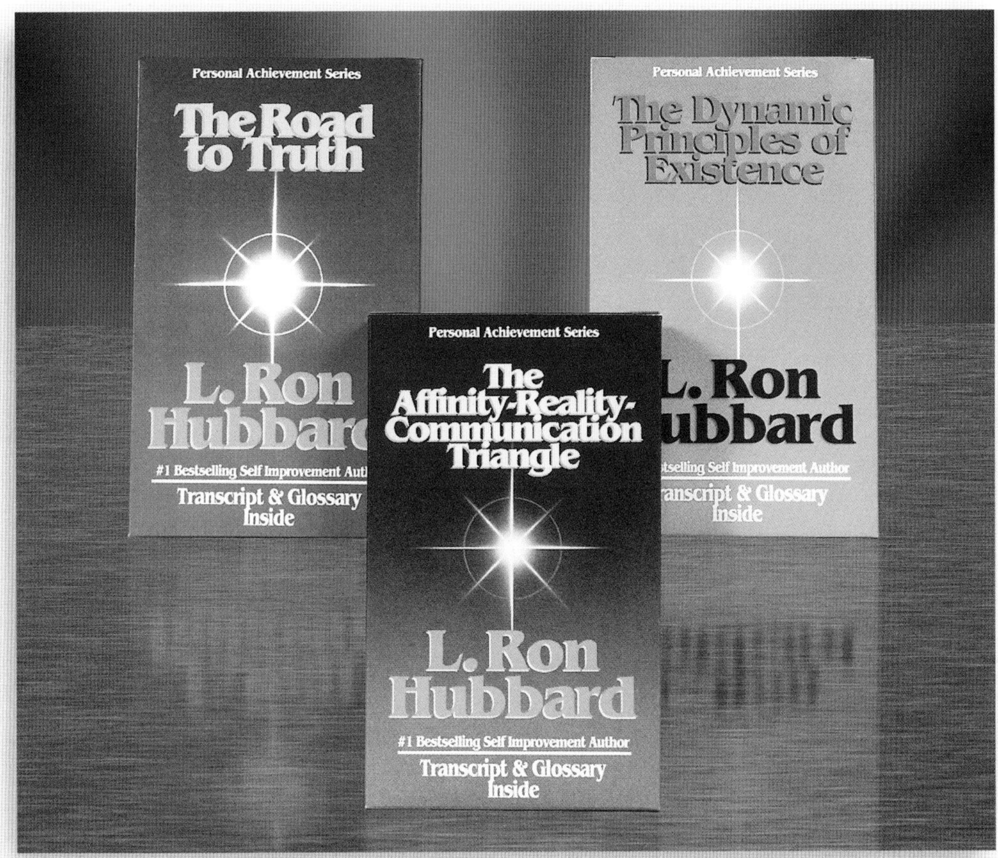

The Personal Achievement Series Lectures

There are nearly 3,000 lectures by L. Ron Hubbard on Scientology. Those which provide introductory Scientology materials form this series, and the hour-long lectures listed here are recommended for additional study about ARC.

The Affinity-Reality-Communication Triangle

Amplifies the data given on the ARC triangle and explains in detail, with many entertaining and thoughtful examples, how ARC can be used to resolve problems and improve personal relationships.

The Road to Truth

Explains man's attempts to find truth and the traps and half-truths he has fallen into along the way. Attainment of truth is a road everyone is aware of and Mr. Hubbard tells how it can be traveled.

The Dynamic Principles of Existence

Some people are more interested in life than others, and generally have more fulfilling lives as a result. Discusses how being a knowing part of and participant in any and all the activities of life is a key to happiness.

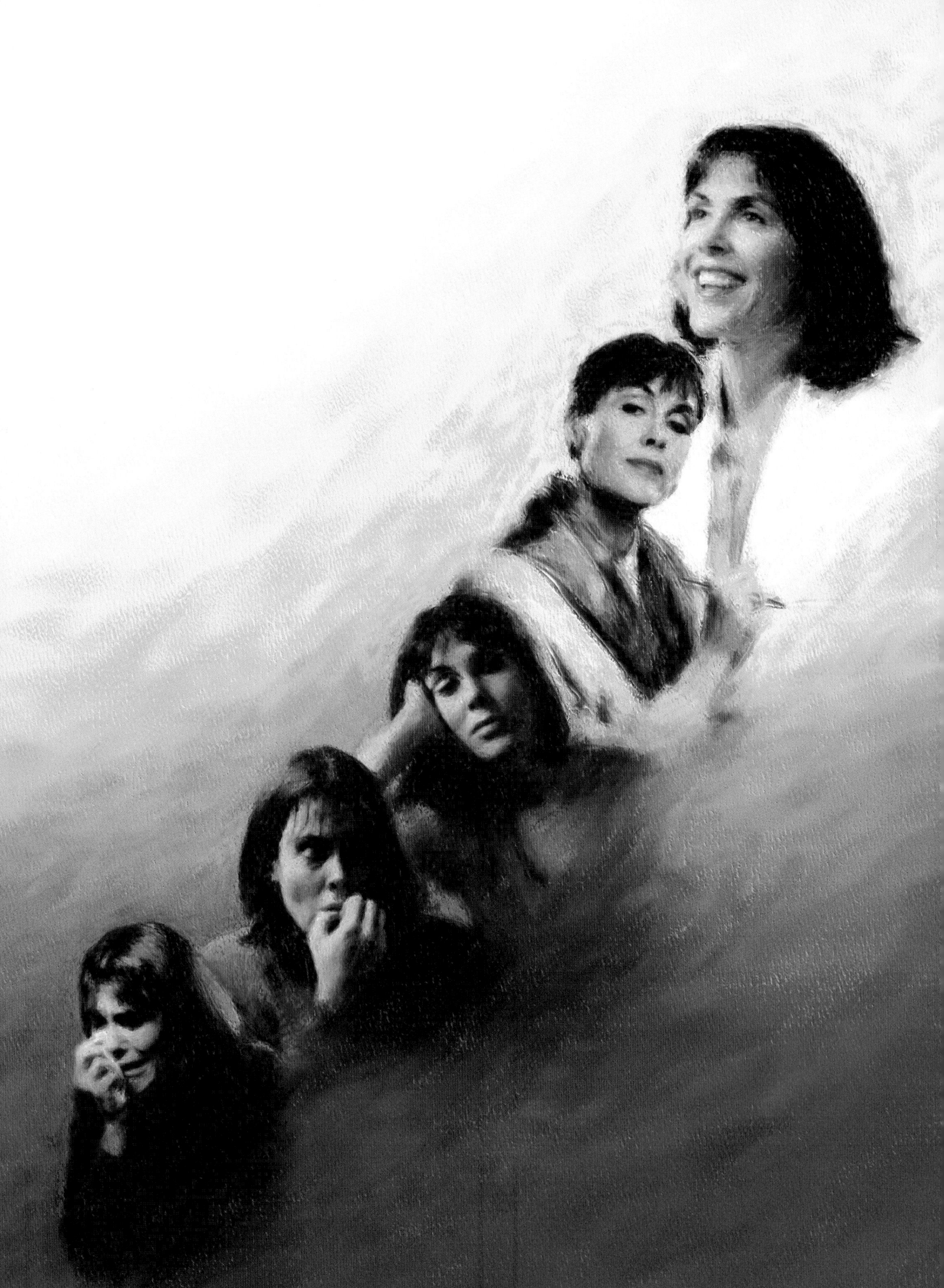

Chapter 4

THE EMOTIONAL TONE SCALE

How often have you heard someone say, "I don't understand him"? Sometimes irrational, unforeseen acts seem to be the norm among our fellows.

The fact is, there has never been a workable method to invariably predict human behavior—until now.

L. Ron Hubbard developed just such a method, and it is applicable to all men, without exception.

With this data, it is possible to accurately predict the behavior of a potential spouse, a business partner, employee or friend—before you commit to a relationship. The risks involved in human interaction can be avoided entirely or minimized when you can infallibly predict how people will behave.

By understanding and using the information in this chapter, all aspects of human relationships will become more productive and more fulfilling. You'll know who to associate with, who to avoid, and you will be able to help those who are mired in uncomfortable situations with others. Imagine knowing, after a very short time, how people will behave in any given circumstance. You can. Each and every time.

The Tone Scale

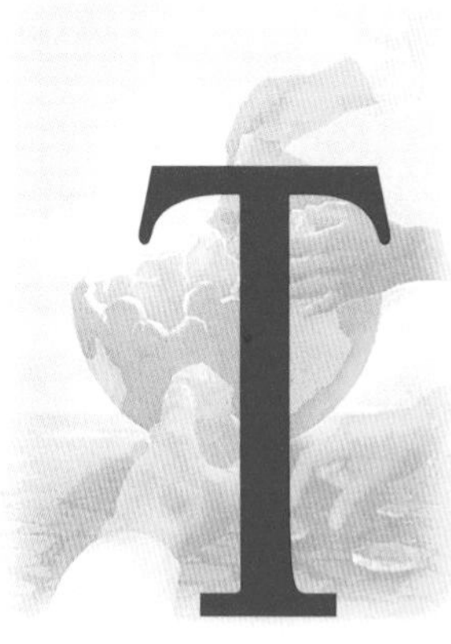

The Tone Scale—a vital tool for any aspect of life involving one's fellows—is a scale which shows the successive emotional tones a person can experience. By "tone" is meant the momentary or continuing emotional state of a person. Emotions such as fear, anger, grief, enthusiasm and others which people experience are shown on this graduated scale.

Skillful use of this scale enables one to both predict and understand human behavior in all its manifestations.

This Tone Scale plots the descending spiral of life from full vitality and consciousness through half-vitality and half-consciousness down to death.

By various calculations about the energy of life, by observation and by test, this Tone Scale is able to give levels of behavior as life declines.

These various levels are common to all men.

When a man is nearly dead, he can be said to be in a chronic *apathy*. And he behaves in a certain way about other things. This is 0.05 on the Tone Scale.

When a man is chronically in *grief* about his losses, he is in grief. And he behaves certain ways about many things. This is 0.5 on the scale.

When a person is not yet so low as grief but realizes losses are impending, or is fixed chronically at this level by past losses, he can be said to be in *fear*. This is around 1.0 on the scale.

An individual who is fighting against threatened losses is in *anger*. And he manifests other aspects of behavior. This is 1.5.

The person who is merely suspicious that loss may take place or who has become fixed at this level is resentful. He can be said to be in *antagonism*. This is 2.0 on the scale.

Above antagonism, the situation of a person is not so good that he is enthusiastic, not so bad that he is resentful. He has lost some goals and cannot immediately locate others. He is said to be in *boredom,* or at 2.5 on the Tone Scale.

At 3.0 on the scale, a person has a *conservative,* cautious aspect toward life but is reaching his goals.

At 4.0 the individual is *enthusiastic,* happy and vital.

Very few people are natural 4.0s. A charitable average is probably around 2.8.

You have watched this scale in operation before now. Have you ever seen a child trying to acquire, let us say, a nickel? At first he is happy. He simply wants a nickel. If refused, he then explains why he wants it. If he fails to get it and did not want it badly, he becomes bored and goes away. But if he wants it badly, he will get antagonistic about it. Then he will become angry. Then, that failing, he may lie about why he wants it. That failing, he goes into grief. And if he is still refused, he finally sinks into apathy and says he doesn't want it. This is negation.

A child threatened by danger also dwindles down the scale. At first he does not appreciate that the danger is posed at him and he is quite cheerful. Then the danger, let us say it is a dog, starts to approach him. The child sees the danger but still does not believe it is for him and keeps on with his business. But his playthings "bore" him for the moment. He is a little apprehensive and not sure. Then the dog comes nearer. The child "resents him" or shows some antagonism. The dog comes nearer still. The child becomes angry and makes some effort to injure the dog. The dog comes still nearer and is more

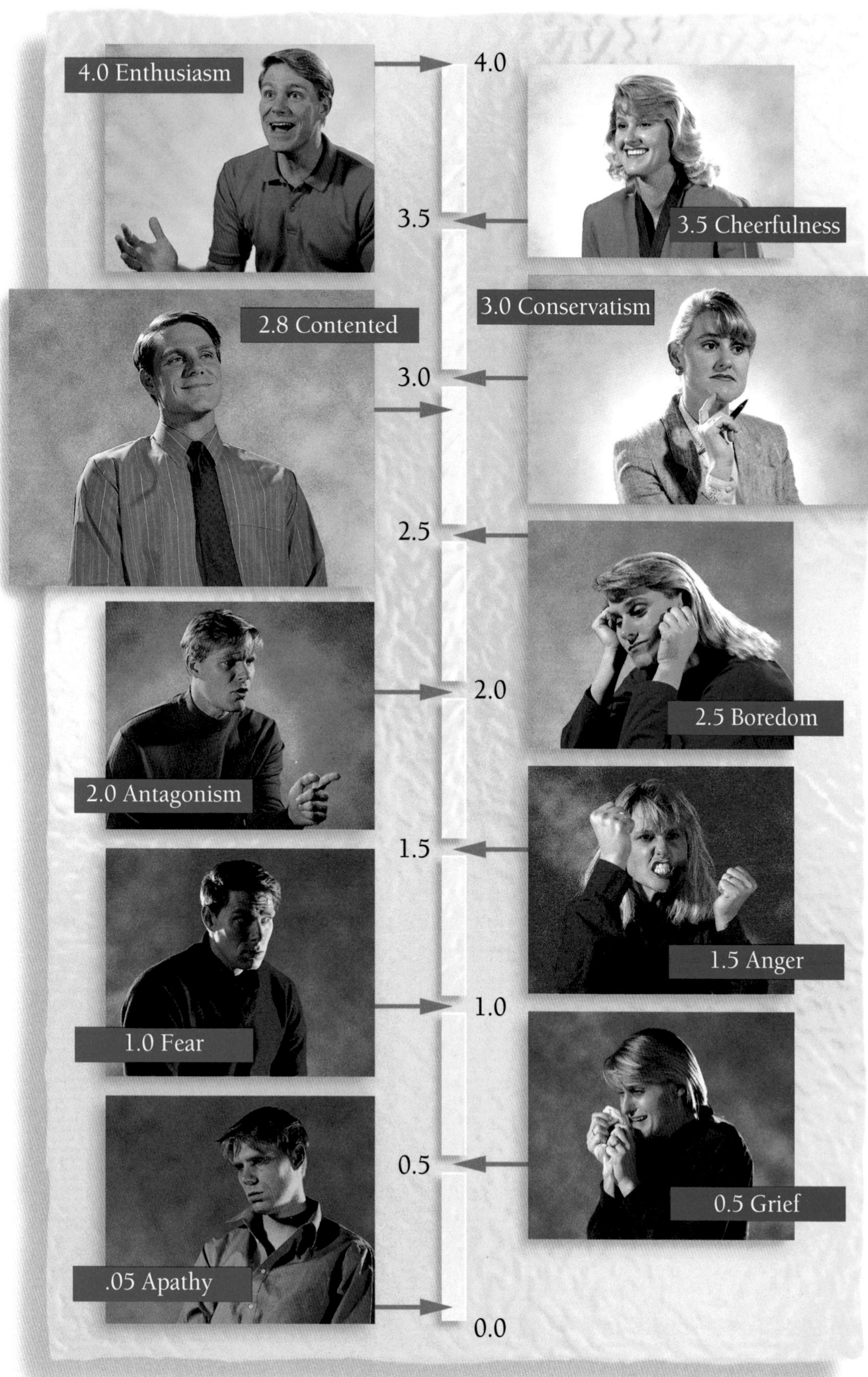
4.0 Enthusiasm
4.0
3.5
3.5 Cheerfulness
2.8 Contented
3.0 Conservatism
3.0
2.5
2.0
2.5 Boredom
2.0 Antagonism
1.5
1.5 Anger
1.0
1.0 Fear
0.5
0.5 Grief
.05 Apathy
0.0

Every person has a chronic or habitual tone. He or she moves up or down the Tone Scale as he experiences success or failure. These are temporary, or acute, tone levels. A primary goal of Scientology is to raise a person's chronic position on the Tone Scale.

threatening. The child becomes afraid. Fear unavailing, the child cries. If the dog still threatens him, the child may go into an apathy and simply wait to be bitten.

Objects or animals or people which assist survival, as they become inaccessible to the individual, bring him down the Tone Scale.

Objects, animals or people which threaten survival, as they approach the individual, bring him down the Tone Scale.

This scale has a chronic or an acute aspect. A person can be brought down the Tone Scale to a low level for ten minutes and then go back up, or he can be brought down it for ten years and not go back up.

A man who has suffered too many losses, too much pain, tends to become fixed at some lower level of the scale and, with only slight fluctuations, stays there. Then his general and common behavior will be at that level of the Tone Scale.

Just as a 0.5 moment of grief can cause a child to act along the grief band for a short while, so can a 0.5 fixation cause an individual to act 0.5 toward most things in his life.

There is momentary behavior or fixed behavior.

The Tone Scale in Full

The full Tone Scale, as can be seen on page 116, starts well below apathy. In other words, a person is feeling no emotion about a subject at all. An example of this was the American attitude concerning the atomic bomb; something about which they should have been very concerned was so far beyond their ability to control and so likely to end their existence that they were below apathy about it. They actually did not even feel that it was very much of a problem.

Feeling apathetic about the atomic bomb would be an advance over the feeling of no emotion whatsoever on a subject which should intimately concern a person. In other words, on many subjects and problems people are actually well below apathy. There the Tone Scale starts, on utter, dead null far below death itself.

Going up into improved tones one encounters the level of body death, apathy, grief, fear, anger, antagonism, boredom, enthusiasm and serenity, in that order. There are many small stops between these tones, but one knowing anything about human beings should definitely know these particular emotions. A person who is in apathy, when his tone is improved, feels grief. A person in grief, when his tone improves, feels fear. A person in fear, when his tone improves, feels anger. A person in anger, when his tone improves, feels antagonism. A person in antagonism, when his tone improves, feels boredom. When a person in boredom improves his tone, he is enthusiastic. When an enthusiastic person improves his tone, he feels serenity. Actually the below apathy level is so low as to constitute a no-affinity, no-emotion, no-problem, no-consequence state of mind on things which are actually tremendously important.

The Tone Scale in Full

40.0	Serenity of Beingness
30.0	Postulates
22.0	Games
20.0	Action
8.0	Exhilaration
6.0	Aesthetic
4.0	Enthusiasm
3.5	Cheerfulness
3.3	Strong Interest
3.0	Conservatism
2.9	Mild Interest
2.8	Contented
2.6	Disinterested
2.5	Boredom
2.4	Monotony
2.0	Antagonism
1.9	Hostility
1.8	Pain
1.5	Anger
1.4	Hate
1.3	Resentment
1.2	No Sympathy
1.15	Unexpressed Resentment
1.1	Covert Hostility
1.02	Anxiety
1.0	Fear
.98	Despair
.96	Terror
.94	Numb

Sympathy	.9
Propitiation	.8
Grief	.5
Making Amends	.375
Undeserving	.3
Self-abasement	.2
Victim	.1
Hopeless	.07
Apathy	.05
Useless	.03
Dying	.01
Body Death	0.0
Failure	-0.01
Pity	-0.1
Shame	-0.2
Accountable	-0.7
Blame	-1.0
Regret	-1.3
Controlling Bodies	-1.5
Protecting Bodies	-2.2
Owning Bodies	-3.0
Approval from Bodies	-3.5
Needing Bodies	-4.0
Worshiping Bodies	-5.0
Sacrifice	-6.0
Hiding	-8.0
Being Objects	-10.0
Being Nothing	-20.0
Can't Hide	-30.0
Total Failure	-40.0

Characteristics on the Tone Scale

The area below apathy is an area without pain, interest, or anything else that matters to anyone, but it is an area of grave danger since one is below the level of being able to respond to anything and may accordingly lose everything without apparently noticing it.

A workman who is in very bad condition and who is actually a liability to the organization may not be capable of experiencing pain or any emotion on any subject. He is below apathy. We have seen workmen who would hurt their hand and think nothing of it and go right on working even though their hand was very badly injured. People working in medical offices and hospitals in industrial areas are quite amazed sometimes to discover how little attention some workmen pay to their own injuries. It is an ugly fact that people who pay no attention to their own injuries and who are not even feeling pain from those injuries are not and never will be, without some attention from a Scientologist, efficient people. They are liabilities to have around. They do not respond properly. If such a person is working a crane and the crane suddenly goes out of control to dump its load on a group of men, that subapathy crane operator will simply let the crane drop its load. In other words, he is a potential murderer. He cannot stop anything, he cannot change anything and he cannot start anything and yet, on some automatic response basis, he manages some of the time to hold down a job, but the moment a real emergency confronts him he is not likely to respond properly and accidents result.

Where there are accidents in industry they stem from these people in the subapathy tone range. Where bad mistakes are made in offices which cost firms a great deal of money, lost time and cause other personnel difficulties, such mistakes are found rather uniformly to stem from these subapathy people. So do not think that one of these states of being unable to feel anything, of being numb, of being incapable of pain or joy is any use to anyone. It is not. A person who is in this condition cannot control things and in actuality is not *there* sufficiently to be controlled by anyone else and does strange and unpredictable things.

Just as a person can be chronically in subapathy, so a person can be in apathy. This is dangerous enough but is at least expressed. Communication from the person himself, not from some training pattern is to be expected.

People can be chronically in grief, chronically in fear, chronically in anger, or in antagonism, or boredom, or actually can be "stuck in enthusiasm." A person who is truly able is normally fairly serene about things. He can, however, express other emotions. It is a mistake to believe that a total serenity is of any real value. When a situation which demands tears cannot be cried about, one is not in serenity as a chronic tone. Serenity can be mistaken rather easily for subapathy, but of course only by a very untrained observer. One glance at the physical condition of the person is enough to differentiate. People who are in subapathy are normally quite ill.

On the level of each of the emotions we have a communication factor. In subapathy an individual is not really communicating at all. Some social response or training pattern or, as we say, "circuit" is communicating. The person himself does not seem to be there and isn't really talking. Therefore his communications are sometimes strange to say the least. He does the wrong things at the wrong time. He says the wrong things at the wrong time.

Naturally when a person is stuck on any of the bands of the Tone Scale—subapathy, apathy, grief, fear, anger, antagonism, boredom, enthusiasm or serenity—he voices communications with that emotional tone. A person who is always angry about something is stuck in anger. Such a person is not as bad off as somebody in subapathy, but he is still rather dangerous to have around since he will make trouble, and a person who is angry does not control things well. The communication characteristics of people at these various levels on the Tone Scale are quite fascinating. They say things and handle communication each in a distinct characteristic fashion for each level of the Tone Scale.

There is also a level of reality for each of the levels of the Tone Scale. Reality is an intensely interesting subject since it has to do, in the main, with relative solids. In other words, the solidity of things and the emotional tone of people have a definite connection. People low on the Tone Scale cannot tolerate solids. They cannot tolerate a solid object. The thing is not real to them; it is thin or lacking weight. As they come upscale, the same object becomes more and more solid and they can finally see it in its true level of solidity. In other words, these people have a definite reaction to mass at various points on the scale. Things are bright to them or very, very dull. If you could look through the eyes of the person in subapathy you would see a very watery, thin, dreamy, misty, unreal world indeed. If you looked through the eyes of an angry man you would see a world which was menacingly solid, where all the solids posed a brutality toward him, but they still would not be sufficiently solid or sufficiently real or visible for a person in good condition. A person in serenity can see solids as they are, as bright as they are, and can tolerate an enormous heaviness or solidity without reacting to it. In other words, as we go up the Tone Scale from the lowest to the highest, things can get more and more solid and more and more real.

Observing the Obvious

The Tone Scale is an extremely useful tool to help predict the characteristics and behavior of a person. But to do this well you must be able to recognize a person's position on the scale at a glance.

The Tone Scale is very easy to apply on a casual basis for some acute tone. "Joe was on a 1.5 kick last night." Sure, he turned red as a beet and threw a book at your head. Simple. Mary breaks into sobs, and grabs for the Kleenex, easily recognizable as grief. But how about a person's chronic tone level? This can be masked by a thin veneer of social training and responses. Such is called a social tone. It is neither chronic, nor acute, but is a reflection of the person's social education and mannerisms adopted to present himself to others. How sharp and how certain are you about that? Take a person that you are familiar with. What, exactly, is his chronic tone?

There is a word "obnosis" which has been put together from the phrase, "observing the obvious." The art of observing the obvious is strenuously neglected in our society at this time. Pity. It's the only way you ever see anything; you observe the obvious. You look at the isness of something, at what is actually there. Fortunately for us, the ability to obnose is not in any sense "inborn" or mystical. But it is being taught that way by people outside of Scientology.

How do you teach somebody to see what is there? Well, you put up something for him to look at, and have him tell you what he sees. An individual can practice this on his own or in a group situation, such as a class. One simply selects a person or object and observes what is *there.* In a classroom situation, for instance, a student is asked to stand up in the front of the room and be looked at by the rest of the students. An Instructor stands by, and asks the students:

"What do you see?"

The first responses run about like this:

"Well, I can see he's had a lot of experience."

"Oh, can you? Can you really see his experience? What do you see there?"

"Well, I can tell from the wrinkles around his eyes and mouth that he's had lots of experience."

"All right, but what do you see?"

"Oh, I get you. I see wrinkles around his eyes and mouth."

"Good!"

The Instructor accepts nothing that is not plainly visible.

A student starts to catch on and says, "Well, I can really see he's got ears."

"All right, but from where you're sitting can you see both ears right now as you're looking at him?"

"Well, no."

"Okay. What do you see?"

"I see he's got a left ear."

"Fine!"

No guesses, no assumptions will do. For example, "He's got good posture."

"Good posture by comparison with what?"

"Well, he's standing straighter than most people I've seen."

"Are they here now?"

"Well, no, but I've got memories of them."

"Come on. Good posture in relation to what, that you can see right now."

"Well, he's standing straighter than you are. You're a little slouched."

"Right this minute?"

"Yes."

"Very good."

The goal of such drilling is to get a student to the point where he can look at another person, or an object, and see exactly what is there. Not a deduction of what might be there from what he does see there. Just what is there, visible and plain to the eye. It's so simple, it hurts.

You can get a good tip on chronic tone from what a person does with his eyes. At apathy, he will give the appearance of looking fixedly, for minutes on end, at a particular object. The only thing is, he doesn't see it. He isn't aware of the object at all. If you dropped a bag over his head, the focus of his eyes would probably remain the same.

Moving up to grief, the person does look "downcast." A person in chronic grief tends to focus his eyes down in the direction of the floor a good bit. In the lower ranges of grief, his attention will be fairly fixed, as in apathy. As he starts moving up into the fear band, you get the focus shifting around, but still directed downward.

At fear itself, the very obvious characteristic is that the person can't look at you. People are too dangerous to look at. He's supposedly talking to you, but he's looking over in left field. Then he glances at your feet briefly, then over your head (you get the impression a plane's passing over), but now he's looking back over his shoulder. Flick, flick, flick. In short, he'll look anywhere but at you.

Then, in the lower band of anger, he will look away from you, deliberately. He looks *away* from you; it's an overt communication break. A little further up the line and he'll look directly at you all right, but not very pleasantly. He wants to locate you—as a target.

Then, at boredom, you get the eyes wandering around again, but not frantically as in fear. Also, he won't be avoiding looking at you. He'll include you among the things he looks at.

Equipped with data of this sort, and having gained some proficiency in the obnosis of people, a person can next go out into the public to talk to strangers and spot them on the Tone Scale. Usually, but only as a slight crutch in approaching people, a person doing this should have a series of questions to ask each person, and a clipboard for jotting down the answers, notes, etc. The real purpose of their talking to people at all is to spot them on the Tone Scale,

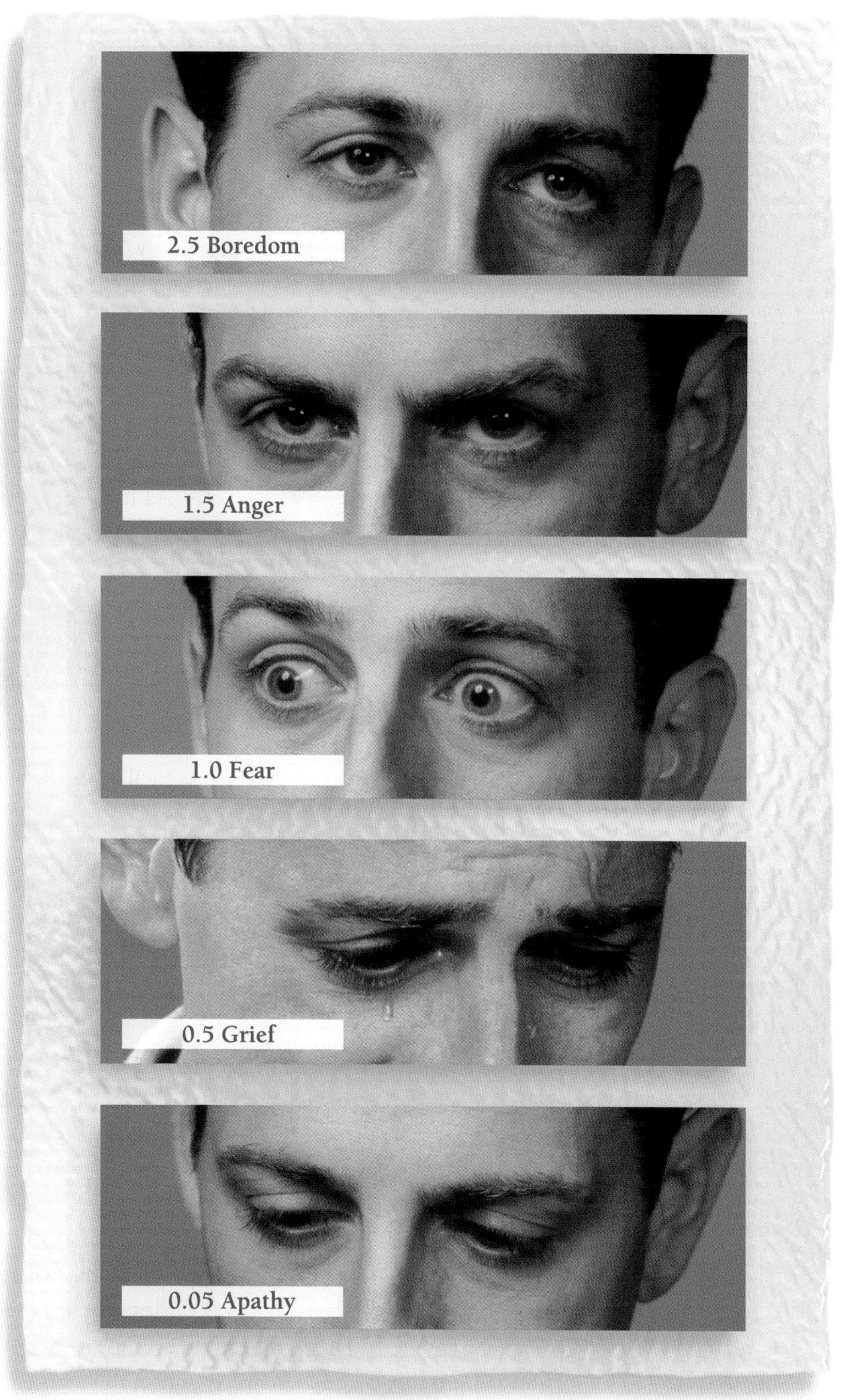

What a person does with his eyes can help you spot his position on the Tone Scale.

chronic tone and social tone. They are given questions calculated to produce lags and break through social training and education, so that the chronic tone juts out.

Here are some sample questions used for this drill: "What's the most obvious thing about me?" "When was the last time you had your hair cut?" "Do you think people do as much work now as they did fifty years ago?"

At first, the persons doing this merely spot the tone of the person they are interviewing—and many and various are the adventures they have while doing this! Later, as they gain some assurance about stopping strangers and asking them questions, these instructions are added: "Interview at least fifteen people. With the first five, match their tone, as soon as you've spotted it. The next five, you drop below their chronic tone, and see what happens. For the last five, put on a higher tone than theirs."

What can a person gain from these exercises? A willingness to communicate with anyone, for one thing. To begin with, a person can be highly selective about the sort of people he stops. Only old ladies. No one who looks angry. Or only people who look clean. Finally, they just stop the next person who comes along, even though he looks leprous and armed to the teeth. Their ability to confront people has come way up, and a person is just somebody else to talk to. They become willing to pinpoint a person on the scale, without wavering or hesitating.

They also become quite gifted and flexible at assuming tones at will, and putting them across convincingly, which is very useful in many situations, and lots of fun to do.

Being able to recognize the tone level of people at a single glance is an ability which can give a tremendous advantage in one's dealings with others. It is a skill well worth the time and effort to acquire.

The Hubbard Chart of Human Evaluation

The whole subject of how to accurately judge our fellows is something that man has wanted to be able to do for a long time. In Scientology we have a chart which shows a way one can precisely evaluate human behavior and predict what a person will do.

This is the Hubbard Chart of Human Evaluation, a foldout copy of which is on page 130.

The chart displays the degree of ethics, responsibility, persistence on a given course, handling of truth and other identifying aspects of a person along the various levels of the Tone Scale.

You can examine the chart and you will find in the boxes, as you go across it, the various characteristics of people at these levels. Horribly enough these characteristics have been found to be constant. If you have a 3.0 as your rating, then you will carry across the whole chart at 3.0.

If you can locate two or three characteristics along a certain level of this scale, you can look in the number column opposite those characteristics and find the level. It may be 2.5, it may be 1.5. Wherever it is, simply look at *all* the columns opposite the number you found and you will see the remaining characteristics.

The only mistake you can make in evaluating somebody else on this Tone Scale is to assume that he departs from it somewhere and is higher in one department than he is in another. The characteristic may be masked to which you object—but it is there.

Look at the top of the first column and you get a general picture of the behavior and physiology of the person. Look at the second column for the physical condition. Look at the third column for the most generally expressed emotion of the person. Continue on across the various columns. Somewhere you will find data about somebody or yourself of which you can be sure. Then simply examine all the other boxes at the level of the data you were certain about. That band, be it 1.5 or 3.0, will tell you the story of a human being.

Of course, as good news and bad, happy days and sad ones, strike a person, there are momentary raises and lowerings on this Tone Scale. But, as mentioned, there is a chronic level, an average behavior for each individual.

As an individual is found lower and lower on this chart, so is his alertness, his consciousness lower and lower.

The individual's chronic mood or attitude toward existence declines in direct ratio to the way he regards the physical universe and organisms about him.

It is not a complete statement to say, merely, that one becomes fixed in his regard for the physical universe and organisms about him, for there are definite ways, beyond consciousness, which permit this to take place. Manifestation, however, is a decline of consciousness with regard to the physical environment of an individual. That decline of consciousness is a partial cause of a gradual sag down this chart, but it is illustrative enough for our purposes in this volume.

The position of an individual on this Tone Scale varies through the day and throughout the years but is fairly stable for given periods. One's position on the chart will rise on receipt of good news, sink with bad news. This is the usual give and take with life. Everyone however has a *chronic* position on the chart which is unalterable save for Scientology processing.

Scientology processing is a very unique form of personal counseling which helps an individual look at his own existence and improves his ability to confront what he is and where he is. Processing thus raises the chronic tone of that individual.

On the other hand, on an acute basis, necessity level (lifting oneself by one's bootstraps as in emergencies) can raise an individual well up this chart for brief periods.

One's environment also greatly influences one's position on the chart. Every environment has its own tone level. A man who is really a 3.0 can begin to act like a 1.1 (covert hostility) in a 1.1 environment. However, a 1.1 usually acts no better than about 1.5 in an environment with a high tone. If one lives in a low-toned environment he can expect, eventually, to be low-toned. This is also true of marriage—one tends to match the tone level of one's marital partner.

This Tone Scale is also valid for groups. A business or a nation can be examined as to its various standard reactions and these can be plotted. This will give the survival potential of a business or a nation.

This chart can also be used in employing people or in choosing partners. It is an accurate index of what to expect and gives you a chance to predict what people will do before you have any great experience with them. Also, it gives you some clue as to what can happen to you in certain environments or around certain people, for they can drag you down or boost you high.

However, don't use this chart as an effort to make somebody knuckle under. Don't tell people where they are on it. It may ruin them. Let them take their own examinations.

A Tone Scale Test

Probably the most accurate index of a person's position on the Tone Scale is speech.

Unless a person talks openly and listens receptively he cannot be considered very high on the Tone Scale.

In column 10 of the Hubbard Chart of Human Evaluation, "Speech: Talks—Speech: Listens," there are double boxes: one set referring to talking, the other to listening. It may not have occurred to some people that communication is both outflow and inflow. An observation of how a person both listens and talks will give an accurate indication of his position on the Tone Scale.

It is interesting to note that with this column one can conduct what we call a "two-minute psychometry" on someone. *Psychometry* is the measurement of mental traits, abilities and processes. The way to do a two-minute psychometry is simply to start talking to the person at the highest possible tone level, creatively and constructively, and then gradually drop the tone of one's conversation down to the point where it achieves response from the

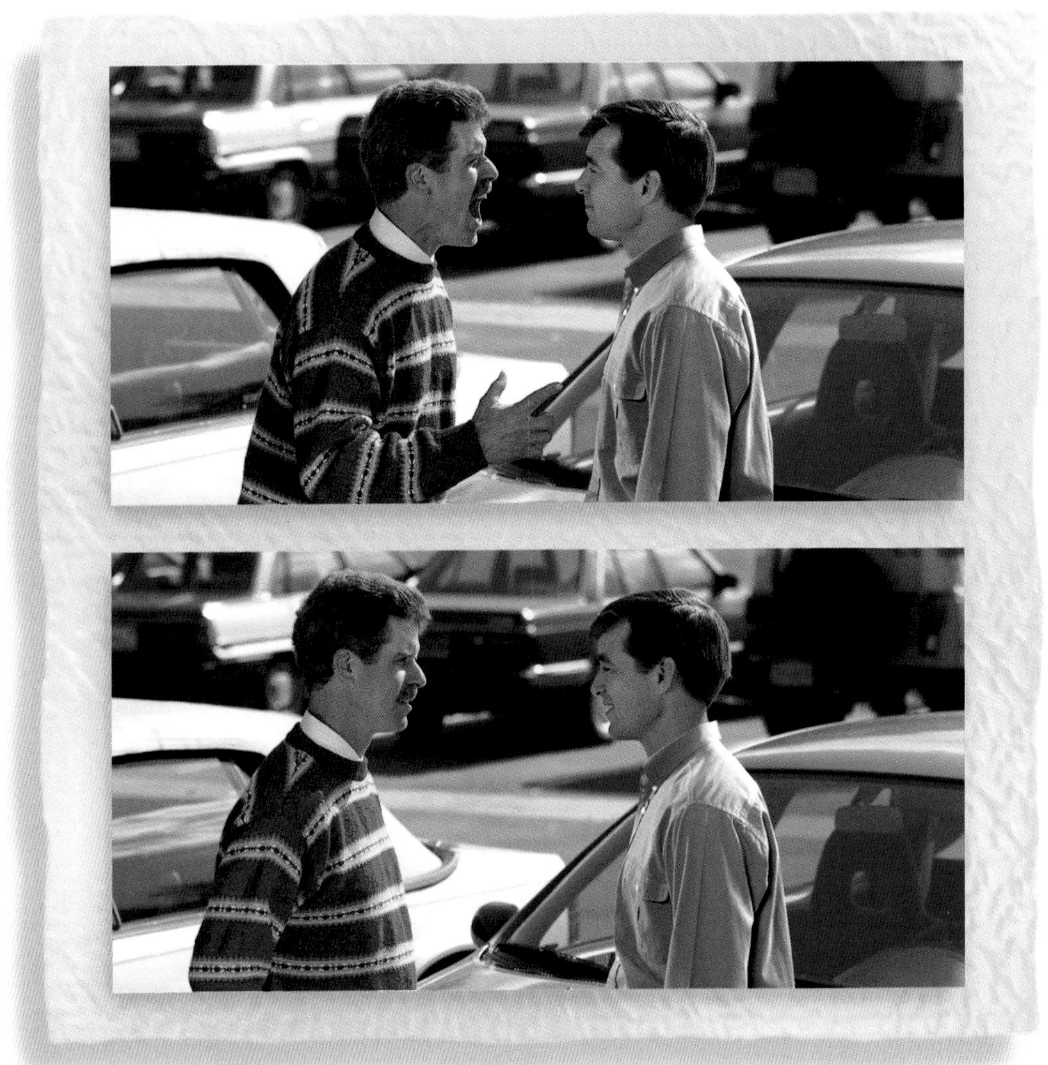

An individual can be lifted only about half a point on the Tone Scale by conversation.

By responding to a person's anger with boredom, a person's tone can be lifted.

person. An individual best responds to his own tone band; and an individual can be lifted only about half a point on the Tone Scale by conversation. In doing this type of "psychometry," one should not carry any particular band of conversation too long, not more than a sentence or two, because this will have a tendency to raise slightly the tone of the person and so spoil the accuracy of the test.

Two-minute psychometry, then, is done, first, by announcing something creative and constructive and seeing whether the person responds in kind; then, giving forth some casual conversation, perhaps about sports, and seeing if the person responds to that. Getting no response start talking antagonistically about things about which the person knows—but not, of course, about the person—to see if he achieves a response at this point. Then give forth with a sentence or two of anger against some condition. Then indulge in a small amount of discreditable gossip and see if there is any response to that. If this does not work, then dredge up some statements of hopelessness and misery. Somewhere in this range the person will agree with the type of conversation that is being offered—that is, he will respond to it in kind. A conversation can then be carried on along this band where the person has been discovered, and one will rapidly gain enough information to make a good first estimate of the person's position on the chart.

This two-minute psychometry by conversation can also be applied to groups. That speaker who desires to command his audience must not talk above or below his audience's tone more than half a point. If he wishes to lift the audience's tone, he should talk about half a point above their general tone level. An expert speaker, using this two-minute psychometry and carefully noting the responses of his audience, can, in two minutes, discover the tone of the audience—whereupon, all he has to do is adopt a tone slightly above theirs.

The Tone Scale and the Chart of Human Evaluation are the most important tools ever developed for the prediction of human behavior. Employ these tools and you will at all times know who you are dealing with, who to associate with, who to trust. ■

HUBBARD CHART OF HUMAN EVALUATION

Tone Scale	1 Behavior and Physiology	2 Medical Range	3 Emotion	4 Sexual Behavior Attitude Toward Children	5 Command over Environment	6 Actual Worth to Society Compared to Apparent Worth	7 Ethic Level	8 Handling of Truth
4.0	Excellent at projects, execution. Fast reaction time (relative to age).	Near accident-proof. No psychosomatic ills. Nearly immune to bacteria.	Eagerness, exhilaration.	Sexual interest high but often sublimated to creative thought. Intense interest in children.	High self-mastery. Aggressive toward environ. Dislikes to control people. High reasoning, volatile emotions.	High worth. Apparent worth will be realized. Creative and constructive.	Bases ethics on reason. Very high ethic level.	High concept of truth.
3.5	Good at projects, execution, sports.	Highly resistant to common infections. No colds.	Strong interest.	High interest in opposite sex. Constancy. Love of children.	Reasons well. Good control. Accepts ownership. Emotion free. Liberal.	Good value to society. Adjusts environ to benefit of self and others.	Heeds ethics of group but refines them higher as reason demands.	Truthful.
3.0	Capable of fair amount of action, sports.	Resistant to infection and disease. Few psychosomatic ills.	Mild interest. Content.	Interest in procreation. Interest in children.	Controls bodily functions. Reasons well. Free emotion still inhibited. Allows rights to others. Democratic.	Any apparent worth is actual worth. Fair value.	Follows ethics in which trained as honestly as possible. Moral.	Cautious of asserting truths. Social lies.
2.5	Relatively inactive, but capable of action.	Occasionally ill. Susceptible to usual diseases.	Indifference. Boredom.	Disinterest in procreation. Vague tolerance of children.	In control of function and some reasoning powers. Does not desire much ownership.	Capable of constructive action; seldom much quantity. Small value. "Well adjusted."	Treats ethics insincerely. Not particularly honest or dishonest.	Insincere. Careless of facts.
2.0	Capable of destructive and minor constructive action.	Severe sporadic illnesses.	Expressed resentment.	Disgust at sex; revulsion. Nagging of and nervousness about children.	Antagonistic and destructive to self, others, and environ. Desires command in order to injure.	Dangerous. Any apparent worth wiped out by potentials of injury to others.	Below this point: authoritarian. Chronically and bluntly dishonest when occasion arises.	Truth twisted to suit antagonism.
1.5	Capable of destructive action.	Depository illnesses (arthritis). (Range 1.0 to 2.0 interchangeable.)	Anger.	Rape. Sex as punishment. Brutal treatment of children.	Smashes or destroys others or environ. Failing this, may destroy self. Fascistic.	Insincere. Heavy liability. Possible murderer. Even when intentions avowedly good will bring about destruction.	Below this point: criminal. Immoral. Actively dishonest. Destructive of any and all ethics.	Blatant and destructive lying.
1.1	Capable of minor execution.	Endocrine and neurological illnesses.	Unexpressed resentment. Fear.	Promiscuity, perversion, sadism, irregular practices. Use of children for sadistic purposes.	No control of reason or emotions, but apparent organic control. Uses sly means of controlling others, especially hypnotism. Communistic.	Active liability. Enturbulates others. Apparent worth outweighed by vicious hidden intents.	Sex criminal. Negative ethics. Deviously dishonest without reason. Pseudoethical activities screen perversion of ethics.	Ingenious and vicious perversions of truth. Covers lying artfully.
0.5	Capable of relatively uncontrolled action.	Chronic malfunction of organs. (Accident-prone.)	Grief. Apathy.	Impotency, anxiety, possible efforts to reproduce. Anxiety about children.	Barest functional control of self only.	Liability to society. Possible suicide. Utterly careless of others.	Nonexistent. Not thinking. Obeying anyone.	Details facts with no concept of their reality.
0.1	Alive as an organism.	Chronically ill. (Refusing sustenance.)	Deepest apathy.	No effort to procreate.	No command of self, others, environ. Suicide.	High liability, needing care and efforts of others without making any contribution.	None.	No reaction.

9 Courage Level	10 Speech: Talks Speech: Listens	11 Subject's Handling of Written or Spoken Comm When Acting as a Relay Point	12 Reality (Agreement)	13 Ability to Handle Responsibility	14 Persistence on a Given Course	15 Literalness of Reception of Statements	16 Method Used by Subject to Handle Others	17 Hypnotic Level	18 Ability to Experience Present Time Pleasure	19 Your Value as a Friend	20 How Much Others Like You	21 State of Your Possessions	22 How Well Are You Understood	23 Potential Success	24 Potential Survival	**Tone Scale**
High courage level.	Strong, able, swift and full exchange of beliefs and ideas.	Passes theta comm, contributes to it. Cuts entheta lines.	Search for different viewpoints in order to broaden own reality. Changes reality.	Inherent sense of responsibility on all dynamics.	High creative persistence.	High differentiation. Good understanding of all comm, as modified by Clear's education.	Gains support by creative enthusiasm and vitality backed by reason.	Impossible to hypnotize without drugs.	Finds existence very full of pleasure.	Excellent.	Loved by many.	In excellent condition.	Very well.	Excellent.	Excellent. Considerable longevity.	4.0
Courage displayed on reasonable risks.	Will talk of deep-seated beliefs and ideas. — Will accept deep-seated beliefs, ideas; consider them.	Passes theta comm. Resents and hits back at entheta lines.	Ability to understand and evaluate reality of others and to change viewpoint. Agreeable.	Capable of assuming and carrying on responsibilities.	Good persistence and direction toward constructive goals.	Good grasp of statements. Good sense of humor.	Gains support by creative reasoning and vitality.	Difficult to trance unless still possessed of a trance engram.	Finds life pleasurable most of the time.	Very good.	Well loved.	In good condition.	Well.	Very good.	Very good.	3.5
Conservative display of courage where risk is small.	Tentative expression of limited number of personal ideas. — Receives ideas and beliefs if cautiously stated.	Passes comm. Conservative. Inclines toward moderate construction and creation.	Awareness of possible validity of different reality. Conservative agreement.	Handles responsibility in a slipshod fashion.	Fair persistence if obstacles not too great.	Good differentiation of meaning of statements.	Invites support by practical reasoning and social graces.	Could be hypnotized, but alert when awake.	Experiences pleasure some of the time.	Good.	Respected by most.	Fairly good.	Usually.	Good.	Good.	3.0
Neither courage nor cowardice. Neglect of danger.	Casual pointless conversation. — Listens only to ordinary affairs.	Cancels any comm of higher or lower tone. Devaluates urgencies.	Refusal to match two realities. Indifference to conflict in reality. Too careless to agree or disagree.	Too careless. Not trustworthy.	Idle, poor concentration.	Accepts very little, literally or otherwise. Apt to be literal about humor.	Careless of support from others.	Can be a hypnotic subject, but mostly alert.	Experiences moments of pleasure. Low intensity.	Fair.	Liked by a few.	Shows some neglect.	Sometimes misunderstood.	Fair.	Fair.	2.5
Reactive, unreasoning thrusts at danger.	Talks in threats. Invalidates other people. — Listens to threats. Openly mocks theta talk.	Deals in hostile or threatening comm. Lets only small amount of theta go through.	Verbal doubt. Defense of own reality. Attempts to undermine others. Disagrees.	Uses responsibility to further own ends.	Persistence toward destruction of enemies. No constructive persistence below this point.	Accepts remarks of tone 2.0 literally.	Nags and bluntly criticizes to demand compliance with wishes.	Negates somewhat, but can be hypnotized.	Occasionally experiences some pleasure in extraordinary moments.	Poor.	Rarely liked.	Very neglected.	Often misunderstood.	Poor.	Poor.	2.0
Unreasonable bravery, usually damaging to self.	Talks of death, destruction, hate only. — Listens only to death and destruction. Wrecks theta lines.	Perverts comm to entheta regardless of original content. — Stops theta comm. Passes entheta and perverts it.	Destruction of opposing reality. "You're wrong." Disagrees with reality of others.	Assumes responsibility in order to destroy.	Destructive persistence begins strongly, weakens quickly.	Accepts alarming remarks literally. Brutal sense of humor.	Uses threats, punishment and alarming lies to dominate others.	Negates heavily against remarks, but absorbs them.	Seldom experiences any pleasure.	Definite liability.	Openly disliked by most.	Often broken. Bad repair.	Continually misunderstood.	Usually a failure.	Early demise.	1.5
Occasional underhanded displays of action, otherwise cowardly.	Talks apparent theta, but intent vicious. — Listens little; mostly to cabal, gossip, lies.	Relays only malicious comm. — Cuts comm lines. Won't relay.	Doubt of own reality. Insecurity. Doubt of opposing reality.	Incapable, capricious, irresponsible.	Vacillation on any course. Very poor concentration. Flighty.	Lack of acceptance of any remarks. Tendency to accept all literally avoided by forced humor.	Nullifies others to get them to level where they can be used. Devious and vicious means. Hypnotism, gossip. Seeks hidden control.	In a permanent light trance, but negates.	Most gaiety forced. Real pleasure out of reach.	Dangerous liability.	Generally despised.	Poor. In poor condition.	No real understanding.	Nearly always fails.	Brief.	1.1
Complete cowardice.	Talks very little and only in apathetic tones. — Listens little; mostly to apathy or pity.	Takes little heed of comm. Does not relay.	Shame, anxiety, strong doubt of own reality. Easily has reality of others forced on him.	None.	Sporadic persistence toward self-destruction.	Literal acceptance of any remark matching tone.	Enturbulates others to control them. Cries for pity. Wild lying to gain sympathy.	Very hypnotic. Any remark made may be a "positive suggestion."	None.	Very great liability.	Not liked. Only pitied by some.	In very bad condition generally.	Not at all understood.	Utter failure.	Demise soon.	0.5
No reaction.	Does not talk. — Does not listen.	Does not relay. Unaware of comm.	Complete withdrawal from conflicting reality. No reality.	None.	None.	Complete literal acceptance.	Pretends death so others will not think him dangerous and will go away.	Is equivalent to a hypnotized subject when "awake."	None.	Total liability.	Not regarded.	No realization of possession.	Ignored.	No effort. Complete failure.	Almost dead.	0.1

Fold Out

Test Your Understanding

Answer the following questions about the Tone Scale. Refer back to it to check your answers. If you need to, review the chapter. Going over the material several times will increase your certainty and help you better apply it.

- ❑ *What is the Tone Scale?*
- ❑ *How can the Hubbard Chart of Human Evaluation be used to predict a person's behavior?*
- ❑ *What do the levels below 0.05 on the Tone Scale indicate about a person who is in one of them?*
- ❑ *How can obnosis be applied to help improve an immediate situation?*
- ❑ *How can emotion be used to raise a person on the Tone Scale?*

Practical Exercises

The following exercises will help you understand this chapter and increase your ability to actually apply the knowledge it contains.

1 Using the Hubbard Chart of Human Evaluation, consider five people you know and determine the chronic tone level for each. (Do not tell the person what you determined his tone level to be.)

2 Practice obnosis. Look around your environment and practice seeing what is there. Notice things which are plainly obvious. Don't allow any assumption into your observation. Continue to practice obnosis until you are sure you can do it without adding in any assumptions.

3 Spot the tone levels of different people. Go to a place where there are lots of people. Pick out a person and notice his or her tone level. Do this again and again with different people. Observe people in conversation or engaging in some activity and note their tone levels. Continue doing this until you are confident you can spot the tone level of people by observing them. (Do not tell the people you observe what tone level you think them to be in, however.)

4 Practice spotting the tone levels of people by engaging them in conversation. Take a clipboard and paper and interview people on the street. Ask them some sample questions such as "What's the most obvious thing about me?" "When was the last time you had a haircut?" "Do you think people do as much work now as they did fifty years ago?" Other questions of a similar nature can be used to gain responses from the person. Determine the person's tone level based on his responses. Is there a social tone sitting atop his chronic tone? Repeat the interview with other people, noting the person's tone level each time. Keep this up until you can approach anyone and engage him in conversation and determine his chronic tone level. (Important note: Do not tell the person what tone level you observe him to be in, or evaluate his tone level for him.)

5 When you have gained assurance at Exercise 4, interview more people. Interview at least fifteen people. With the first five, match their tone as soon as you have spotted it. With the next five, drop below their chronic tone and see what happens. For the last five, put on a higher tone than theirs. Note down your observations from doing this. Practice this with more people until you are confident you can spot a person's tone level and then match it, drop below it or assume a tone above it.

6 Do a two-minute psychometry on a person. Engage a person in a conversation and, using the technique given in the chapter, determine what tone level the person responds to. Repeat this with other people until you are confident you can spot what tone level a person will respond to.

7 Practice raising a person's tone level. Engage a person in conversation. Once you have determined his tone level, adopt a tone one-half to one full tone above his. Note what happens to his tone level. Repeat this with other people until you are confident you can raise a person on the Tone Scale.

RESULTS FROM APPLICATION

Knowledge of the Tone Scale and the ability to use it has given people a new freedom when dealing with others that could not otherwise exist for them. It has given them the ability to predict the behavior of others and deal with them successfully no matter whether a person be in apathy, grief, fear, anger, antagonism, boredom, cheerfulness or enthusiasm. The skill to bring another up the Tone Scale is easily achieved with this knowledge.

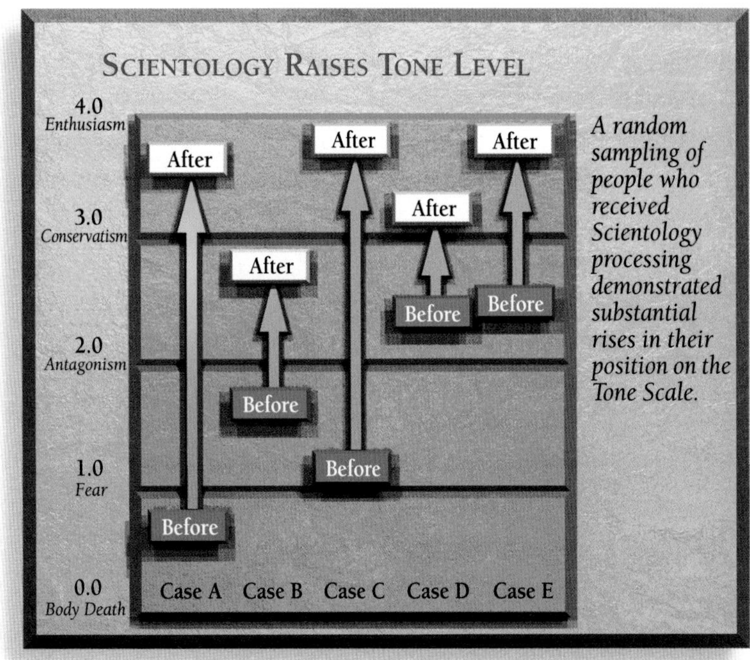

A random sampling of people who received Scientology processing demonstrated substantial rises in their position on the Tone Scale.

Many people have found that the actions, reactions and behavior of others become highly predictable when one can observe where they are on the scale. Life is less confusing or mysterious. The health, survival potential and longevity of an individual or group can also be predicted. How another will treat his property or yours becomes obvious.

People from all walks of life: artists, performers, actors, executives, foremen and teachers all swear that use of this technology puts them in the driver's seat in life. Being able to predict the behavior of others makes life a game that you can win, as shown in the following accounts.

Knowing how people in different tone levels react made all the difference to a Southern California contractor. He experienced a huge increase in his general competence upon learning this data.

"I had always been driven crazy trying to be logical in dealing with people in the lower bands of the Tone Scale, especially people in antagonism. Once I knew the data on the Tone Scale, I was no longer bothered by certain customers, particularly the antagonistic ones, I had to service. Running my business became a breeze and my personal sales statistics tripled in just a few weeks. I was much more causative in dealing with people."

Dismayed when first asked to do a sales course, a woman who worked in a telecommunications company in Florida was amazed that she could do such a job successfully. She had her own considerations about salesmen and didn't want to be "one of those annoying salespeople who call you at the most inopportune time to tell you about something you have no interest in." However, she had the good fortune to do a sales course that included data on the emotional Tone Scale.

*"I **really** enjoyed this course and the gains I got from it! I had heard about the emotional Tone Scale before, but I had no idea really how to use it. And I realized that 'bad' salesmen don't have this data, so no wonder they are annoying! Using the technology, I can now go in at the right tone level and make my sales boom!"*

In Denmark, a girl was having a problem with a friend. Something was bothering him that he would not communicate about. She tried to talk to him, but he still wouldn't say what was wrong. His reticence was creating a big upset between them. She decided to write him a very cheerful letter but, to her surprise, it had no effect on him. When she asked him about it, he told her that he couldn't even remember what it said! She eventually solved this dilemma using the Tone Scale.

"I finally realized that my communication was too high for his tone level, and thus it resulted in no communication. So I wrote him another letter which was closer to his tone level, and amazingly enough it got across to him very much! He started talking to me and we are friends again.

"If I hadn't had the technology on the Tone Scale I would have given up. This made me brave enough to write him another letter. Otherwise, I would have gone into apathy about it and would have lost a very good friend. Instead, using the Tone Scale and communication, I brought him up the scale and salvaged our friendship!"

A girl in Scandinavia had just broken up with her boyfriend. Although not particularly happy, she did, however, have the data on the Tone Scale. She decided to use this tool to turn around her life:

*"I had a lot of very good friends but no prospects for a boyfriend. A new guy joined our group of friends. We got in communication shortly after he joined the group and I realized that we had almost identical communication levels. He seemed like a very nice guy. I would mention that something needed to get handled and I would turn around and he would be busy handling it. He would say that we needed rolls for dinner and I was already on my way to the bakery. I would mention something and he would let me know that he just thought of this. We matched perfectly on the Tone Scale. I looked at this and was laughing to myself, as he was in no way the type of guy I would earlier have looked for. Priorly, I had always looked at appearance only which led to a hit-and-miss experience. This guy, however, was a **real** match and within weeks we decided to get married and we did."*

SUGGESTIONS FOR FURTHER STUDY

L. Ron Hubbard wrote a considerable amount about the Tone Scale and the Hubbard Chart of Human Evaluation. Many of his writings and hundreds of his lectures amplify the data in this chapter and provide a complete understanding of this basic of human relationships. Anyone desiring greater ability to interact with people is advised to study the following:

Self Analysis

The first book ever written which provides definite techniques to improve memory, speed reaction time, handle psychosomatic illness and reduce stress. The reader assesses his condition with a battery of tests before starting and then launches into an analysis of his past guided by specific and easily followed directions. Offers the means to self-discovery through a series of more than twenty Scientology processes designed to give an individual the clearest look he has ever had into his past.

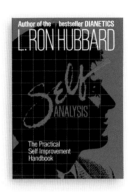

Special Course in Human Evaluation

A one-week course which contains different written materials and ten of Mr. Hubbard's lectures on the Tone Scale and how to use it in different aspects of life. With the data and demonstrations and exercises, this course results in someone who, through the application of the Tone Scale and the Hubbard Chart of Human Evaluation, can accurately evaluate and predict human behavior. (Delivered in Scientology organizations.)

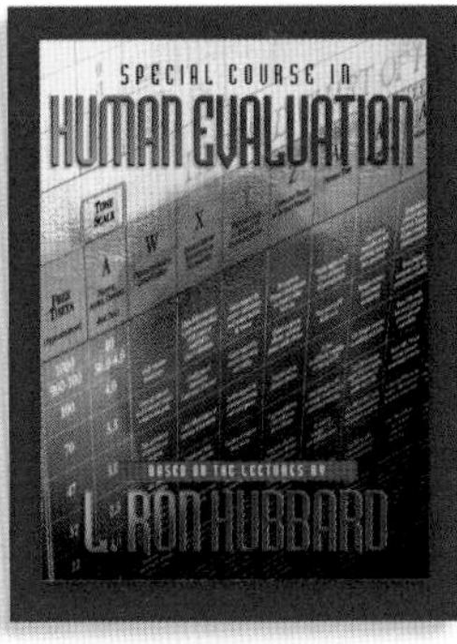

Science of Survival

Built around a more advanced version of the Hubbard Chart of Human Evaluation than contained in this chapter, this authoritative text contains the most complete description of human behavior ever written. A chapter is devoted to each column of the chart and clarifies the seeming confusion of human conduct into definite categories.

One can use the book to accurately predict what another will do in any situation in life, even those with whom one has not had extensive prior experience. Developed for use by Scientology practitioners, this Tone Scale technology has been used for more than fifty years by persons in a wide range of professions. Millions of other people use the book simply to understand people better and improve their relationships.

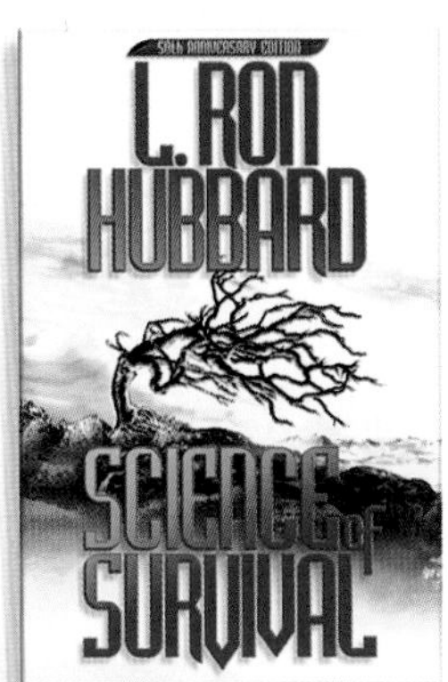

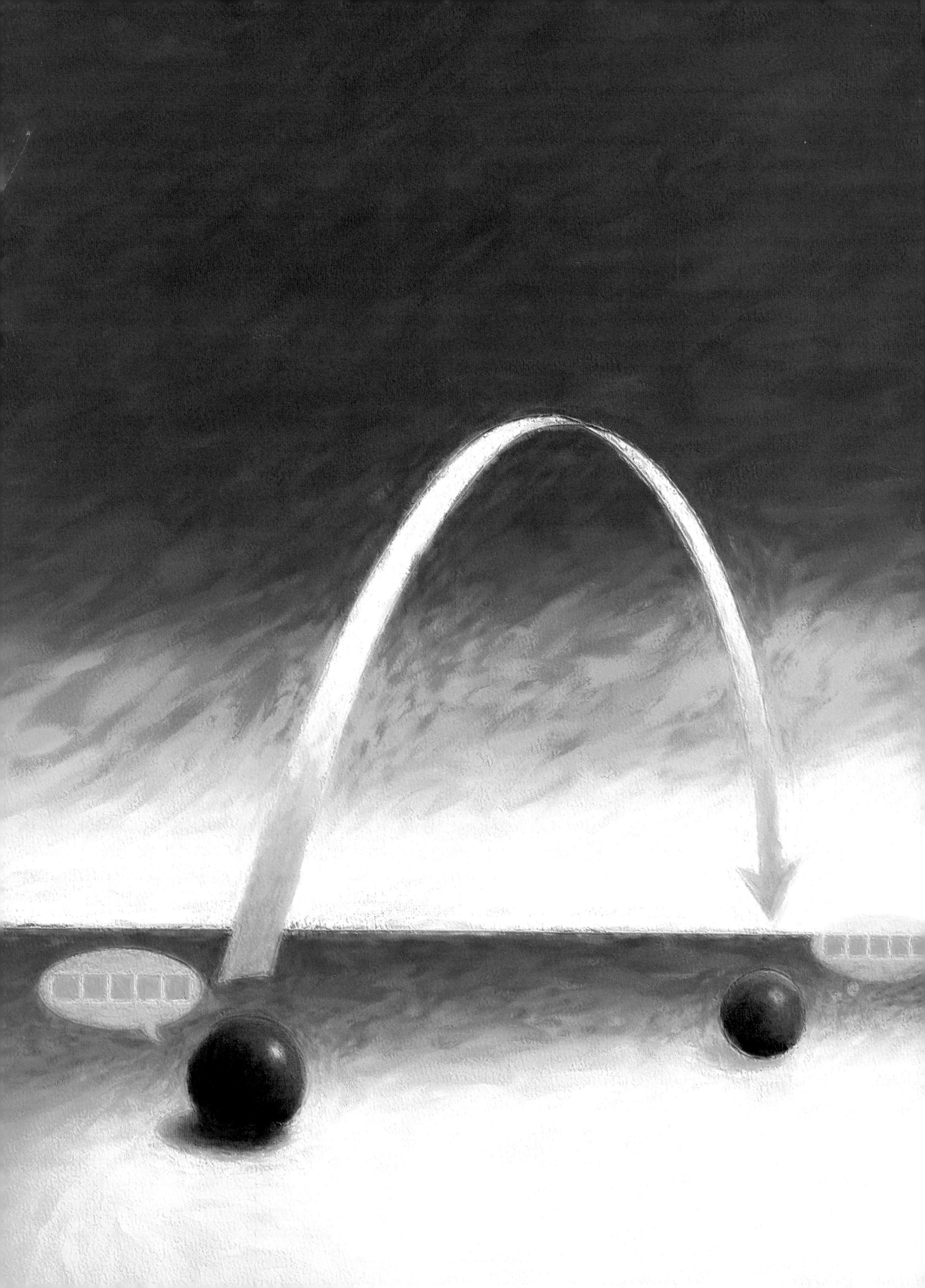

Chapter 5

Communication

A man is as alive as he can communicate," L. Ron Hubbard wrote. And communication is a facet of life which he explored very deeply indeed, ultimately writing hundreds of thousands of words about this vital subject. Communication skills are essential in **any** *sphere of human interaction. In fact, when all is said and done, on whatever level, communication is the sole activity all people share.*

The benefits of effective communication are too numerous to list, for they enhance all aspects of life from the personal to the professional. The **ability** *to communicate is vital to the success of any endeavor.*

In this chapter you will learn what good communication consists of and how to recognize the bad, what the component parts of communication are and how to utilize them, and why more communication, not less, brings the individual greater freedom.

Also included in this chapter are numerous drills that Mr. Hubbard developed which improve one's communication level and have great practical application to life. A thorough understanding of this data will provide you with tools you can use forever.

What Is Communication?

How does one talk so that another person listens and understands? How does one listen? How does one know if he has been heard and understood?

These are all points about communication that have never before been analyzed or explained.

People have known that communication is an important part of life but until now no one has ever been able to tell anyone *how* to communicate.

Until Scientology, the subject of communication had received no emphasis or study. Any attention given to it was mechanical and the province of engineers. Yet all human endeavor depends utterly on a full knowledge of the real basics of communication.

To master communication, one must understand it.

In Scientology, communication *has* been defined—an accomplishment that has led to a much deeper understanding of life itself.

Communication, in essence, is the shift of a particle from one part of space to another part of space. A *particle* is the thing being communicated. It can be an object, a written message, a spoken word or an idea. In its crudest definition, this *is* communication.

This simple view of communication leads to the full definition:

Communication is the consideration and action of impelling an impulse or particle from source-point across a distance to receipt-point, with the intention of bringing into being at the receipt-point a duplication and understanding of that which emanated from the source-point.

Duplication is the act of reproducing something exactly. *Emanated* means "came forth."

The formula of communication is cause, distance, effect, with intention, attention and duplication *with understanding.*

The definition and formula of communication open the door to understanding this subject. By dissecting communication into its component parts, we can view the function of each and thus more clearly understand the whole.

Any communication involves a particle which can be in one of four categories: an object…

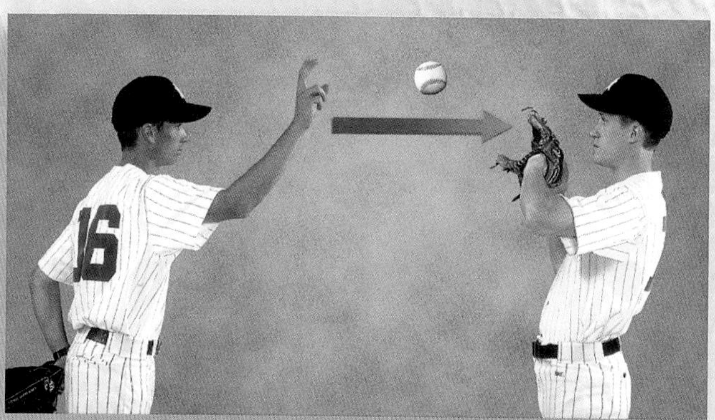

…a written message…

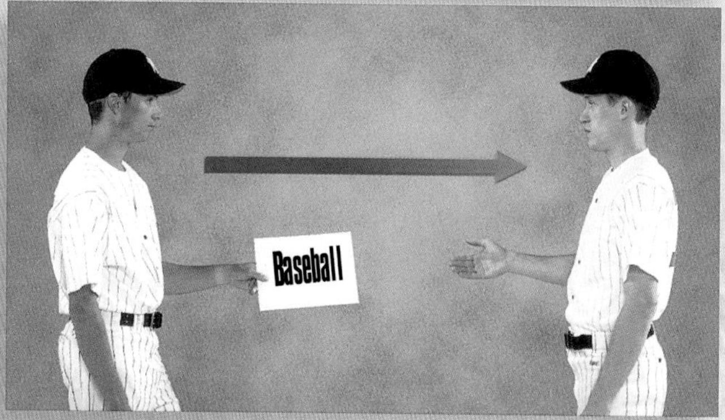

…a spoken word…

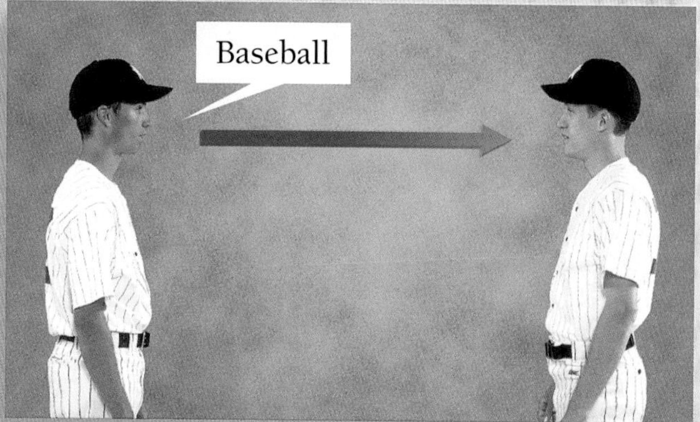

…or an idea.

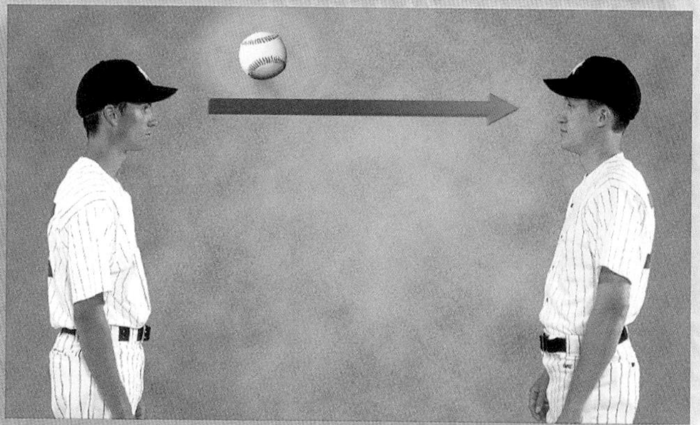

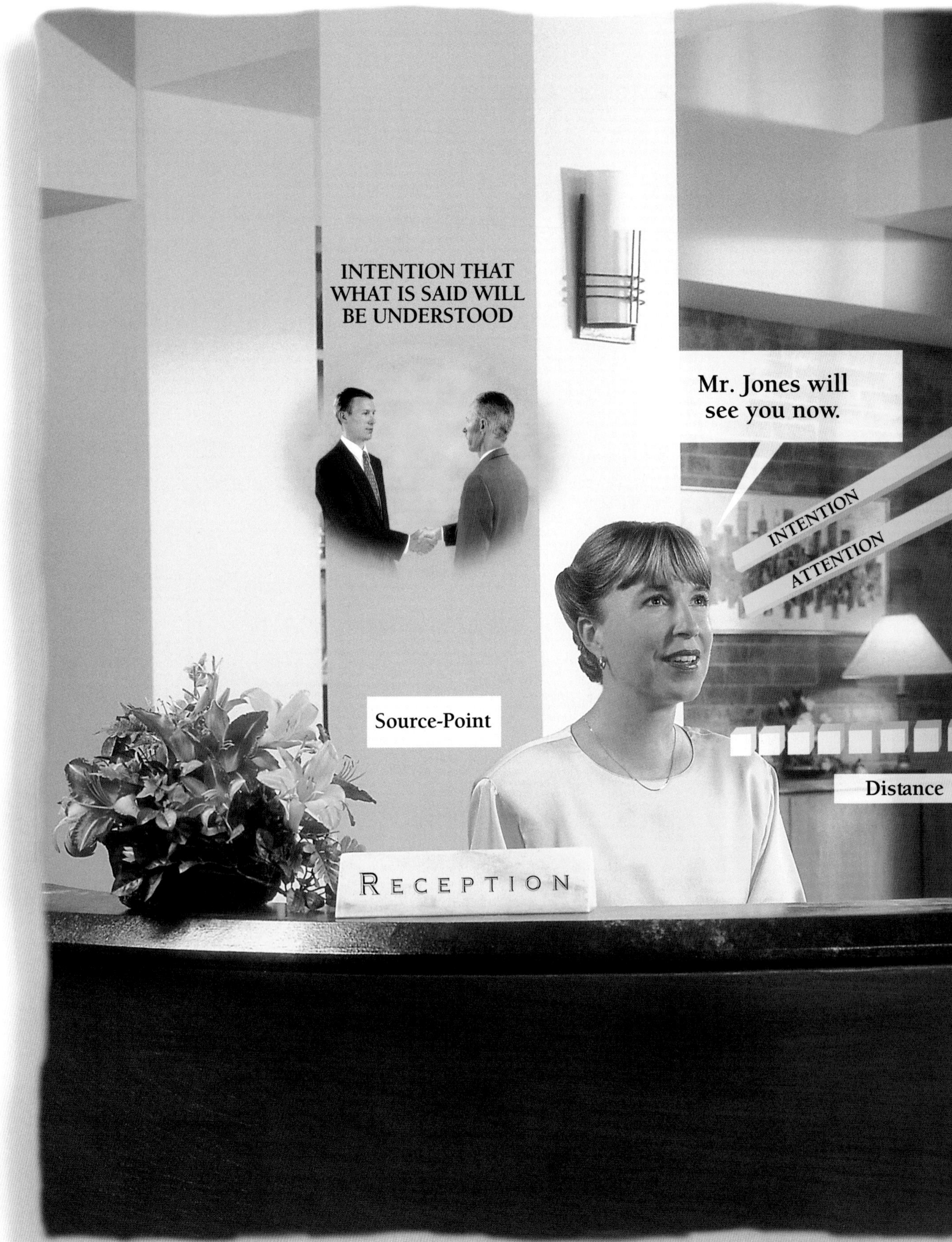
INTENTION THAT
WHAT IS SAID WILL
BE UNDERSTOOD
Mr. Jones will
see you now.
INTENTION
ATTENTION
Source-Point
Distance
RECEPTION

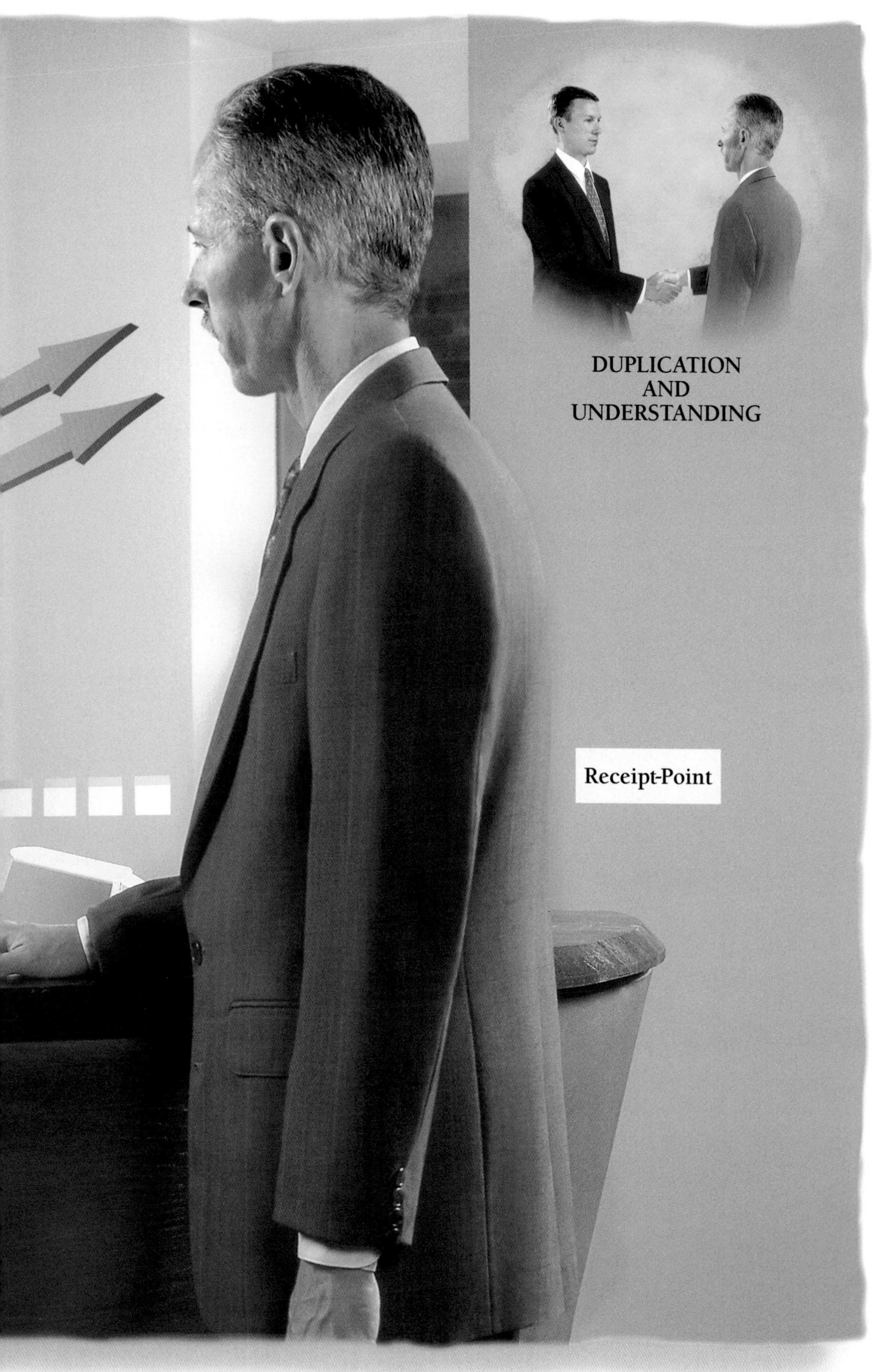

Any successful communication contains all the elements shown here. Any failure to communicate can be analyzed against these components to isolate what went wrong.

FACTORS OF COMMUNICATION

Let us now more closely examine several components of communication by looking at two life units, one of them "A" and the other "B." "A" and "B" are terminals—by terminal we mean a point that receives, relays and sends communication.

First there is "A's" *intention.* This, at "B" becomes *attention,* and for a true communication to take place, a *duplication* at "B" must take place of what emanated from "A."

"A" of course, to emanate a communication, must have given attention originally to "B," and "B" must have given to this communication some intention, at least to listen or receive, so we have both cause and effect having intention and attention.

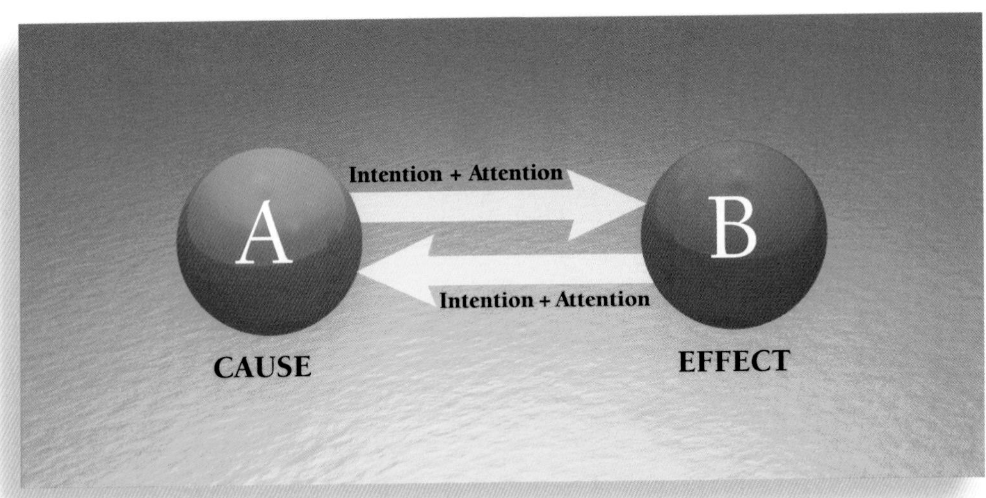

Now, there is another factor which is very important. This is the factor of duplication. We could express this as reality, or we could express it as agreement. The degree of agreement reached between "A" and "B" in this communication cycle becomes their reality, and this is accomplished mechanically by duplication. In other words, the degree of reality reached in this communication cycle depends upon the amount of duplication. "B" as effect, must to some degree duplicate what emanated from "A" as cause, in order for the first part of the cycle to take effect.

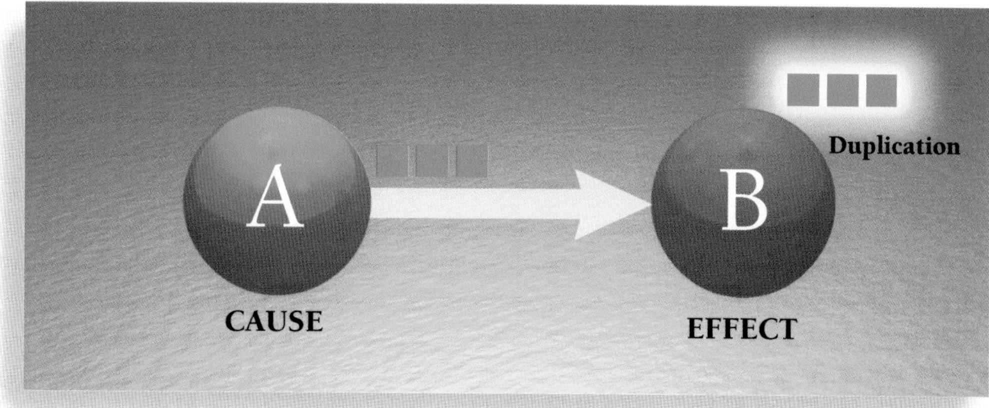

Then "A," now as effect, must duplicate what emanated from "B" for the communication to be concluded. If this is done there is no detrimental consequence.

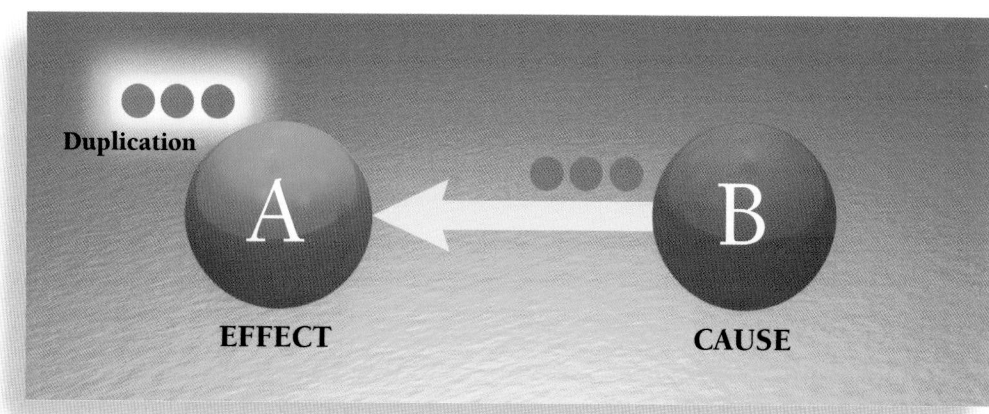

If this duplication does not take place at "B" and then at "A" we get what amounts to an unfinished cycle of action. If, for instance, "B" did not vaguely duplicate what emanated from "A," the first part of the cycle of communication was not achieved, and a great deal of randomity (unpredicted motion), explanation, argument might result. Then if "A" did not duplicate what emanated from "B" when "B" was cause on the second cycle, again an uncompleted cycle of communication occurred with consequent unreality. Now naturally, if we cut down reality, we will cut down affinity—the feeling of love or liking for something or someone. So, where duplication is absent, affinity is seen to drop.

A complete cycle of communication will result in high affinity. If we disarrange any of these factors we get an incomplete cycle of communication and we have either "A" or "B" or both *waiting* for the end of cycle. In such a wise the communication becomes harmful.

An unfinished cycle of communication generates what might be called *answer hunger.* An individual who is waiting for a signal that his communication has been received is prone to accept any inflow. When an individual has, for a very long period of time, consistently waited for answers which did not arrive, any sort of answer from anywhere will be pulled in to him, by him, as an effort to remedy his scarcity for answers.

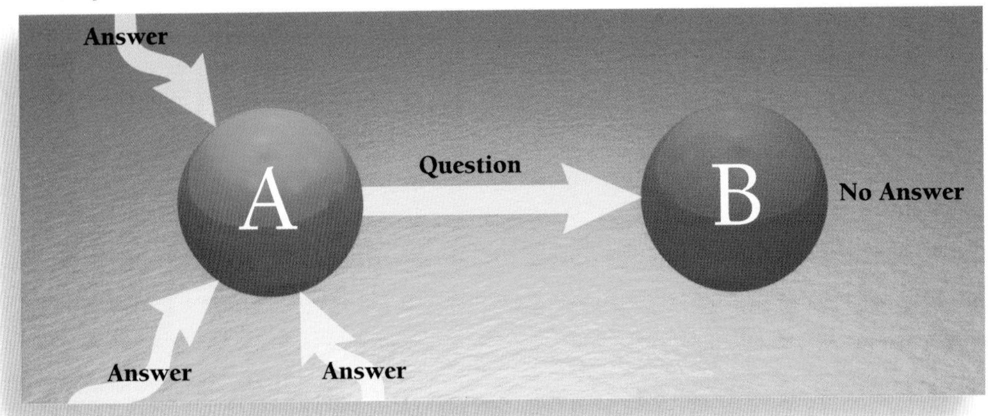

Uncompleted cycles of communication bring about a scarcity of answers. It does not much matter what the answers were or would be as long as they vaguely approximate the subject at hand. It does matter when some entirely unlooked-for answer is given, as in compulsive or obsessive communication, or when no answer is given at all.

Communication itself is detrimental only when the emanating communication at cause was sudden and non sequitur (illogical) to the environment. Here we have violations of attention and intention.

The factor of interest also enters here but is far less important. Nevertheless, it explains a great deal about human behavior. "A" has the intention of interesting "B." "B," to be talked to, becomes interest*ing*.

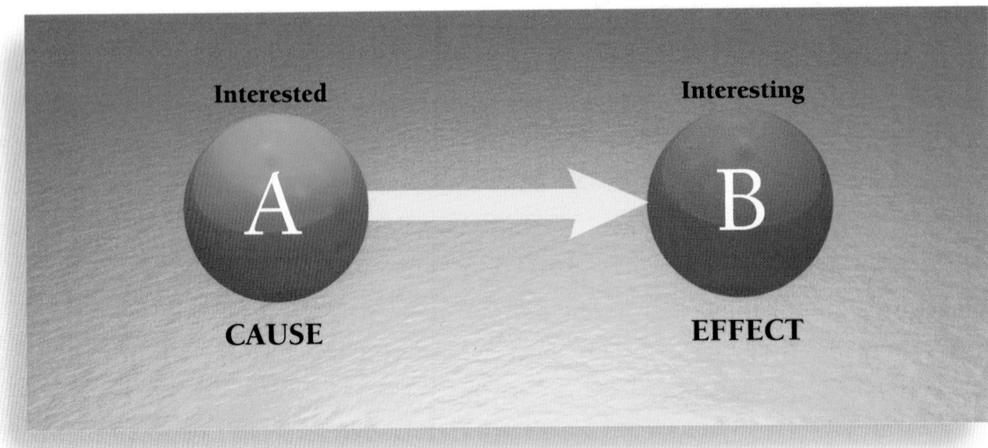

Similarly "B," when he emanates a communication, is interest*ed* and "A" is interest*ing.*

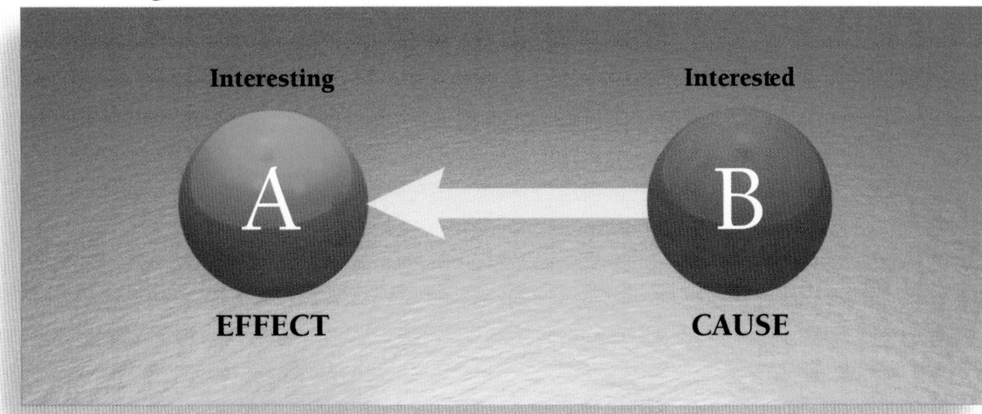

Here we have, as part of the communication formula (but a less important part), the continuous shift from being interested to being interesting on the part of either of the terminals, "A" or "B." Cause is interest*ed,* effect is interest*ing.*

Of some greater importance is the fact that the intention to be received on the part of "A" places upon "A" the necessity of being duplicatable.

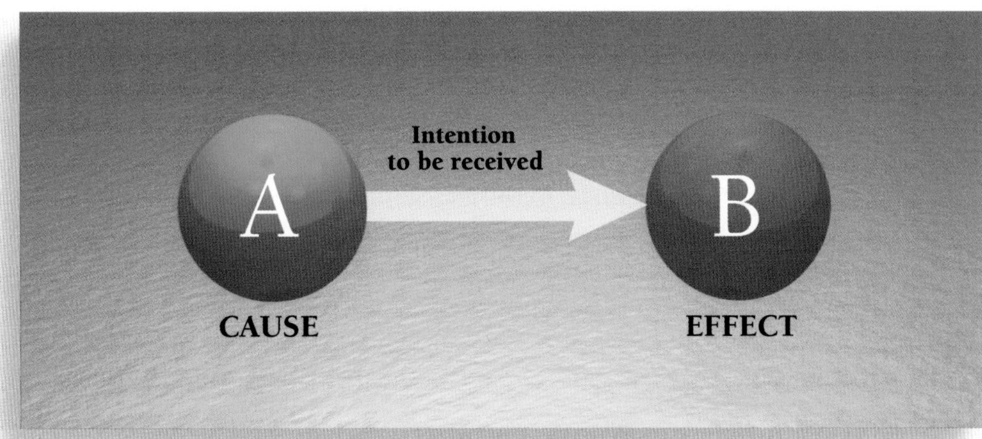

If "A" cannot be duplicatable in any degree, then of course his communication will not be received at "B," for "B," unable to duplicate "A," cannot receive the communication.

As an example of this, "A," let us say, speaks in Chinese, where "B" can only understand French. It is necessary for "A" to make himself duplicatable by speaking French to "B" who only understands French. In a case where "A" speaks one language and "B" another, and they have no language in common, we have the factor of mimicry possible and a communication can yet take place. "A," supposing he had a hand, could raise his hand. "B," supposing he had one, could raise his hand. Then "B" could raise his other hand, and "A" could raise his other hand, and we would have completed a cycle of communication by mimicry.

Basically, all things are considerations. We consider that things are, and so they are. The idea is always senior to the mechanics of energy, space, time, mass. It would be possible to have entirely different ideas about communication than these. However, these happen to be the ideas of communication which are in common in this universe, and which are utilized by the life units of this universe.

Here we have the basic agreement upon the subject of communication in the communication formula as given here. Because ideas are senior to this, a being can get, in addition to the communication formula, a peculiar idea concerning just exactly how communication should be conducted, and if this is not generally agreed upon, can find himself definitely out of communication.

Let us take the example of a modernistic writer who insists that the first three letters of every word should be dropped or that no sentence should be finished. He will not attain agreement among his readers.

There is a continuous action of natural selection, one might say, which weeds out strange or peculiar communication ideas. People, to be in communication, adhere to the basic rules as given here, and when anyone tries to depart too widely from these rules, they simply do not duplicate him and so, in effect, he goes out of communication.

Now we come to the problem of what a life unit must be willing to experience in order to communicate. In the first place the primary source-point must be willing to be duplicatable. It must be able to give at least some attention to the receipt-point. The primary receipt-point must be willing to duplicate,

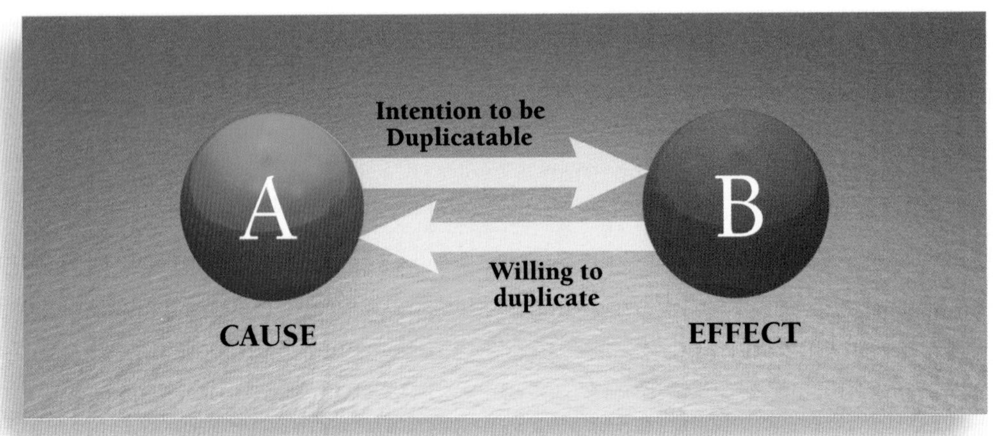

must be willing to receive and must be willing to change into a source-point in order to send the communication, or an answer to it, back. And the primary source-point in its turn must be willing to be a receipt-point.

As we are dealing basically with ideas and not mechanics, we see, then, that a state of mind must exist between a cause- and effect-point whereby each one is willing to be cause or effect at will, is willing to duplicate at will, is willing to be duplicatable at will, is willing to change at will, is willing to experience the distance between, and, in short, willing to communicate.

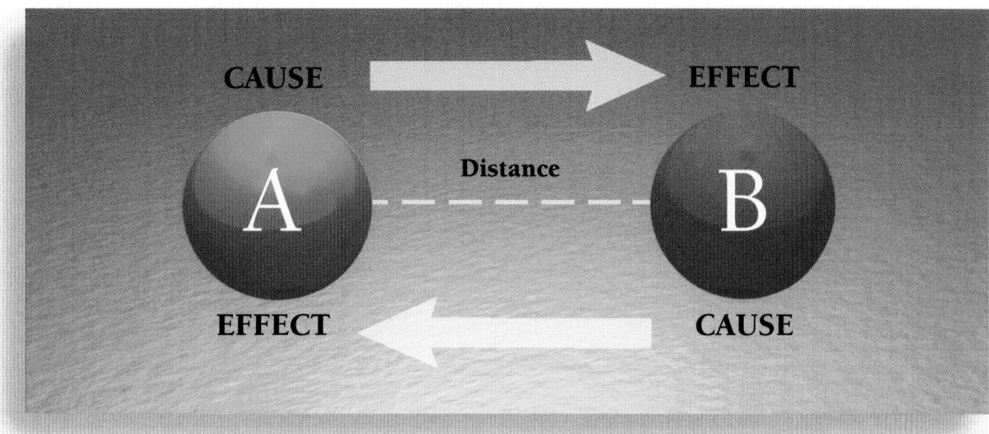

Where we get these conditions in an individual or a group we have sane people.

Where an unwillingness to send or receive communications occurs, where people obsessively or compulsively send communications without direction and without trying to be duplicatable, where individuals in receipt of communications stand silent and do not acknowledge or reply, we have factors of irrationality.

Some of the conditions which can occur in an irrational line are a failure to be duplicatable before one emanates a communication, an intention contrary to being received, an unwillingness to receive or duplicate a communication, an unwillingness to experience distance, an unwillingness to change, an unwillingness to give attention, an unwillingness to express intention, an unwillingness to acknowledge, and, in general, an unwillingness to duplicate.

It might be seen by someone that the solution to communication is not to communicate. One might say that if he hadn't communicated in the first place he wouldn't be in trouble now. Perhaps there is some truth in this, but a man is as dead as he can't communicate. He is as alive as he can communicate.

Two-way Communication

A cycle of communication and two-way communication are actually two different things. If we examine closely the anatomy of communication—the actual structure and parts—we will discover that a cycle of communication is not a two-way communication in its entirety.

If you will inspect Graph A below, you will see a cycle of communication:

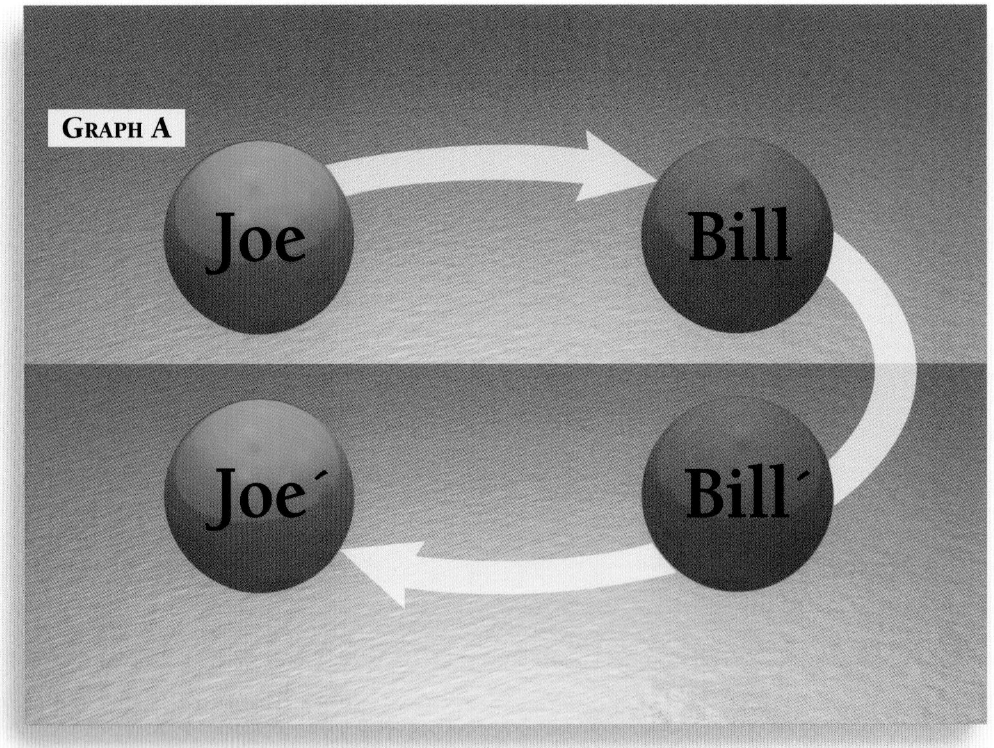

Here we have Joe as the originator of a communication. It is his primary impulse. This impulse is addressed to Bill. We find Bill receiving it, and then Bill originating an answer or acknowledgment as Bill´, which acknowledgment is sent back to Joe´. Joe has said, for instance, "How are you?" Bill has received this, and then Bill (becoming secondary cause) has replied to it as Bill´ with "I'm okay," which goes back to Joe´ and thus ends the cycle.

Now what we call a two-way cycle of communication may ensue as in Graph B below:

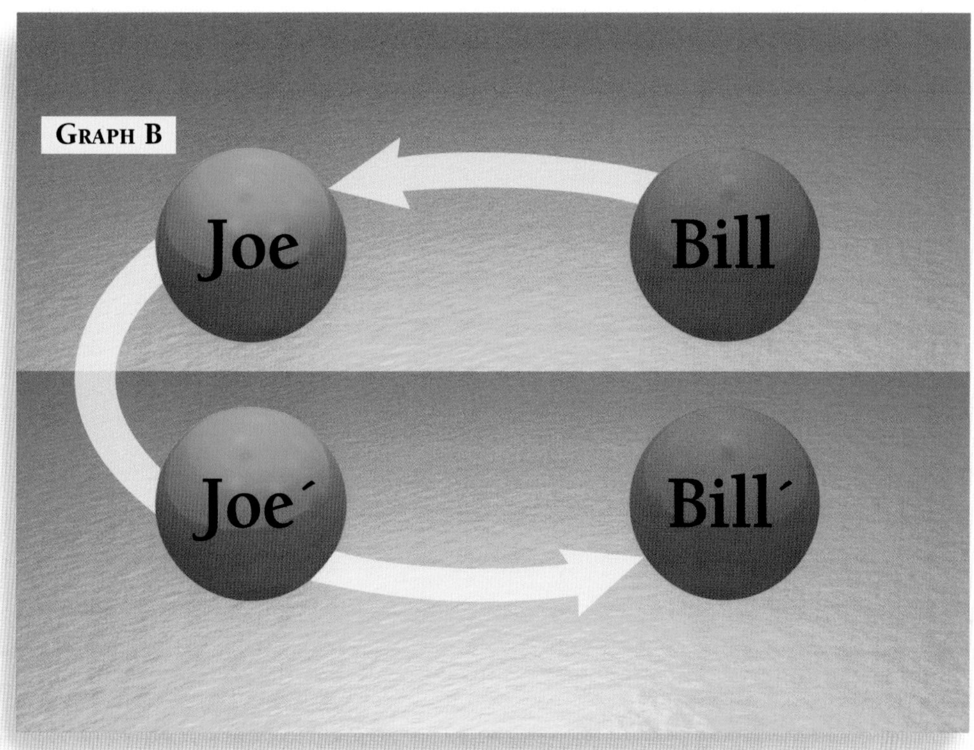

Here we have Bill originating a communication. Bill says, "How's tricks?" Joe receives this, and then as Joe´ or secondary cause, answers "Okay, I guess," which answer is then acknowledged in its receipt by Bill´.

In both of these graphs we discover that in Graph A the acknowledgment of the secondary cause was expressed by Joe´ as a nod or a look of satisfaction. And again, in Graph B Joe´'s "Okay, I guess" is actually acknowledged by Bill´ with a nod or some expression signifying the receipt of the communication.

If both Joe and Bill are "strong, silent men," they would omit some portion of these cycles. The most flagrant omission and the one most often understood as "communication lag" would be for Joe in Graph A to say, "How are you?" and for Bill to stand there without speaking. (By "communication lag" is meant the length of time intervening between the asking of a question and the reply to that specific question by the person asked.)

Here we have Joe causing a communication, and Bill′ failing to continue the cycle. We do not know or inquire, and we are not interested in, whether or not Bill as the receipt-point ever did hear it. We can assume that he was at least present, and that Joe spoke loudly enough to be heard, and that Bill's attention was somewhere in Joe's vicinity. Now, instead of getting on with the cycle of communication, Joe is left there with an incompleted cycle and never gets an opportunity to become Joe′.

There are several ways in which a cycle of communication could not be completed, and these could be categorized as:

1. Joe failing to emanate a communication,

2. Bill failing to hear the communication,

3. Bill′ failing to reply to the communication received by him, and

4. Joe′ failing to acknowledge by some sign or word that he has heard Bill′.

We could assign various reasons to all this, but our purpose here is not to assign reasons why they do not complete a communication cycle. Our entire purpose is involved with the noncompletion of this communication cycle.

Now, as in Graph A, let us say we have in Joe a person who is compulsively and continually originating communications whether he has anybody's attention or not, and whether or not these communications are germane (pertinent) to any existing situation. We discover that Joe is apt to be met, in his communicating, with an inattentive Bill who does not hear him, and thus an absent Bill´ who does not answer him, and thus an absent Joe´ who never acknowledges.

Let us examine this same situation in Graph B. Here we have, in Bill, an origination of a communication. We have the same Joe with a compulsive outflow. Bill says, "How are you?" and the cycle is not completed because Joe, so intent upon his own compulsive line, does not become Joe´ and never gives Bill a chance to become Bill´ and acknowledge.

Now let us take another situation. We find Joe originating communications, and Bill a person who never originates communications. Joe is not necessarily compulsive or obsessive in originating communications, but Bill is inhibited in originating communications. We find that Joe and Bill, working together, then get into this kind of an activity: Joe originates communication, Bill hears it, becomes Bill´, replies to it, and permits Joe a chance to become Joe´. This goes on quite well, but will sooner or later hit a jam on a two-way cycle, which is violated because Bill never originates communication.

A two-way cycle of communication would work as follows: Joe, having originated a communication and having completed it, may then wait for Bill to originate a communication to Joe, thus completing the remainder of the two-way cycle of communication. Bill does originate a communication, this is heard by Joe, answered by Joe´ and acknowledged by Bill´.

Thus we get the normal cycle of a communication between two terminals, for in this case Joe is a terminal and Bill is a terminal and communication can be seen to flow between two terminals. The cycles depend on Joe originating communication, Bill hearing the communication, Bill becoming Bill´ and answering the communication, Joe´ acknowledging the communication, then Bill originating a communication, Joe hearing the communication, Joe´ answering the communication and Bill´ acknowledging the communication.

If they did this, regardless of what they were talking about, they would never become in an argument and would eventually reach an agreement, even if they were hostile to one another. Their difficulties and problems would be cleared up and they would be, in relationship to each other, in good shape.

A two-way communication cycle breaks down when either terminal fails, in its turn, to originate communications. We discover that the entire society has vast difficulties along this line. They are so used to canned entertainment and so inhibited in originating communications by parents who couldn't communicate, and by education and other causes, that people get very low on communication origin. Communication origin is necessary to start a communication in the first place.

Thus we find people talking mainly about things which are forced upon them by exterior causes. They see an accident, they discuss it. They see a movie, they discuss it. They wait for an exterior source to give them the occasion for a conversation. But in view of the fact that both are low on the origin of communication—which could also be stated as low on imagination—we discover that such people, dependent on exterior primal impulses, are more or less compulsive or inhibitive in communication, and thus the conversation veers rapidly and markedly and may wind up with some remarkable animosities (hostile feelings) or misconclusions.

Let us suppose that lack of prime or original cause impulse on Joe's part has brought him into obsessive or compulsive communication, and we find that he is so busy outflowing that he never has a chance to hear anyone who speaks to him, and if he did hear them, would not answer them. Bill, on the other hand, might be so very, very, very low on primal cause (which is to say, low on communication origination) that he never even moves into Bill′, or if he does, would never put forth his own opinion, thus unbalancing Joe further and further into further and further compulsive communication.

As you can see by these graphs, some novel situations could originate. There would be the matter of obsessive answering as well as inhibitive answering. An individual could spend all of his time answering, justifying or explaining—all the same thing—no primal communication having been originated at him. Another individual, as Joe′ in Graph A or Bill′ in Graph B, might spend all of his time acknowledging, even though nothing came his way to acknowledge. The common and most noticed manifestations, however, are obsessive and compulsive origin, and nonanswering acceptance, and nonacknowledgment of answer. And at these places we can discover stuck flows.

As the only crime in the universe seems to be to communicate, and as the only saving grace of a person is to communicate, we can readily understand that an entanglement of communication is certain to result. What we should understand—and much more happily—is that it can now be resolved.

Flows become stuck on this twin cycle of communication where a scarcity occurs in:

1. origination of communication,

2. receipt of communication,

3. answering a communication given,

4. acknowledging answers.

Thus it can be seen that there are only four parts which can become problematic in both Graph A and Graph B, no matter the number of peculiar manifestations which can occur as a result thereof.

COMMUNICATION TRAINING DRILLS

Now that you have discovered the component parts of communication and its formula, how do you use this knowledge? How do you put into practice what you have just studied on the formula of communication? How do you apply the laws of communication so easily and naturally that they almost seem to be a part of you? How, in fact, do you become effective in communication?

In Scientology there are drills that enable anyone to improve his or her level of communication skill. A *drill* is a method of learning or training whereby a person does a procedure over and over again in order to perfect that skill. These communication drills, called *Training Routines* or *TRs* for short, deal with the various parts of the communication formula.

The TRs were originally developed to train Scientology practitioners in technical application, as a high level of communication skill is vital for this activity. However, by drilling each part of the communication formula with these TRs, *any* person's ability to master the communication cycle and thus better communicate with others can be vastly improved.

By doing these drills you will learn how to make your communication understood by others and how to truly understand what they say to you, how to be what is sometimes called "a good listener," how to guide a communication cycle you are having with another person and how to recognize and rectify failures in the communication cycles of others.

These are all skills of immeasurable value in day-to-day life. No matter what your occupation or what kind of activities you are involved in, the ability to communicate with ease and certainty is essential.

The TRs cannot be done alone; you must do them with the help of another person. The way that this is done is that you pair up with another person and do the drills together. This is done on a turnabout basis: when you are doing the drill, the other person helps you become skilled on that drill. Then you switch around and help the other person while he or she does the drill. The action of helping another through the drill is called *coaching.*

The drills give directions for the roles of *student* and *coach.* When you are practicing the drill you are called the *student,* and the person helping you get through the drill is called the *coach.*

It makes no difference whether you start out first as student and your partner as coach, or vice versa. You both take turns being student then coach, to get each other through the drills. By helping each other through the TRs on this alternating basis, you are both able to learn how to fully use the communication cycle.

So, before you embark on doing the TRs, find another person to do the drills with you on this turnabout basis of *student* and *coach.*

It is very important that both you and your partner read through and understand all these drills *before* beginning to practice them. Also, another section follows the drills which explains how to coach someone correctly. This too should be thoroughly studied and understood before the drills are started, as coaching is a very precise procedure. It is vital that proper coaching is done in order to achieve the best possible gains from the TRs.

Each of the TRs has a *Number* and a *Name,* which are simply designations to refer to them by.

The *Commands* are the spoken directions used in starting, continuing and stopping the drill in coaching, and the questions or statements used while doing the TR.

Each drill also states the *Position* you are to sit in.

The particular communication skill that you are aiming to achieve on each TR is stated under its *Purpose.*

The *Training Stress* outlines how that drill is to be done and gives the important points to stress or emphasize in coaching.

Patter is included in some of the drills to show how the various commands or questions are used during the procedure. In Scientology, the word *patter* simply means the special vocabulary of a drill.

When done diligently and exactly as written, these drills lead to successful communication—for anyone.

Do the following:

1. Read all the way through the drills on the following pages, as well as the section entitled *Coaching*.

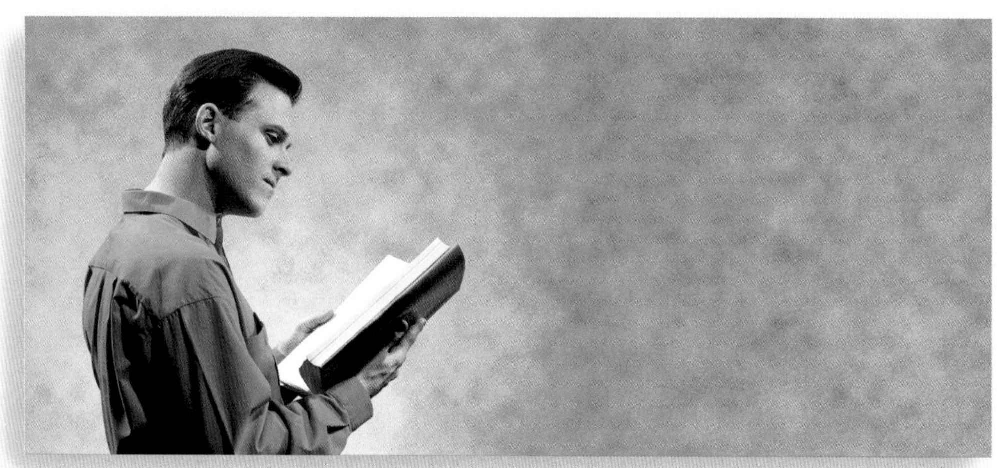

2. Find someone to work with as a partner so you can get each other through the drills.

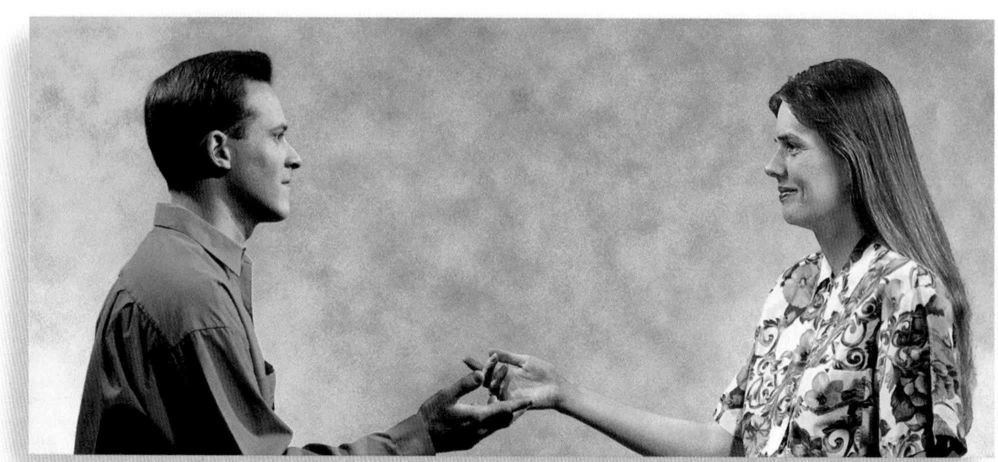

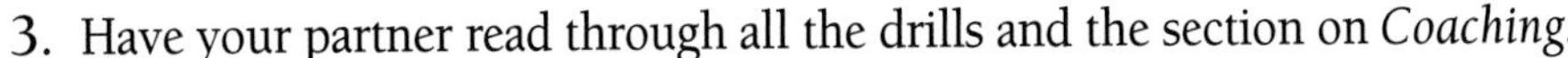

3. Have your partner read through all the drills and the section on *Coaching*.

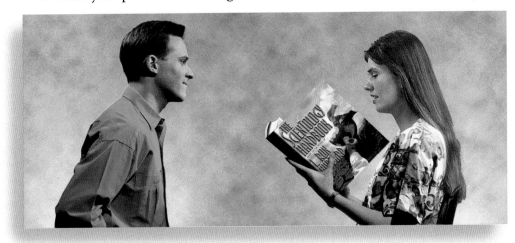

4. Decide which of you will coach first.

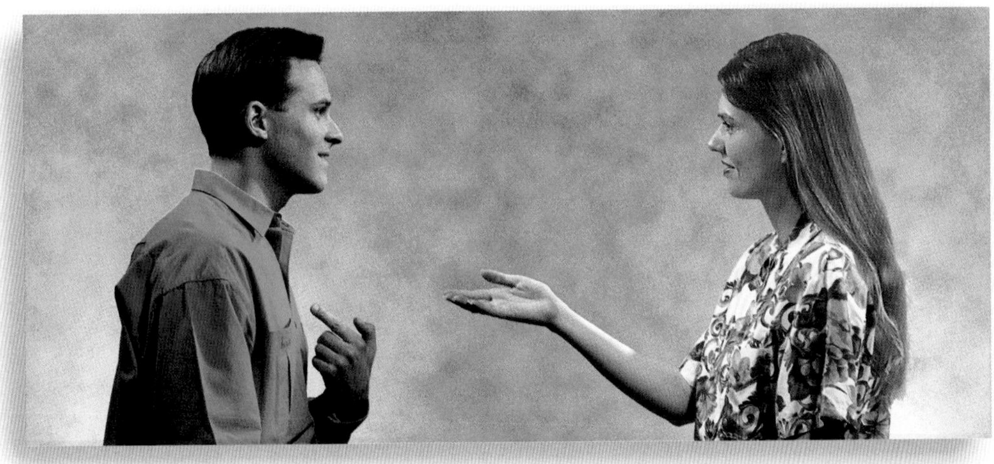

5. Then start the first TR!

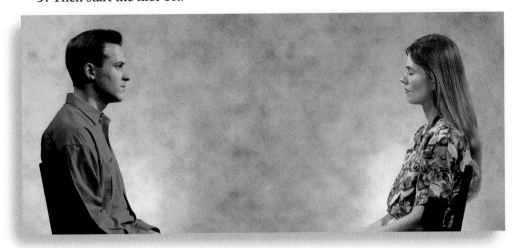

Number: TR 0 Be There

Name: Be There

Commands: The coach says "Start" to begin the drill. The coach uses "That's it" to end the drill or to point out an error to the student. Example: Student falls asleep; coach says, "That's it. You went to sleep. Start."

In this and all drills, when the student has achieved the purpose of the drill, the coach says, "Pass."

Although there is actually little coaching involved in this drill, some is required. The coach starts the drill and keeps the student at it until he passes.

Position: Student and coach sit facing each other a comfortable distance apart—about three feet. The student has his eyes closed.

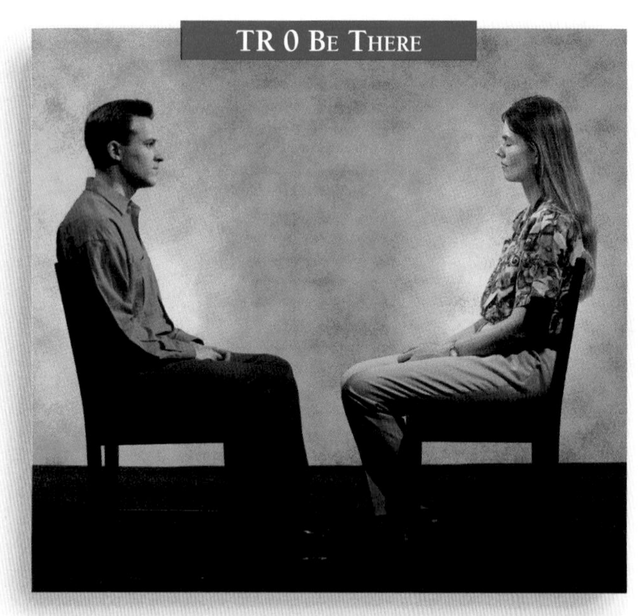

Purpose: To train student to be there comfortably. The idea is to get the student able to *be* there comfortably in a position three feet in front of another person, to *be* there and not do anything else but *be* there.

In order to start a communication, you must be in a place from which to communicate. If you are not *there,* you will not be able to properly start a communication. Being there is a requisite to good communication; there is nothing more complex to it than that.

The student's eyes are closed in this drill to make it easy to be there, as the first step. With eyes closed, one does not have the added requirement of confronting another person, but can simply become accustomed to being there in a relaxed manner.

Training Stress: Student and coach sit facing each other. The student has his eyes closed. There is no conversation. This is a silent drill. There is *no* twitching, moving, "system" or methods used or anything else added to *be* there. Doing something with his body, or forcing his back against the chair in an effort to stay alert, are examples of systems or methods being used instead of simply being there.

One will usually see blackness or an area of the room when one's eyes are closed. *Be there comfortably.*

It is the task of the coach to keep the student alert and doing the drill.

Sit in an upright position in a straight-backed chair. Do the drill until there is no tendency or desire to squirm, twitch, move or change position. If such "turn on," then continue the drill until they are flattened. *Flattened* means the drill has been continued until it no longer produces a reaction.

The student is to do this drill until he is fully convinced, without reservations, that he can continue to sit quietly and comfortably for an indefinite period without any compulsion to twitch or shift about or having to repress such compulsions.

When he can *be* there comfortably and has reached a *major stable win,* the drill is passed.

People commonly experience many improvements while doing TRs, such as an improved ability to confront and to communicate, heightened perceptions, and so on. These are called *wins* as the student has desired to improve his communication skills and his awareness, and each achievement toward accomplishing that is itself a *win*. A *major stable win* means the student has reached the point where he can do that drill, and his skill and ability to do it is stable. A major stable win is a significant, lasting gain.

Number: TR 0 Confronting

Name: Confronting

Confronting is defined as being able to face. When we say one is confronting, we mean that he is facing without flinching or avoiding. The ability to confront is actually the ability to be there comfortably and perceive.

Commands: Coach: "Start," "That's it," "Flunk."

The coach has several terms he uses. The first of these is "Start," at which moment the drill begins. Every time the student does not hold his position, slumps, goes unconscious, twitches, starts his eyes wandering, or in any way demonstrates an incorrect position, the coach says "Flunk" and corrects the difficulty. He then says "Start" again and the drill goes on. When the coach wishes to make comments, he says "That's it," straightens up this point and then again says "Start."

Position: Student and coach sit facing each other a comfortable distance apart—about three feet. Both are looking at each other.

Purpose: To acquire the skill of being able to sit quietly and look at someone without strain.

This drill is the next level of skill up from *TR 0 Be There.* Now he must also confront.

Communication is not really possible in the absence of confront. Have you ever tried to talk to someone who won't look at you? That person is not confronting you. Lack of confront is a barrier to real communication.

Nervous twitches, tensions, all stem from an unwillingness to confront. When that willingness is repaired, these disabilities tend to disappear.

Training Stress: Student and coach sit facing each other, neither making any conversation or effort to be interesting. They sit and look at each other and say and do nothing for some hours. Student must not speak, fidget, giggle or be embarrassed or fall asleep.

It will be found the student tends to confront *with* a body part, rather than just confront. Confronting with a body part can cause the body part to hurt or feel uncomfortable. The solution is just to confront and be there.

The basic rule is that anything which the student is holding tense is the thing *with* which he is confronting. If the student's eyes begin to smart, he is confronting with them. If his stomach begins to protrude and becomes tense, he is confronting with his stomach. If his shoulders or even the back of his head become tense, then he is confronting with the shoulders or the back of his head. An expert coach would in this case give a "That's it," correct the student and then start the drill session anew.

A blink is not a flunk on TR 0 and "blinkless" is not a requirement. The coach should not put any attention on whether somebody is blinking—only on whether or not the person is confronting.

However, wide-eyed staring is unnatural and means the student is trying to confront with his eyes. In such a case the student's eyes will water, become red and will hurt if he continues. A student having excessive trouble with his eyes should be returned to *TR 0 Be There* and master this drill before again attempting to do *TR 0 Confronting.*

TR 0 CONFRONTING

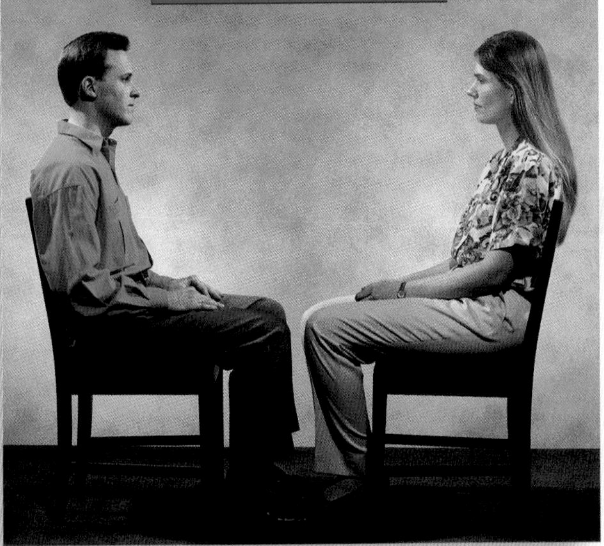

As with *TR 0 Be There,* the student does not use any system or method of confronting other than just *be* there. The drill is misnamed if confronting means to *do* something. The whole action is to accustom the student to comfortably *be there* three feet in front of another without apologizing or moving or being startled or embarrassed or defending self.

Continue the drill until any twitches, flinches or other manifestations no longer exist or have to be suppressed (kept from being known or seen). Anything that turns on will flatten.

Student passes when he can just *be* there and confront and he has reached a *major stable win.*

Number: TR 0 Bullbait

Name: Confronting, Bullbaited

The term *bullbait* means to find certain actions, words, phrases, mannerisms or subjects that cause a student doing the drill to become distracted by reacting to the coach. The word *bullbait* is derived from an English and Spanish sport of *baiting* which meant to set dogs upon a chained bull.

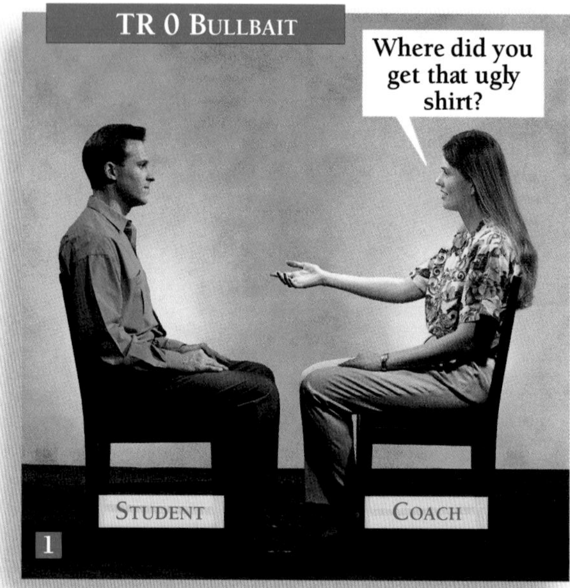

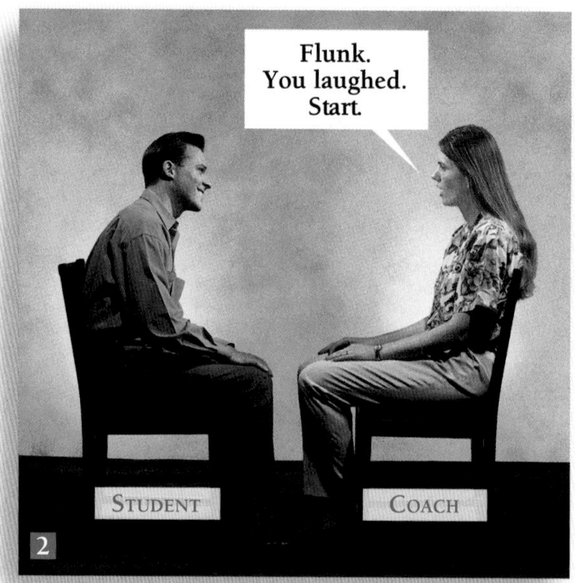

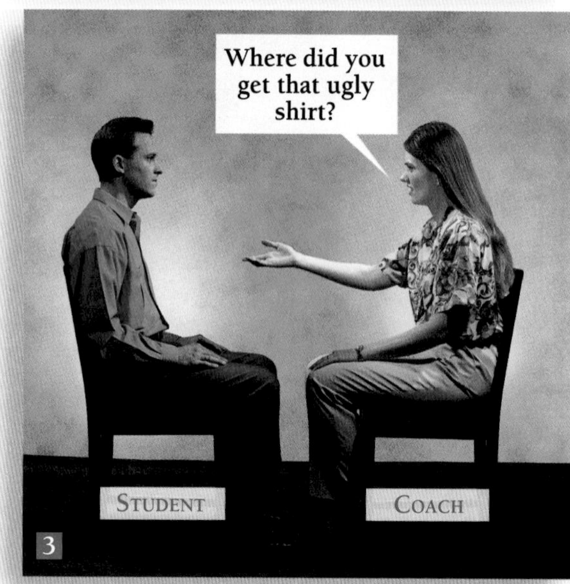

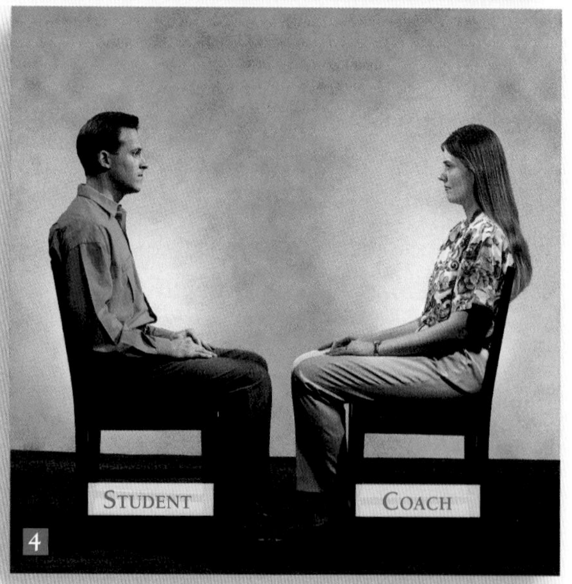

In the photographs above, the coach finds a button on the student (1) and flunks him for breaking his confront (2). She resumes the drill and repeats the phrase which made him react (3), repeating it until the student can comfortably confront it,

It will be found that people have certain things that cause them to react in some way. In Scientology we call this a *button:* an item, word, phrase, subject or area that causes response or reaction in an individual.

For example, the coach says something to the student like, "You have big ears." The student reacts by laughing uncontrollably. The coach has thus found a button on that student. This is bullbaiting.

Commands: Coach: "Start," "That's it," "Flunk."

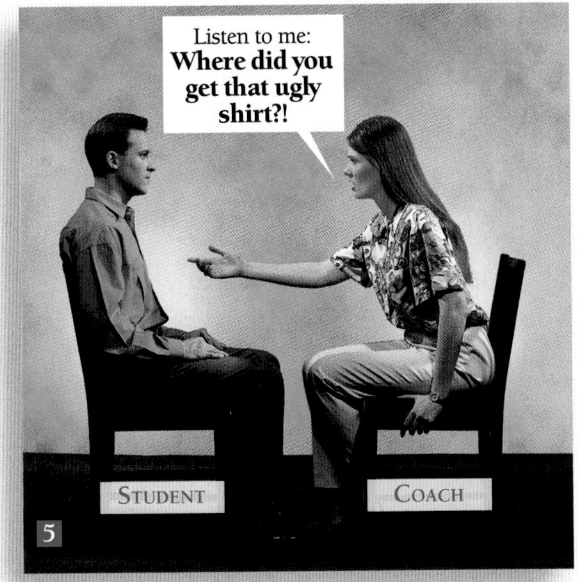

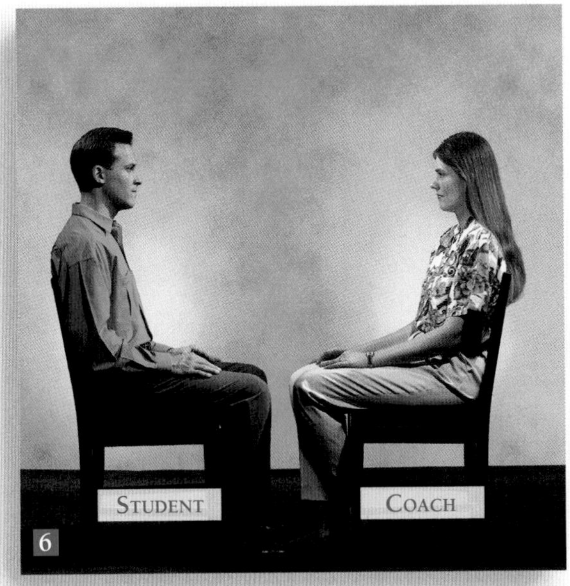

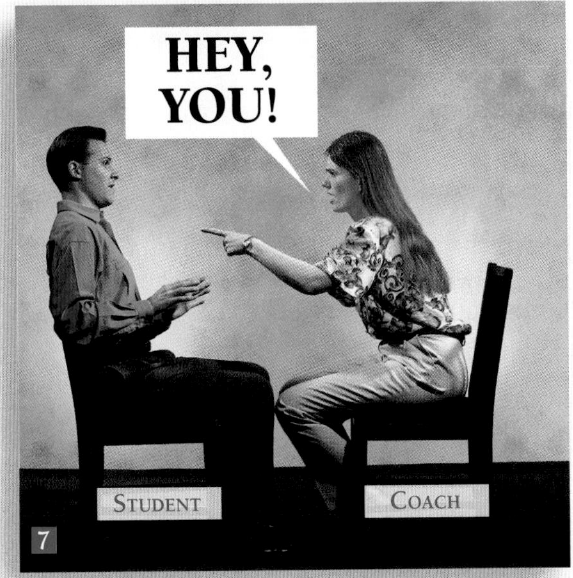

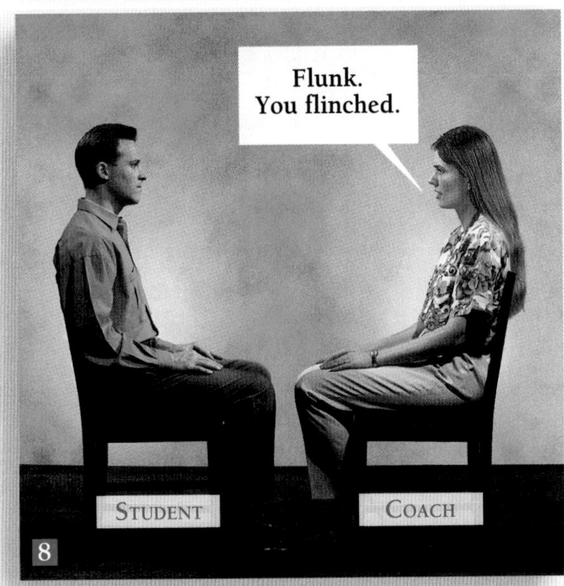

without reacting to it (4, 5, 6). She continues bullbaiting, trying to find another button. When she does so (7), she flunks the student with the reason why (8) and would now proceed to flatten the new button.

Position: Student and coach sit facing each other a comfortable distance apart—about three feet.

Purpose: To acquire the skill of being able to sit quietly and look at someone without strain and without being thrown off, distracted or made to react in any way to what the other person says or does.

In the previous drill, a student learns how to confront with the coach just sitting silently. In *TR 0 Bullbait* the student's ability to confront is increased further and he learns not to be thrown off by the actions of the coach.

This enhances the ability to be there and deliver a communication to another, in any social or life situation, without being distracted by anything.

For example, have you ever had the experience of talking to someone and becoming tongue-tied or flustered when the other person brought up some other subject? Have you ever reacted uncontrollably to something another said even though you didn't want to? This drill can increase your ability to be more causative and in control, in all aspects of communication.

Training Stress: After the student has passed *TR 0 Confronting* and can just *be* there comfortably, "bullbaiting" can begin. Anything added to *being there* is sharply flunked by the coach. Twitches, blinks, sighs, fidgets, anything except just being there is promptly flunked, with the reason why.

Patter as a Coach: Student coughs. Coach: "Flunk! You coughed. Start." This is the whole of the coach's patter as a coach.

Patter as a Confronted Subject: The coach may say anything or do anything except leave the chair. However, the coach must be realistic in his coaching, giving real conditions and circumstances that could come up in everyday life. The coach may not touch the student.

The student's buttons can be found and tromped on hard until they no longer produce a reaction. Any words not coaching words may receive *no* response from the student. If student responds, the coach is instantly a coach (and follows the patter above).

Student passes when he can *be* there comfortably without being thrown off or distracted or made to react in any way to anything the coach says or does and has reached a *major stable win.*

Number: TR 1

Name: Getting Your Communication Across

Purpose: To acquire the skill of getting one specific communication across to a listener and understood.

Have you ever seen someone who just keeps talking, without ever knowing whether or not his communications are being received? Making oneself understood is an important part of the communication formula.

Commands: A phrase (with the "he said's" omitted) is picked out of the book *Alice in Wonderland* and read to the coach. It is repeated until the coach is satisfied it arrived where he is.

Position: Student and coach are seated facing each other a comfortable distance apart.

Training Stress: The communication goes from the book to the student and, as his own, to the coach. It must not go from book to coach. It must sound natural not artificial. Diction (the manner of pronouncing words) and elocution (the mannerisms and art of public speaking) have no part in it. Loudness may have.

The coach must have received the communication (or question) clearly and have understood it before he says "Good."

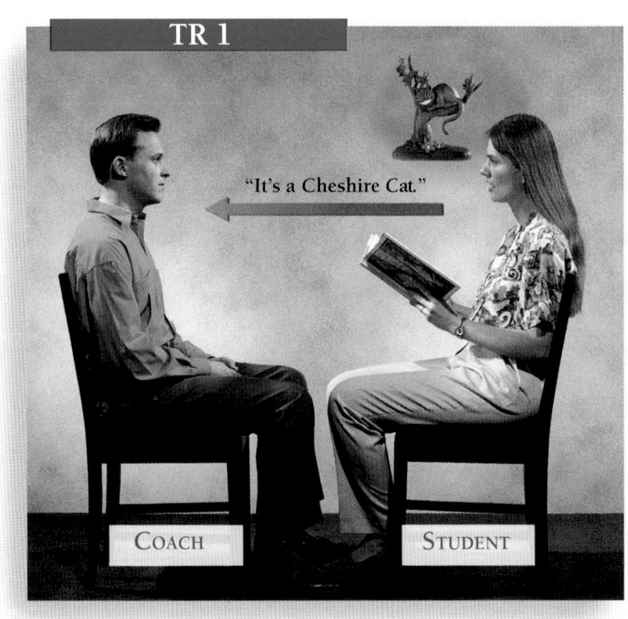

There is no special significance to using the book *Alice in Wonderland.* In this drill you say things from a book instead of making them up.

Any idea is yours that you make yours. When you take an idea out of a book, it becomes your idea, and then as your idea you relay it to another person. The drill is coached this way. The communication is not from the book to the coach. It is from the book to the student, and then the student, making it his own idea, expresses that idea to the coach in such a way that it arrives at the coach.

We know at once a person can't communicate when he cannot take this first basic step of taking an idea, owning it and then communicating it to someone else.

In coaching we want the student to find a phrase in *Alice in Wonderland* and then, taking that as his own idea, communicate it directly to the coach. He can say the same phrase over and over, if he wishes, in any way he wishes to say it, until the coach tells him that he thinks the communication has arrived.

It is the intention that communicates, not the words. When the intention to communicate to a person goes across, the communication will arrive.

The intention must communicate, and it must be communicated in one unit of time. It isn't repeated from the last time it was repeated. It is new, fresh, communicated in present time. Once a communication is relayed across successfully, then he can find another communication and communicate that.

Patter: The coach says "Start," says "Good" without a new start if the communication is received or says "Flunk" if the communication is not received. "Start" is not used again. "That's it" is used to terminate for a discussion or to end the activity. If the drill session is terminated for a discussion, coach must say "Start" again before it resumes.

This drill is passed only when the student can put across a communication naturally, without strain or artificiality or elocutionary bobs and gestures, and when the student can do it easily and relaxedly.

Number: TR 2

Name: Acknowledgments

An *acknowledgment* is something said or done to inform another that his statement or action has been noted, understood and received.

Purpose: To acquire the skill of totally, completely and finally acknowledging a statement, observation or comment in such a way that the person making it is happy with the fact that it has been wholly received and understood and feels no need to repeat or continue it.

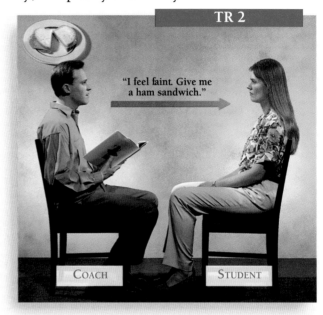

Acknowledgment is a control factor in the cycle of communication. This is true of any communication cycle in any type of situation. The formula of control is start, change and stop. If you can start something, change it and then stop it, you are in control of it. An acknowledgment is a "stop." Therefore, if one acknowledges the communications of others properly, he can control communication.

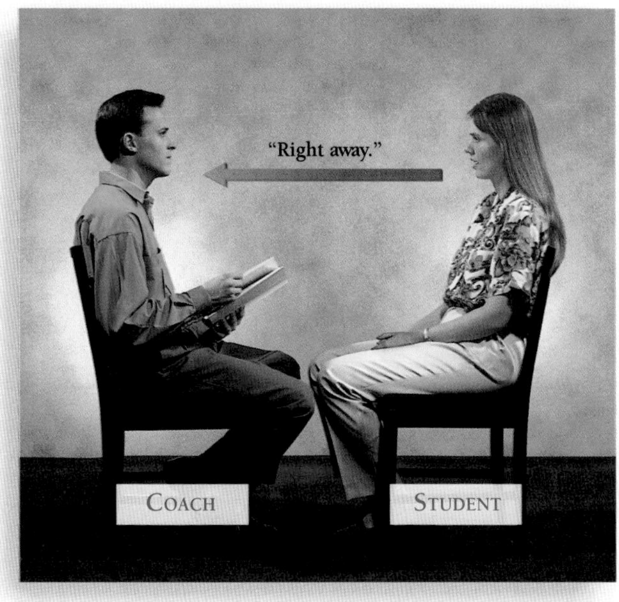

If you said to someone, "Keep going" or "Keep talking," you would not be acknowledging him. The perfect acknowledgment communicates only this: *I have heard your communication.* It signalizes that the person's communication to you has been received. It isn't the word that ends a cycle of communication, it's the intention that ends it.

In life, it is actually very therapeutic for a person to know that he has been acknowledged.

Commands: The coach reads lines from *Alice in Wonderland,* omitting the "he said's," and the student thoroughly acknowledges them. The student says "Good," "Fine," "Okay," "I heard that," *anything* only so long as it is appropriate to the person's communication—in such a way as actually to convince the person who is sitting there that he has heard it. The coach repeats any line he feels was not truly acknowledged.

Position: Student and coach are seated facing each other at a comfortable distance apart.

Training Stress: The student must acknowledge in such a way that the coach is convinced there is no need to repeat himself, that it has been received and understood, totally and finally.

The student does this by *intending* that the communication cycle ends at that point and ending it there. Anything the student does to make that come about is legitimate provided that it does not dismay or upset the coach. The student acknowledges in a manner appropriate to the coach's communication and convinces the coach that he has received it.

Ask the student from time to time what *was* said. Curb over- and under-acknowledgment. Let the student do anything at first to get acknowledgment across, then even him out. Teach him that an acknowledgment is a stop, not the beginning of a new cycle of communication or an encouragement to another to go on and that an acknowledgment must be appropriate for the person's communication. The student must not develop the habit of robotically using "Good," "Thank you" as the only acknowledgments.

Another point of this drill is to teach further that one can fail to get an acknowledgment across or can fail to stop a person with an acknowledgment or can take a person's head off with an acknowledgment which is overdone.

Patter: The coach says "Start," reads a line and says "Flunk" every time the coach feels there has been an improper acknowledgment. The coach repeats the same line after each time he says "Flunk." "That's it" may be used to terminate for discussion or terminate the drill session. "Start" must be used to begin again after a "That's it."

This drill is passed only when the student can totally, completely and finally acknowledge a statement, observation or comment in such a way that the person making it is happy with the fact that it has been wholly received and understood and feels no need to repeat it or continue it.

Number: TR 2 1/2

Name: Half-Acknowledgments

A *half-acknowledgment* is a way of keeping a person talking by giving him the feeling that he is being heard.

Purpose: To acquire the skill to encourage someone who is talking to continue talking.

It is not uncommon to communicate with someone who has apparently finished talking but hasn't really completed saying what he intended to say. Consequently, you could acknowledge him before he has completed and end up chopping his communication. In instances such as this, you have to be alert and observe when the person has more to say and not only let the communication flow to its complete end, but encourage the person to continue talking so he can actually complete his communication.

You may, for instance, find yourself in a conversation with someone and want him to continue talking because you want to know more about what he is saying. The use of a half-acknowledgment is a method to encourage this.

Commands: The coach reads lines from *Alice in Wonderland,* omitting "he said's," and the student half-acknowledges the coach in such a way as to cause the coach to continue talking. The coach should give partial statements that would require a half-acknowledgment from the student. The coach repeats any line he feels was not half-acknowledged.

Position: The student and coach are seated facing each other a comfortable distance apart.

Training Stress: Teach the student that a half-acknowledgment is an encouragement to a person to *continue* talking. Curb overacknowledgment that stops a person from talking. Teach him further that a half-acknowledgment is a way of keeping a person talking by giving the person the feeling that he is being heard.

The student nods or gives half-acknowledgments in such a way as to cause the coach to continue talking. The student must not use direct statements such as "go on" or "continue" to accomplish his purpose. Smiling, nodding and other means are employed. The coach must feel persuaded to continue to talk.

Any positive acknowledgments that would end off the communication flow and any failure to look or act in a manner that invites the coach to continue to talk are flunked and the drill is started again.

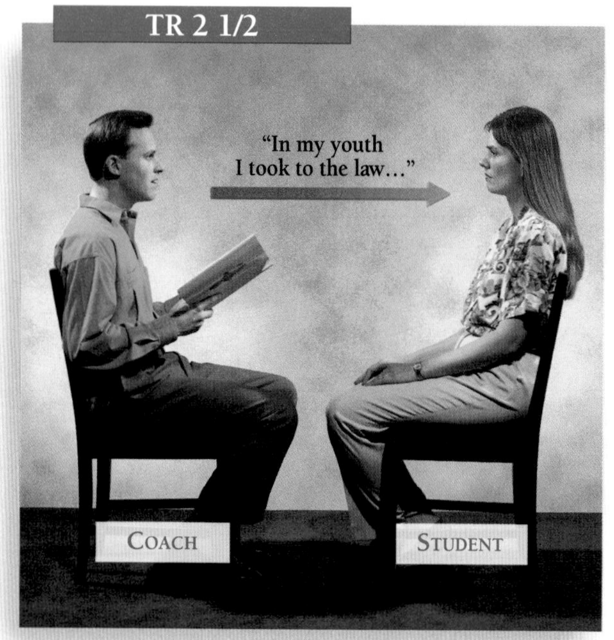

TR 2 1/2
"In my youth
I took to the law..."

Patter: The coach says "Start," reads a line and says "Flunk" every time the coach feels there has been an improper half-acknowledgment. The coach repeats the same line each time after saying "Flunk," until the student gives a proper half-acknowledgment. "That's it" may be used to terminate for discussion or terminate the drill session. If the drill session is terminated for discussion, the coach must say "Start" again to resume it.

The drill is passed when the student is confident that he can cause at will another person to continue to talk.

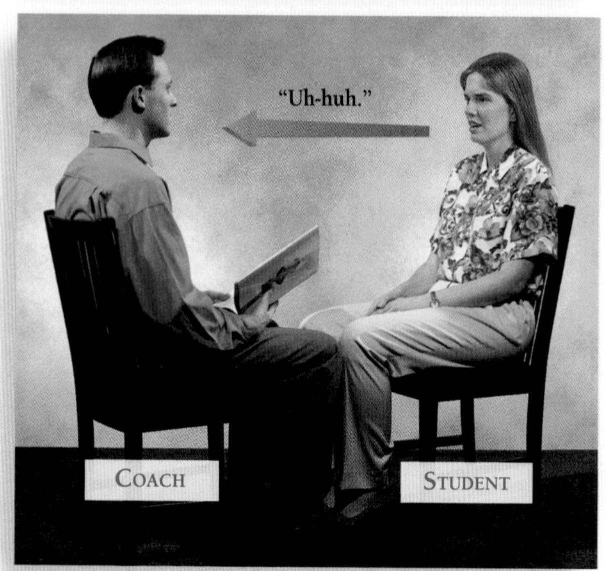

"...and argued each case
with my wife."

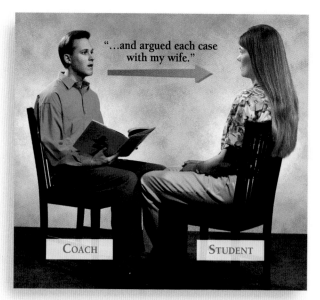

"Uh-huh."

Number: TR 3

Name: Getting a Question Answered

Purpose: To acquire the skill of getting a single exact question answered despite diversions.

Have you ever asked a question and not gotten an answer? This can be upsetting, as the communication cycle is incomplete and is left suspended.

In social or other situations, it is important to be able to get your question answered and complete cycles of communication. This drill gives you that ability.

Commands: Either "Do fish swim?" or "Do birds fly?"

Position: Student and coach seated a comfortable distance apart.

Training Stress: One question and student acknowledgment of its answer in one unit of time which is then finished. To keep the student from straying into variations of question.

The student is flunked if he or she fails to get an answer to the question asked, if he or she fails to repeat the exact question, if he or she Q-and-As with excursions taken by the coach.

Q and A is short for "Question and Answer." It means to not get an answer to one's question, to fail to complete something or to deviate from an intended course of action. Example: Question: "Do birds fly?" Answer: "I don't like birds." Question: "Why not?" Answer: "Because they're dirty." This is Q and A—the original question has not been answered and has been dropped and the person who asked the question has deviated. One could say that he "Q-and-Aed."

Each time a question is repeated it exists, theoretically and purely, in its own moment of time and is uttered itself in present time with its own intention.

When a student is being a machine, simply repeating a question over and over again, there is no intention there. Therefore, when one is repeating a question, it must be expressed in present time as itself with its intention. If a question is always uttered in present time it could be said over and over again without any problem. If a question is repeated over and over with no new intention it becomes arduous.

Patter: The coach uses "Start" and "That's it" as in earlier TRs. The coach is not bound after starting to answer the student's question, but may give a commenting-type answer that doesn't really answer the question, in order to throw the student off. Often the coach should answer the actual question asked by the student. Example:

Student: "Do fish swim?"

Coach: "Yes."

Student: "Good."

Somewhat less often the coach attempts to pull the student into a Q and A or upset the student. Example:

Student: "Do fish swim?"

Coach: "Aren't you hungry?"

Student: "Yes."

Coach: "Flunk."

When the question is not answered, the student must repeat the question until he gets an answer. Anything except question and acknowledgment is flunked. Unnecessary repeating of the question is flunked. A poor delivery of the question (e.g., lack of intention) is flunked. A poor acknowledgment is flunked. A Q and A is flunked (as in example). Student upset or confusion is flunked. Student failure to utter the next question without a long communication lag is flunked.

A choppy or premature acknowledgment is flunked. Lack of an acknowledgment (or with a distinct communication lag) is flunked. Any words from the coach except an answer to the question, "Start," "Flunk," "Good" or "That's it" should have no influence on the student except to get him to repeat the question again.

"Start," "Flunk," "Good" and "That's it" may not be used to fluster or trap the student. Any other statement under the sun may be. The coach should not use introverted statements such as, "I just had a realization." "Coach divertive" statements should all concern the student, not the coach, and should be designed to throw the student off and cause the student to lose control or track of what the student is doing. The student's job is to keep the drill going in spite of anything, using only question or acknowledgment. If the student does anything else than the above, it is a flunk and the coach must say so.

When the student can consistently get his question answered despite diversions, he has passed this drill.

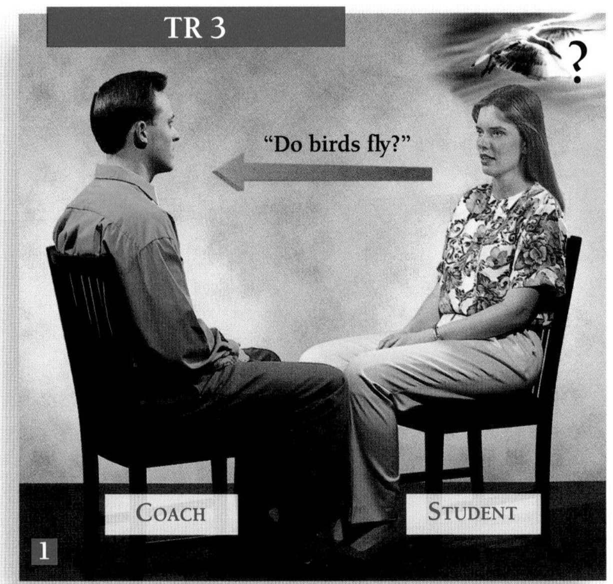

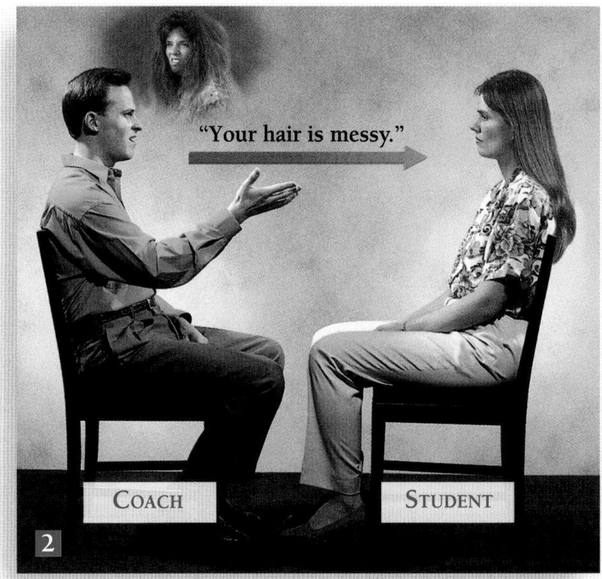

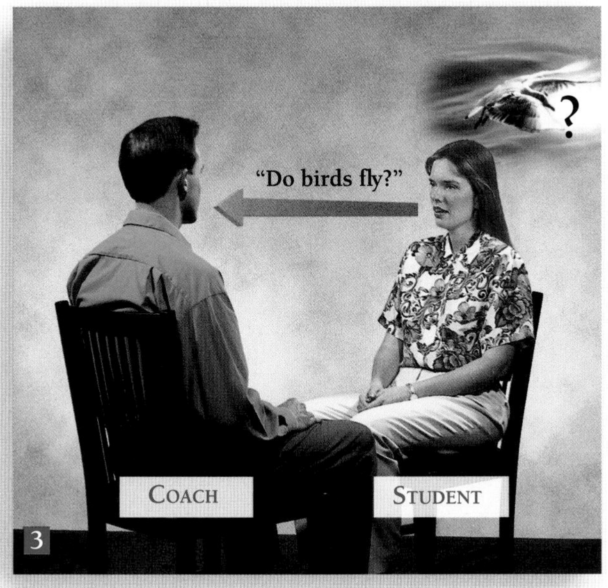

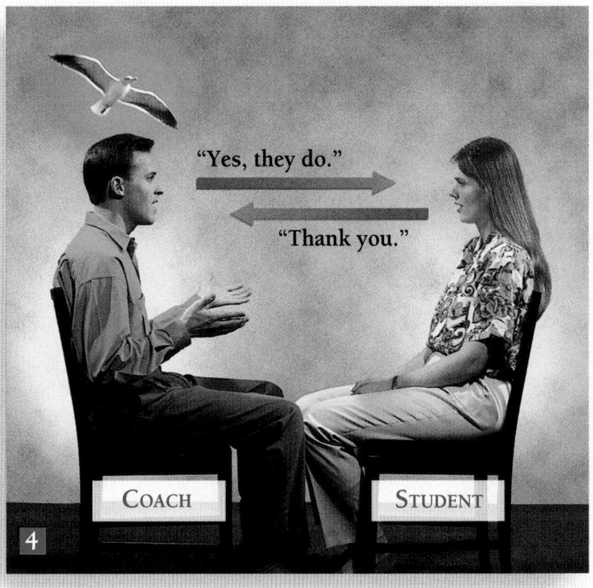

Number: TR 4

Name: Handling Originations

Definition: As used in this drill, the word *origination* means something voluntarily said or done unexpectedly by a person concerning himself, his ideas, reactions or difficulties.

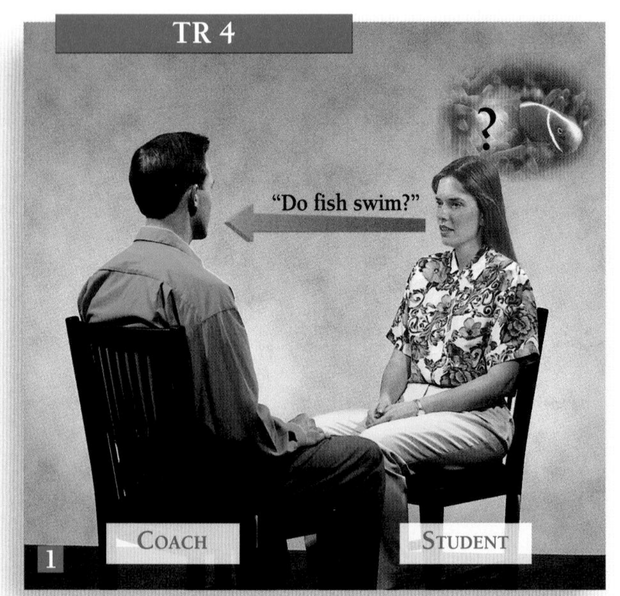

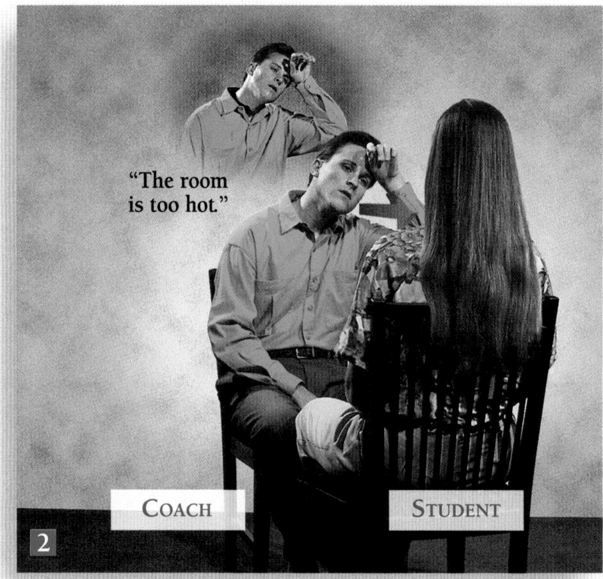

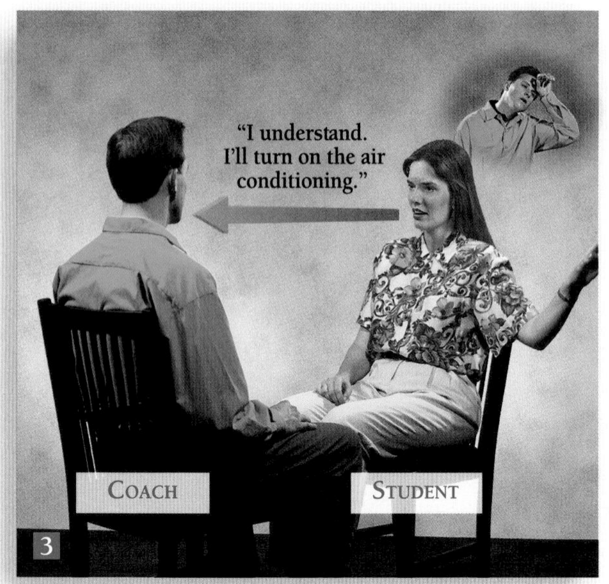

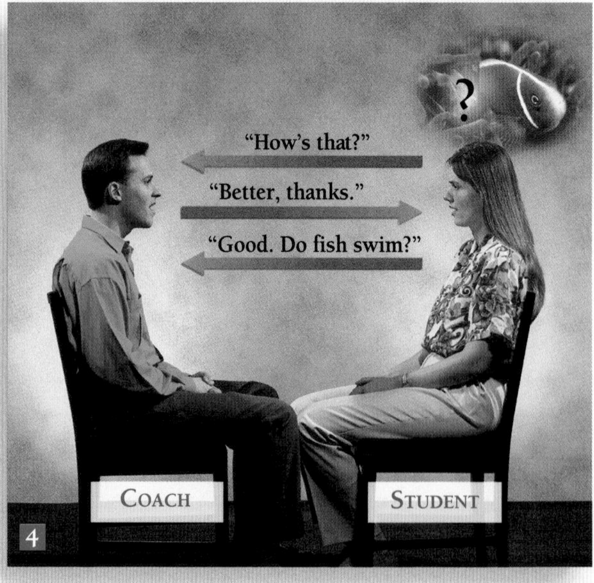

Purpose: To teach the student not to be tongue-tied or startled or thrown off by the originations of another and to maintain good communication throughout an origination.

People frequently say the most astonishing things and take you completely by surprise.

Almost every argument you have had was because you did not handle an origination. If a person walks in and says he just passed with the highest mark in the whole school, and you say how hungry you are, you'll find yourself in a fight. He feels ignored.

Handling an origination merely tells the person you've heard what he said. This might be called a form of acknowledgment, but it isn't; it is the communication formula in reverse. The person you were speaking to is now the cause-point of the communication and is speaking to you. Thus you now have to handle this origination and once again resume your role as cause-point to complete the original communication cycle.

Commands: The student asks the coach, "Do fish swim?" or "Do birds fly?" Coach answers, but now and then makes startling comments from the prepared Origination Sheet provided on page 182. Student must handle originations to satisfaction of coach.

Position: Student and coach sit facing each other at a comfortable distance apart.

Training Stress: The student is taught to hear origination and do three things. (1) Understand it; (2) Acknowledge it; and (3) Return the person to the original cycle of communication so that it can be completed. If the coach feels abruptness or too much time consumed or lack of comprehension, he corrects the student into better handling.

Patter: All originations concern the coach, his ideas, reactions or difficulties, none concern the student. Otherwise the patter is the same as in earlier training routines. The student's patter is governed by: (1) Clarifying and understanding the origination, (2) Acknowledging the origination, (3) Repeating the question. Anything else is a flunk.

The student must be taught to prevent upsets and differentiate between a vital problem that concerns the person and a mere effort to divert him. Flunks are given if the student does more than (1) Understand; (2) Acknowledge; (3) Return the person to the original cycle of communication.

Coach may throw in remarks personal to student as on TR 3. Student's failure to differentiate between these comments (by trying to handle them) and coach's originations about self is a flunk.

Student's failure to persist is always a flunk in any TR but here more so. Coach should not always read from the Origination Sheet to originate, but can make up his own origination, and not always look at student when about to comment. By *originate* is meant to make a statement or remark referring to the state of the coach or his fancied worries, feelings, attitudes, etc. By *comment* is meant a statement or remark aimed only at student or room. Originations are handled, comments are disregarded by the student. Example:

Student: "Do birds fly?"

Coach: "Yes."

Student: "Thank you."

Student: "Do birds fly?"

Coach: "I went fishing yesterday."

Student: "Thanks for letting me know. Do birds fly?"

Coach: "Yes, they do."

Student: "Very good."

When the student can smoothly handle originations without being startled or thrown off and can maintain good communication throughout an origination, he has passed this drill.

COACHING

Coaching is a technology in itself, a vital part of Scientology study. It should be thoroughly understood by both you and your partner before starting to drill any of the TRs.

Good coaching can make the difference between getting through a drill with excellent results for a student or not getting through the drill at all.

In order to help you to do the best you possibly can as far as being a coach is concerned, below you will find a few data that will assist you:

1. Coach with a purpose.

Have for your goal when you are coaching someone that the student is going to get the training drill correct; be purposeful in working toward obtaining this goal. Whenever you correct the student as a coach, just don't do it with no reason, with no purpose. Have the purpose in mind for the student to get a better understanding of the training drill and to do it to the best of his ability.

2. Coach with reality.

Be realistic in your coaching. When you give an origination to a student, really make it an origination, not just something that the sheet said you should say, so that it is as if the student was having to handle it exactly as you say under real conditions and circumstances. This does not mean, however, that you really feel the things that you are giving the student, such as saying to him, "My leg hurts." This does not mean that your leg should hurt, but you should say it in such a manner as to get across to the student that your leg hurts. Another thing about this is do not use any experiences from your past to coach with. Be inventive in the present.

3. Coach with an intention.

Behind all your coaching should be your intention that by the end of the drill the student will be aware that he is doing better at the end of it than he did at the beginning. The student must have a feeling that he has accomplished something in the training drill, no matter how small it is. It is your intention and always should be while coaching that the student you are coaching be a more able person and have a greater understanding of that on which he is being coached.

4. In coaching take up only one thing at a time.

For example, using TR 4, if the student arrives at the goal set up for TR 4, then check over, one at a time, the earlier TRs. Is he confronting you? Does he originate the question to you each time as his own and did he really intend for you to receive it? Are his acknowledgments ending the cycles of communication, etc. But only coach these things one at a time, never two or more at a time. Make sure that the student does each thing you coach him on correctly before going on to the next training step. The better a student gets at a particular drill or a particular part of a drill you should demand, as a coach, a higher standard of ability. This does not mean that you should be "never satisfied." It does mean that a person can always get better, and once you have reached a certain level of ability, then work toward a new plateau.

If you do find that the student is having a hard time on one of the drills, the first thing to do is have him read over the text of the drill and find any words he did not fully understand and look them up in a dictionary. If this does not remedy the situation, check if it is one of the *earlier* drills that he is hung up on. If you find this to be the case, you should go back to the earlier one he is hung up on and get him through that drill to a pass. Once you have done that, start on the next drill and do that one to a pass and come up again through the later ones.

As a coach, you should always work in the direction of better and more precise coaching. Never allow yourself to do a sloppy job of coaching because you would be doing your student a disservice, and we doubt that you would like the same disservice when you are the one being a student.

In coaching, never give an opinion as such, but always give your directions as a direct statement, rather than saying, "I think" or "Well, maybe it might be this way," etc.

When a coach, you are primarily responsible for the drill and the results that are obtained on the student.

Once in a while the student will start to rationalize and justify what he is doing if he is doing something wrong. He will give you reasons why and "becauses." Talking about such things at great length does not accomplish very much. The only thing that does accomplish the goals of the TR and resolves any differences is doing the drill. You will get further by doing it than by talking about it.

In the TRs, the coach should coach with the material given under "Training Stress" and "Purpose."

These drills occasionally have a tendency to upset the student. There is a possibility that during a drill a student may become angry or upset. Should this occur, the coach must help the student through the upset rather than ending the drill and leaving the student in distress. In such an instance, just leaving the student sitting there will in fact leave him more upset than getting him through the drill. The intention of the drill is to teach the student to communicate, and any upset is purely incidental to the drill and plays no part in it.

There is a small thing that most people forget to do and that is telling the student when he has gotten the drill right or he has done a good job on a particular step. Besides correcting wrongnesses, there is also complimenting rightness.

You very definitely "flunk" the student for anything that amounts to "self-coaching" (where the student attempts to correct himself). The reason for this is that the student will tend to introvert (look inward) and will look too much at how he is doing and what he is doing rather than just doing it.

As a coach, keep your attention on the student and how he is doing and don't become so interested in what you yourself are doing that you neglect the student and are unaware of his ability or inability to do the drill correctly. It is easy to become "interesting" to a student, to make him laugh and act up a bit. But your main job as a coach is to see how good he can get in each training drill and that is what you should have your attention on; that, and how well he is doing.

To a large degree the progress of the student is determined by the standard of coaching. Good results produce better people.

Once coaching is understood by you and your partner, you are ready to drill on the TRs. Doing these drills exactly as described is key to successfully mastering them.

It takes hours and hours of practice on these drills to perfect them, but it is time well spent. Each of the TRs is done until the student has achieved the purpose of the drill and can *do* that TR.

A student can spend many hours on any TR before reaching a point where he really acquires the skill of that TR and maintains it. This is particularly true of *TR 0 Be There, TR 0 Confronting* and *TR 0 Bullbait.*

There is one TR which has a specific time requirement for passing: on *TR 0 Confronting,* the student is to do the drill until he has reached a point where he can do it comfortably for two hours straight.

The coach works with the student on a particular TR to a point where the student achieves an increased ability to do the drill well. However, it is better to go through the TRs several times, from *TR 0 Be There* to *TR 4* in sequence, getting tougher each time, than to stay on one forever or for the coach to be so tough at the start that the student goes into a decline.

With tough but fair coaching conducted on a proper gradient, the student will complete these TRs with certainty in his ability to apply the communication formula in any situation he may be called upon to face.

This is one of the most valuable abilities he will ever learn.

Origination Sheet

Coach uses these now and then in Training Routine Number 4
Handling Originations

I have a pain in my stomach.

The room seems bigger.

My body feels heavy.

I had a twitch in my leg.

I feel like I'm sinking.

The colors in the room are brighter.

My head feels lopsided.

I feel wonderful.

I have an awful feeling of fear.

You are the first person who ever listened to me.

I just realized I've had a headache for years.

This is silly.

I feel all confused.

I've got a sharp pain in my back.

I feel lighter somehow.

I can't tell you.

I feel terrible—like I'd lost something, or something.

WOW—I didn't know that before.

The room seems to be getting dark.

I feel awfully tense.

You surely have a nice office here.

I feel warm all over.

By the way, I won that tennis tournament yesterday.

My head feels like it has a tight band round it.

Continued...

When are you going to get a haircut?

I feel like I was all hemmed in somehow.

Who is going to win the cup final?

This chair is so comfortable I could go to sleep.

I keep thinking about that cop who blew his whistle at me this morning.

How long do we have to do this?

My face tingles.

I'm getting sleepy.

I'm starving. Let's go to lunch.

Suddenly, I'm so tired.

Everything is getting blurry.

Is this room rocking?

I just realized how wrong I've been all my life.

I feel like there is a spider's web on my face.

My left knee hurts.

I feel so light!

Isn't it getting hotter in here?

I just remembered the first time I went swimming.

My back has been aching like this for years.

Are you married?

I feel so lonesome.

I feel like I can't talk.

My body is starting to shake all over.

My ribs hurt.

Everything seems to be getting dark.

Don't you get tired of listening to someone like me?

COMMUNICATION IS LIFE

One's ability to communicate can spell the difference between success or failure in all aspects of living. You will notice that those people you know who are successful in their endeavors generally have a high ability to communicate; those who are not, do not.

Communication is not just a way of getting along in life, it is the heart of life. It is by thousands of percent the senior factor in understanding life and living it successfully.

We instinctively revere the great artist, painter or musician, and society as a whole looks upon them as not quite ordinary beings. And they are not. But the understanding and skilled use of communication is not only for the artist, it is for anyone.

In examining the whole subject of communication, one is apt to discover, if he takes a penetrating look, that there are very few people around him who are actually *communicating,* but that there are a lot of people who think they are communicating who are not.

The apparency sometimes is that it is better not to communicate than to communicate, but that is never really the case. Communication is the solvent for any human problem. An understanding of communication itself was not available before Scientology.

A thorough knowledge of the communication formula and an understanding of how any difficulties in its application can be recognized and corrected are vital tools to successful living. The knowledge and drills contained in this chapter will start one on the road to success. A professional level of skill can be attained in Scientology churches on the Hubbard Professional TR Course. Here, expert supervision and complete data on the subject are available to those wishing to perfect their ability to communicate.

Communication is life.

Without it we are dead to all.

To the degree we can communicate, we are alive. ■

TEST YOUR UNDERSTANDING

Answer the following questions about the information contained in this chapter. Refer back to it to check your answers. If you need to, review the chapter. Going over the material several times will increase your certainty and help you better apply it.

- ❑ *What is communication?*
- ❑ *How do intention and attention relate to successful communication?*
- ❑ *What is duplication and why is it important in communication?*
- ❑ *What is the cycle of communication?*
- ❑ *How does acknowledgment apply to the cycle of communication?*
- ❑ *What is two-way communication?*
- ❑ *What are TRs and how do they relate to communication?*
- ❑ *What is a coach?*
- ❑ *Why is it important to be able to handle originations?*

PRACTICAL EXERCISES

Here are exercises relating to communication. Doing these exercises will help increase your understanding of the knowledge contained in this chapter.

1 Look around and observe examples of the different parts of communication; note which parts are used and not used in conversations you observe (including intention, attention, duplication, understanding, and whether the people involved are factually being source-point or receipt-point). Continue to observe communications around you until you can easily identify the various parts of communication and identify any parts which are absent or not being used correctly.

2 Notice acknowledgments in communication. Observe two people talking, and pay particular attention to the use of acknowledgment by each person. Note any lack of acknowledgment as well. What differences do you observe in communication when acknowledgment is present compared to when it is not present?

3 Observe two-way communication between two people. Note whether the communication is smooth or not, and observe the different elements of good communication or their absence. Observe other two-way communication cycles, repeating this same exercise.

4 Do each of the TRs. Work with another person as your partner and do the drills, beginning with *TR 0 Be There*. Do each drill exactly as stated in the chapter with the proper use of coaching, until you and your partner both complete each drill to a pass.

RESULTS FROM APPLICATION

The success level of a person is directly linked to his communication level. People who understand the basics of good communication make others around them feel comfortable, understood and recognized. In short, they make others feel worthwhile and important.

The stories below bear testimony to the fact that a person is as alive as he can communicate, and that communication is the universal solvent.

In Europe, a mother had been having great difficulty communicating with her sixteen-year-old daughter. Their relationship became even more strained when she discovered that her daughter had been taking drugs. Here is what she had to say about a Scientology communication course they participated in together as part of a drug withdrawal program:

"This course only took a few hours a day. At that time my daughter and I were not really talking with each other. It was mostly just 'hellos' and 'goodbyes.' The communication course not only helped us to begin to communicate again, but taught us some very valuable things about communicating with another person. We learned how to be relaxed around other people, how to effectively talk as well as listen, how to confront our problems and problems in general, and not run away. The things we learned in those few hours will stay with us a lifetime."

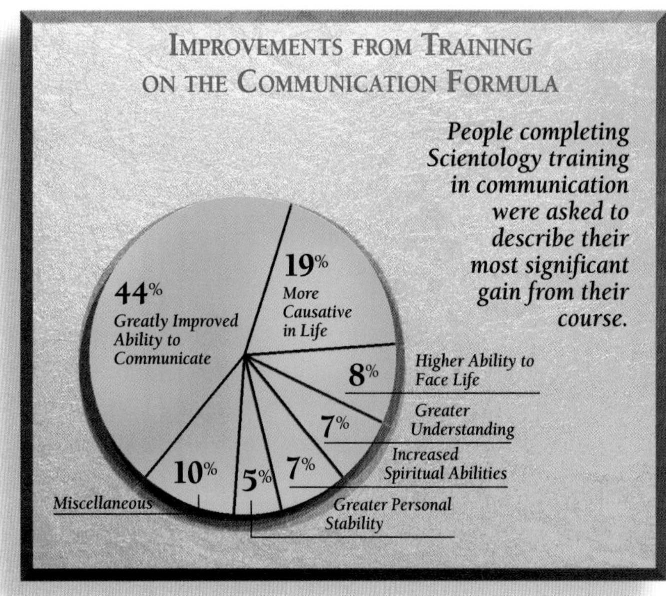

A volunteer nurse in South Africa was traveling in a taxi with several other people when they were held up by an angry man brandishing a knife. At that moment she asked herself, "What data could I apply now that I learned in the Scientology workshops I attended?" She had learned about communication, and determined that all she had to do was face the man *and* the situation and use her communication skills. She then proceeded to quietly talk to the man, telling him not to do something that he would later regret, just for the sake of a little money. This made sense to the criminal and he gave the money back to everyone in the taxi. She was proud that she had been able to handle the situation by using the communication skills she acquired in the Scientology workshops.

Being extremely depressed, a young man from Hawaii was literally looking for a high building to jump from. Luckily, he didn't find one high enough before a friend advised him to instead take a course in Scientology on communication. He went ahead and did the course, despite being barely literate. As he put it:

"I went from someone who wanted to be a nail to someone who is a hammer. It ***totally*** *changed my life! My friends could not believe the miraculous change in me."*

Growing up as a teenager was very difficult for a young woman from Los Angeles as she was not able to communicate to her parents as she would have liked to. She related:

"I loved my parents, but sometimes my communication would not get across to them. I, of course, blamed them for this. After learning the communication formula, and learning what two-way communication was, I was very surprised to find that it was quite easy to talk to my parents. We can now talk about most anything and there is understanding between us, where there wasn't before. The love between us has grown and I like it very much. What a difference this has made in my life. Thank you, Mr. Hubbard."

In New York City, a girl who had just learned about L. Ron Hubbard's technology on communication was walking home with her husband one night when they heard sudden screeching brakes and a thump. They swiftly walked over to the scene of the accident—a man had been hit by a car driven by a drunk driver. The wife said that just by knowing and using the communication formula and how to control a situation, she was able to handle a lot of confusion:

"The man was obviously in pain. My husband immediately began using basic Scientology techniques to assist the man and told me to start putting order into the environment. So I got the drunken driver and the other four unruly, intoxicated men out of their car and got them under control. By then a crowd of nearly fifty people had gathered and within ten minutes, using what I had learned about communication, I had them under control too. When the police showed up, there was virtually nothing left for them to do. I told one of them what we had done and then another cop, who hadn't heard our communication cycle, asked me to step behind the rope. The cop I had spoken to told him, 'Not her, she's the one that did our job!' The driver was carted off to jail and the man who was hit was doing much better on his way to the hospital. We were taken to the police station and filed reports as witnesses and were thanked by the New York Police Department. The sergeant told us that he wished a lot more people could do what we did. This stuff works!"

Communication was a big problem to a woman living on the West Coast. She was painfully shy and life was pretty miserable as a result. Her own description of the situation was:

"Before I learned about the formula of communication, I didn't speak to anyone I didn't know very *well. I used to prop up the wall at parties. I had to ask someone else's opinion before I made any decision in my life. I had had one boyfriend for four weeks only, and I was twenty-five years old! Now I am a lot more sure of myself. I make my own decisions which are always correct and I feel able to speak freely to anyone I meet. I am a lot closer to my family and last month I got engaged to be married. Knowing and using the communication formula has really changed my life."*

The Scientology communication course gave a man from southern California tremendous gains, enhancing his relationship with his family and improving his job performance.

"I experienced **immediate** *benefit from the TRs, both in my relationships with my wife and kids, and in my job. I am applying* **all** *of the drills with fantastic results. I communicated 'eyeball to eyeball' with my wife for the first time in six months without any arguments. We were both* **thrilled**! *I have started to* **listen** *effectively to my kids, and taught them how to acknowledge others in conversation. There was a* **marked** *change in their behavior as a result. And I experienced tremendous increased effectiveness in my job! You know, there is really something here!"*

José knew that he needed better communication skills to handle his life so he enrolled on a communication course and was amazed at the immediate change from doing the Training Routines.

"After I started to apply the TRs, I realized some of the mistakes I had been making in my attempted communication to others. I soon learned the difference between 'talking' and 'communicating.' I can now approach persons whom I used to avoid. I now purposefully communicate with these individuals. I can also tactfully instigate, cause to continue, and terminate conversations with anyone. And my wife and I now engage in quality communication, instead of just 'talking' with each other. That is a big success!"

SUGGESTIONS FOR FURTHER STUDY

The subject of communication occupies a prominent place in the legacy of L. Ron Hubbard's research. He often lectured on the application of communication to benefit others seeking to improve and wrote several books and hundreds of shorter articles on the subject. This chapter could only touch upon some of the most basic principles. There are, however, many other materials available for the interested reader. Those listed below are recommended for further data about communication and practice in its application so as to become skilled in its use.

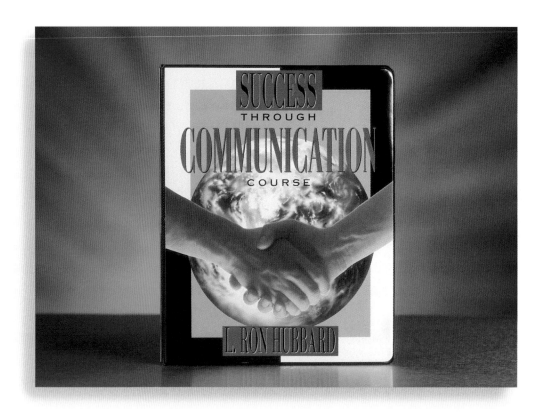

Success Through Communication Course

A week-long course which thoroughly teaches communication skills to train a person to guide and control communication in social or other situations. Contains eighteen separate drills, each one of which deals with a different aspect of good communication. Students learn effective ways to listen, make themselves understood, get their questions answered, handle communication upsets, start and maintain a conversation, get another person talking and much more. This course is for anyone who wants to communicate better. The skills taught here are used by thousands to bring greater success in relationships, careers and many other dealings with people. (Delivered in Scientology organizations.)

The New Hubbard Professional TR Course

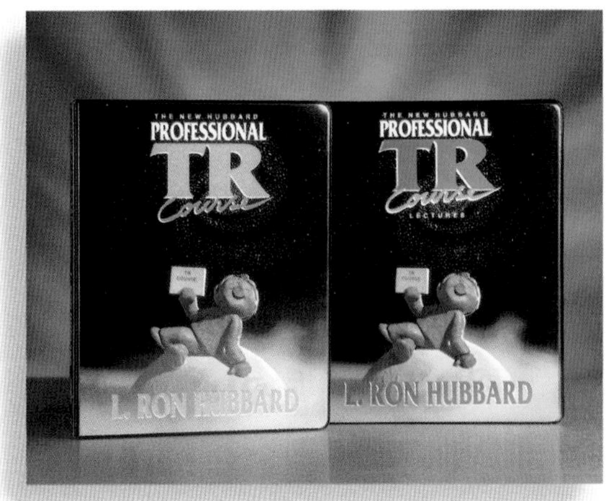

This is the premier course on Scientology communication technology. Here, the full theory on communication is covered, including extensive writings by Mr. Hubbard on the subject, films which provide visual explanations of all aspects of communication as well as superb demonstrations of how to correctly do the TRs, and seven taped lectures wherein Mr. Hubbard demonstrates the correct use of the TRs and proper handling of the cycle of communication. Additionally, the course contains special exercises which vastly increase a person's subjective understanding of communication, helping him to perfect his communication skills. These elements, plus supervision of the student's TR drilling by trained organization staff, result in a course graduate who can handle anyone with communication alone and whose communication can stand up faultlessly to any situation no matter how rough. (Delivered in Scientology organizations.)

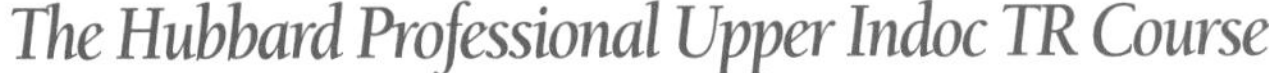

The Hubbard Professional Upper Indoc TR Course

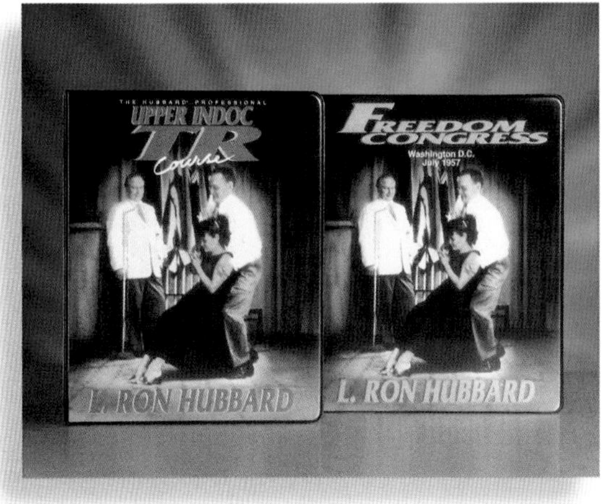

The ability to control things and direct people and situations is key to any success in life, and can be learned by a student who has completed the Hubbard Professional TR Course. Upper Indoc TRs (*indoc* is short for "indoctrination," meaning to teach) are the most advanced communication drills in Scientology. On this course one studies the theory of these drills, which includes eleven lectures and demonstrations of the TRs by Mr. Hubbard, and a film which shows how to do each Upper Indoc TR. The student then learns a high level of skill in starting, changing and stopping communication cycles and life situations through drilling and mastery of these TRs. It is not possible to successfully do anything in life if one cannot control objects, situations and communication. This course teaches that skill. (Delivered in Scientology organizations.)

Dianetics 55!

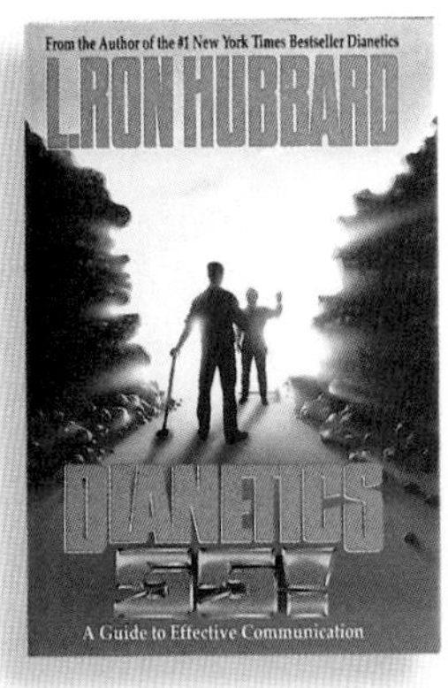

Contains Mr. Hubbard's most thorough exposition on communication, going into great detail on all its aspects. This work is *the* manual on communication and vital to success in virtually any activity in life. The quality of one's life is closely linked to his ability to communicate and this book provides Mr. Hubbard's most concentrated researches on the area.

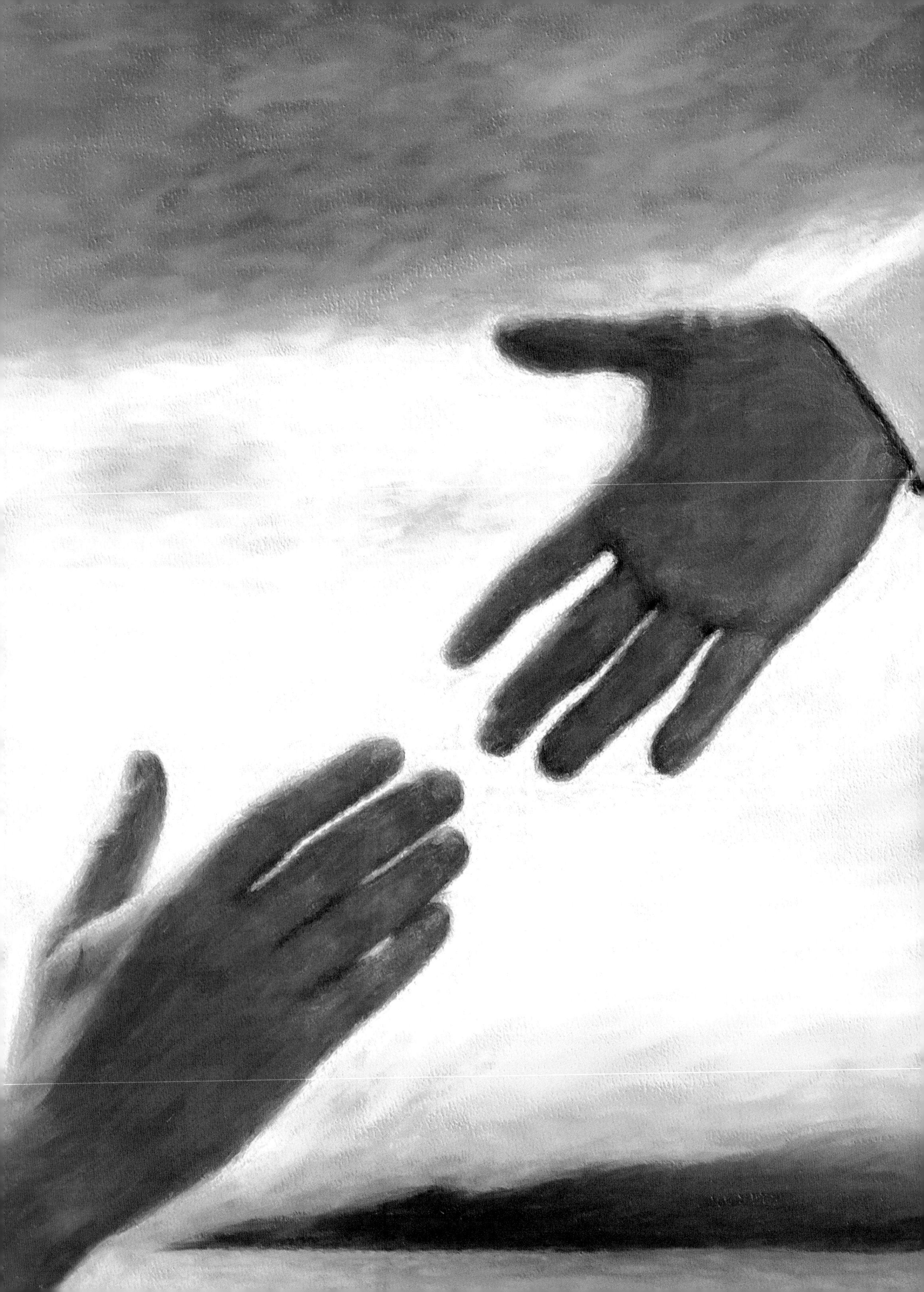

Chapter 6

Assists for Illnesses and Injuries

People sometimes get hurt in the business of living. The human body is subject to disease, injuries and various mishaps of accidental or intentional character.

Throughout the ages, religions have attempted to relieve man's physical suffering. Methods have ranged from prayer to the laying on of hands, and many superstitions arose to account for their occasional effectiveness. It has been a commonly held belief, however, no matter the method used, that the spirit can have an effect on the body.

Today, medicine treats the body when there is something wrong with it. But it overlooks almost totally the relationship of the spiritual being to his body and the effect the former has on the latter.

The fact is, after any necessary medical treatment, the individual himself has an enormous capacity to influence the body and its well-being or lack of it.

L. Ron Hubbard developed numerous applications of his discoveries for the mental and spiritual aspects of a person's physical difficulties. And as more and more techniques evolved, a new body of technology came into use, called "Assists."

The ways assists can be applied are almost limitless. They always help and often have miraculous results. Dozens of assists exist today for a wide array of conditions, and several of the most basic and widely used are included in this chapter.

Factors of Assists

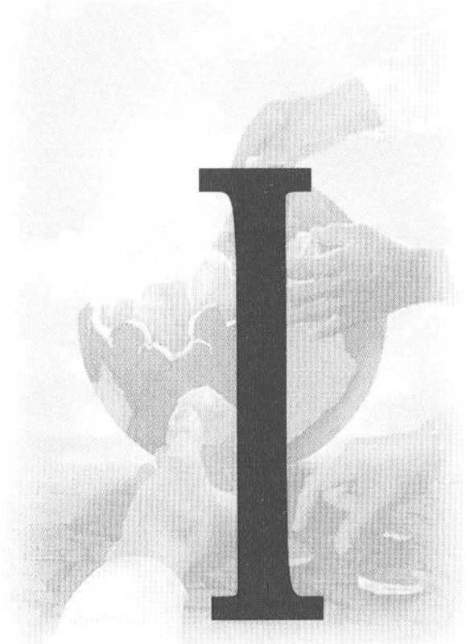

In Scientology an *assist* is an action undertaken to help a person confront physical difficulties. If a child has fallen and hurt himself, an assist can help him overcome the trauma. If a person has a toothache or has had a tooth pulled, an assist can help relieve the pain. When people are ill, assists can ease the discomfort and speed recovery. Even broken bones respond to assists. These and many other conditions can be improved by application of procedures classified under this heading of "Assists."

An assist, then, can be described as a Scientology process which is done to alleviate a present time discomfort. A *process* is an exact series of directions or sequence of actions taken to accomplish a desired result. There are many processes contained in the materials of Scientology, but assists make up a class of processes in themselves.

All Scientology processes address and handle a wide range of conditions affecting the *spirit,* the being himself.

The spirit in Scientology is called the *thetan,* by which is meant the person himself—not his body or his name, the physical universe, his mind or anything else—it is that which is aware of being aware; the identity which *is* the individual. The term *thetan* was coined to eliminate any possible confusion with older, invalid concepts. It comes from the Greek letter *theta* which the Greeks used to represent *thought* or perhaps *spirit,* to which an *n* is added to make a noun in the modern style used to create words in engineering.

Probably the greatest discovery of Scientology and its most forceful contribution to the knowledge of mankind has been the isolation, description and handling of the human spirit. In Scientology it can be demonstrated that that thing which is the person, the personality, is separable from the body and the mind at will and without causing bodily death or mental derangement.

In ages past there has been considerable controversy concerning the human spirit or soul, and various attempts to control man have been effective in view of his almost complete ignorance of his own identity. As you know that you are where you are at this moment, so you would know if you, a spirit, were detached from your mind and body. Man had not discovered this before because, lacking the technologies of Scientology, he had very little reality upon his detachment from his mind and body; therefore, he conceived himself to be at least in part a mind and a body. The entire cult of communism was based upon the fact that one lives only one life, that there is no hereafter and that the individual has no religious significance. Man at large has been close to this state for at least the last century. The state is of a very low order, excluding as it does all self-recognition.

The thetan (spirit) is described in Scientology as having no mass, no wavelength, no energy and no time or location in space except by consideration or postulate. (A postulate, simply put, is a decision that something will happen.)

The spirit, then, is not a *thing*. It is the *creator* of things.

By spiritual means, but means which are as precise as mathematics, a host of bad conditions of life may be remedied in Scientology. Illness and malfunction can be divided into two general classes. First, those resulting from the operation of the spirit directly upon the communication networks of life or the body and, second, those occasioned by the disruption of structure through purely physical causes.

The term *psychosomatic* means the mind making the body ill or illnesses which have been created physically within the body by derangement of the mind. *Psycho* refers to mind and *somatic* refers to body.

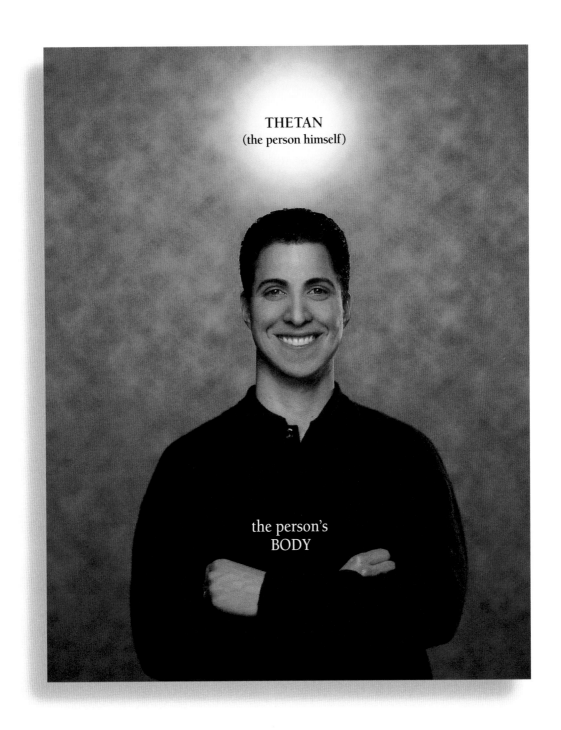

It can be demonstrated that a person is not a body, but is, in fact, a spiritual being, called in Scientology a thetan.

Unhappiness, inability to heal and psychosomatic illnesses (which include some 70 percent of the illnesses of man) are best handled by immediate address of the thetan. Illnesses caused by recognizable bacteria and injury in accident are best treated by physical means. These fall distinctly into the field of medicine and are not the province of Scientology, even though accidents and illness and bacterial infection are predetermined in almost all cases by spiritual malfunction and unrest. And conditions in accidents are definitely prolonged by any spiritual malfunction.

Thus we have the field of medicine addressing the immediate injury, such surgical matters as birth and acute infection, and such things as bruises and scrapes resulting from accidents, as well as the administration of drugs and antibiotics to prevent the demise of the patient in a crisis. This is the role of medicine.

Where tendency to disease or injury exists, or where disease or injury is being prolonged, or where unhappiness and worry causes mental or physical upset, we are dealing in the realm of Scientology. For such things are best healed, or best prevented, or best remedied by immediate and direct recourse to the thetan and its action on the body.

The only truly therapeutic agent in this universe is the spirit. In Scientology this has been demonstrated with more thoroughness and exists with more certainty than the physical sciences or mathematics. A Scientologist *can* help make an individual well and happy simply by addressing the human spirit.

Helping an Individual Heal Himself

Injuries, operations, delivery of babies, severe illnesses and periods of intense emotional shock all deserve to be handled with thorough and complete assists.

An assist in no way intrudes upon the role of medicine. Medical examination and diagnosis should be sought where needed, and where treatment is routinely successful, medical treatment should be obtained. As an assist can at times cover up an actual injury or broken bone, no chances should be taken, especially if the condition does not easily respond. In other words, where something is merely thought to be a slight sprain, to be on the safe side an X-ray should be obtained, particularly if it does not at once respond. An assist is not a substitute for medical treatment and does not attempt to cure injuries requiring medical aid, but is complementary (adds) to it. It is even doubtful if full healing can be accomplished by medical treatment alone and it is certain that an assist greatly speeds recovery. In short, one should realize that physical healing does not take into account the being and the repercussion on the spiritual existence of the person.

Injury and illness are *predisposed* (made more likely to occur) by the spiritual state of the person. They are *precipitated* (brought on) by the being himself as a manifestation of his current spiritual condition. And they are *prolonged* (extended in time beyond normal limits) by any failure to fully handle the spiritual factors associated with them.

The causes of *predisposition, precipitation* and *prolongation* are addressed with assists.

Certainly life is not very tolerable to a person who has been injured or ill, to a woman who has just delivered a baby, to a person who has just suffered a heavy emotional shock. And there is no reason a person should remain in such a low state, particularly for weeks, months or years, when he or she could be remarkably *assisted* to recover in hours, days or weeks.

It is in fact a sort of practiced cruelty to insist by neglect that a person continue on in such a state when one can learn and practice and obtain relief for such a person.

One does not have to be a medical doctor to take someone to a medical doctor. And one does not have to be a medical doctor to observe that medical treatment may not be helping the patient. And one does not have to be a medical doctor to handle things caused spiritually by the being himself.

Just as there are two sides to healing—the spiritual and the structural or physical—there are also two states that can be spiritually attained. The first of these states might be classified as "humanly tolerable." Assists come under this heading. The second is "spiritually improved."

Any minister (and this has been true as long as there has been a subject called religion) is bound to relieve his fellow being of anguish. There are many ways a minister can do this.

An assist is not engaging in healing. It is certainly not engaging in treatment. What it is doing is *assisting the individual to heal himself or be healed by another agency by removing his reasons for precipitating and prolonging his condition and lessening his predisposition to further injure himself or remain in an intolerable condition.*

This is entirely outside the field of "healing" as envisioned by the medical doctor and by actual records of results is very, very far beyond the capability of psychology, psychiatry and "mental treatment" as practiced in those fields.

In short, the assist is strictly and entirely in the field of the spirit and is the traditional province of religion, though not restricted to religion only.

A person applying Assist Technology should realize the power which lies in his hands and his potential skills when trained. He has this to give in the presence of suffering: he can make life tolerable. He can also shorten a term of recovery and may even make recovery possible when it might not be otherwise.

When confronted by someone who has been injured or ill, operated upon or who has suffered a grave emotional shock, one or more of the following assists should be used to help the person.

Contact Assist

There is a basic principle in Scientology which consists of putting an injured body member exactly on and in the place it was injured. Doing this can have a therapeutic effect and is called a Contact Assist. This is the most common assist for accidents and injuries.

Theory

One of the basics of life's reactions is to avoid places where one has been hurt. This is a survival factor but it is not analytical (based on rational thought). For example, if one ran into a table and injured himself, he would tend to avoid coming near that spot again. He would think he was avoiding the table, but actually he is avoiding the exact location of the accident. Even if the table were taken away, he would continue to avoid the *location* where he was injured. This is the basic reason for a Contact Assist.

When the exact spot of the accident or injury is available, always do a Contact Assist. It can be followed by other types of assists, but the Contact Assist should always be done first if the physical objects and location are available.

Procedure

1. Remember that first aid and physical actions often have to be taken before a Contact Assist can be begun. First aid always comes first. Look over the situation from the standpoint of how much first aid is required, and when you have solved that situation, then render the assist. An assist will not shut off a pumping artery, but a tourniquet will.

2. Take the person to the exact spot where the accident occurred. If the object was hot, you let it cool first; if the current was on, you turn it off before doing the assist.

3. Tell the person, "We are now going to do a Contact Assist."

4. Have the person get into the same position he was in before the accident happened. If he had a tool in his hand, or was using one, he should be going through the same motions with it.

5. Tell the person to move slowly through the accident just like it happened. Have him duplicate exactly what happened at the time of the injury by making him touch the exact spot with his injured body part. You have him gently touch the thing that hurt him. If he pricked his finger on a thorn in the rose garden, you get him to gently touch the same part of the same finger that was pricked to the same exact thorn. If he closed his hand in a door, you would have him go back and, with his injured hand, touch the *exact spot* on the *same* door, duplicating the same motions that occurred at the time of the injury. There are hardly any commands involved with it; the less you say, the better off you are.

6. Repeat this over and over again until the exact somatic *turns on* and *blows off*—appears and then disappears. (In Scientology we use the word *somatic* to designate any body sensation, illness, pain or discomfort. *Soma* means "body" in Greek.)

In addition to the somatic blowing, the person will also have a realization about something: his injury or the circumstances related to how he got hurt or the environment. Such a realization is called a *cognition.*

You have to get him to touch the exact point to produce the exact phenomenon of the somatic blowing. When this occurs and he has a cognition, end the assist by telling the person, "End of assist."

Don't Force the Person

A Contact Assist must sometimes be done on a gradient—with a gradual approach. Let's say a child stubbed his shin on the lawn mower and now doesn't want to come nearer than one hundred feet from that lawn mower. You would make him do a Contact Assist with his shin and body at that point (one hundred feet from the same lawn mower), having him go through the motions of the accident. Gradually, gradient by gradient, you narrow the distance that he is willing to approach it and eventually he will go up and do a Contact Assist on the lawn mower.

You must never forcibly drag the person up to the spot where the injury or accident occurred. If you try to force the person, you could overwhelm him which could have a bad effect on him.

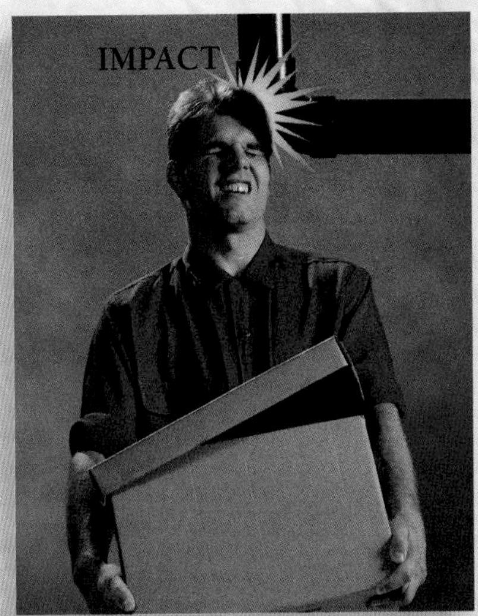

When one has an accident or injury a Contact Assist should be done.

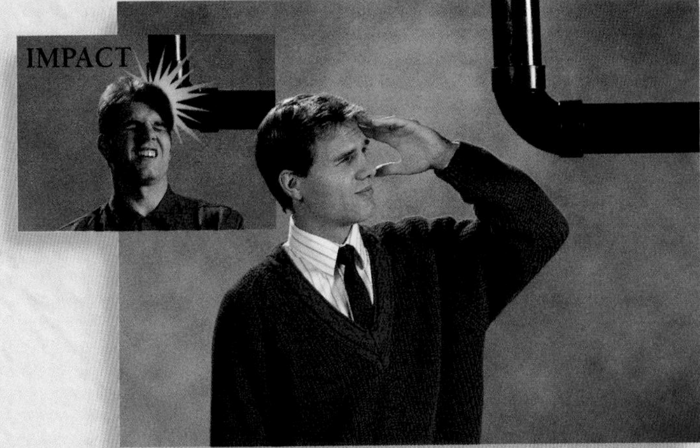

One of the basics of life's reactions is to avoid places where one has been hurt.

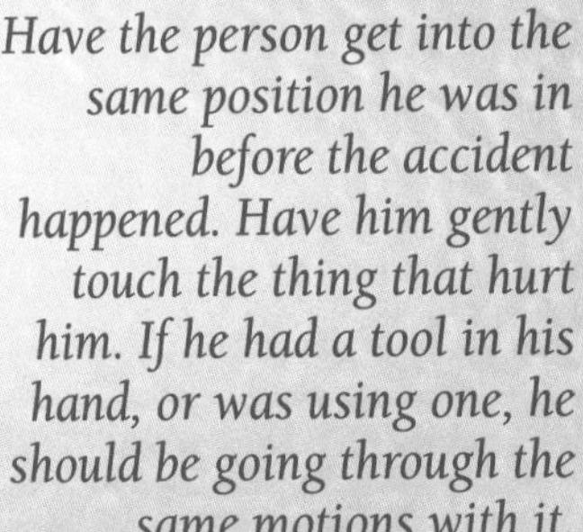

Have the person get into the same position he was in before the accident happened. Have him gently touch the thing that hurt him. If he had a tool in his hand, or was using one, he should be going through the same motions with it.

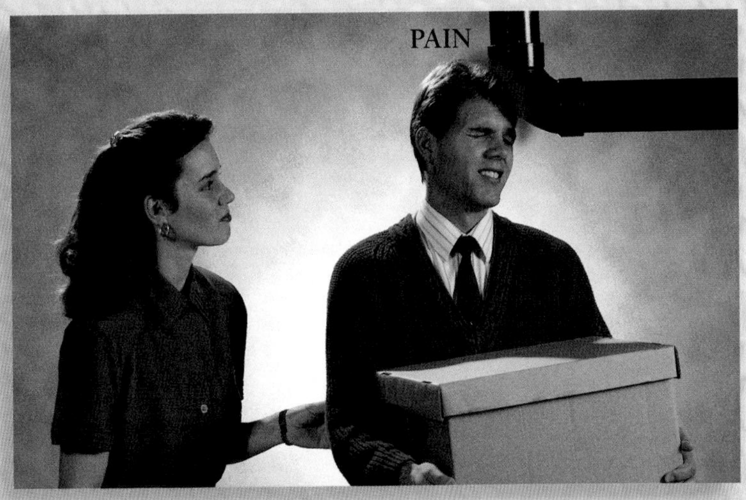

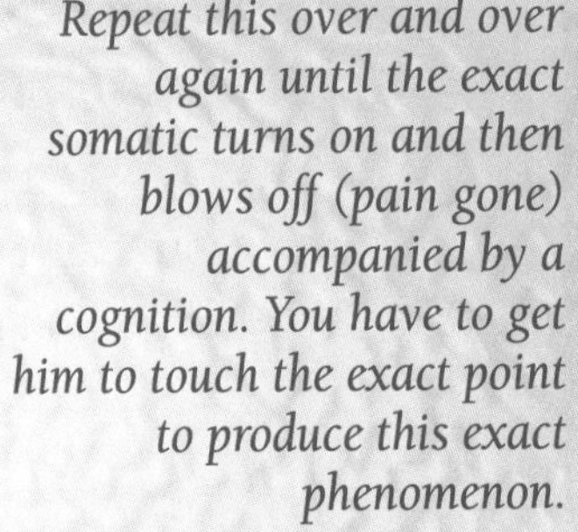

Repeat this over and over again until the exact somatic turns on and then blows off (pain gone) accompanied by a cognition. You have to get him to touch the exact point to produce this exact phenomenon.

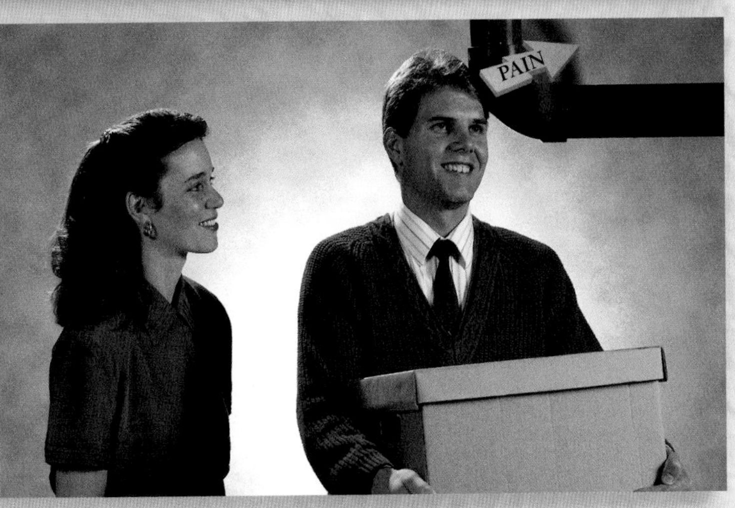

Contact Assists can be done solo (by oneself) but one must be sure to do it until the somatic blows.

Any type of injury can and should be handled with a Contact Assist. It is always the best type of injury assist when the exact spot is available and should precede any other assist actions. Contact Assists have unlimited use. They're sometimes miraculous—but they always help.

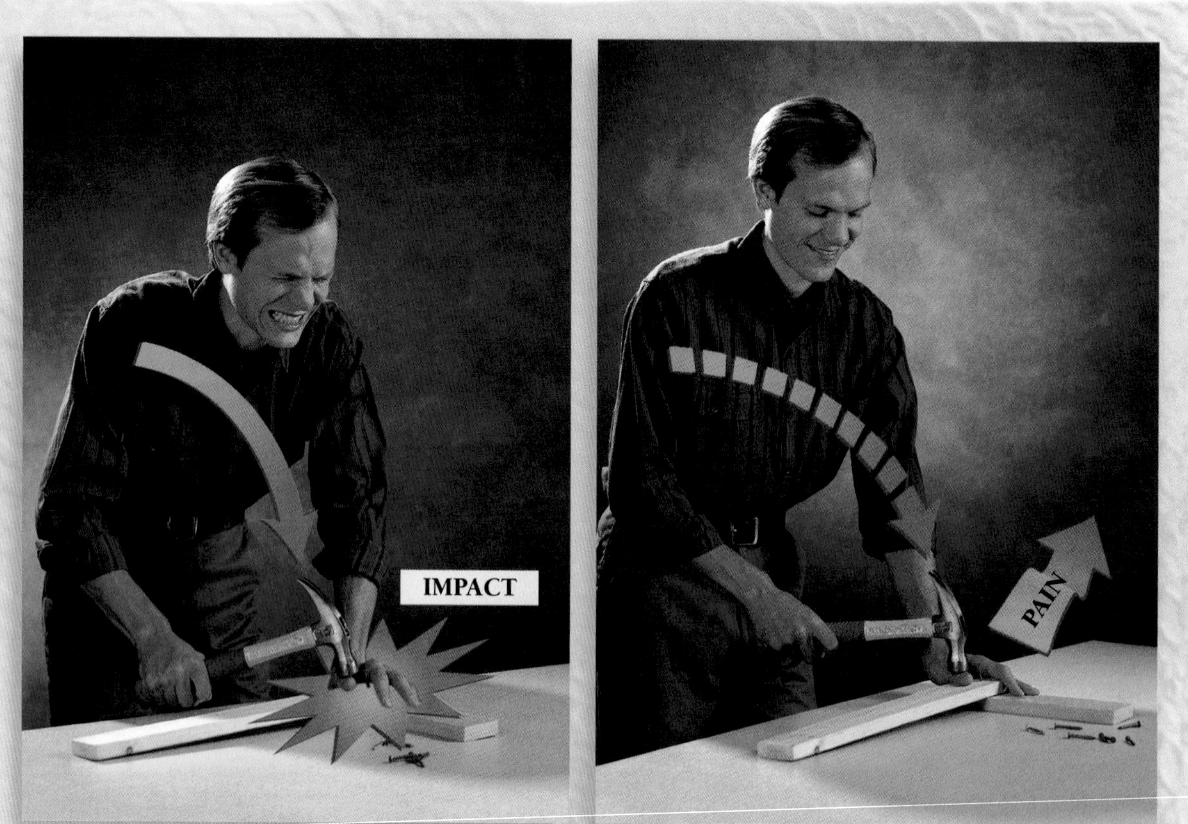

If a person is injured, he can do a Contact Assist on himself. He gently duplicates exactly what happened at the time of the injury, taking care to continue until the pain dissipates.

TOUCH ASSIST

The Touch Assist is the most widely used and probably best known assist. It was first developed in the early 1950s and has been in use ever since.

The application of Touch Assists is not limited to injuries. They are not just for the banged hand or the burned wrist. They can be done on a dull pain in the back, a constant earache, an infected boil, an upset stomach. In fact, the number of things this simple but powerful process can be applied to is unlimited!

Theory

The purpose of a Touch Assist is to reestablish communication with injured or ill body parts. It brings the person's attention to the injured or affected body areas. This is done by repetitively touching the ill or injured person's body and putting him into communication with the injury. His communication with it brings about recovery. The technique is based on the principle that the way to heal anything or remedy anything is to put somebody into communication with it.

Every single physical illness stems from a failure of the being to communicate with the thing or area that is ill. Prolongation of a chronic injury occurs in the absence of physical communication with the affected area or with the location of the spot of injury in the physical universe.

When attention is withdrawn from injured or ill body areas, so are circulation, nerve flows and energy. This limits nutrition to the area and prevents the drain of waste products. Some ancient healers attributed remarkable flows and qualities to the "laying on of hands." Probably the workable element in this was simply heightening awareness of the affected area and restoring the physical communication factors. For example, if you do a Touch Assist on somebody who has a sprained wrist, you are putting him back into communication with that wrist as completely as possible.

In addition to control and direction of the person's attention, a Touch Assist also handles the factors of *location* and *time.* If a person has been

A Touch Assist helps handle the factors of time and location when a person has been injured. Part of his attention is stuck in the past moment and place of the impact.

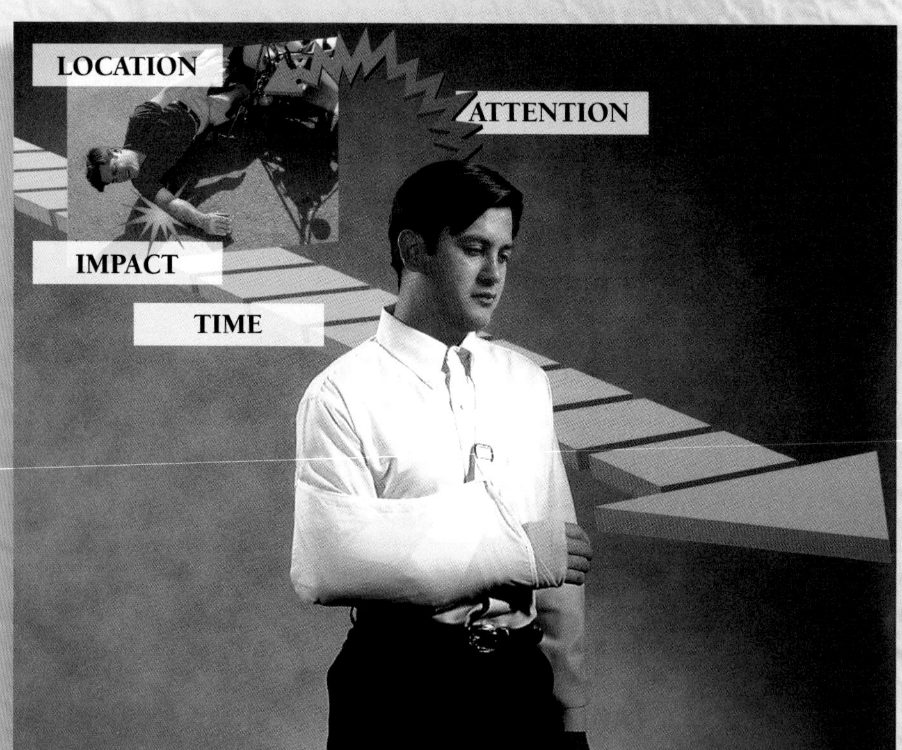

The assist restores the person to the present and thus permits healing to occur.

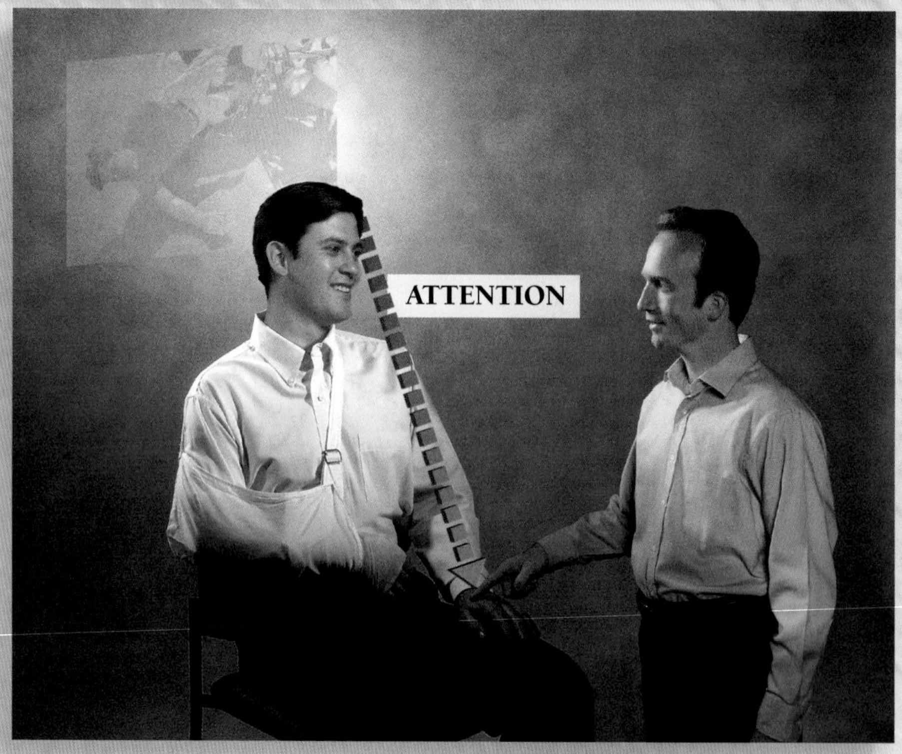

injured, his attention avoids the injured or affected part but at the same time is stuck in it. He is also avoiding the *location* of the injury, and the person himself and the injured body part are stuck in the *time* of the impact. A Touch Assist permits healing to occur by restoring the person to the present and his whereabouts to some degree.

Procedure

0. Administer any first aid that may be needed *before* you begin the assist. For example, if the person has a bleeding wound it should be dressed as the first action.

1. Have the person sit down or lie down—whatever position will be more comfortable for him.

2. Tell him that you are going to be doing a Touch Assist and explain briefly the procedure.

Tell the person the command you will be using and ensure he understands it. The command used is "Feel my finger."

Tell the person that he should let you know when he has done the command.

3. Give the command "Feel my finger," then touch a point, using moderate finger pressure.

Do *not* touch and then give the command; that would be backwards.

Touch with only *one* finger. If you used two fingers the person could be confused about which he was supposed to feel.

4. Acknowledge the person by saying "Thank you" or "Okay" or "Good," etc.

5. Continue giving the command, touching and acknowledging when the person has indicated he has done the command.

When doing a Touch Assist on a particular injured or affected area, you approach the area on a gradient and recede from it on a gradient.

You approach the injury or affected area, go away from it, approach it, go away from it, approach it closer, go away from it further, approach to a point where you are actually touching the injured or affected part and go away further. You try to follow the nerve channels of the body, which include the spine, the limbs and the various relay points like the elbows, the wrists, the back sides of the knees and the fingertips. These are the points you head for. These are all points in which the shock wave can get locked up. What you are trying to do is get a communication wave flowing again through the body, because the shock of injury stopped it.

No matter what part of the body is being helped, the areas touched should include the extremities (hands and feet) and the spine.

The touching must be balanced to both left and right sides of the body. When you have touched the person's right big toe, you next touch the left big toe; when you have touched a point a few inches to one side of the person's spine, you next touch the spot the same distance from the spine on the opposite side. This is important because the brain and the body's communication system interlock. You can find that a pain in the left hand runs out (dissipates) when you touch the right hand, because the right hand has got it locked up.

In addition to handling the left and right sides of the body, the body's *back* and *front* sides must also be addressed. In other words, if attention has been given to the front of the body, attention must also be given to the back.

The same principle applies in handling a particular body *part.* For instance, you might be handling an injury on the front of the right leg. Your Touch Assist would include the front of the right leg, the front of the left leg, the back of the right leg and the back of the left leg, in addition to the usual actions of handling the extremities and spine.

6. Continue the assist until the person feels better. You will notice an improvement in the person from what he says or how he looks. These are called *indicators.*

Indicators are conditions or circumstances arising during an assist which indicate whether it is running well or badly. When a bad condition, such as an injured hand, improves, that is a *good indicator*. If the pain in his hand lessened, that would be a good indicator.

A Touch Assist is continued until the person being helped has *good indicators,* meaning he feels better, the pain has diminished, he is happier about it, etc. He will also have a cognition.

7. When this occurs, tell the person, "End of assist."

You may have to give Touch Assists day after day to achieve a result. On first doing a Touch Assist you might only get a small improvement. Giving another Touch Assist on the following day, you could expect a bit more improvement. Next day you may get a somatic blowing off completely. It might take many more days than this, with a Touch Assist given each day, before such a result is achieved; the point is that the number of Touch Assists you can do on the same thing is unlimited.

Uses

Use on Injuries

Never do a Touch Assist as the first action on an injured person when you can do a Contact Assist. If the exact location where the injury occurred is available, do a Contact Assist. The Contact Assist can then be followed by a Touch Assist or any other assist action.

Use on Animals

Touch Assists can be used to good results on animals. In doing a Touch Assist on a sick or injured dog or cat, you should wear thick gloves, as they may snap and scratch.

Persons on Drugs

A Touch Assist can be done on a person who has been given painkillers or other drugs. This isn't optimum but it is sometimes necessary under emergency conditions.

Communication with the body lessens when one is ill or injured. A Touch Assist helps restore a person's ability to communicate fully with an ill or injured body part.

Tell the person, "Feel my finger," and touch a spot on his body. Acknowledge him when he does so.

Follow the nerve channels of the body. The touching must be balanced to both sides of the body.

A Touch Assist must include the extremities and the spine. A correctly done Touch Assist can speed the thetan's ability to heal or repair a condition with his body.

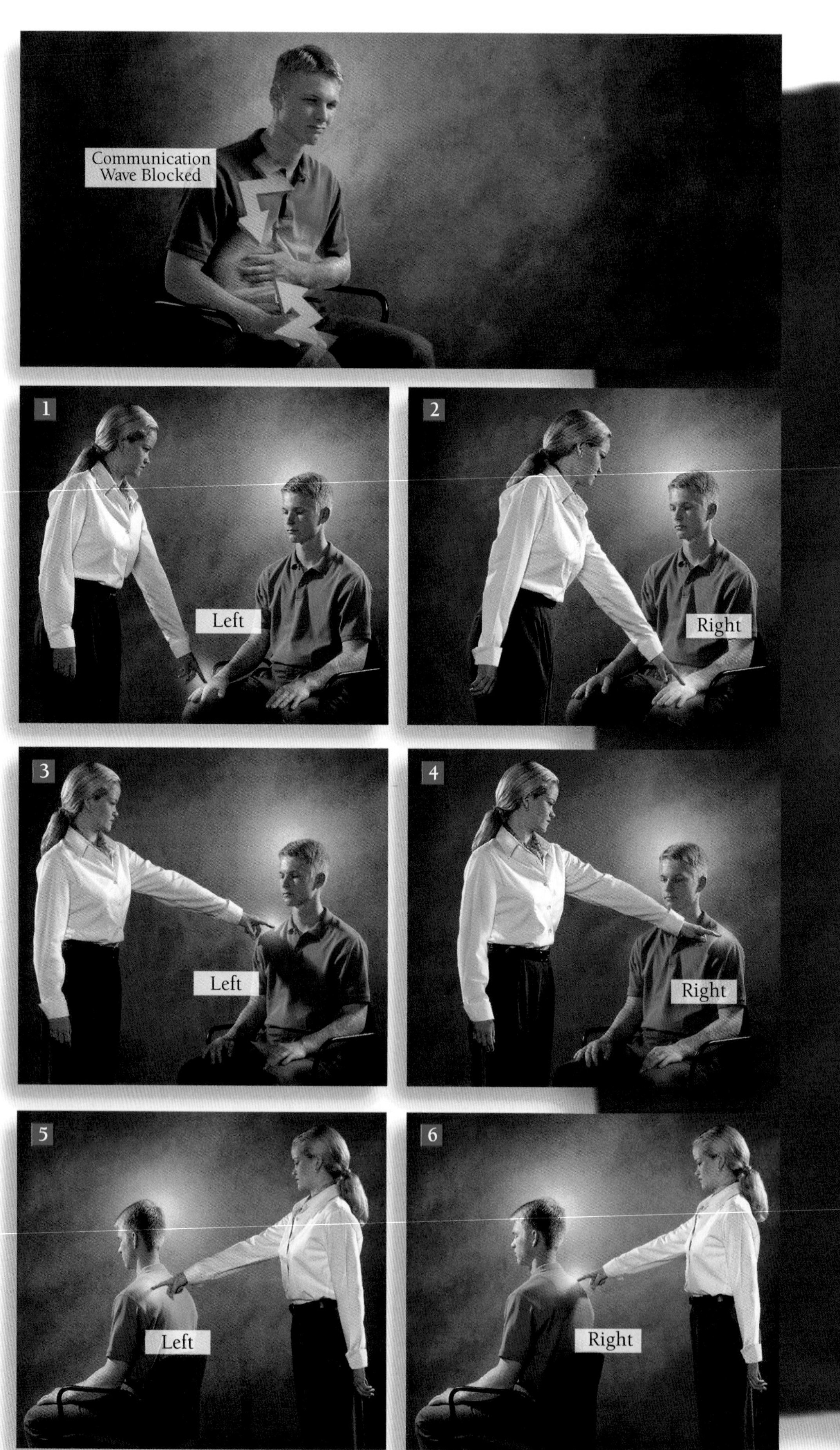

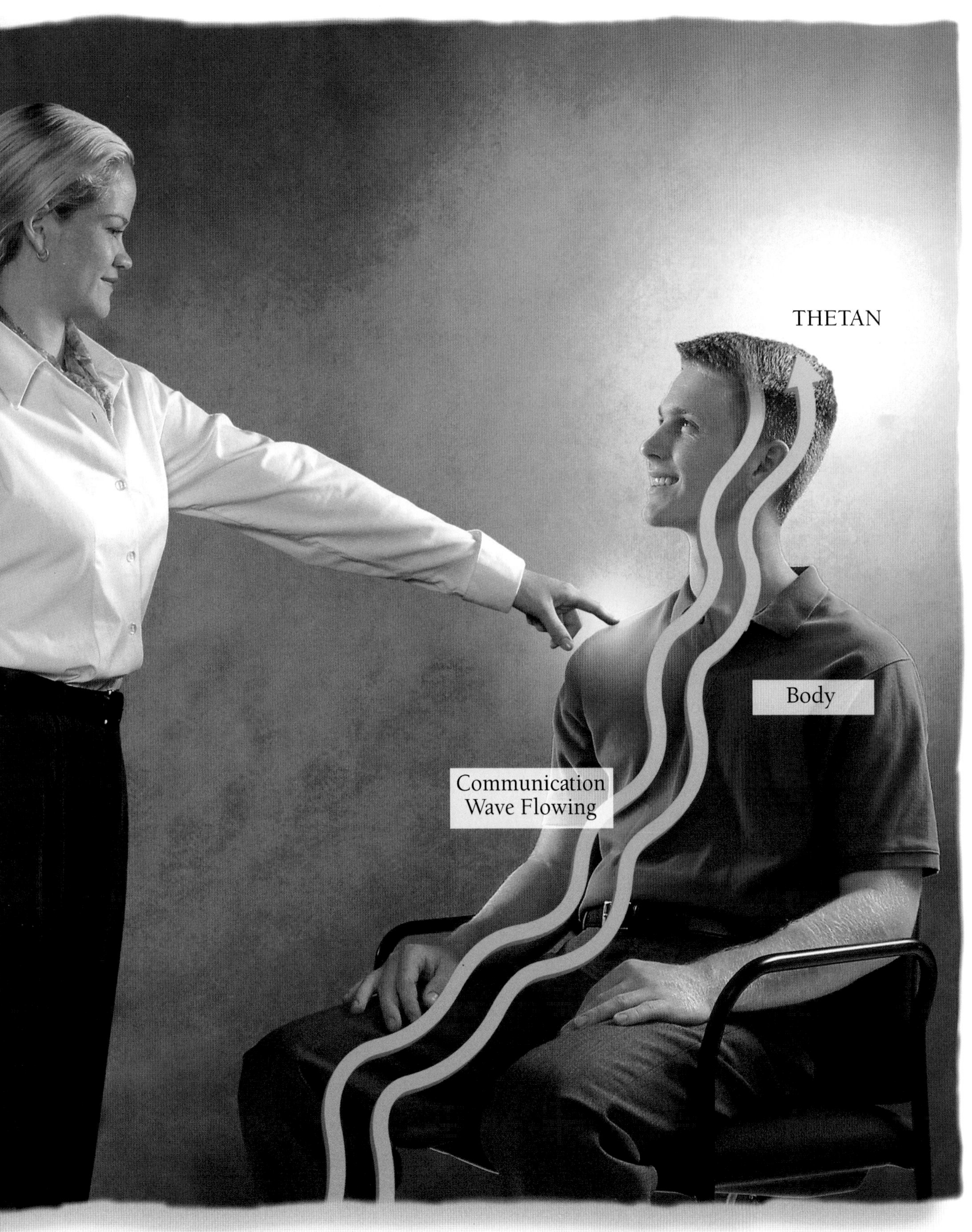
THETAN
Body
Communication
Wave Flowing

Where a person has been injured, your objective should be to get to him and give him a Touch Assist *before* anyone gives him a painkiller. If the body has been very badly damaged, the person may still be in agony after your assist, but you will have gotten some of the shock off. At this point a medical doctor could administer a painkiller and repair the physical damage. Of course, if the person needs immediate treatment for excessive pain, you would not prevent it from being administered and would then deliver the Touch Assist when the person was more comfortable.

Headaches

Do not do a Touch Assist on a person who has a headache. Research has shown that headaches are often the result of mental phenomena that a Touch Assist would be the incorrect handling for.

Head Injuries

If a person has received an actual *injury* to the head such as being poked in the eye or hit on the head with a bat, he can be given a Touch Assist. The same applies to injuries to the teeth or painful dental work.

The Touch Assist is easy to learn and can get quite remarkable results. It has the advantage of being easy to teach others. So use it well to help those around you, and teach them to help others in turn.

Nerve Assist

Among the many types of assists in Scientology is one which can straighten joints and the spine.

This is called a Nerve Assist.

Chiropractic spinal adjustment is often successful. But sometimes the spine goes out of place again and has to be adjusted time after time. The Nerve Assist was actually developed as a favor to chiropractors, many of whom now use it.

In our theory, it is nerves that hold the muscles tense, which then hold the spine out of place.

There are twelve big nerves which run down a person's spine, spreading out from the spine across both sides of the shoulders and back. These twelve nerves branch out into smaller nerve channels and nerve endings. Nerves affect the muscles and can, if continually tensed, pull the spine and other parts of the body structure out of place.

Nerves carry the shock of impacts. Such a shock should dissipate, but it seldom does entirely. Nerves give orders to muscles. With an impact, a surge of energy starts down the nerve channels. Then, from the small ends of the nerve channels, the energy surge reverses and the result is a bulge of energy which stops midway along the channel. This gives what is called a "standing wave." It is just standing there, not going anywhere.

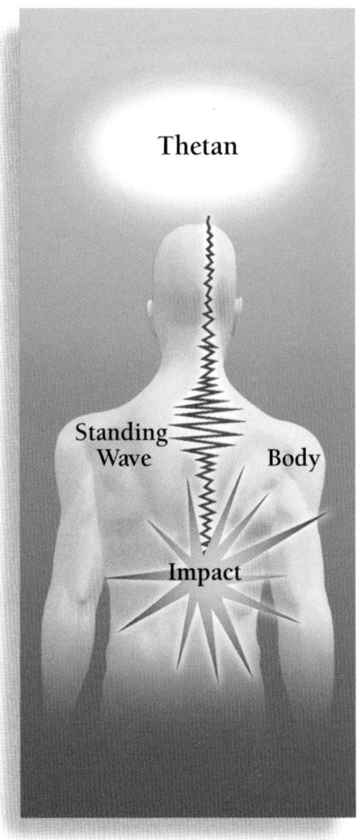

Standing waves of energy form when the shock of an impact locks up in a nerve channel.

The Nerve Assist consists of gently releasing the standing waves in the nerve channels of the body, improving communication with the body and bringing the being relief.

Procedure

1. Have the person lie face down on a bed or cot. Then, with your two index fingers, stroke down close to the spine on either side, fairly rapidly but not very forcefully. This action is then repeated twice.

2. Then reverse your original action, following the same channels with your two fingers back *up* the spine. This is done three times.

3. Now, with your fingers spread fan-like, stroke the nerve channels, using both hands at the same time. Stroke away from the spine and to the sides of the body following the nerve channels as represented in the top illustration on the opposite page. Once you have covered the whole back in this way (working down from the top of the spine to the bottom of the spine), repeat this step two more times.

4. Now reverse the direction of your strokes so they go back up to the spine.

5. Now have the person turn over so he is lying face up. Using both hands, continue to parallel the nerve channels around to the front of the body.

(Note: In following the nerve channels around to the front of the body, stroke only as far as the points of the arrows in the bottom illustration opposite. The nerve channels being handled do not extend across the chest or abdomen, so stroking is not done across those areas.)

6. Then reverse your direction on those same nerve channels.

(Note: In following the nerve channels in step 6, begin stroking at the spots indicated by the points of the arrows in the bottom illustration opposite, stroking towards the back.)

7. Now stroke down the arms and legs.

The person is again turned face down, lying on his stomach, and you start over at step 1.

This procedure is continued until the person has a cognition or expresses some relief, and has very good indicators. He may also experience a bone going into place, often accompanied by a dull popping sound. At this point the Nerve Assist should be ended off for that session.

The Nerve Assist should be repeated daily until *all* the standing waves are released.

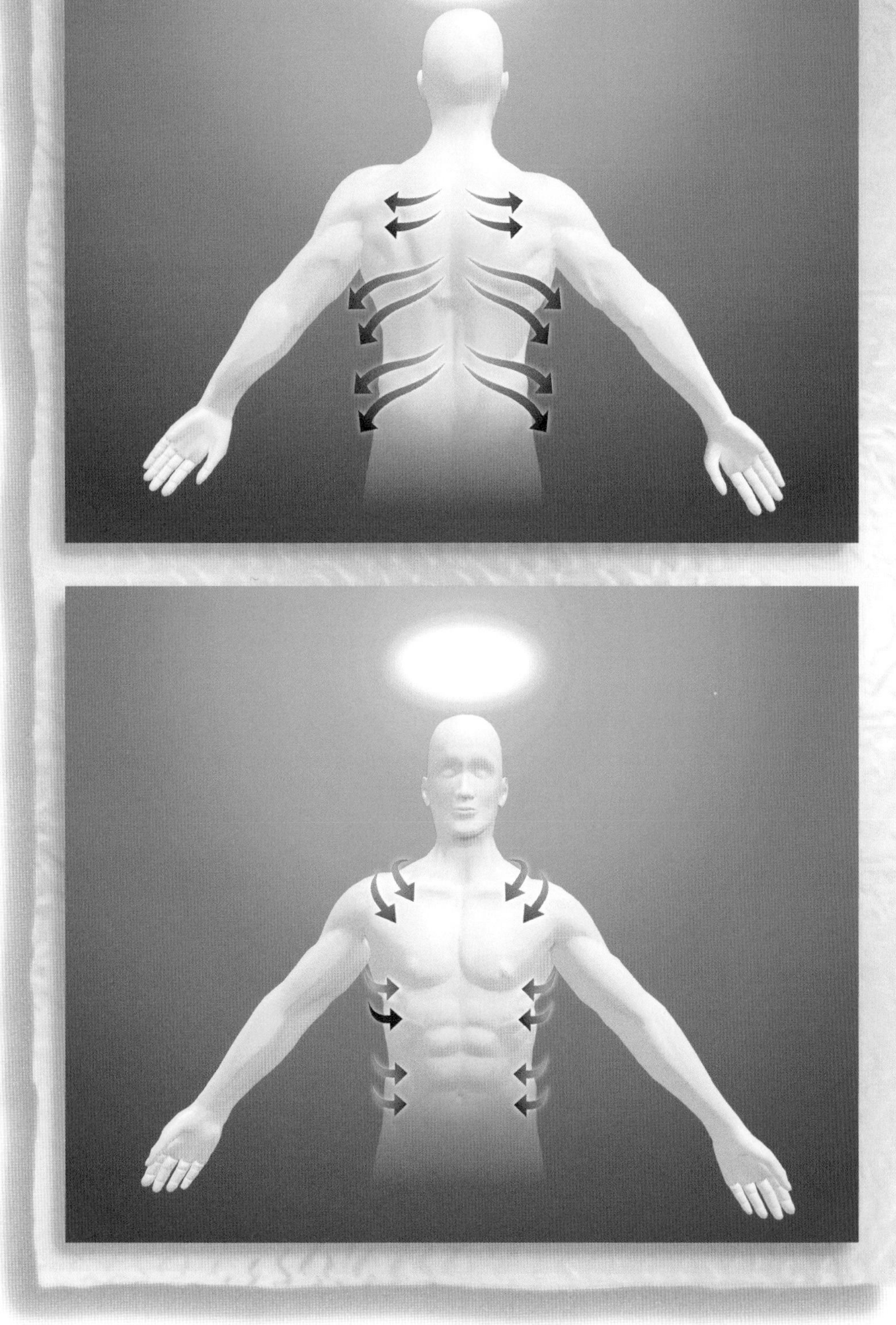

Stroke along the nerve channels which branch out from the spine, around to the front of the body.

When the person is lying face up, stroke only as far as shown by the arrows.

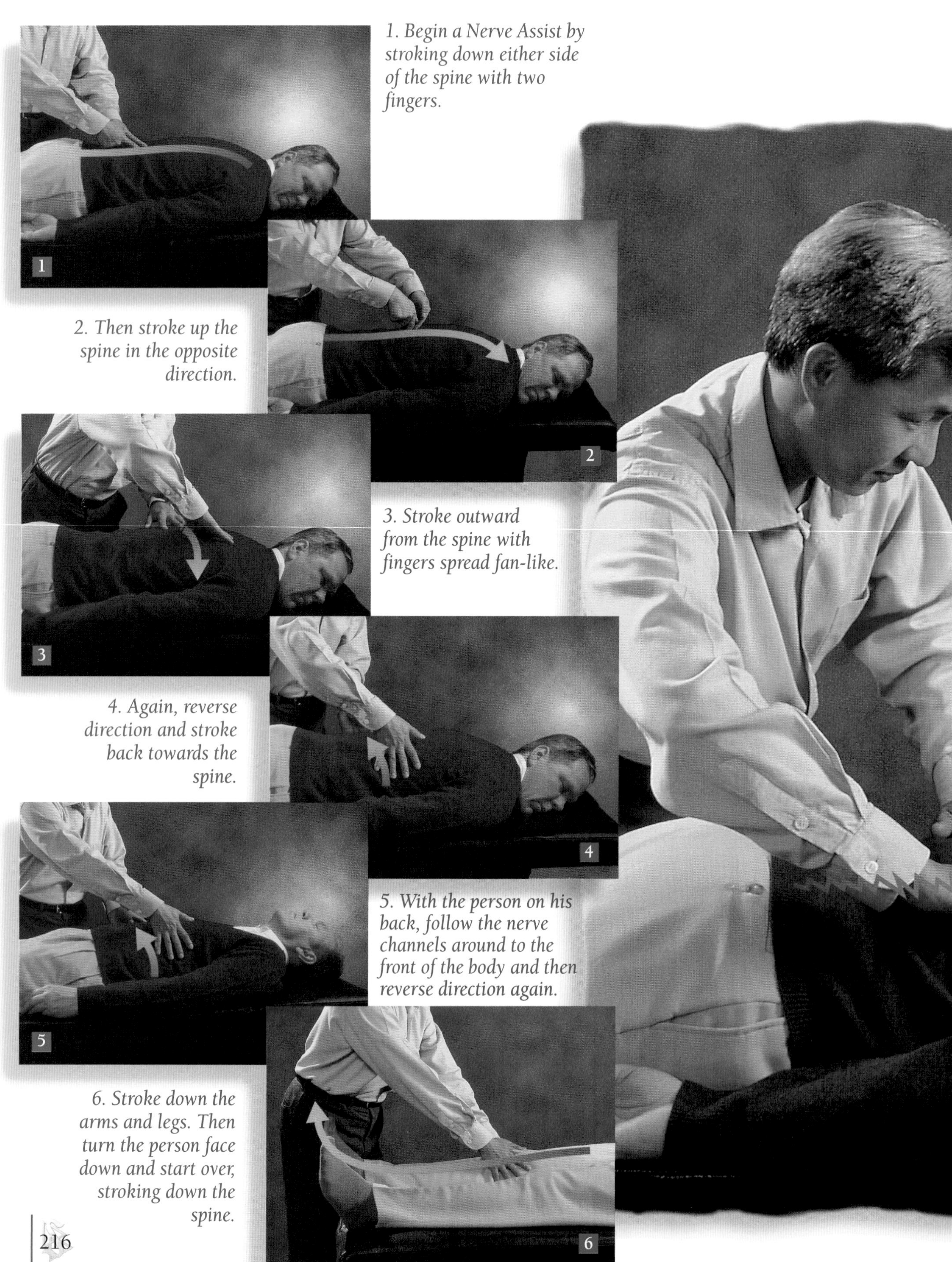

1. Begin a Nerve Assist by stroking down either side of the spine with two fingers.

2. Then stroke up the spine in the opposite direction.

3. Stroke outward from the spine with fingers spread fan-like.

4. Again, reverse direction and stroke back towards the spine.

5. With the person on his back, follow the nerve channels around to the front of the body and then reverse direction again.

6. Stroke down the arms and legs. Then turn the person face down and start over, stroking down the spine.

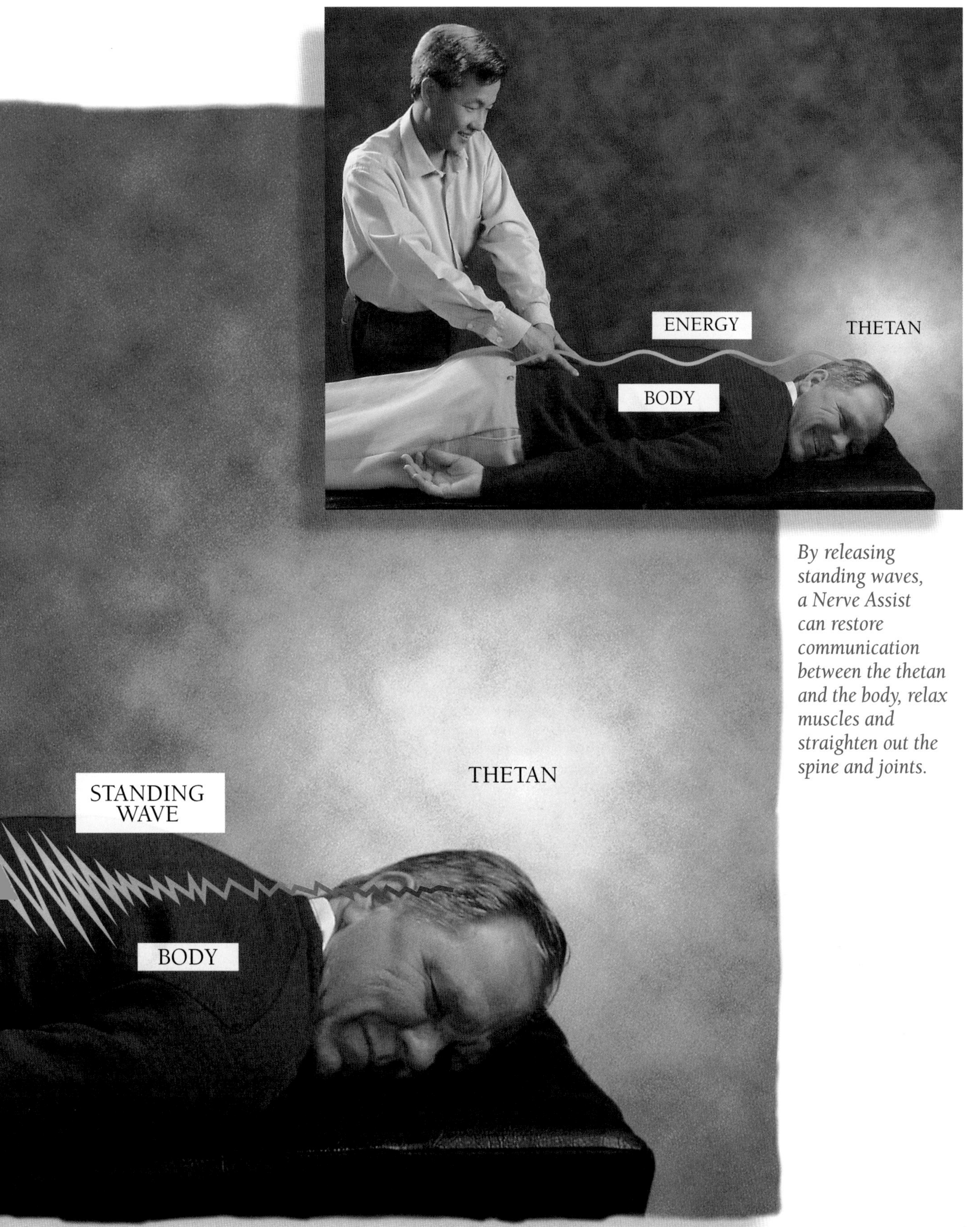

By releasing standing waves, a Nerve Assist can restore communication between the thetan and the body, relax muscles and straighten out the spine and joints.

The Body Communication Process

The Body Communication Process is used when a person has been chronically out of communication with his body, such as after an illness or injury, or when the person has been dormant for a long period of time.

The Body Communication Process does not in any way replace or alter Touch Assists or Contact Assists. Where a person has been injured or has specific areas of the body where an assist is needed, the Touch Assist or the Contact Assist should be used.

This process may be done only *after* any necessary medical attention or other necessary assists have been done. It is not done in place of these.

The purpose of the process is to enable the being to reestablish communication with his body.

Procedure

1. The individual lies on his back on a couch, bed or cot. Doing this assist on the clothed body with shoes removed gives satisfactory results. Any constricting articles such as neckties or tight belts should be removed or loosened. It is not necessary to remove any clothing except for heavy or bulky garments.

Where more than one session of this process is given, the body position may be varied to advantage by having the person lie face downward during alternate sessions.

2. Use the command "Feel my hands." ("Feel my hand" on the occasion where only one hand is applied.)

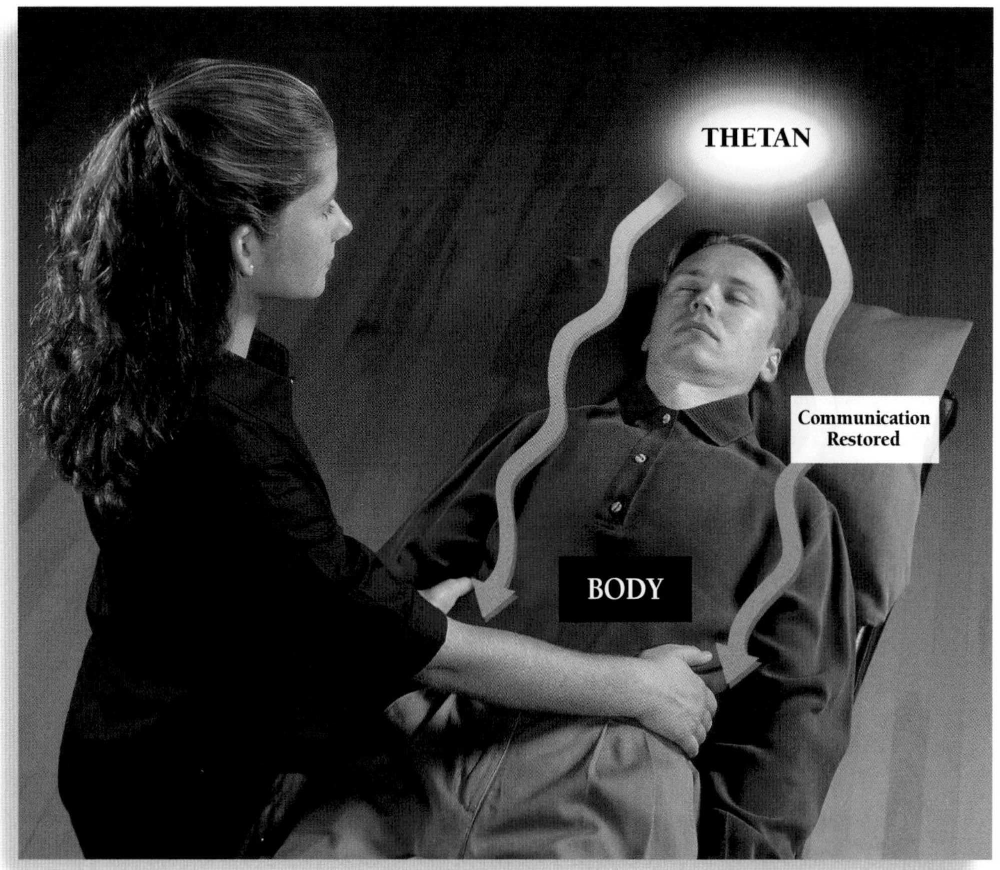

By placing the hands in different positions and getting the person to feel them, someone who is ill or injured can be brought back into better communication with the body.

3. Explain the purpose of this process to the person and tell him briefly what you are going to do.

4. Have the person close his eyes. Then place your hands on the individual's shoulders with a firm but gentle grip, using an agreed-upon firmness, and give the command.

5. When the person replies that he has, acknowledge him.

6. Place your hands in different positions on the body, giving the command and acknowledging the person each time after he has responded. Touch the chest, front of chest, sides of chest, both sides of the abdomen at the waist, then one hand going around the abdomen in a clockwise direction.

(Clockwise because this is the direction of flow of the large bowel.) Continue with both hands on the small of the back, one on each side and lifting firmly; one hand placed over each hip with firmer pressure on these bony parts, then down one leg to the knee with both hands and down the other leg to the knee with both hands, then back to the other leg and down over the calf, the lower calf, the ankle, the foot and the toes and down the other leg from the knee to the toes.

Then work upward in a flow towards the shoulders, down each arm and out to the fingers, both hands behind the neck, one on each side, sides of the face, forehead and back of the head, sides of the head, then away toward the extremities of the body.

An infinite variety of placing of the hands is available avoiding, of course, the genital areas or buttocks in both sexes and a woman's breasts. The process proceeds up and down the body, toward the extremities.

7. The process is continued until the person has a good change, a cognition and very good indicators. At this point the assist may be ended. Tell the person, "End of assist."

The assist should not be continued past a cognition and very good indicators.

Locational Processing Assist

One of the easiest assists to render is Locational Processing. A Locational is done by directing a person's attention off the painful area of his body or his difficulties and out onto the environment.

Say you wanted to render an assist on somebody who had a very indefinite difficulty. That is the hardest one to render an assist on. The person has a pain but he cannot say where. He doesn't know what has happened to him. He just *feels* bad. Use Locational Processing as such. You will find out that this process will work when other processes fail.

Procedure

1. Tell the person you are going to do a Locational Assist and briefly explain the procedure.

2. Tell him the command to be used and ensure he understands it. The command is "Look at that _______ (object)."

3. Point to an object and tell the person, "Look at that _______ (object)."

4. When the person has done so, acknowledge him.

5. Continue giving the command, directing the person's attention to different objects in the environment. Be sure to acknowledge the person each time after he has complied.

For instance, you say, "Look at that tree." "Thank you." "Look at that building." "Good." "Look at that street." "All right." "Look at that lawn." "Very good." You point each time to the object.

6. Keep this up until the person has good indicators and a cognition. You can end the assist at this point. Tell the person, "End of assist."

A Locational Assist is a very easy assist to deliver. It can be done on specific injuries or when a person is ill or if the person has a very indefinite difficulty. Doing a Locational Assist can help him considerably.

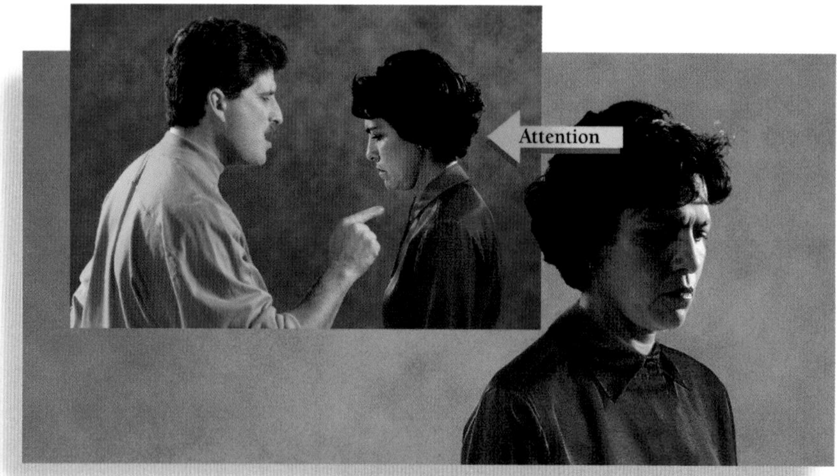

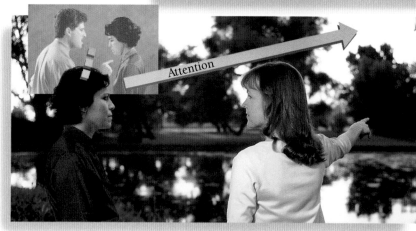

An upset can be addressed with an assist. The woman's attention is stuck on a recent argument.

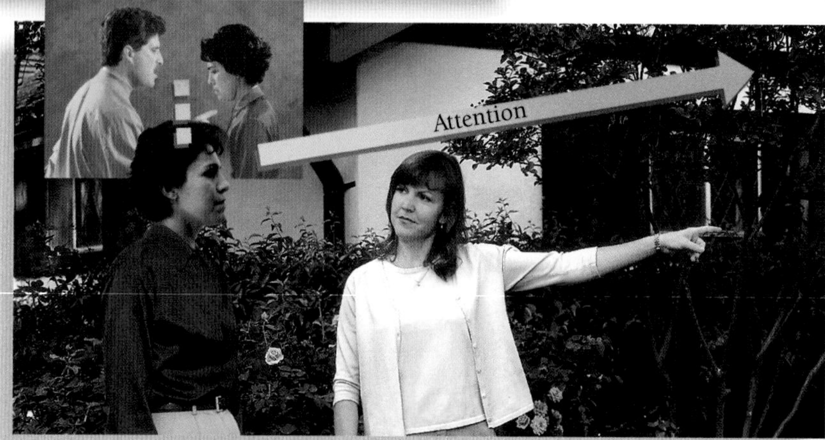

Locational Processing directs the person's attention to things in the environment.

Tell the person, "Look at that _______ (object)." Acknowledge when she has done so.

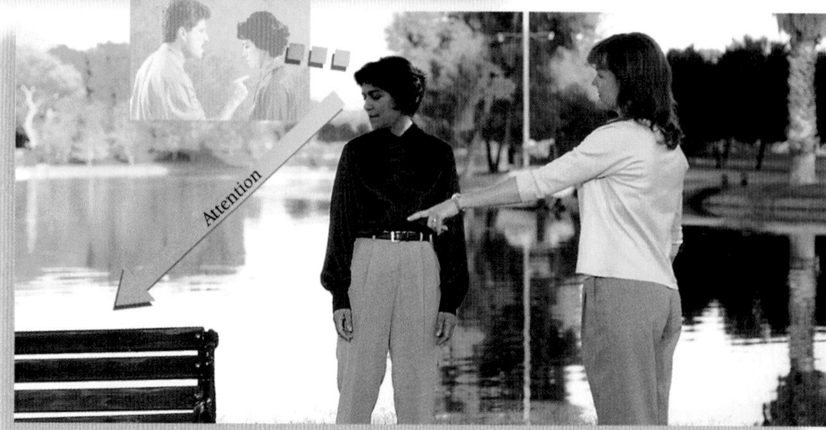

Continue directing the person's attention to things in the environment.

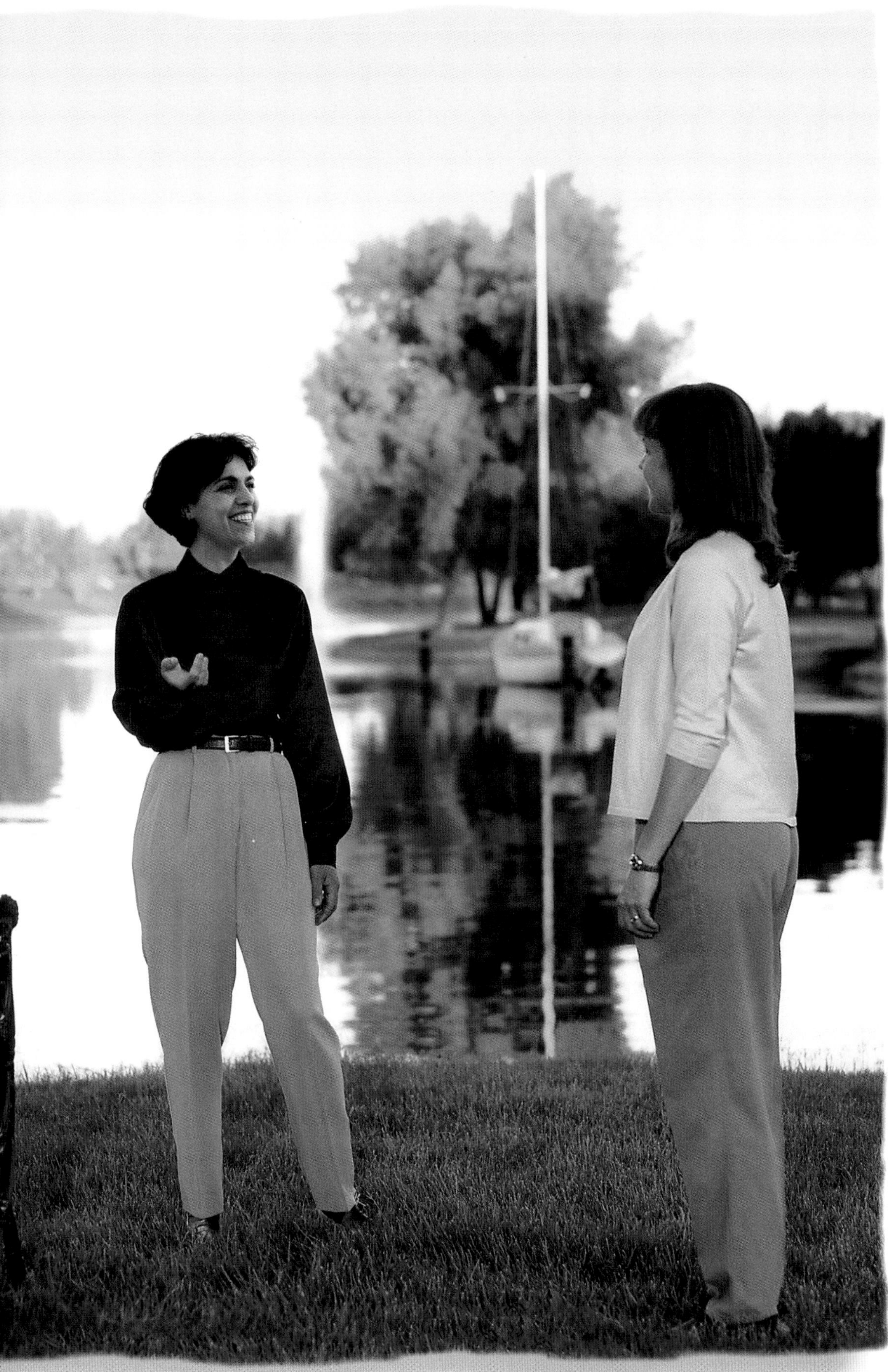

Locational Processing can unstick attention from the upset, leaving her more able to solve the problem.

HOW TO MAKE A PERSON SOBER

There is an interesting use of Locational Processing as a way to make a person sober. It can make a drunk person sober in a very few minutes. As society currently has no technology for handling the drunk, who is an embarrassment to his family, his friends and often to himself, this process has social value and may serve as a line of cooperation and assistance to the police.

Procedure

Use the command:

"Look at that _______ (room object)."

A drunk is usually considered somewhat unconfrontable and he himself certainly cannot confront. One thing he cannot confront is an empty glass. He always refills it if it is empty.

Repeat the command, each time pointing out a room object, as often as required to bring the person to sobriety. Do not get distracted into answering the frequent comment, "What object?" Just get the command carried out, acknowledge and give the next command.

Run until the person is no longer drunk.

Do not ever get angry with or strike a drunk, whatever the provocation.

This process is not intended to handle the condition of alcoholism. There are more advanced Scientology procedures that can be done to handle the conditions that caused a person to be alcoholic. But one can do a lot of good for the person and those around him by using this assist to bring him back to sobriety.

We are not particularly in the business of handling the drunk. But we are in the field of helping our fellow men. In a society where the only alternative is a night in jail and a fine, which is not desired by either the police or the intoxicated person, we can assist both and handle the situation in a matter of minutes.

Unconscious Person Assist

A person who is unconscious, even someone who has been in a long-continued coma, can be helped using a process called an Unconscious Person Assist. With this assist you can help to get the person into communication with you and his surroundings, and so bring him from unconsciousness back to life and livingness. It is an easy assist to learn and to do.

Theory

The theory of why assists work includes three factors. The first is control and direction of attention. The second is location. The third is time. The injured or ill person *remains* ill or injured because there is something wrong with each of these three factors. His *attention* is not under any control, he is *located* thoughtwise elsewhere and he is not in present *time.* He is in the past. The problem of someone who wishes to help with an assist is how to control the person's attention, get the person located *here* and into present time. By having the unconscious person touch nearby things like a pillow, the floor or his body (without hurting an injured body part), you can help bring his attention under control and bring him into present time. The process is feather-light, but it can reach a long way down.

Procedure

1. Take the person's hand gently in your hand and tell him, "I am going to assist you to recover."

2. Give the command "Feel that _________(object)." Gently move the person's hand and press it against an object, and give him a very short time to feel it. Use the bedspread, pillow, bed, etc. You do not wait for any response, but you do give the person a moment to feel the object. (Don't fall for the belief that "unconscious" people are unable to think or be aware in any way. A thetan is seldom unconscious regardless of what the body is doing or not doing.)

3. Acknowledge the person.

4. Give the next command and move the person's hand to touch another object.

For example:

"Feel that bedspread."

(Person giving the assist places the unconscious person's hand on bedspread.)

(Pause)

"Thank you."

"Feel that pillow."

(Person giving the assist moves the unconscious person's hand and places it on pillow.)

(Pause)

"Thank you."

And so on.

5. Continue giving commands, moving his hand to the next object and acknowledging.

6. When the person has regained consciousness, you end off by saying, "End of assist."

If you are handling a person in a coma, you may not get him back to consciousness in a single assist session. What you look for in such a case as a signal to end the session is an improvement in the person's condition. There are various indicators which will tell you you've gotten an improvement. The person's breathing may be easier; his skin tone may improve; he may simply look better or more comfortable than when you started that session. Watch very carefully for such indicators. They show you are making progress. When you have an improvement on a person in a coma, end off by saying "That's it for today" and let the person know when you will see him for the next session.

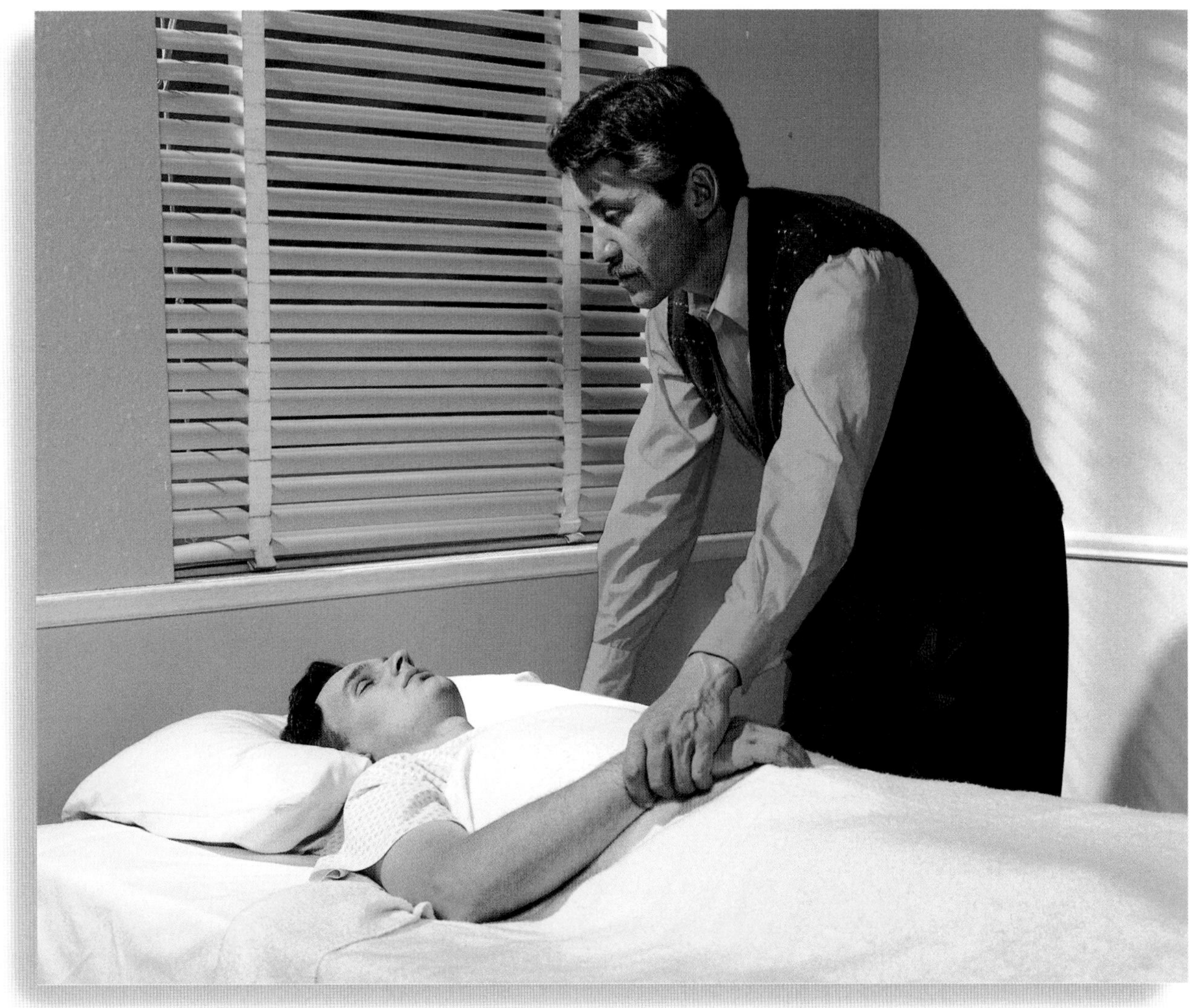

Having the unconscious person touch nearby things like a pillow, a blanket or his body can help bring his attention under control and bring him into present time and back to life and livingness.

Hand Signal System

A signal system can be arranged with an unconscious person in order to question him and get "yes" or "no" answers. The signal system is simple: clasp the person's hand gently in yours so that he can squeeze it. Tell him, "You can answer me by squeezing my hand. Squeeze once for 'Yes' and twice for 'No.'" You can then ask simple questions to find out if you have gotten an improvement: "Can you hear me?" or "Do you know where you are?" The person will usually respond, if faintly, even while unconscious. If there is no response or a negative response, continue with the assist session.

This system is especially useful when giving an assist to someone who is in a coma. Say you notice a change in the person during the assist, such as his eyelids quiver or squint slightly. The signal system can be used at that point to ask the person, "Do you feel any better?" or "Do you know where you are?" If you find he's improved, you end off that session, otherwise continue on until he does have an improvement.

Another example of the use of this system would be in starting an assist session on someone in a coma whom you've been giving regular assist sessions to. At the start of such a session you can establish the hand-squeeze signal system and ask the person, "Are you doing any better today?" or "Are you doing better than when I was here last?" Whatever response you get (short of the person coming back to consciousness right then and there), you still go ahead with the Unconscious Person Assist until you have an improvement for that session.

You may have to put in control on the environment before the assist can be started. For instance, if you were doing the assist in a hospital you would need to ensure that the medical staff would not interrupt you when giving the assist.

The assist is complete when you have the person back to consciousness. This may happen rather rapidly or it may sometimes require many sessions before it is achieved. Your job is to keep at it, taking each session to an improvement for the person. When the person is conscious again the assist is ended, but this is not the end of your handling of him. It means you can now move on to other assist actions and processing.

This simple assist can bring back life and livingness to an unconscious person. When done correctly, the result can be the greatest magic anybody ever saw!

Assists and the Environment

An assist carries with it a certain responsibility. A person goes through life and casts his shadow upon many people. You will quite likely find yourself in situations where a stranger would benefit from an assist.

Your approach under these circumstances should be straightforward and positive. Be professional and definite. You don't even need to ask for permission, just do it. If you are going to help some stranger out, help him out. Don't stand around explaining to bystanders what you are going to do or waiting for somebody's permission. If you are at the scene of a commotion and act as though you are the one in charge, you will be in charge. This is part and parcel of the knowledge of how to do an assist. If you do this well, the assists you render will amount to something.

Say, for example, there is a serious accident and a crowd of people are pressing around. The police are trying to push the people back. Well, push the people back and then lean over the victim and give him an assist. If you are enough *there,* everybody else will realize that you are the *one* that is *there.* Such things as panic, worry, wonder, upset, looking dreamily into the far distance, wondering what is wrong or what should be done are no part of your makeup if you are rendering an assist. Cool, calm and collected should be the keynote of your attitude. Realize that to take control of any given situation it is only necessary to be there more than anybody else. There is no magic involved. Just *be* there. The other people at the scene aren't. And if you are there enough, then somebody else will pull himself out of it and go on living.

Where you are giving an assist to a person, put things in the environment into an orderly state as the first step, unless you need to give immediate first aid.

First aid *always* precedes an assist. You should look the situation over from the standpoint of how much first aid is required. Maybe you will find somebody with a temperature of 106 degrees who needs to lie down and be cooled off before any assist is done and though antibiotics are much overrated, he might be better off with a shot of these antibiotics than with an assist at that time.

A good example would be a situation where somebody is washing dishes in the kitchen. Suddenly, there is a horrendous crash and the person falls down and hits the floor, but as she is going down, she grabs a butcher knife and cuts her hand. One of the first things you would do is wrap a bandage around her hand to stop the bleeding. Another part of the first aid would be to pick up the dishes and put them back on the sink and sweep the pieces together into a more orderly semblance. This is the first step toward restoring control.

Then you would give her an assist. To remove her from the scene of the accident is not as desirable as doing the assist on her there. Perhaps this is contrary to what you believe, but it is true, and is why you bring some order into the environment first. You manifest order in a much wider sphere than a cut hand in order to bring about a healing of the cut hand. If you understand that your responsibility always extends much wider than the immediate zone of commotion, you will be more successful. If you bring order to the wider environment, you also bring it to the narrower environment.

If you know you are going into a zone of accidents and you are going to be in the vicinity of a great deal of destruction and chaos, you would be very foolish not to have first aid training. Keep in mind that you may often have to find some method of controlling, handling and directing personnel who get in your way before you can render an assist. In circumstances such as these, an assist requires that you control the entire environment and personnel associated with the assist, if necessary.

As someone who knows and practices the technology of Scientology, you have every right and responsibility to relieve suffering when you see it. Religion exists in no small part to handle the upsets and anguish of life. These include spiritual duress (hardship) by reason of physical conditions.

Ministers long before Christ's Apostles had as a part of their duties the ministering to the spiritual anguish of their people. They have concentrated upon spiritual uplift and betterment. But where physical suffering impeded this course, they have acted. To devote themselves only to the alleviation of physical duress is of course to attest that the physical body is more important

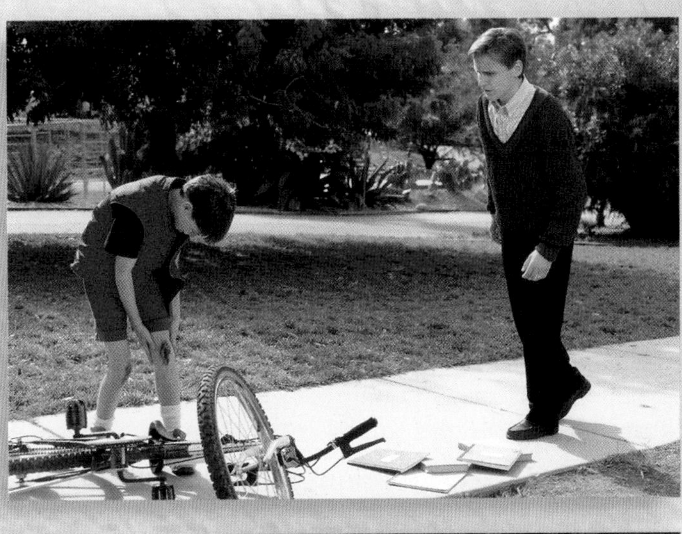

The area around an injured person is often chaotic and disorderly.

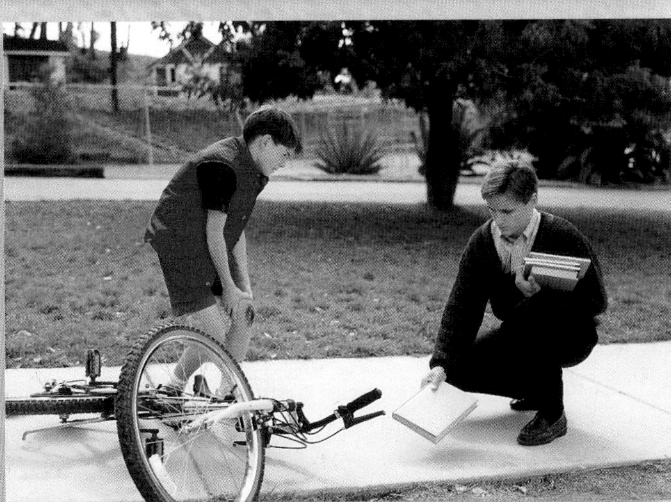

Putting order into it can lessen the confusion and reestablish control.

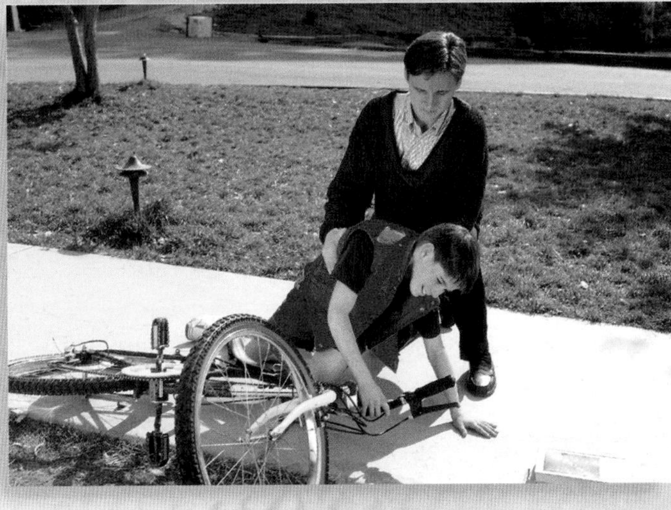

An assist will produce a better result when some attention is paid to the environment first.

than the spiritual beingness of the person which, of course, it is not. But physical anguish can so distract a being that he deserts any aspirations of betterment and begins to seek some cessation of his suffering. The specialty of the medical doctor is the curing of physical disease or nonoptimum physical conditions. In some instances he can do so. It is no invasion of his province to assist the patient to greater healing potential. And ills that are solely spiritual in nature are not medical.

The "psych-iatrist" and "psych-ologist" on the other hand took their very names from religion since *psyche* means soul. They, by actual statistics, are not as successful as priests in relieving mental anguish. But they modernly seek to do so by using drugs or hypnotism or physical means. They damage more than they help.

Those with spiritual knowledge have a responsibility to those about them to relieve suffering. There are many ways to do this without drugs or hypnotism or shock or surgery or violence.

The primary method of relieving suffering is the *assist.*

As the knowledge of how to do them exists and as the skill is easily acquired, we should not neglect those who will benefit from them.

If you truly want to help your fellows, that exact skill and those results are very well worth having. ■

TEST YOUR UNDERSTANDING

Answer the following questions about assists. Refer back to the chapter to check your answers. If you need to, review the chapter. Going over the material several times will increase your certainty and help you obtain better success in applying it.

- ❑ *What is an assist?*
- ❑ *What is the basis on which a Contact Assist works?*
- ❑ *Think of five situations where a Touch Assist would be beneficial.*
- ❑ *How does a Nerve Assist work?*
- ❑ *When would you use a Locational Processing Assist?*
- ❑ *How would you do an Unconscious Person Assist?*

PRACTICAL EXERCISES

Here are exercises you can do to practice giving assists. Doing these exercises will help you become proficient in helping others with assists.

1 Find someone who has suffered an injury. Go with him to the exact location of the injury and render a Contact Assist to the person until the exact somatic turns on and then blows off and the person has a cognition.

2 Find someone who needs a Touch Assist and give him one until he has good indicators and a cognition.

3 Find someone who needs a Nerve Assist and give him one until he has a cognition or expresses some relief and has very good indicators.

4 Find someone who needs the Body Communication Process and give him one until he has a good change, a cognition and very good indicators.

5 Find someone who has an injury or who just feels bad, and give him or her a Locational Processing Assist until the person has good indicators and a cognition.

6 Practice helping people with assists. Deliver any of the assists you have learned to friends, relatives, associates or even strangers. For instance, visit a hospital and give assists to people who are ill or injured or recovering from operations. Render assistance to someone in an emergency room. The more assists you deliver, the more skilled you will become and the more people you will help.

Results from Application

There is no way to accurately estimate the number of people who have been helped over the years by L. Ron Hubbard's Assist Technology. Although not a substitute for medical treatment, many people recover faster from minor or major accidents, illnesses, upsets, losses and a wide range of conditions affecting their well-being. If assists were universally used, it is estimated that health care costs could be reduced by up to one-third, a huge reduction of what is becoming an increasingly staggering burden.

Many cases have been reported where, because of an assist, the expense of a trip to the doctor or hospital was saved. And doctors have been astonished at the speed of recovery they have witnessed after assists were delivered to patients under their care.

It bears repeating here that assists do not invade the province of medicine or healing. But the results from assists demonstrate conclusively the improvement the individual can make in his own state of well-being. The following stories are not claims made by the Church of Scientology, but relate the experiences of individuals. By reading them one can gain an appreciation of just how effective assists can be.

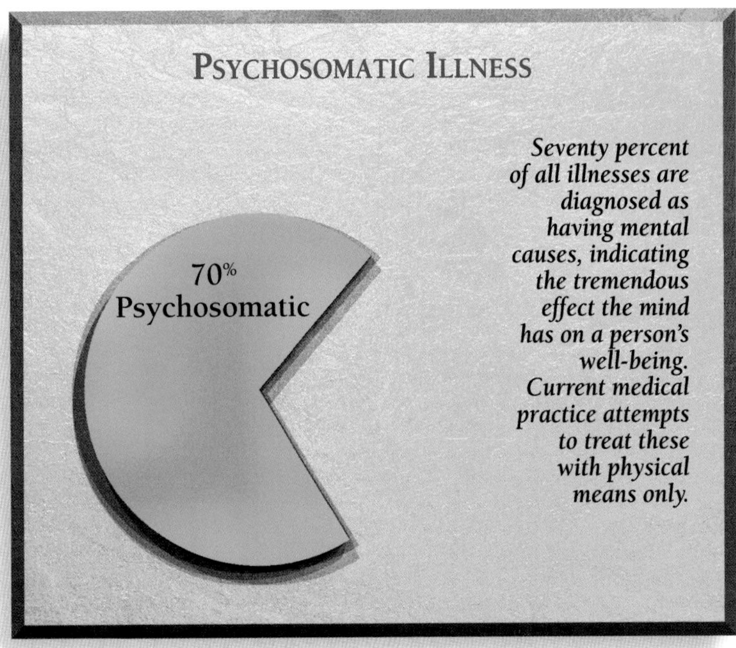

Psychosomatic Illness
70%
Psychosomatic
Seventy percent of all illnesses are diagnosed as having mental causes, indicating the tremendous effect the mind has on a person's well-being. Current medical practice attempts to treat these with physical means only.

In Los Angeles, a man was suffering from an inflammation in his elbow so bad he could not move it. He was only able to hold it as if it were in a sling. His brother gave him a Touch Assist and said this about the results:

"After only a few minutes I was amazed to watch the swelling go down and the whole injured area turn beet red as though a rash were forming. My brother started laughing and said, 'It's working already, my arm feels hot and it feels like the blood is flowing through it again.' We continued, and after the assist he had full mobility of his arm and was practically dancing. Four hours later he called me to say 'thanks'—he realized he had forgotten to tell me in all the excitement."

A computer programmer living in Los Angeles suffered a chronic kidney problem. The condition worsened until it became life-threatening and he was hospitalized. For seventeen months he underwent intensive care, including major surgery. The man's condition became critical to the point the doctors were convinced he had only a few hours to live and he was put on a life-support system. His wife learned how to deliver assists and gave him assists continuously during this crisis period. The man later described his experience in these words:

"I was very ill for months. I was under intensive care for weeks with a bleeding ulcer infection and kidney failure. My heart stopped three times and I died three times. I was unconscious for over a week, and I basically did not want to live. The doctors were going to give up on me and stop the treatment. The nurses did not expect me to live. But my wife came to the hospital every day to give me assists.

"As a result of the assists, I soon started becoming aware of my environment and had a determination to survive. The assists made life seem bright enough to continue living. I am now recovered and would not have lived if it weren't for the help many people gave me using the procedures developed by L. Ron Hubbard."

Remarkable recovery from a severe injury was made by a man in San Francisco, through the use of Assist Technology. Even to this day, he expresses awe about his recovery:

"I was working as a chimney sweep and had an accident in which I fell three stories, landing on my feet and breaking both of my heels. I went to the hospital where they prescribed painkillers and wanted to keep me overnight. Instead, I went home and my wife gave me a Touch Assist which handled the agony I was in, allowing me to sleep that night without painkillers. I received Touch Assists daily and by the end of that week, I was able to hobble around on crutches on my tiptoes. Then I received another type of assist after which something felt 'different' and when I stood up, I found I could easily stand on my feet without my crutches! This was amazing to me, as prior to this assist, the thought of putting all my weight on my feet was unthinkable. I was even able to walk down the hall! My recovery time was considerably cut down by the assists and in a short while I was running again and in great health. The speed and thoroughness of my recovery was a miracle to me and I am very thankful to Mr. Hubbard for developing this technology and making it available to all of us."

The life of a South African woman was completely changed by assists she received from a friend. The woman was helpless and in chronic pain from severe arthritis. Her friend found it hard to believe that such a simple procedure opened the door to complete recovery.

"I had success applying Touch Assist technology to a woman from South Africa. She was in her seventies and had severe and painful arthritis in her hands. She had to spend at least an hour every

morning just to get dressed, including soaking her hands in hot water and doing other things to reduce the pain and to make her fingers at least a little bit mobile. All I did for about a week was give her a Touch Assist two or three times a day. Gradually her arthritis improved and after a week there was a vast improvement in this condition. She was able to do things like tie her shoes and button her blouse, which she could not do before the assists started. She was much more cheerful and very happy about the progress and greatly reduced pain. With additional assists she recovered fully from the arthritis."

A California man was able to save the life of a young mother who had been badly hurt in a car accident. He was amazed at the effectiveness of the assist:

"I was driving down a boulevard when I saw a huge car accident. There was a lady lying in the street unconscious and as no one was helping her and the people there were in fear of doing anything, I moved the crowd back and told them to be quiet. I had to kneel down and almost lie on the ground to get near her to help her. I then gave her the commands one gives an unconscious person—I thought she was alive but it was hard to tell, there was blood pouring out of her mouth. I continued to give her the commands and while I was doing this two doctors came up and both stood about six feet from me. They were very hesitant to get involved and one offered help if needed but they clearly did not want to interrupt something that they could see was helping the lady. After some time she started to move and then to talk, then she wanted to see her child—she got very insistent about seeing her kid to be sure her kid was okay. I had her child brought over, the child was fine and the lady calmed down. By then, the ambulance had come to take her to the hospital and she was fully conscious. She was very thankful for the help."

Through a ten-minute assist, a woman from England was able to produce a miracle that enabled another woman to successfully give birth to her baby when it had been medically declared impossible.

"A Danish friend had experienced a very difficult time at the birth of her first child and her doctor had advised against having more children. But she and her husband really wanted to have another baby. She had had two miscarriages, and had undergone a surgical procedure to help her carry a baby to full term. She got pregnant again, but was very worried that she would miscarry. One day while I was visiting her home, the familiar symptoms of another miscarriage began and she was in tears of despair. With her agreement I immediately administered a Touch Assist. After only about ten minutes of the assist, her face flushed and she exclaimed that it felt as if a huge weight had suddenly left her body. The pain and bleeding stopped and she started to laugh with relief. She had no more trouble with the pregnancy and a

few months later gave birth to a healthy baby girl without any unusual medical assistance, to the complete surprise of her doctor."

A girl from Switzerland was able to help her mother recover from a bad fall. She said:

"Last week I went to visit my mom and when I got there she was a bit scratched up and I found out that she had just fallen down on the concrete pretty badly. She then showed me her hand and wrist which were all blue and swelling. I immediately took her to the place she had fallen and I had her duplicate the exact same motion that happened when she fell and hurt her hand. At first it was hurting, then suddenly, she felt tingling in her hand and the pain went away. We looked at her hand and the blue reduced and my mom said that her hand was much better. During the rest of the day she kept saying that her hand was much better and after that it was healed. This was the result of the Contact Assist we did."

In San Diego, a man badly injured in a car accident was helped with miraculous results. The man who rendered the assistance recounted the experience:

"I came upon what was a very bad car wreck with two vehicles totally smashed from impact and rolling over and over. I ran to the first person I saw. He was sitting behind the wheel of one of the cars, unconscious, with windshield glass in his face and arms. He looked like he was dead and not breathing. I got myself into the car and told him to 'Feel my hand.' His eyes immediately popped open and he said 'What happened?' I told him that he had been in a car wreck and told him that I was a Scientology minister-in-training and I was going to give him an assist and got his agreement to do as I asked.

"I then proceeded to give him a locational and all the bleeding stopped. A nurse had shown up and started to dab him with a cloth, but all she was doing was pushing the glass into his face which started the bleeding again. I pointed this out and she left. I had by this time gotten the man out of the car and continued with the locational. He brightened way up and originated calling his wife to let her know that he was all right and would be home after he went to the hospital.

"By now the police had shown up and ambulances had come. The officer in charge had sent all the ambulances with the other people involved in the wreck and told me that the person I was working with looked well enough not to have to go to the hospital and that he would not call another ambulance right away. This amazed me as the guy had glass splinters all through his face and arms. I walked over to a police car that had just driven up, opened the back door and placed the injured person in the back and sent the police car to the emergency room at the hospital.

"I saw the technology work that night and realized for myself that one can be in control of the situation providing he knows and uses the technology. It works."

Suggestions for Further Study

The assists in this chapter, while the most used, are only a fraction of the technology L. Ron Hubbard developed in the area. The books and courses listed here are available to any person wishing the complete data on the subject.

Assists Processing Handbook

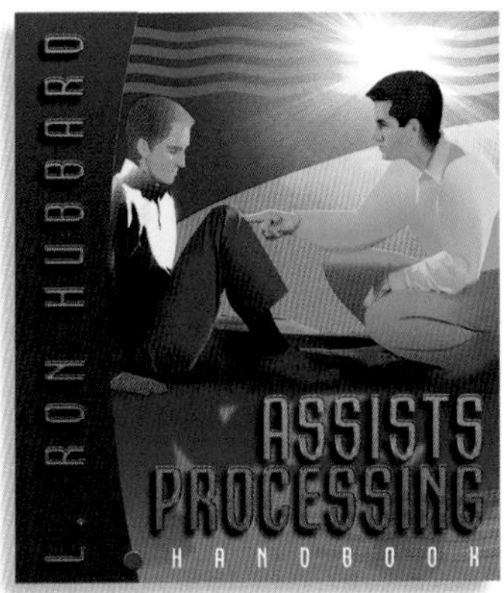

The complete collection of more than 130 different assists developed by L. Ron Hubbard for use in a wide variety of circumstances. Gives detailed instructions for assists to handle toothaches, a fight with a spouse, nosebleeds, newborn babies, people with fevers, even a person in a coma. *All* Mr. Hubbard's technology on assists is contained in this volume. Complete with reference tables which list the range of assists for different situations encountered. Scientology organizations deliver a course based on the book—the Hubbard Assists Processing Auditor Course—which thoroughly trains a person to skillfully apply all assists.

Hubbard Qualified Scientologist Course

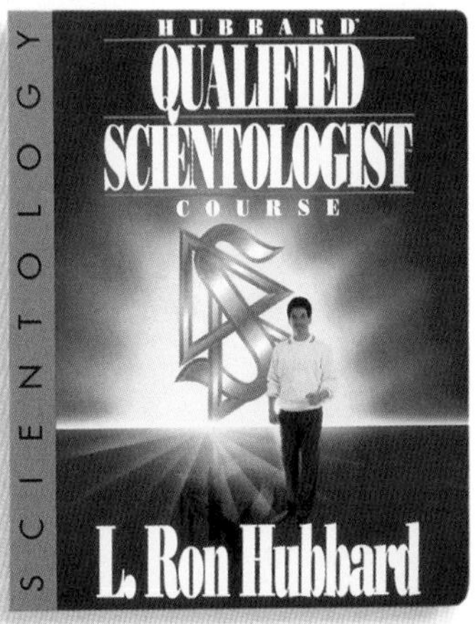

Provides a broad spectrum of Scientology basics, expanding the knowledge of assists contained in this chapter. Students become experienced in the application of assists and other Scientology procedures to help others. In addition to material on assists, the course also contains many other Scientology fundamentals. These give the student a firm grounding in Scientology's philosophic principles. (Delivered in Scientology organizations.)

Hubbard New Era Dianetics Auditor Course

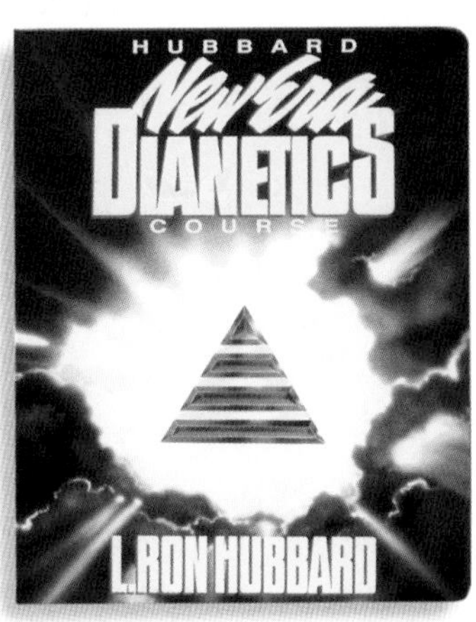

A New Era Dianetics Auditor is a skilled practitioner who can bring individuals to a higher awareness of their spiritual capabilities and greater well-being through exact application of carefully researched processes. This course teaches the ultimate and most powerful refinement of Dianetics technology developed by L. Ron Hubbard in more than forty years of research. Contains all New Era Dianetics technology including advanced assist auditing techniques, and five of Mr. Hubbard's lectures. In a three-week full-time course of study, an auditor becomes adept at applying this technology to alleviate the source of psychosomatic illnesses and a host of other conditions. (Delivered in Scientology organizations.)

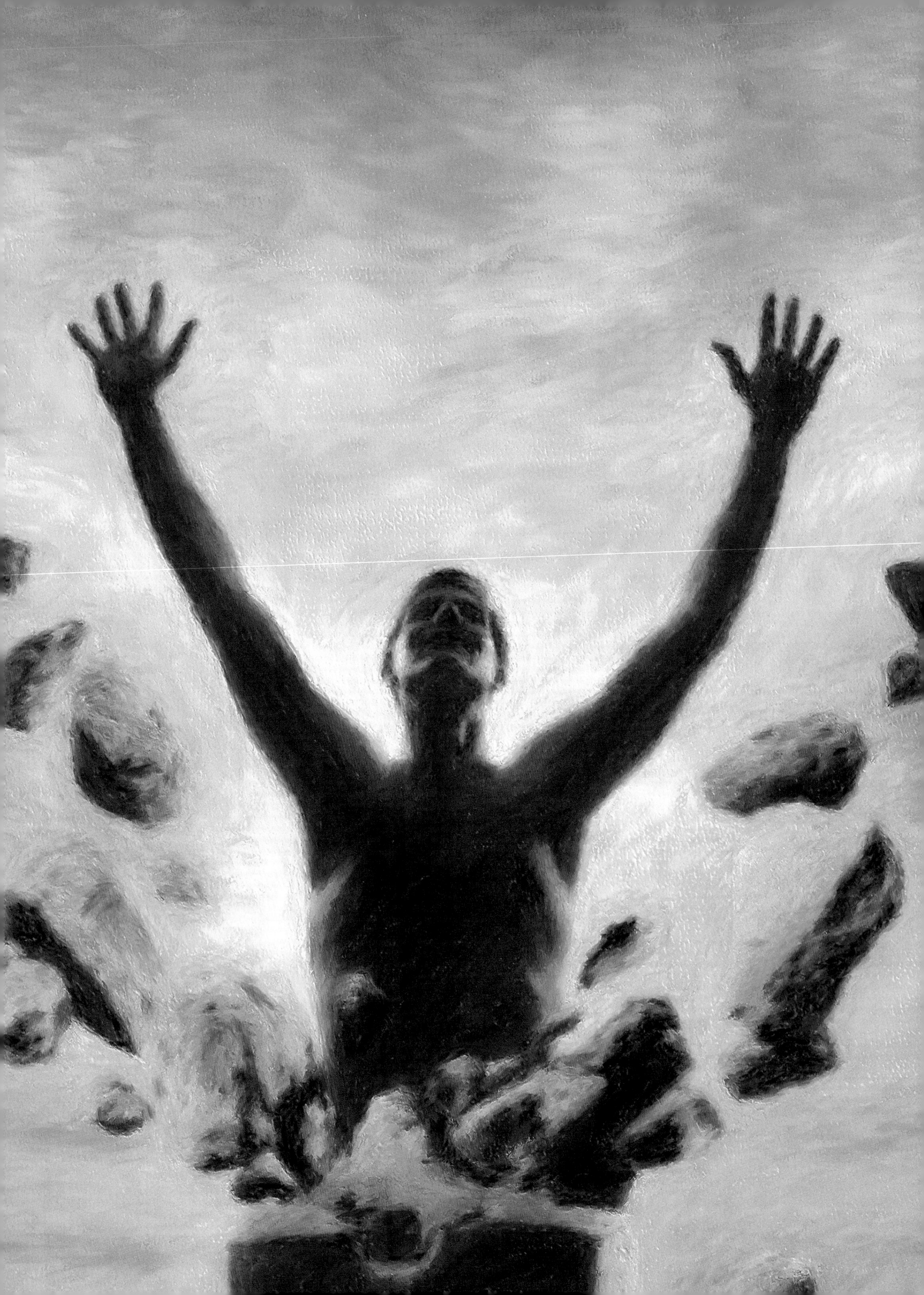

Chapter 7

Answers to Drugs

To say that drugs have become the major affliction of society is not stating the situation too strongly. No sector of life is untouched by this epidemic. Crime and violence are the most obvious byproducts, but amorality, aborted educations and, indeed, ruined lives are no less serious and just as widespread.

And the problem is not limited to street drugs; the effects of medical and psychiatric drugs, whether painkillers, tranquilizers or "antidepressants," are as disastrous.

L. Ron Hubbard addressed this problem, not with the objective of resolving the physical ills of individuals but as a continuation of his quest to free man as a spirit and handle, along this route, any barrier that needed to be resolved. Drugs were such a barrier.

Until Mr. Hubbard developed a workable drug rehabilitation program, there was no solution. Psychiatric-inspired programs had many more failures than successes and some only created worse addictions. Other people, more well-intentioned, found that good intentions weren't enough. They lacked a technology that worked.

Mr. Hubbard's program provides that technology. From helping the person discover why he took drugs in the first place, to eliminating the mental and spiritual damage done by drugs, to detoxifying the body of long-term drug residues, to providing the person with tools that will enable him to stay off drugs for good, it is without doubt the most thorough and effective program in the world. Today, for the first time, as hundreds of thousands will attest, those addicted to drugs and alcohol can free themselves of this tyranny and face life with renewed vigor and hope. This chapter contains some of the elementary principles of this program and provides the first real understanding of substance abuse problems.

THE REASON BEHIND THE DRUG PROBLEM

People have used drugs for as long as they have tried to ease pain and avoid problems. Since the early 1960s, however, drugs have been in very widespread use. Before that time they were rare. A worldwide spread of drugs occurred during that decade, and a large percentage of people became drug-takers.

By drugs (to mention a few) are meant tranquilizers, opium, cocaine, marijuana, peyote, amphetamines and the psychiatrist's gifts to man, LSD and angel dust, which are the worst. Any medical drugs are included. Drugs are drugs. There are thousands of trade names and slang terms for these drugs. Alcohol is also classified as a drug.

Drugs are supposed to do wonderful things but all they really do is ruin the person.

Drug problems do not end when a person stops taking drugs. The accumulated effects of drug-taking can leave one severely impaired, both physically and mentally. Even someone off drugs for years still has "blank periods." Drugs can injure a person's ability to concentrate, to work, to learn—in short, they can shatter a life.

Yet though the dangers and liabilities of drugs are blatantly obvious and increasingly well documented, people continue to take them.

Why?

When a person is depressed or in pain, and where he finds no physical relief from treatment, he will eventually discover for himself that drugs remove his symptoms.

This is also true for pains which are "psychosomatic." The term "psychosomatic" means the mind making the body ill or illnesses caused through the mind. "Psycho" refers to "mind" and "soma" refers to "body."

In almost all cases of psychosomatic pain, illness or discomfort the person has sought some cure for the upset.

When he at last finds that only drugs give him relief, he will surrender to them and become dependent upon them, often to the point of addiction.

Years before, had there been any other way out, most people would have taken it. But when they are told there is no cure, that their pains are "imaginary," life tends to become insupportable. They then can become chronic drug-takers and are in danger of addiction.

The time required to make an addict varies, of course. The complaint itself may only be "sadness" or "weariness." The ability to face life, in any case, is reduced.

Any substance that brings relief or makes life less a burden physically or mentally will then be welcome.

In an unsettled and insecure environment, psychosomatic illness is very widespread.

So before any government strikes too heavily at spreading drug use, it should recognize that it is a symptom of failed psychotherapy. The social scientist, the psychologist and psychiatrist and health ministers have failed to handle spreading psychosomatic illness.

It is too easy to blame the drug problem on "social unrest" or the "pace of modern society."

The hard, solid fact is that until now there has been no effective psychotherapy in broad practice. The result is a drug-dependent population.

Drug users have been found to have begun taking drugs because of physical suffering or hopelessness.

The user, driven by pain and environmental hopelessness, continues to take drugs. Though he doesn't want to be an addict, he doesn't feel that there is any other way out.

However, with proper treatment, drug dependency *can* be fully handled.

As soon as he can feel healthier and more competent mentally and physically without drugs than he does on drugs, a person ceases to require drugs.

Drug addiction has been shrugged off by psychiatry as "unimportant" and the social problem of drug-taking has received no attention from psychiatrists—rather the contrary, since they themselves introduced and popularized LSD. And many of them are pushers.

Government agencies have failed markedly to halt the increase in drug-taking and there has been no real or widespread cure.

The liability of the drug user, even after he has ceased to use drugs, is that he "goes blank" at unexpected times, has periods of irresponsibility and tends to sicken easily.

Scientology technology has been able to eradicate the major damage in persons who have been on drugs as well as make further addiction unnecessary and unwanted.

Scientology has no interest in the political or social aspects of the various types of drugs or even drug-taking as such. Drugs, however, pose a growing threat to mental and spiritual advancement—which is the true mission of Scientology.

Thus, Scientology contains an exact technology which not only gets a person painlessly off drugs but handles their physical, mental and spiritual effects *and* locates and fully resolves the reason underlying a person's drug-taking. Nothing else can do this with certainty.

When a person can find no solution to a problem, whether the problem be anything from physical suffering to hopelessness…

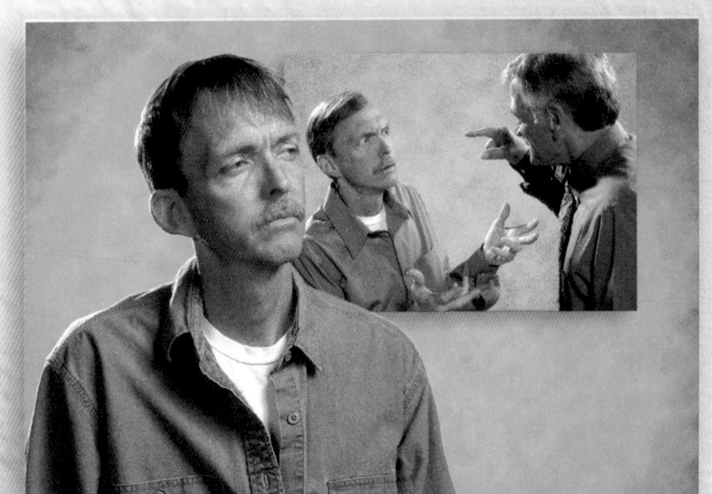

…he sooner or later finds that drugs relieve symptoms.

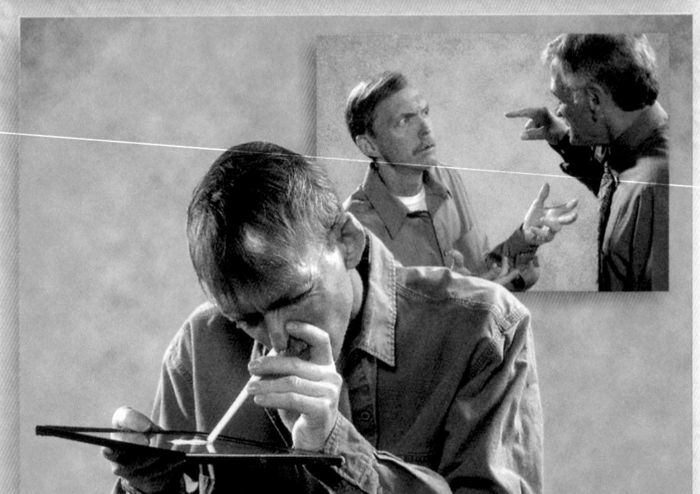

The problem, however, is not gone, but only masked by the drugs. Until the problem itself is effectively resolved, the person will be dependent on drugs or even addicted to them.

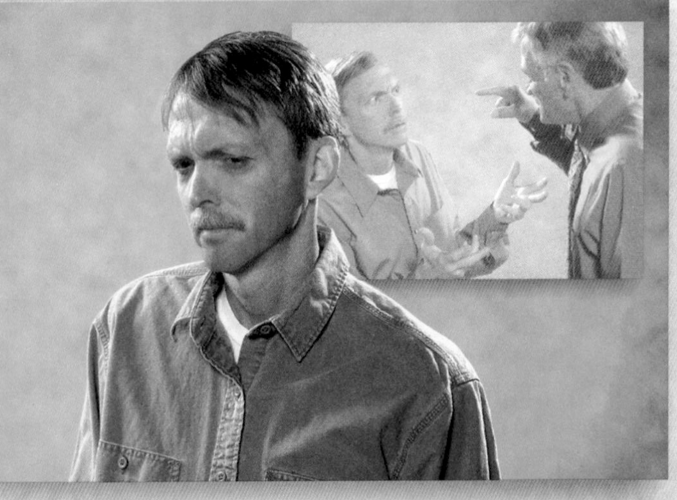

Drugs and Their Effects on the Mind

Drugs essentially are poisons. The degree they are taken determines the effect. A small amount gives a stimulant (increases activity). A greater amount acts as a sedative (suppresses activity). A larger amount acts as a poison and can kill one.

This is true of any drug. Each requires a different amount.

Caffeine is a drug, so coffee is an example. One hundred cups of coffee would probably kill a person. Ten cups would probably put him to sleep. Two or three cups stimulates. This is a very common drug. It is not very harmful as it takes so much of it to have an effect. So it is known as a stimulant.

Arsenic is known as a poison. Yet a tiny amount of arsenic is a stimulant, a good-sized dose puts one to sleep and a few grains kills one.

But there are many drugs which have another liability: they directly affect the mind.

In order to have a good understanding of the mental effects of drugs, it is necessary to know something about what the mind is. The *mind* is not a brain. It is the accumulated recordings of thoughts, conclusions, decisions, observations and perceptions of a person throughout his entire existence. In Scientology it has been discovered that the *mind* is a communication and control system between a thetan and his environment. By *thetan* is meant the person himself, the spiritual being—not his body or his name, the physical universe, his mind, or anything else.

The most obvious portion of the mind is recognizable by anyone not in serious condition. This is the *mental image picture.*

Various phenomena connect themselves with this entity called the mind. Some people closing their eyes see only blackness, some people see pictures.

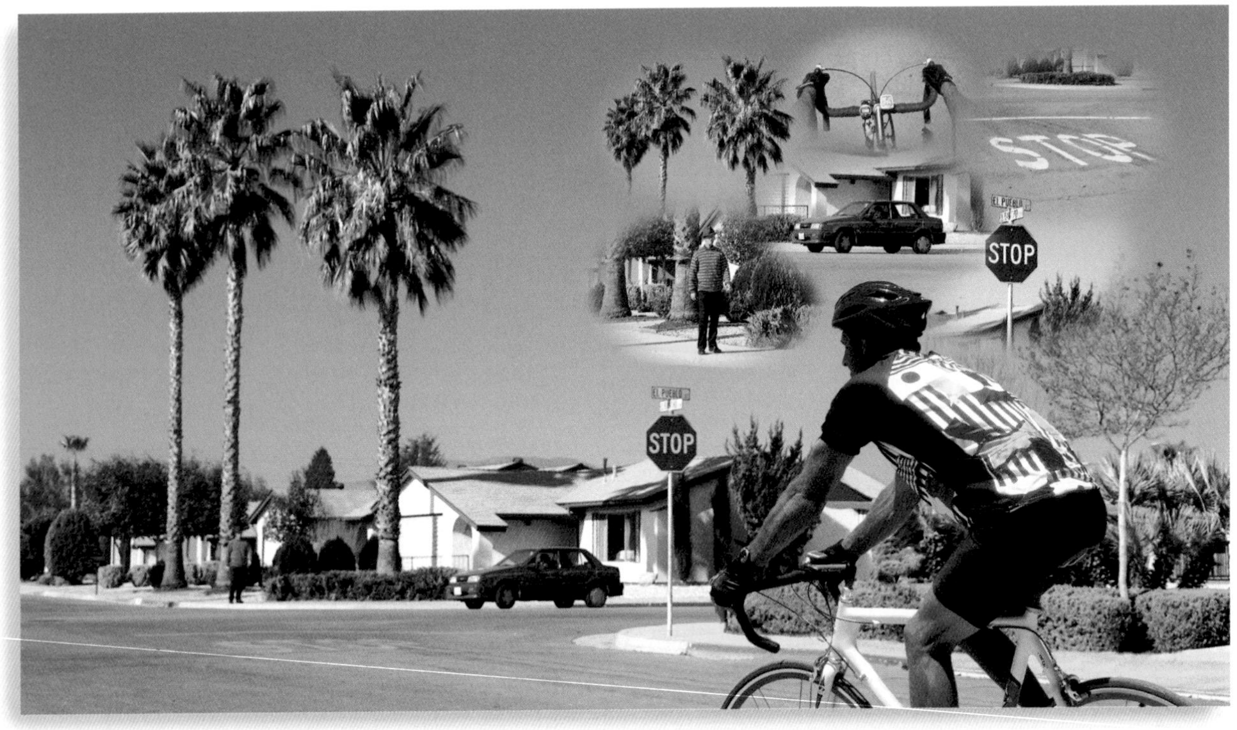

The mind is a communication and control system between a thetan and his environment. The mind is not a brain.

The thetan receives, by the communication system called the mind, various impressions, including direct views of the physical universe. In addition to this he receives impressions from past activities and, most important, he himself conceives things about the past and future which are independent of immediately present stimuli.

A person who has taken drugs, in addition to the physical factors involved, retains mental image pictures of those drugs and their effects. Mental image pictures are three-dimensional color pictures with sound and smell and all other perceptions, plus the conclusions or speculations of the individual. They are mental copies of one's perceptions sometime in the past, although in cases of unconsciousness or lessened consciousness they exist *below* the individual's awareness. For example, a person who had taken LSD would retain "pictures" of that experience in his mind, complete with recordings of the sights, physical sensations, smells, sounds, etc., that occurred while he was under the influence of LSD.

Let us say an individual took LSD one day while at a fairground with some friends, and the day's experiences included feeling nauseated and dizzy, getting into an argument with a friend, feeling an emotion of sadness, and later feeling very tired. He would have mental image pictures of that entire incident.

At a later time, if this person's environment were to contain enough similarities to the elements in that past incident, he may experience a reactivation of that incident. As a result he could feel nauseated, dizzy, sad and very tired—all for no apparent reason. This is known as *restimulation:* the reactivation of a past memory due to similar circumstances in the present approximating circumstances of the past.

Such mental image pictures can also be reactivated by drug residuals, as the presence of these drugs in the tissues of the body can simulate the earlier drug experiences.

Using the above example of the person who took LSD, sometime later—perhaps years afterward—the residuals of the drug that are still in his body tissues can cause a restimulation of that LSD incident. The mental image pictures are reactivated, and he experiences the same sensations of nausea, dizziness and tiredness, and he feels sad. He does not know why. He might also perceive mental images of the persons he was with and the accompanying sights and sounds and smells.

These are the effects on the mind of *past* drug usage. However, the *current* use of drugs creates a similar and more immediate effect on the mind.

When a person uses a drug such as marijuana, peyote, opium, morphine or heroin, mental image pictures of past times can "turn on" or restimulate below the individual's conscious awareness, causing him to perceive something different than what is actually going on.

Thus, right there before your eyes, apparently in the same room as you are, doing the same things, the drug-taker is really only partially there and partially in some past events.

He *seems* to be there. Really he isn't "tracking" fully with present time.

What is going on to a rational observation is *not* what is going on to him.

Thus, he does not understand statements made by another but tries to fit them into his composite reality, meaning a reality made up of different components. In order to fit them in, he has to alter them.

Drugs affect the mind by reactivating incidents from a person's past, below his conscious awareness.

This can distort the drug user's perception of what is happening around him.

As a result, the person's actions may appear very odd or irrational.

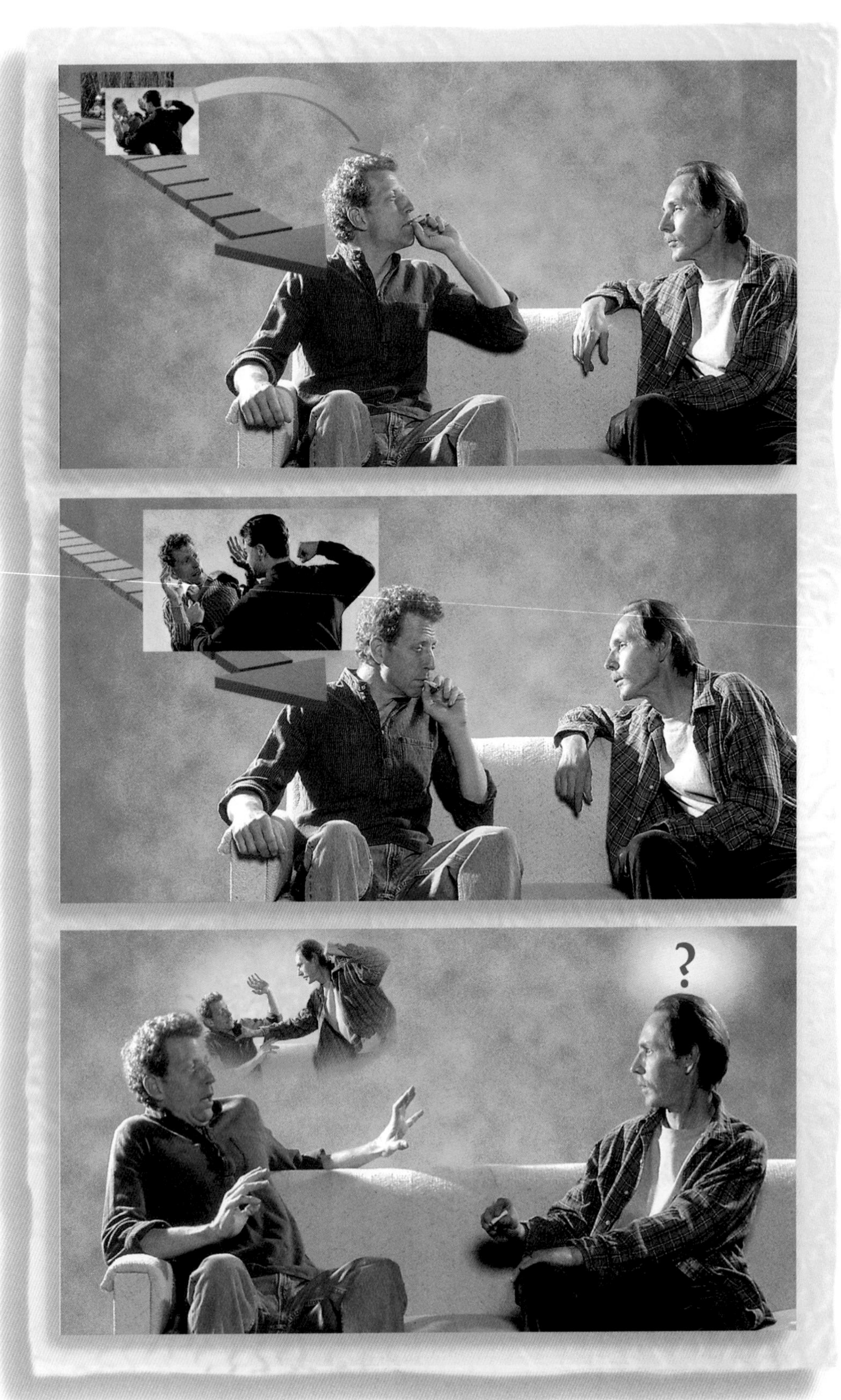

For example, a drug user may be *sure* he is helping one *repair* a floor that needs fixing, but in fact he is hindering the actual operation in progress which consists of *cleaning* the floor. So when he "helps one" mop the floor, he introduces chaos into the activity. Since *he* is *repairing* the floor, a request to "give me the mop" has to be reinterpreted as "hand me the hammer." But the mop handle is longer than a hammer handle so the bucket gets upset.

This can be slight, wherein the person is seen to make occasional mistakes. It can be as serious as total insanity where the events apparent to him are *completely* different than those apparent to anyone else. And it can be all grades in between.

It is not that he doesn't know what is going on. It is that he perceives *something else* going on instead of the present sequence of events.

Thus, others appear to him to be stupid or unreasonable or insane. As *they* don't agree in their actions and orders with what he *plainly sees* is in progress, "they" aren't sensible. Example: A group is moving furniture. To all but one they are simply moving furniture. This one perceives himself to be "moving geometric shapes into a cloud." Thus, this one "makes mistakes." As the group doesn't see inside him and only sees another like themselves, they can't figure out why he "balls things up so."

Such persons as drug-takers and the insane are thus slightly or wholly on an apparently different time track of "present time" events.

A drug may be taken to drive a person out of an unbearable present time or out of consciousness altogether.

In some persons they do not afterwards return wholly to present time.

A thetan can also escape an unbearable present time by dropping into the past, even without drugs.

The drug-taker and the insane alike have not recovered present time, to a greater or lesser degree. Thus they think they are running on a different time track than they are.

These are the underlying facts in odd human behavior.

As what is going on according to the perception and subjective reality of such a person is varied in greater or lesser degree from the objective reality of others, such a person disturbs the environment and disrupts the smooth running of *any* group—from family to business to nation.

We have all known such a person, so it is not uncommon in the current civilization. The sudden remark which makes no sense, totally out of context with what is being spoken about; the blank stare when given an order or remark—behind these lies a whole imaginary world which is jarred by our attempts to get something done in present time.

The repercussions of drugs then, go far beyond their immediate effects and often influence many others besides the user. The consequences can be very harmful. This is true not only of illegal street drugs but also of medical drugs that are supposed to help people.

Painkillers

Doctors and others prescribe painkillers such as aspirin, tranquilizers, hypnotics and soporifics (sleep-inducing drugs) in an understandable wish to relieve pain.

However, it has never been known in chemistry or medicine exactly how or why these things worked. Such compositions are derived by accidental discoveries that "such and so depresses pain."

The effects of existing compounds are not uniform in result and often have very bad side effects.

As the *reason* they worked was unknown, very little advance has been made in biochemistry—the chemistry of life processes and substances. If the reason they worked were known and accepted, possibly chemists could develop some actual painkillers which had minimal side effects.

Pain or discomfort of a psychosomatic nature comes from mental image pictures created by the thetan which press against and affect the body. For example, a mental image picture of a past incident in which an arm was broken can be reactivated in the present, impinging on the body and causing pain in that same arm.

By actual clinical test, the actions of aspirin and other pain depressants are to:

A. *Inhibit the ability of the thetan to create mental image pictures*

and also

B. *To impede the electrical conductivity of nerve channels.*

As a result, the thetan is rendered *stupid,* blank, forgetful, delusive and irresponsible. He gets into a "wooden" sort of state, unfeeling, insensitive, unable and definitely not trustworthy, a menace to his fellows actually.

When the drugs wear off or start to wear off, the ability to create mental image pictures starts to return and *turns on somatics* (body sensations, illnesses or pains or discomforts) *much harder.* One of the answers a person

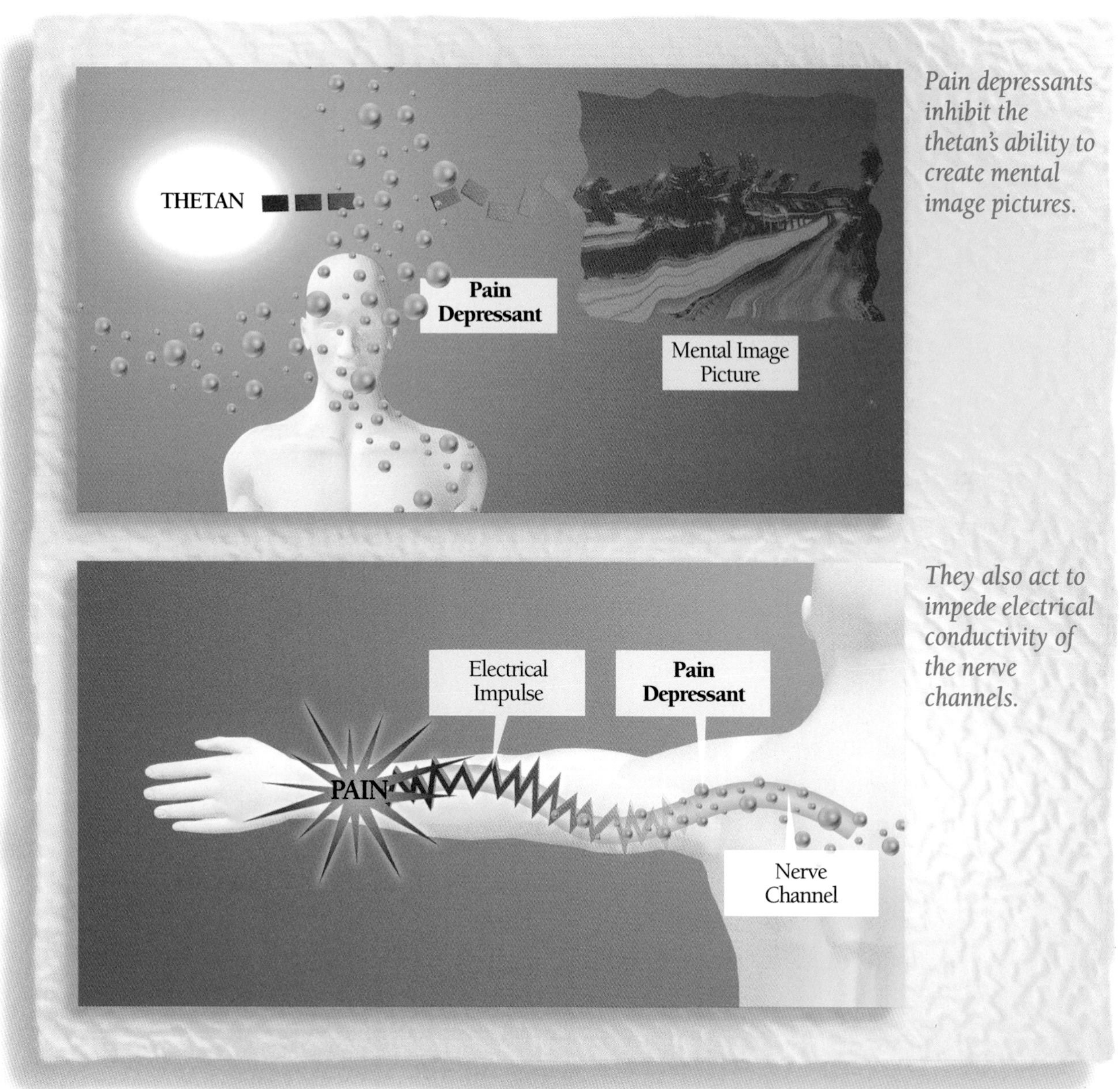

Pain depressants inhibit the thetan's ability to create mental image pictures.

They also act to impede electrical conductivity of the nerve channels.

has for this is *more* drugs. To say nothing of heroin, there are aspirin addicts. The compulsion stems from a desire to get rid of the somatics and unwanted sensations again. The being gets more and more wooden, requiring more and more quantity and more frequent use.

Sexually it is common for someone on drugs to be very stimulated at first. But after the original sexual "kicks," the stimulation of sexual sensation becomes harder and harder to achieve. The effort to achieve it becomes obsessive while it itself is less and less satisfying.

The cycle of drug restimulation of pictures (or creation in general) can be at first to increase creation and then eventually inhibit it totally.

If one were working on the problem of pain relief biochemically, the least harmful pain depressant would be one that inhibited the creation of mental image pictures with minimal resulting "woodenness" or stupidity and which was body-soluble (easily dissolved in the body) so that it passed rapidly out of the nerves and system.

There are unwanted sensations that drugs block off, but there is a whole sector of desirable sensations, and drugs block off all sensations.

The only defense that can be made for drugs is that they give a short, quick oblivion from immediate agony and permit the handling of a person to effect repair. But even then this is applicable to persons who have no other system to handle their pain.

Dexterity, ability and alertness are the main things that prevent getting into painful situations. These all vanish with drugs. So drugs set you up to get into situations which are truly disastrous and keep you that way.

One has a choice between being dead with drugs or being alive without them. Drugs rob life of the sensations and joys which are the only reasons for living anyhow.

HELPING SOMEONE GET OFF DRUGS

When the world went into heavy drug abuse, the problem of drying out became one of the first order. All pre-Scientology efforts to help drug users failed—and had been failing throughout man's history.

However, workable solutions have been developed in Scientology which enable a person not only to cease drug use, but to reach and eradicate the root causes which started him or her down that dark road.

Drugs can extract a dreadful price from the user should he ever try to quit.

What is called *withdrawal symptoms* set in. These are the physical and mental reactions to no longer taking drugs. They are ghastly. No torturer ever set up anything worse.

The person had this problem then:

A. Stay on drugs and be trapped and suffering from here on out, or

B. Try to come off the drugs and be so agonizingly ill meanwhile that he couldn't stand it.

This was a dead-if-you-do, dead-if-you-don't sort of problem.

Medicine did not solve it adequately. Psychotherapy was impossible.

Two approaches now exist to this withdrawal problem, both of which should be used:

1. Nutritionist experiments indicate that vitamins and minerals assist the withdrawal.

2. Light Objective Processes ease the gradual withdrawal and make it possible.

A *process* is an exact series of directions or sequence of actions taken to accomplish a desired result. Its application is called *processing*. There are many processes contained in the materials of Scientology which can be used to help a person direct his attention off himself and onto his environment and the people and things in it—an action which is very therapeutic for someone coming off drugs. These are called Objective Processes. When properly used, they ease the person's symptoms and make drug withdrawal possible with a minimum of discomfort.

Objective refers to outward things, not the thoughts or feelings of the individual. *Objective Processes* deal with the real and observable. They call for the person to spot or find something exterior to himself in order to carry out the procedures.

The Objective Processes referred to here are called "light" Objective Processes in that they are simpler and less advanced than other Objective Processes which exist in Scientology.

The details of how to use these two approaches to getting someone unhooked from drugs follow. If you know someone who is dependent on drugs, you can help him withdraw from them by applying the principles and techniques given here.

On severe cases of drug addiction one should send the person to a qualified medical doctor for examination to determine if there are any special precautions that may need to be taken for that particular person.

Some persons may have been put on some therapeutic drug by a medical doctor and possibly should remain on it. But these are not the usual drugs we are dealing with. It is up to the person and the doctor what should be done in such cases.

Nutritional Data

According to world-renowned nutritionist Adelle Davis, vitamin therapy has had success in handling withdrawal symptoms.

Instead of just telling the person to break off drugs with all that suffering and danger of failure, the patient is given heavy doses of vitamins. The data is repeated here for information.

The Drug Bomb

A vitamin formula called the "drug bomb" has been found effective in combating the effects of withdrawal. It consists of:

1,000 milligrams of niacinamide (*not* nicotinic acid). This helps counteract any mental disturbance.

5,000 IU of vitamin A.

400 IU of vitamin D.

800 IU of vitamin E.

2,000 milligrams of vitamin C.

500 milligrams of magnesium carbonate (to make the vitamin C effective).

25 milligrams of B_6.

200 milligrams of B complex.

300 milligrams of B_1.

100 milligrams of pantothenic acid.

This formula should be given four times a day while a person is coming off drugs, roughly every six hours.

It should *not* be taken on an empty stomach, as it could cause stomach burn. It should be taken after meals or, if taken between meals, with yogurt.

Great caution must be taken to give the dose in such a way that the vitamins will not corrode the stomach. If this is neglected, the person can be given a false duodenal (upper intestine) ulcer and will be unable to continue the treatment. Drug users are usually in terrible physical condition anyway. Thus, the vitamins would have to be in "enteric coated" tablets, meaning an intestinal shielding must be on the pills so they gradually dissolve and don't hit the sensitive upper stomach hard enough to corrode it.

Thus, milk with powdered amino acids in it would have to be given to wash the pills down.

In testing these recommendations, stomach corrosion (wearing away) from the vitamin formula was the main barrier noted.

If the formula is given without any cushion, the person can (a) feel too full after eating, (b) have a stomachache, (c) have a burning sensation, (d) the exterior of the stomach can get sore. These are all stomach ulcer symptoms.

If such symptoms turn on, end off the vitamins. Aluminum hydroxide tablets chewed up and swallowed in milk each time the symptoms start will ease the stomach. Powdered amino acids, yogurt and milk must then be given until the stomach gets better.

The potential benefits of the drug bomb far outweigh any possible drawbacks and so it has much value. The difficulties and agonies of withdrawal are the primary failure point in trying to salvage a being from the insanity of drugs.

Calcium and Magnesium

Used in conjunction with the drug bomb, there is an additional method of alleviating drug withdrawal symptoms which involves use of the minerals calcium and magnesium.

Muscular spasms are caused by lack of calcium. Nervous reactions are diminished by magnesium.

Calcium does not go into solution in the body and is not utilized unless it is in an acid.

Tests for other uses than drug reactions brought about the means of getting calcium into solution in the body along with magnesium so that the results of both could be achieved. The answer was to add vinegar, which would provide the acidic formula needed.

The result was a solution which proved to be highly effective, named the "Cal-Mag Formula."

The use of Cal-Mag, experimental in the early 1970s to help ease withdrawal symptoms, is now long past the experimental stage. Cal-Mag has been used very effectively during withdrawal to help ease and counteract the convulsions, muscular spasms and severe nervous reactions experienced by an addict when coming off drugs.

The Cal-Mag Formula uses a ratio of one part elemental magnesium to two parts elemental calcium, mixed with vinegar in water.

As the formula calls for precise amounts of calcium and magnesium, some further explanation of these quantities should be given here.

The Cal-Mag Formula is made using the compounds calcium gluconate and magnesium carbonate. Both of these come in white, powdery form. Each is a compound of different substances. In other words, calcium gluconate contains other substances besides calcium; it is not all pure calcium but contains only a percentage of pure elemental calcium. Similarly, magnesium carbonate contains other substances besides magnesium, and includes only a percentage of pure elemental magnesium.

But it is the amount of elemental magnesium in correct ratio to the amount of elemental calcium that is important in the preparation of the Cal-Mag Formula. This does *not* mean that you use pure magnesium or pure calcium when you make Cal-Mag. Use only calcium gluconate and magnesium carbonate.

Magnesium Carbonate: The desired compound for Cal-Mag, called magnesium carbonate basic, contains 29 percent magnesium. (This compound is also sometimes called magnesium alba.)

There are different magnesium compounds with different percentages of elemental magnesium, but using any kind other than that recommended here will give varying amounts of magnesium which will violate the needed ratio of one part magnesium to two parts calcium.

It is magnesium carbonate basic, containing 29 percent elemental magnesium which is used in making Cal-Mag. And it is essential to ensure that the magnesium carbonate basic which is used is fresh, not old.

Calcium Gluconate: There is only one kind of calcium gluconate compound and 9 percent of that compound is calcium, so there is no problem in selecting the correct calcium gluconate compound for the Cal-Mag preparation.

The ingredients can be obtained in most health food stores or where vitamins are sold.

To prepare Cal-Mag:

1. Put 1 level tablespoon (15 ml) of calcium gluconate in a normal-sized glass.

2. Add ½ level teaspoon (2.5 ml) of magnesium carbonate.

3. Add 1 tablespoon (15 ml) of cider vinegar (at least 5 percent acidity).

4. Stir it well.

5. Add ½ glass (about 120 ml) of boiling water and stir until all the powder is dissolved and the liquid is clear. (If this doesn't occur it could be from poor grade or old magnesium carbonate.)

6. Fill the remainder of glass with lukewarm or cold water and cover.

You can make larger quantities at one time, simply by multiplying all the ingredients accordingly. The solution will stay good for two days.

It can be made wrongly so that it does not dissolve. Variations from the above produce an unsuccessful mix that can taste pretty horrible.

(Note, again, that the ratio is one part elemental magnesium to two parts elemental calcium. If one wants to work this out precisely, one can work out the elemental amounts. The formula above has been given for the compound amounts.)

Anything from one to three glasses of this a day, with or after meals, *replaces any tranquilizer.* It does not produce the drugged effects of tranquilizers (which are quite deadly).

It has proven effective in helping to handle the muscular spasms, tics and nervous reactions that can occur as a result of drug withdrawal.

It should be mentioned that many health food stores do carry premixed preparations of calcium and magnesium. Before using any of these in place of Cal-Mag, one should read the label to see if the calcium and magnesium are given in correct proportions and check if it contains acid (such as ascorbic acid or citric acid). Otherwise, such preparations are worthless and will not give the same results as the Cal-Mag Formula.

How to Prepare Cal-Mag

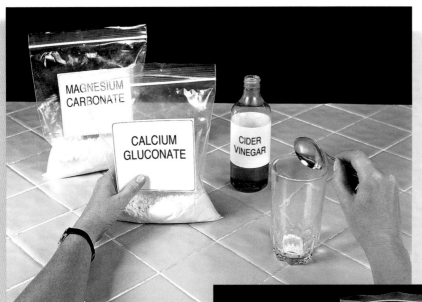

1. Put 1 level tablespoon (15 ml) of calcium gluconate in a normal-sized glass. Use a measuring spoon, not tableware.

2. Add ½ level teaspoon (2.5 ml) of magnesium carbonate. Again, use a proper measuring spoon.

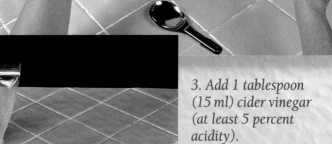

3. Add 1 tablespoon (15 ml) cider vinegar (at least 5 percent acidity).

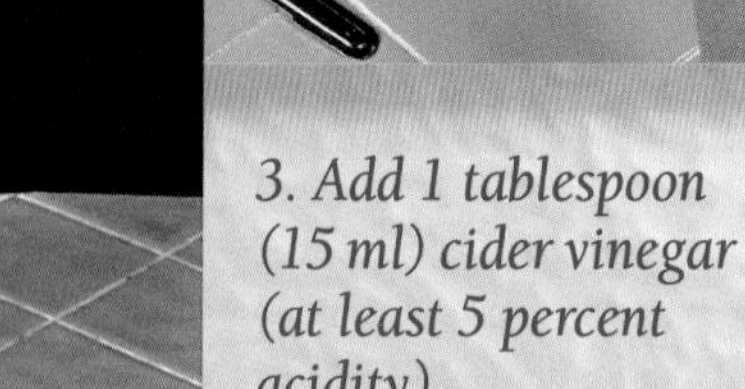

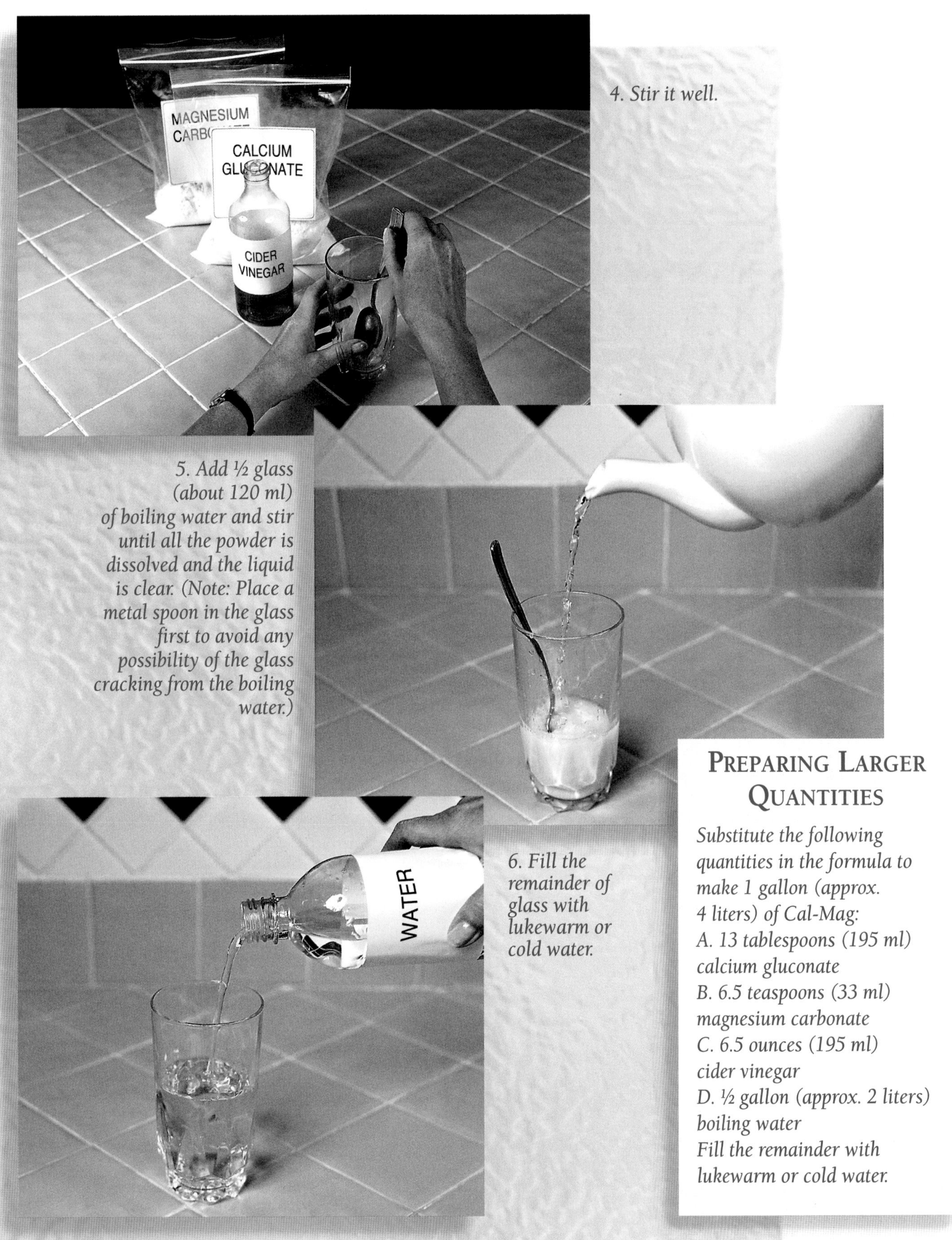

4. *Stir it well.*

5. *Add ½ glass (about 120 ml) of boiling water and stir until all the powder is dissolved and the liquid is clear. (Note: Place a metal spoon in the glass first to avoid any possibility of the glass cracking from the boiling water.)*

6. *Fill the remainder of glass with lukewarm or cold water.*

Preparing Larger Quantities

Substitute the following quantities in the formula to make 1 gallon (approx. 4 liters) of Cal-Mag:
A. 13 tablespoons (195 ml) calcium gluconate
B. 6.5 teaspoons (33 ml) magnesium carbonate
C. 6.5 ounces (195 ml) cider vinegar
D. ½ gallon (approx. 2 liters) boiling water
Fill the remainder with lukewarm or cold water.

Objective Processes

In addition to nutritional handling, the other approach to the drug withdrawal problem consists of Objective Processes.

Because drugs tend to push a person into experiences of the past and stick his attention in these moments, processes which pull more of a person's attention outward help unstick him from the past.

There are many Objective Processes in Scientology which accomplish this.

Objective Processes help a person get into present time and become more aware of his surroundings and other people and away from past problems. The more a person is able to face the present, and not be stuck in the past, the more he can enjoy life. He can be in better communication with his environment as it exists, not as it once was. This is worthwhile for anyone to achieve, but for someone who has been heavily on drugs and suffered their ill effects it can be a revelation.

Five Objective Processes are included here.

It is best to do these processes in a quiet place, free of distraction or interruption and with enough time to do the process until the person being helped has good indicators and has had a cognition. *Indicators* are conditions or circumstances arising during a process which indicate (point out or show) whether it is going well or badly. The person looking brighter or more cheerful, for example, has good indicators. A *cognition* is a new realization about life. It is a "What do you know, I..." statement; something a person suddenly understands or feels.

These processes are given to the person in addition to the drug bomb and Cal-Mag. They are very effective when given several times a day to help get the person through the period of withdrawal from drugs, which usually takes about a week or less. For example, a person could be given one of these processes in the morning, and some hours later he could be given another. A person going through withdrawal often sleeps considerably more than usual, especially at the beginning of such a program. Therefore, one would not go at this too strenuously; giving the person two or three of these Objective Processes each day should be sufficient to get a result.

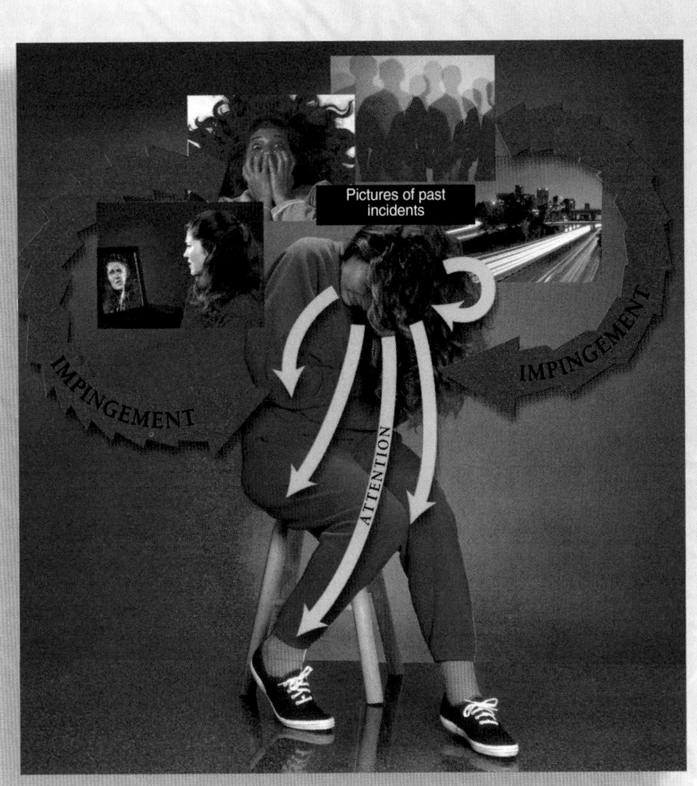

The attention of a person withdrawing from drug use can be very stuck on the body, and past incidents can be reactivated heavily.

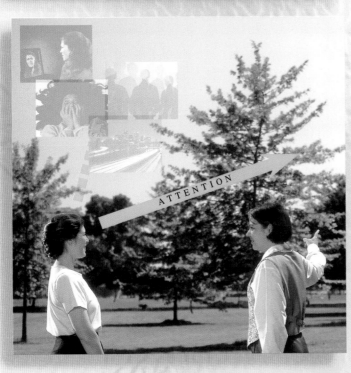

Light Objective Processes can extrovert the person's attention and greatly ease any discomfort. Past incidents drop out of the present and no longer impinge on the person.

"Notice That"

This process directs a person's attention off his body and out onto the environment. The procedure is as follows:

1. Tell the person you are going to process him and briefly explain the procedure.

2. The command used is:

"Notice that _______________ (indicated object)."

Ensure he understands it.

3. Indicate an obvious object by pointing to it. Tell the person, "Notice that _______________ (object)."

4. When the person has done so, acknowledge him by saying, "Thank you" or "Okay" or "Good," etc.

5. Continue giving the command, directing the person's attention to different objects in the environment. Be sure to acknowledge the person each time after he has carried out the command.

For example, say:

"Notice that chair."

"Thank you."

"Notice that window."

"All right."

"Notice that floor."

"Very good."

And so on.

6. Continue the process until the person being helped has good indicators and has had a cognition.

You can end the process at this point. Tell the person, "End of process."

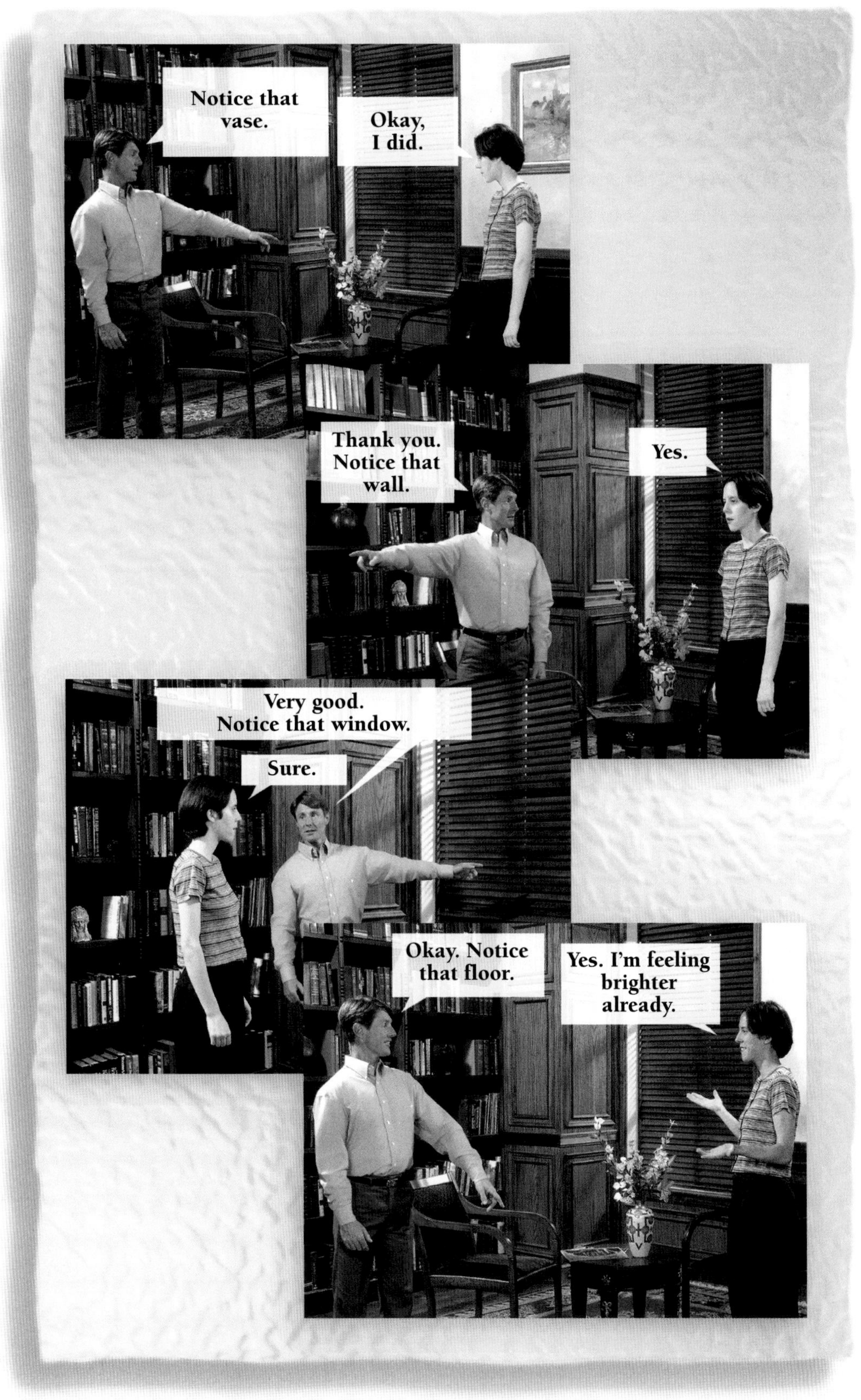
Notice that vase.
Okay, I did.
Thank you. Notice that wall.
Yes.
Very good. Notice that window.
Sure.
Okay. Notice that floor.
Yes. I'm feeling brighter already.

A Havingness Process

Havingness is the feeling that one owns or possesses. It can also be described as the concept of being able to reach or not being prevented from reaching. This process puts a person's attention onto the environment so he can have it. The procedure is as follows:

1. Tell the person you are going to process him and briefly explain the procedure.

2. The command used is:

"Look around here and find something you could have."

Ensure he understands it.

3. Give the command, "Look around here and find something you could have."

4. When the person has done so, acknowledge him by saying, "Thank you" or "Okay" or "Good," etc.

5. Continue giving the command. Be sure to acknowledge the person each time after he has carried out the command.

For example, say:

"Look around here and find something you could have."

"Thank you."

"Look around here and find something you could have."

"Good."

"Look around here and find something you could have."

"All right."

"Look around here and find something you could have."

"Very good."

And so on.

6. Continue the process until the person being helped has good indicators and has had a cognition. You end the process at this point. Tell the person, "End of process."

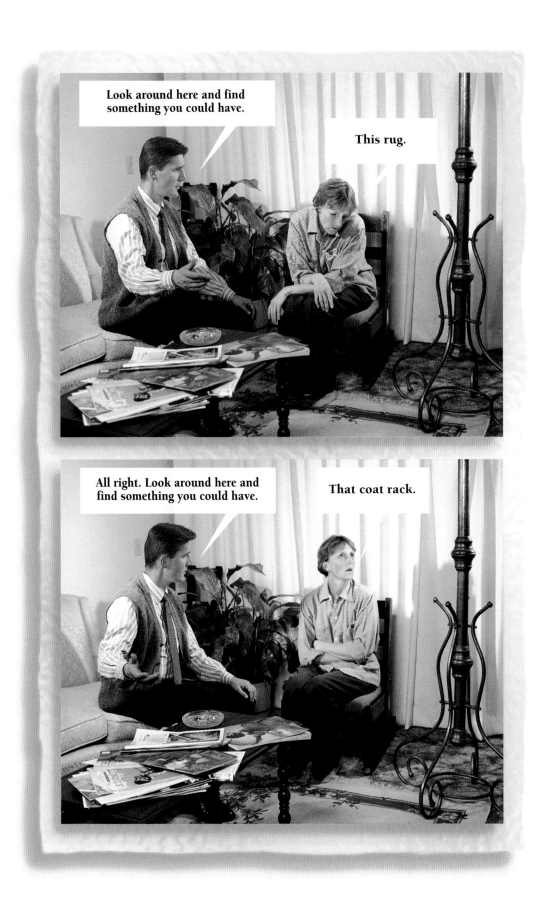
Look around here and find something you could have.
This rug.
All right. Look around here and find something you could have.
That coat rack.

"Touch That"

This process is done with both persons walking about, or if the person being helped is not able to walk, they may be seated at a table with a number of objects scattered on its surface. The procedure is as follows:

1. Tell the person you are going to process him and briefly explain the procedure.

2. The command used is:

"Touch that ______________ (indicated object)."

Choose different objects in the room for the person to touch.

Ensure the person understands the command.

3. Give the command, "Touch that ______________ (indicated object)."

4. When the person has done so, acknowledge him.

5. Continue giving the command. Be sure to acknowledge the person each time after he has carried out the command.

For example, say:

"Touch that table."

"Thank you."

"Touch that chair."

"Good."

And so on.

6. Continue the process until the person being helped has good indicators and has had a cognition. You end the process at this point. Tell the person, "End of process."

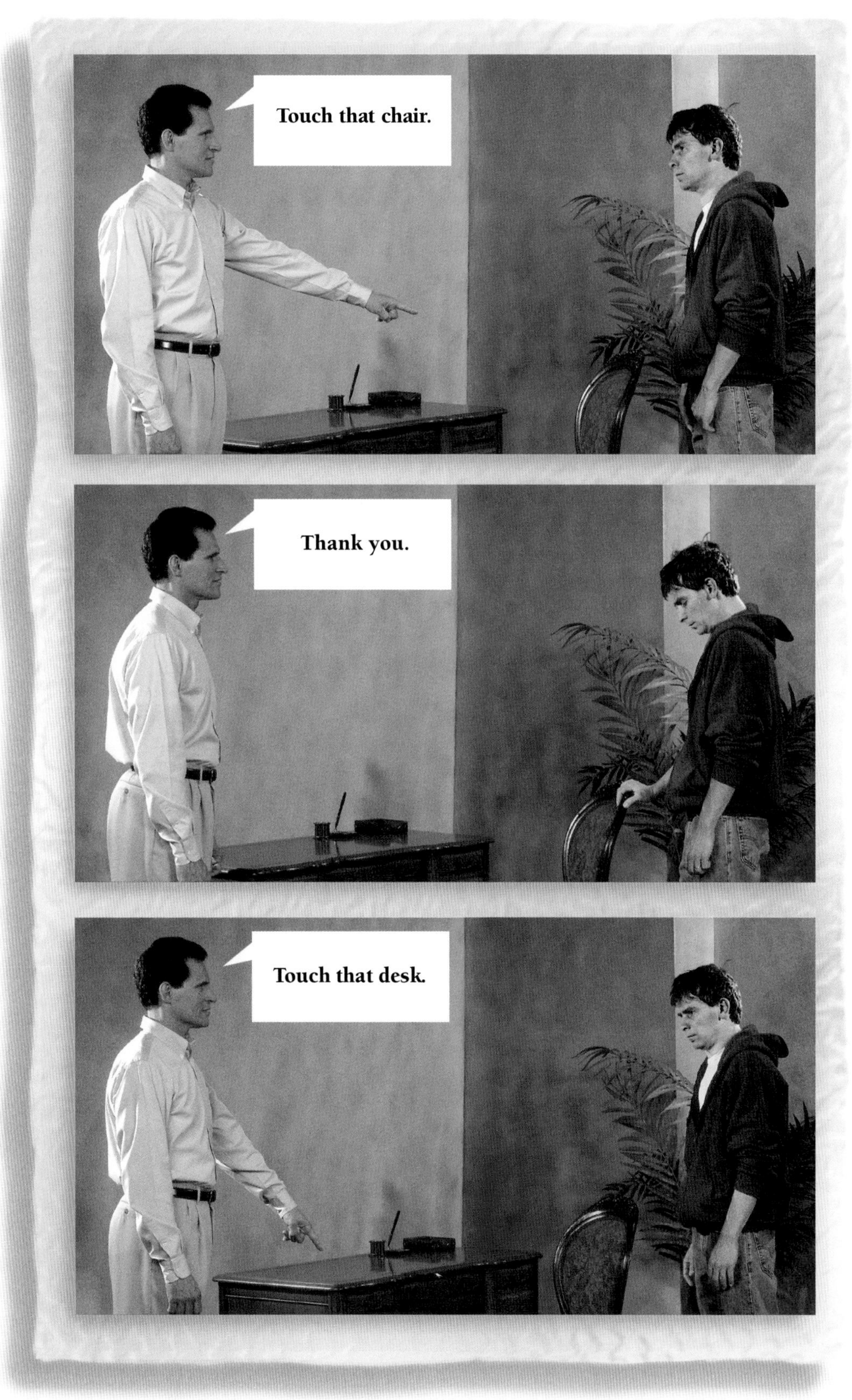
Touch that chair.
Thank you.
Touch that desk.

Touch and Let Go on Room Objects

This is a very good technique and will raise the person's reality on the objects in the room. The procedure is as follows:

1. Tell the person you are going to process him and briefly explain the procedure.

2. The commands used are:

a. "What in the room is really real to you?"

b. "Go over and touch it."

c. "Now let go of it."

Ensure he understands them.

3. Give the command, "What in the room is really real to you?"

4. When the person has answered, acknowledge him.

5. Then give the next command, "Go over and touch it."

6. When the person has done so, acknowledge him.

7. Then give the next command, "Now let go of it."

8. When the person has done so, acknowledge him.

9. Continue giving the commands in this sequence: a, b, c, a, b, c, etc. Be sure to acknowledge the person each time after he has carried out the command.

For example, say:

"What in the room is really real to you?"

"Thank you."

"Go over and touch it."

"Good."

"Now let go of it."

"All right."

"What in the room is really real to you?"

"Very good."

And so on.

10. Continue the process until the person being helped has good indicators and has had a cognition. You end the process at this point. Tell the person, "End of process."

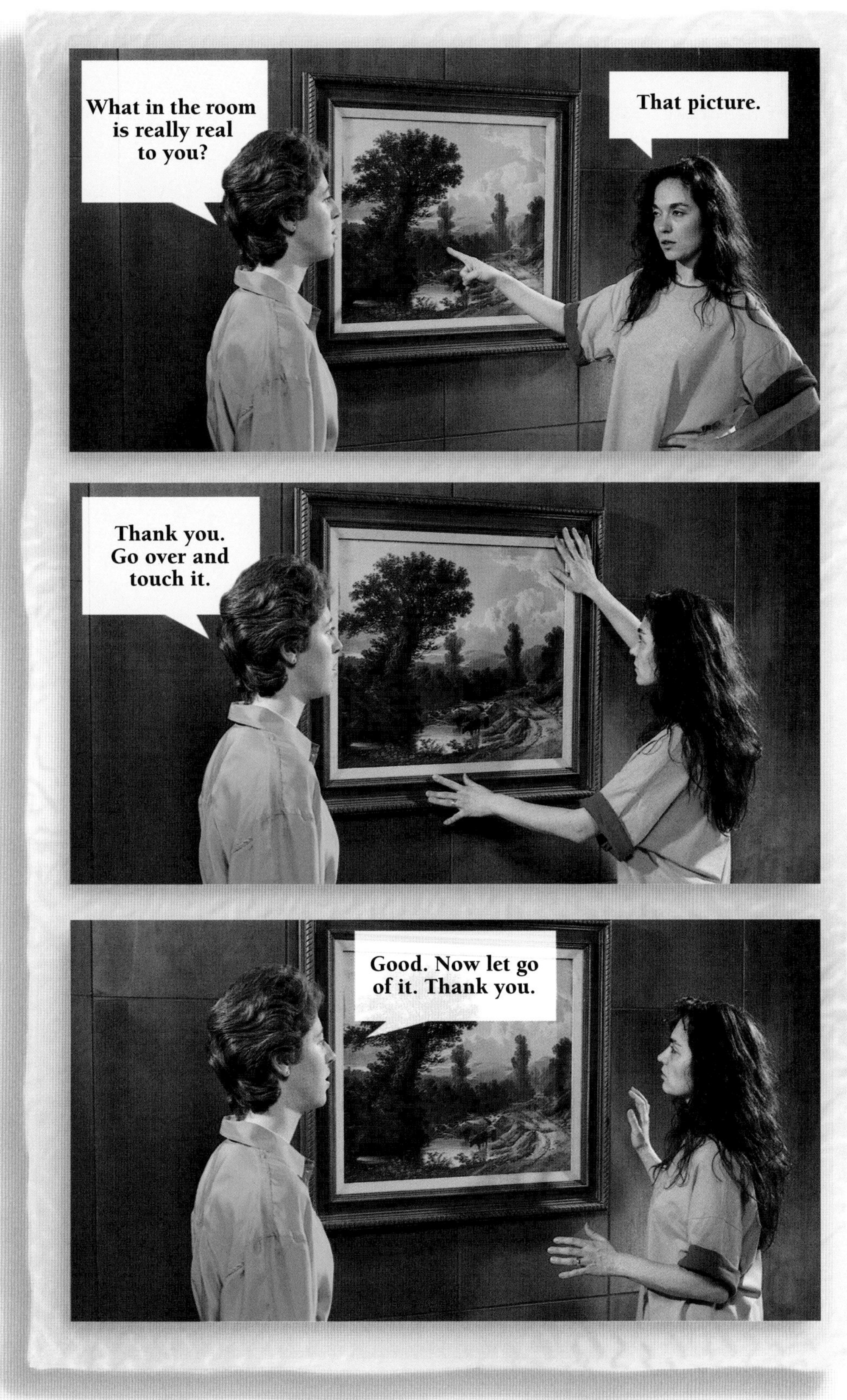
What in the room is really real to you?
That picture.
Thank you. Go over and touch it.
Good. Now let go of it. Thank you.

"Become Curious About That"

This is a basic Objective Process and is very simple. The procedure is as follows:

1. Tell the person you are going to process him and briefly explain the procedure.

2. The command used is:

"Become curious about that."

Ensure he understands it.

3. Indicate an object in the room by pointing at it and say, "Become curious about that."

You don't call the object by name, you just indicate it. You *don't* say, "Become curious about that chair."

4. When the person has done so, acknowledge him by saying, "Thank you" or "Okay" or "Good," etc.

5. Continue the procedure giving the command. Be sure to acknowledge the person each time after he has carried out the command.

For example, say:

"Become curious about that." (Indicate an object.)

"Thank you."

"Become curious about that." (Indicate an object.)

"Good."

"Become curious about that." (Indicate an object.)

"All right."

"Become curious about that." (Indicate an object.)

"Very good."

And so on.

6. Continue the process until the person being helped has good indicators and has had a cognition. You end the process at this point. Tell the person, "End of process."

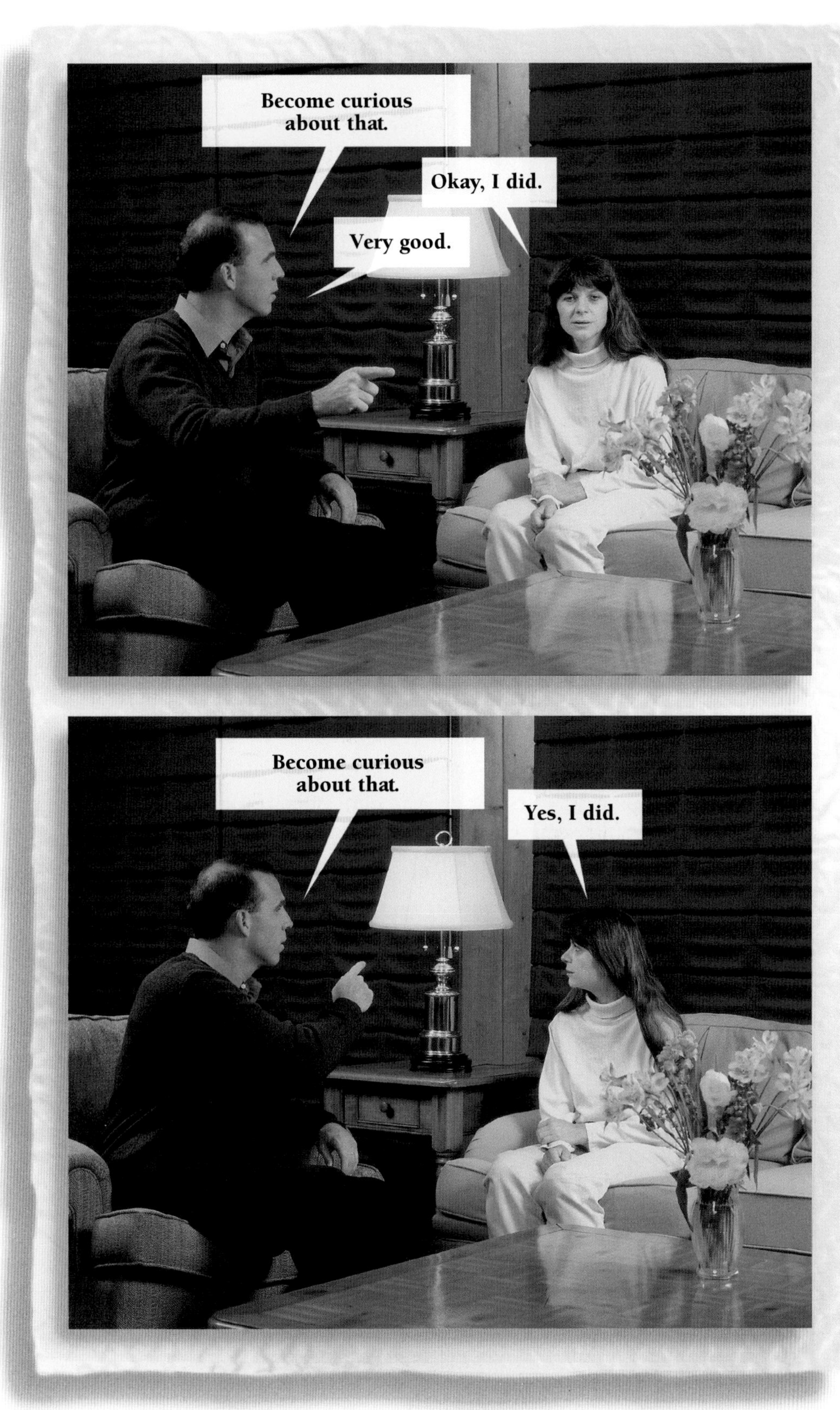
Become curious about that.
Okay, I did.
Very good.
Become curious about that.
Yes, I did.

The Full Resolution

Once a person has been gotten off drugs, other factors must be addressed in order to achieve a full recovery.

This applies to any former drug user, whether the person has recently withdrawn from drugs or stopped using them years earlier. It applies to persons who were never "hard drug users" as well as those who were.

The Purification Program

We live in a chemical-oriented society. One would be hard put to find someone in the present-day civilization who is not affected by this fact. The vast majority of the public is subjected every day to the intake of food preservatives and other chemical poisons including atmospheric poisons, pesticides and the like. Added to this are the pain pills, tranquilizers and other medical drugs used and prescribed by doctors. And we have as well the widespread use of marijuana, LSD, angel dust and other street drugs which contribute heavily to the scene.

In 1977, L. Ron Hubbard discovered that LSD apparently stays in the system for years after the person took it, lodging in the tissues—mainly the fatty tissues of the body—and is liable to go into action again, giving the person unpredictable "trips."

The "restimulation" experienced by people who had been on LSD appeared to act as if they had just taken more LSD.

From subsequent research it appears that not only LSD but other chemical poisons and toxic substances, preservatives and pesticides, as well as medical drugs and the long list of heavy street drugs (angel dust, heroin, marijuana, etc.) can lodge in the tissues and remain in the body for years.

Even medicinal drugs such as diet pills, codeine, Novocain and others have gone into restimulation years after they were taken and had supposedly been eliminated from the body.

Thus it seems that any or all of these hostile biochemical substances can get caught up in the tissues and their accumulation probably disarranges the biochemistry and fluid balance of the body.

The consequences are numerous. Tests show that the learning rate of a person who has been on drugs is much lower than a nondrug person. And the memory of a person who has been on drugs is such as to remove him from fear of consequences.

The being (thetan) of course has mental image pictures of these toxic substances and as long as those substances are in the body, they can restimulate a being. When they are gone from the body, the constant restimulation can cease. So it is actually a spiritual action that is being done.

In Scientology, we have an effective method to cleanse the body of these substances; it is called the Purification program, and it will benefit anyone who lives in this society so inundated with toxins and chemicals.

The Purification program is a tightly supervised regimen which includes:

Exercise

Sauna sweat-out

Nutrition, including vitamins, minerals, etc., as well as oil intake

A properly ordered personal schedule

Exercise: The exercise on this program is in the form of running. The purpose of this is *not* to generate sweat but to get the blood circulating and the system functioning so that impurities held in the system can be released and are pumped out.

Sauna sweat-out: Following the running, the person goes into the sauna to sweat. The impurities can now be dispelled from the body and leave the system through the pores.

Nutrition (including vitamins, minerals and oil intake): When we speak of nutrition we are not talking only about food, but about vitamins and minerals as well, as these are vital to proper nutrition and vital to the effectiveness of this program. We are not, however, talking about "diet" in the overused sense of the word. The person simply eats what he normally eats. He should make sure he gets some vegetables and that the vegetables aren't overcooked.

Toxic substances tend to lock up *mainly,* but not exclusively, in the fat tissue of the body. The theory, then, is that one could replace the fat tissues that hold these toxic accumulations. The body will actually tend to hold on to something it is short of. Thus, if you try to get rid of something it is short of, it won't give it up. So, in the matter of oil, if the person takes some oil, the body might possibly exchange the good oil for the bad fat in the body. That is the basic theory. There are particular vegetable oils which are used for this purpose.

One of the things that toxins and drugs do is create nutritional deficiencies in the body in the form of vitamin and mineral deficiencies. It is easily seen that there is a wide range of toxic substances which create nutritional deficiencies. Alcohol, for example, depends for its effects on a person being able to burn up vitamin B_1. When it burns up all the B_1 in the system the person goes into dt's (delirium tremens) and nightmares.

In the case of other toxic substances the probability exists that other vitamins besides B_1 are burned up. What we seem to have hit on here is that the LSD and street drugs burn up not only B_1 and B complex (which we assume they do) but also create a deficiency in niacin in the body and that they possibly depend on niacin (one of the B complex vitamins) for their effect.

Niacin is essential to nutrition and vital to the effectiveness of the Purification program. It can produce some startling and, in the end, very beneficial results when taken properly on the program, along with the other necessary vitamins and minerals in sufficient and proportionate quantities and along with proper running and sweat-out. Taken in sufficient quantities it appears to break up and unleash LSD, marijuana and other drugs and poisons from the tissues and cells. It can rapidly release LSD crystals into the system. Running and sweating must be done in conjunction with taking niacin to ensure the toxic substances it releases actually do get flushed out of the body.

A properly ordered personal schedule: It is important that a person on this program maintains a properly ordered personal schedule. This means that once one has started on the program he must stick to it sensibly and not skip days or do it in a random fashion. It also means that one should get enough sleep. If one proceeds through the program in an orderly fashion it will be faster and more effective.

The Purification program does not supplant the actions described earlier in this chapter for persons currently on drugs who are apt to experience withdrawal symptoms when taken off of them. The program would be begun only after such technology was applied.

The Harmful Effects of Drugs

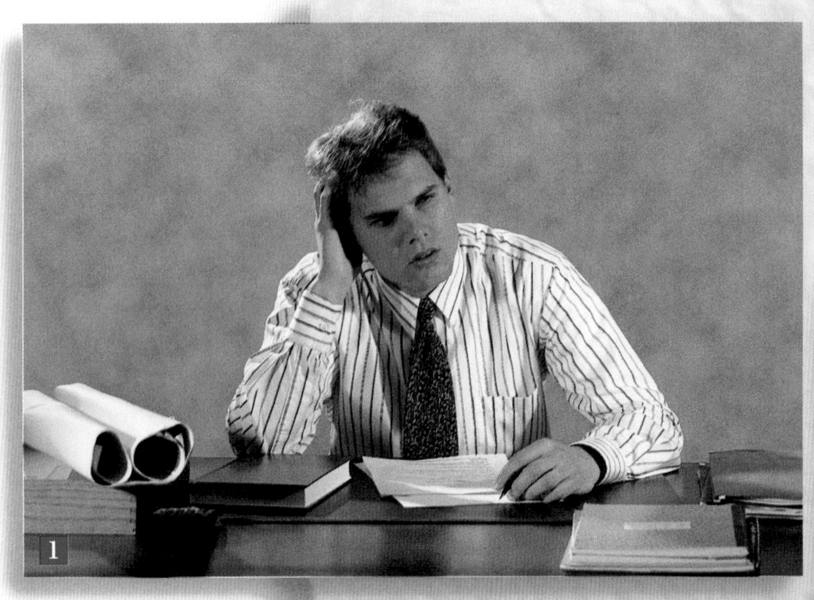

In a drug-ridden world, the individual often finds himself victimized by the harmful effects of drugs, medicine and alcohol, even if taken years before.

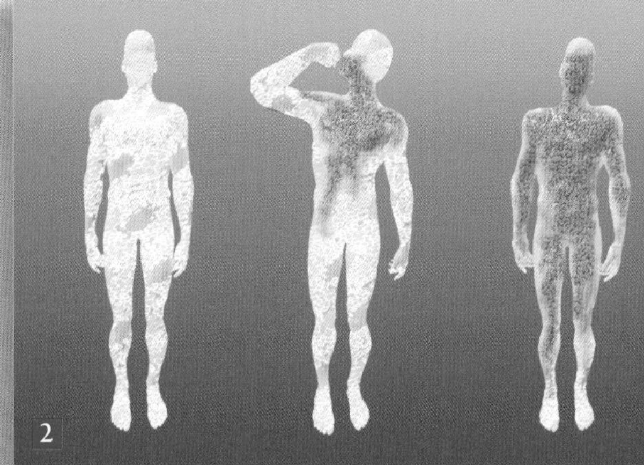

Drugs are essentially poisons and take their toll on a person's body by eating up its stores of vitamins and minerals.

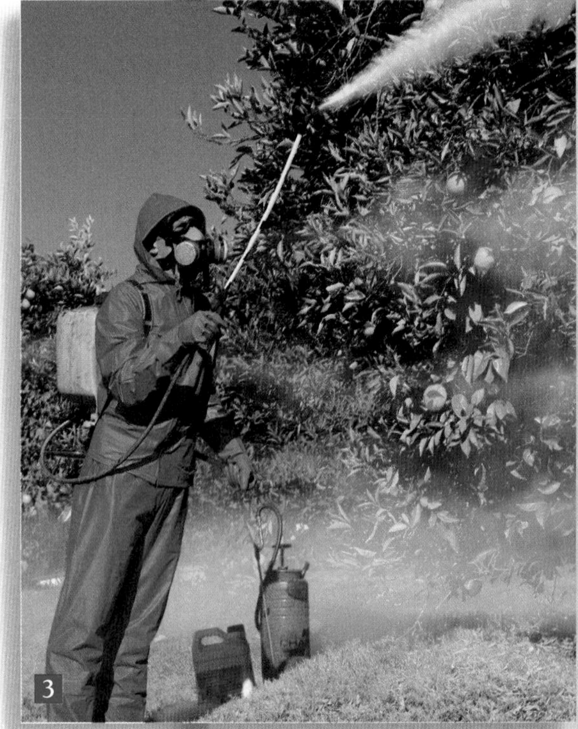

Besides drugs, our world is awash with other substances toxic to human life.

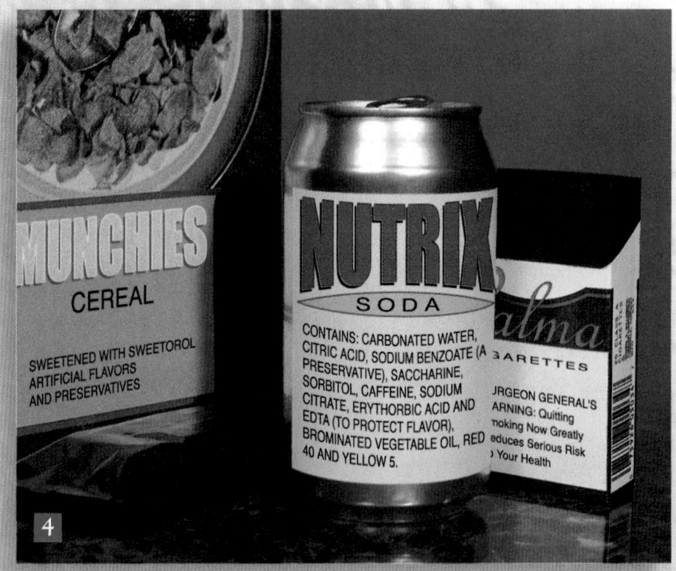

There are literally thousands of artificial substances around that can enter a person's system, many of which are toxic. We live in a chemical-oriented society.

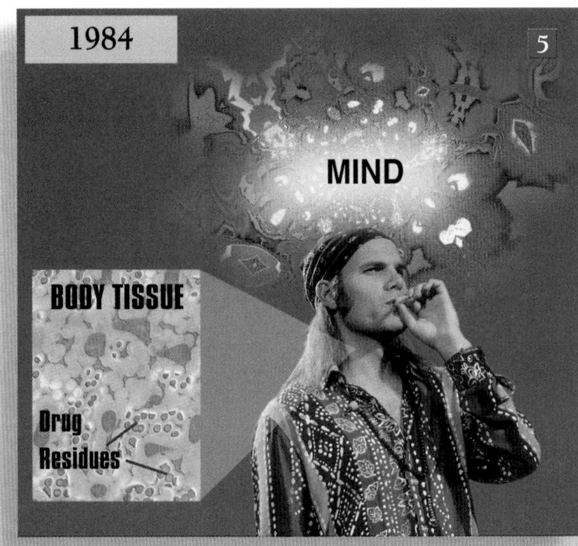

It is a proven fact that drug residues can be trapped in the body.

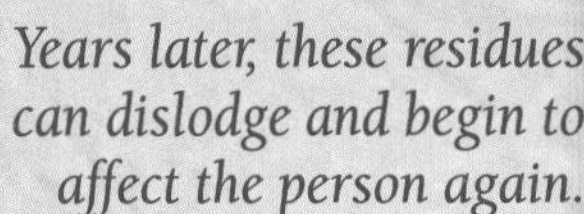

Years later, these residues can dislodge and begin to affect the person again.

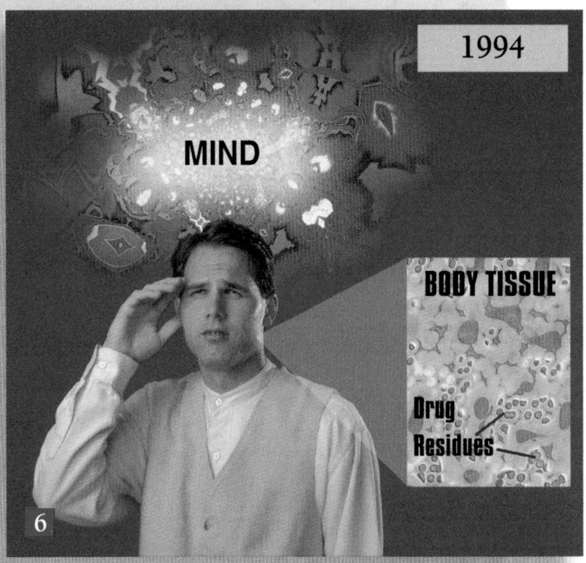

Though a person is no longer taking drugs, he has mental pictures of drugs and drug experiences…

…which can reactivate as long as toxic drug residues are locked in the body. A person's awareness, ability and attitudes can be adversely affected.

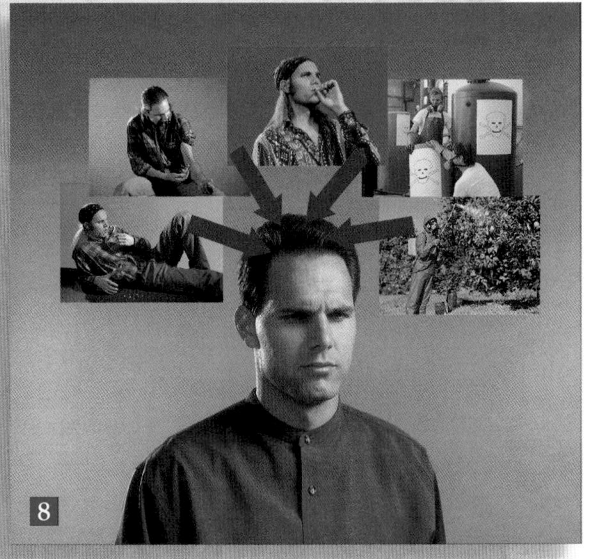

The Purification Program Illustrated

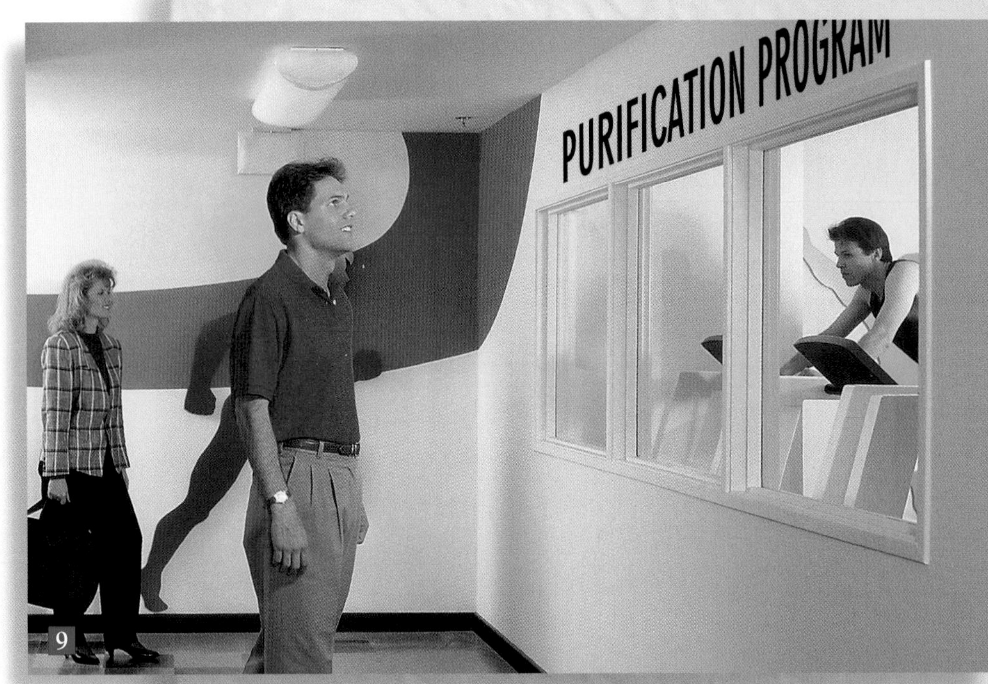

There is however a way out of this trap: the Purification program, an exact regimen which can rid the body of harmful drug residues and other toxic substances.

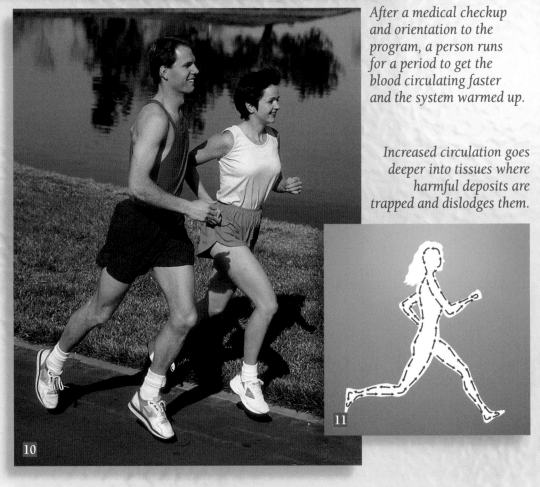

After a medical checkup and orientation to the program, a person runs for a period to get the blood circulating faster and the system warmed up.

Increased circulation goes deeper into tissues where harmful deposits are trapped and dislodges them.

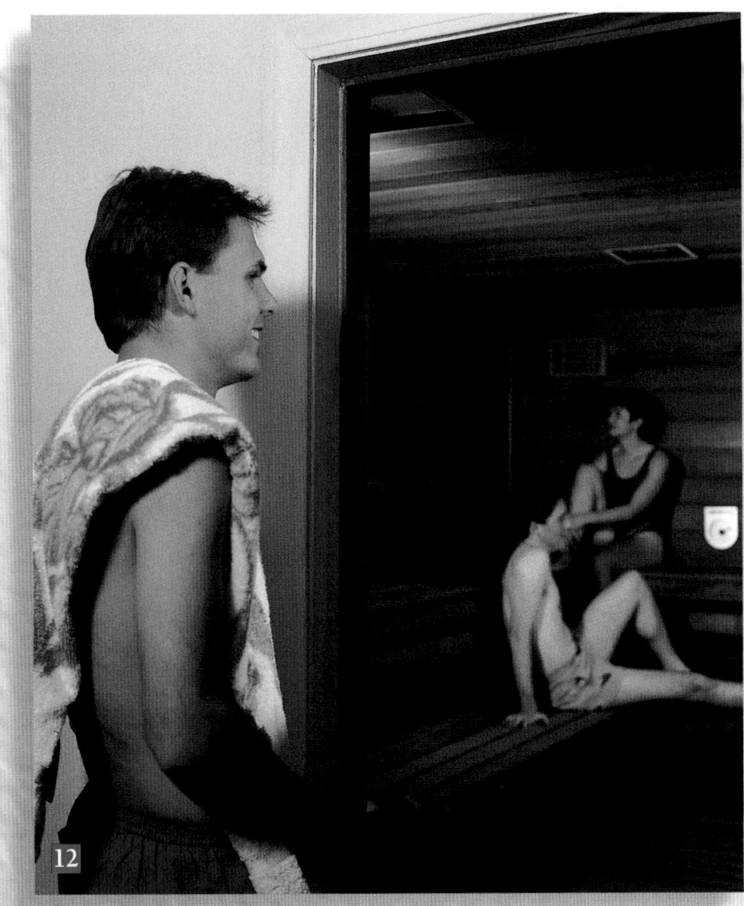

After running, the person sweats out the drug residuals in a sauna. Profuse sweating helps purify the system of these toxic substances.

Nutrition in the form of certain vitamins and minerals is also an important part of the program.

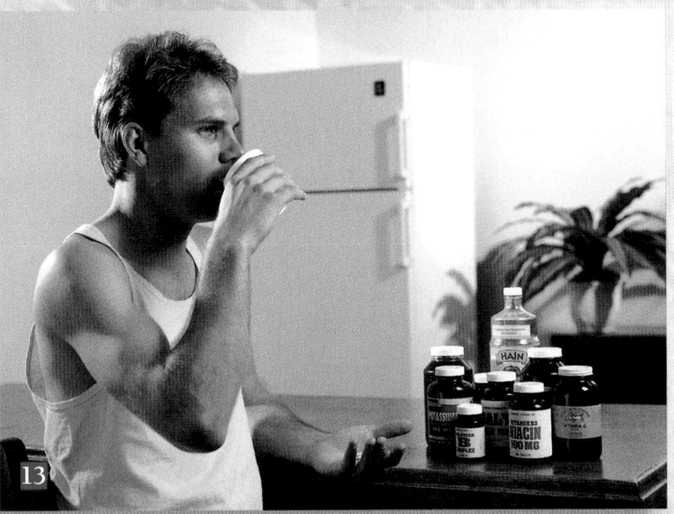

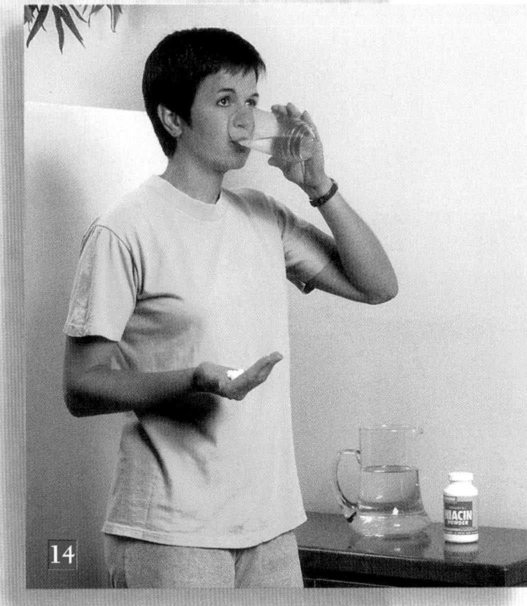

Niacin, one of the B complex vitamins, plays a vital role. It appears to break up and unleash drug and chemical deposits from body tissues and cells.

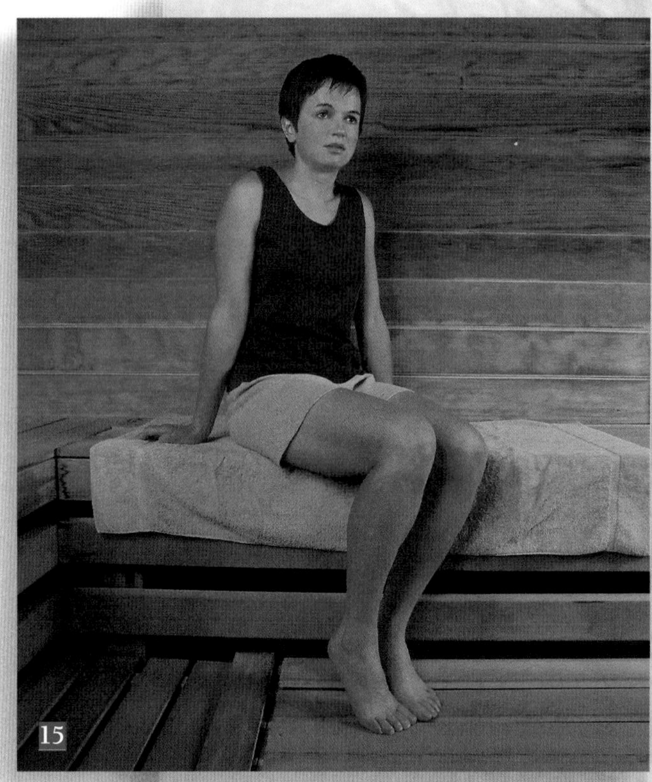

Niacin can produce some dramatic effects, such as a hot flush, as it interacts with deficiencies which already exist in cellular structure.

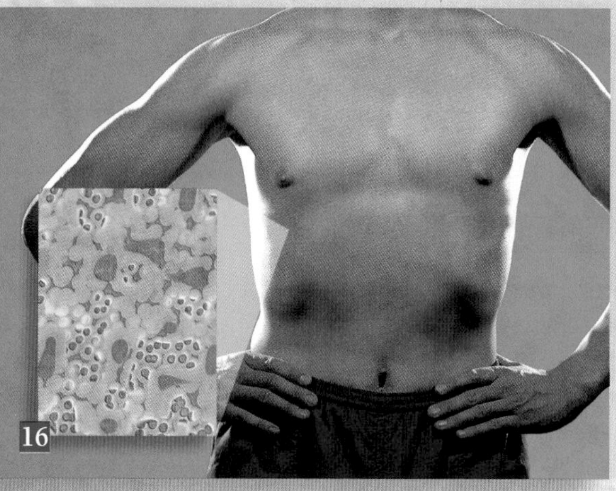

Because drug residues tend to "lock up" in fatty tissues…

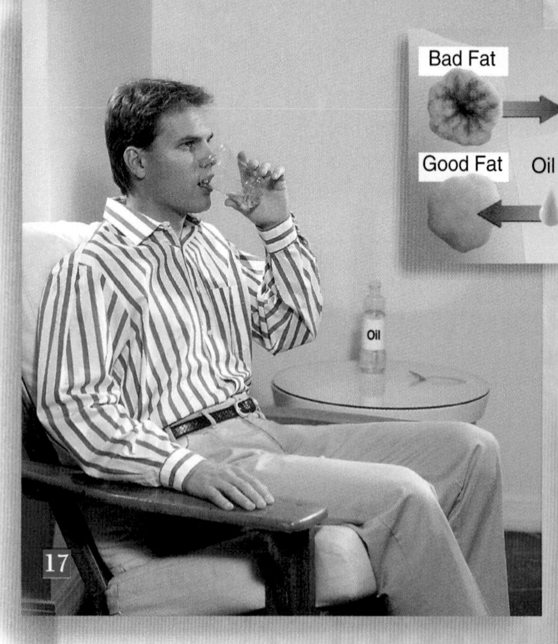

…some oil is taken every day to encourage bad, drug-laden fat to exchange with good oil.

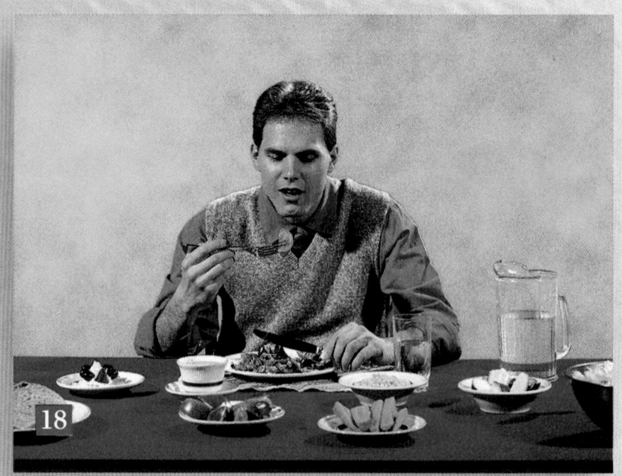

The person continues to eat his regular diet, ensuring he gets plenty of vegetables (which are not overcooked).

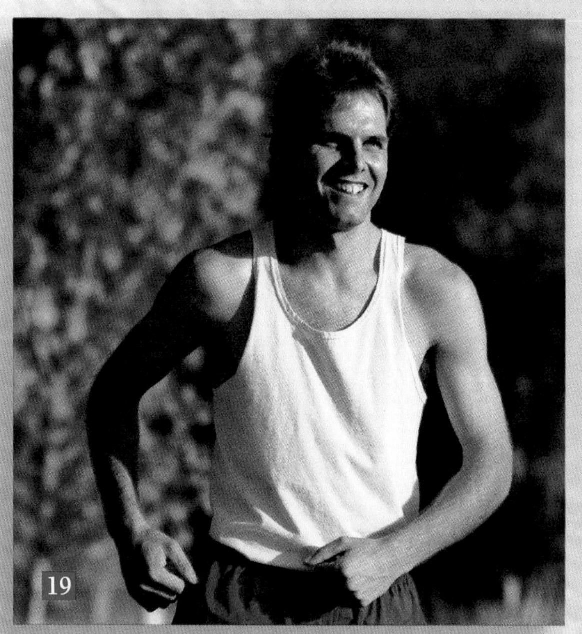
19

The regimen of running…

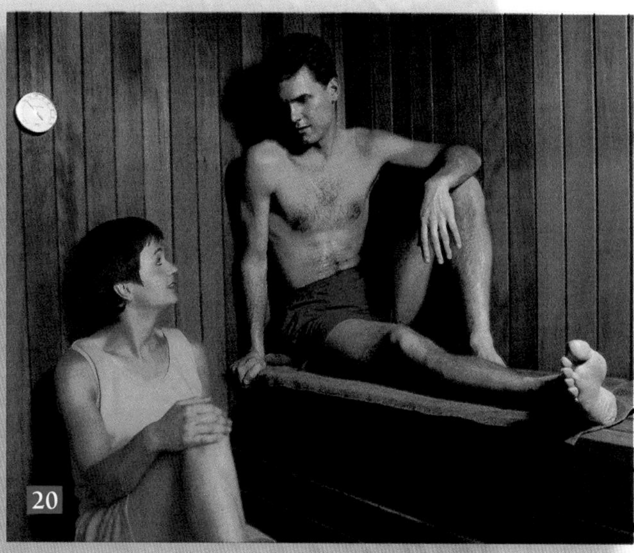
20

…sweating in a sauna, nutrition, and adequate rest is repeated daily…

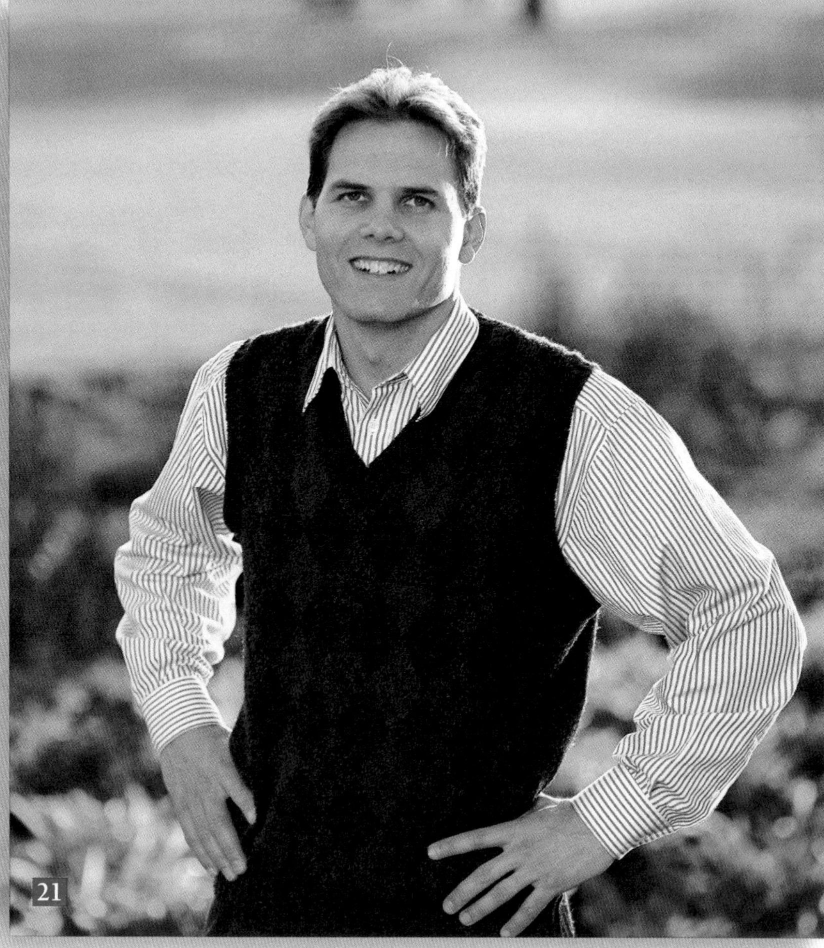
21

…until one no longer feels the effects of past drugs going into restimulation. The Purification program puts a person in a position where he can make real mental and spiritual gains with Scientology processing, because the effects of drugs on the mind and spirit are not constantly being put into restimulation.

The purpose of this program is very simply to clean out and purify one's system of all the accumulated impurities such as drugs, insecticides and pesticides, food preservatives, etc., which by their presence and restimulative effects could prevent or delay freeing the being spiritually through further Scientology processing. For someone who has taken LSD or angel dust this would include getting rid of any residual crystals from the body.

As the person goes through the Purification program, one should be able to see an improvement in his physical well-being as he rids the system of its accumulated impurities. The result of this program is a purified body, free from the impurities, drugs, etc., that had accumulated in it. We are not concerned with handling bodies with the Purification program, however. Our concern is freeing the individual up spiritually.

The Purification program is available under expert supervision in Scientology organizations and missions around the world. Also the book *Clear Body, Clear Mind: The Effective Purification Program* tells one exactly how this program is administered and describes all of its steps.

One should be able to get through the whole program in two weeks at five hours a day. Some will take more and some will take less.

With the Purification program we now have the means to get rapid recovery from the effects of the accumulation of the environmental chemical poisons as well as the medical drugs and street drugs which inhibit a person mentally and spiritually.

With the inclusion of vitamins, minerals and oils we are able to work toward restoring the biochemical balance of the body and make it possible for the body to reconstruct itself from the damage done by drugs and other biochemical substances.

The Drug Rundown

While the Purification program is a vital step in handling the effects of drugs, it is not a full handling in itself.

Complete freedom from drugs and their damaging consequences requires that a person also directly address the mental image pictures that are connected with having taken drugs. While the Purification program gets rid of drug residues that keep mental image pictures in constant restimulation, these pictures still exist. They can be restimulated by perceptions in the environment and affect the person adversely, below his awareness and out of his control, a factor that is both insidious and extremely detrimental.

The processing which directly deals with these pictures is called the Drug Rundown. It is delivered by highly trained practitioners in Scientology churches and missions.

A *rundown* is a series of steps designed to handle a specific aspect of a person's life or difficulties and which has a known end result. The result of the Drug Rundown is freedom from the harmful effects of drugs, alcohol and medicine and freedom from the need to take them.

A person's perceptions and recordings of the physical universe when on drugs are inaccurate, to say the least, as they are a combination of past events, imagination and the actual events which occurred at the time. A person can have pictures from past experiences tangled up with his present time perceptions. In essence, then, the pictures in his mind are scrambled to one degree or another. Thus his memory and his ability to think are both impaired.

The Drug Rundown handles several major aspects of past drug use. First, experiences the person had while taking drugs are directly addressed with precise procedures, which free up attention that became stuck on those experiences so they no longer affect him.

The more a person has had his attention freed from past incidents, the more able he is to deal with his life. He feels brighter, has increased perception, is better able to control himself and the things in his surroundings, and he becomes more able to rationally interact with others.

Normally, a person accurately records in his mind perceptions of the physical universe.

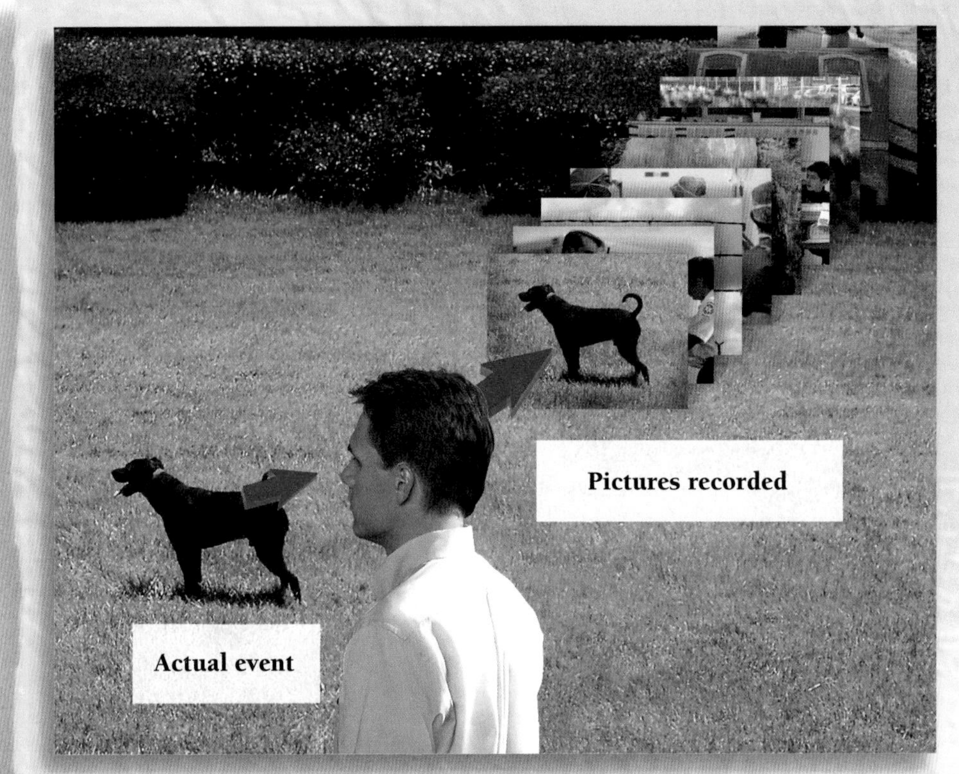

But drugs can tangle these recordings and badly distort what he perceives and, later, his recollection of what actually occurred.

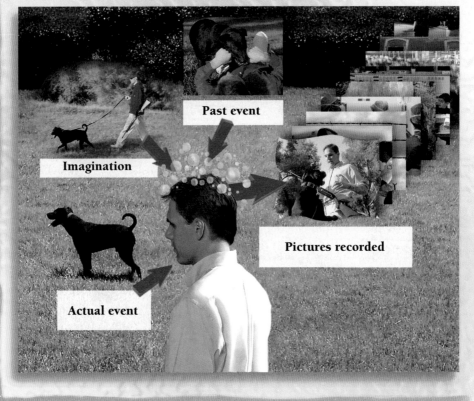

Another factor addressed by the Drug Rundown is that a person who has taken drugs also has a host of unpleasant physical, emotional and mental sensations connected with them. By discovering and examining the source of these, the harmful energy connected with them in the mind is released.

Finally, the processing gets right to the core of the matter and locates the basic reasons a person took drugs. A person originally turned to drugs for a *reason*—some physical suffering or hopelessness. The drug problem is thus essentially spiritual. The being was somehow suffering and drugs became a way to alleviate this.

The person looked upon drugs, alcohol or medicine as a cure for unwanted feelings or conditions—which could cover an almost infinite spectrum, and include anything from physical pains to anxiety to lack of confidence. One, therefore, has to find out what was actually wrong *before* drugs became his solution or "cure."

If this original reason is not addressed, the need or compulsion to take drugs or medicine or alcohol remains. Processing not only effectively deals with the effects of drugs, but enables the person to discover and eradicate the causes which led him to take them in the first place, thereby completely eliminating any desire to use or depend on them in the future.

The Drug Rundown, therefore, deals with and handles the unwanted feelings the person had both during *and* prior to the use of drugs, alcohol or medicine. The compulsion to still use drugs or alcohol is removed so that the person has no need to ever again turn to them.

By completing this processing, the person is at last free from any effects of drugs.

A full resolution of the mental and spiritual damage from past drug use requires *all* these steps.

A person can locate the source of any harmful mental effects of drugs, alcohol and medicine with Drug Rundown processing. The person can become free from those harmful mental effects and, as well, free from the need to take drugs ever again.

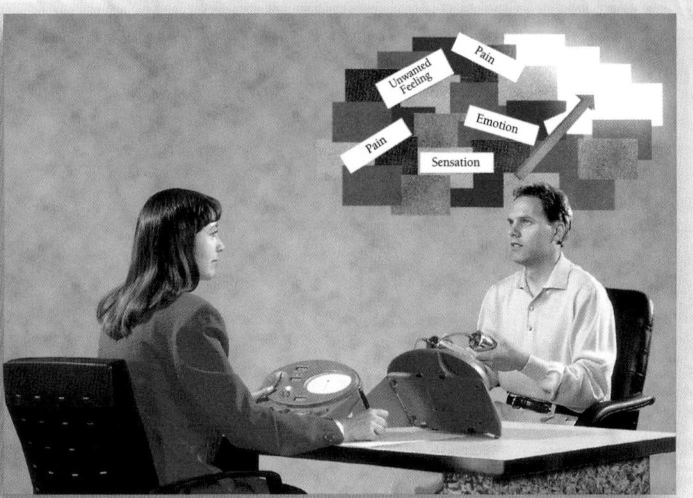

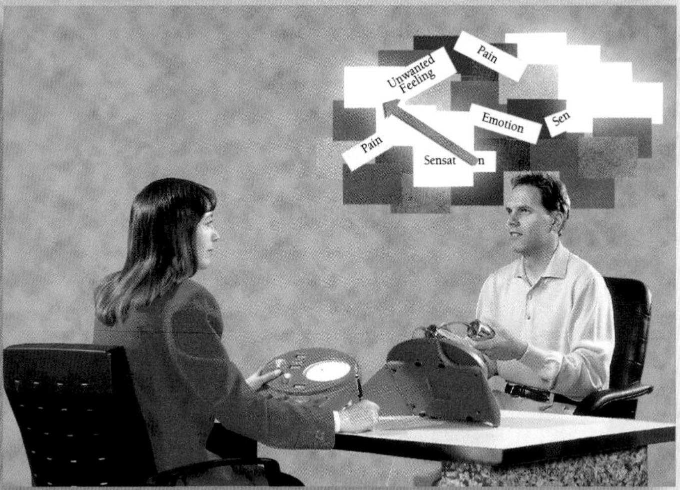

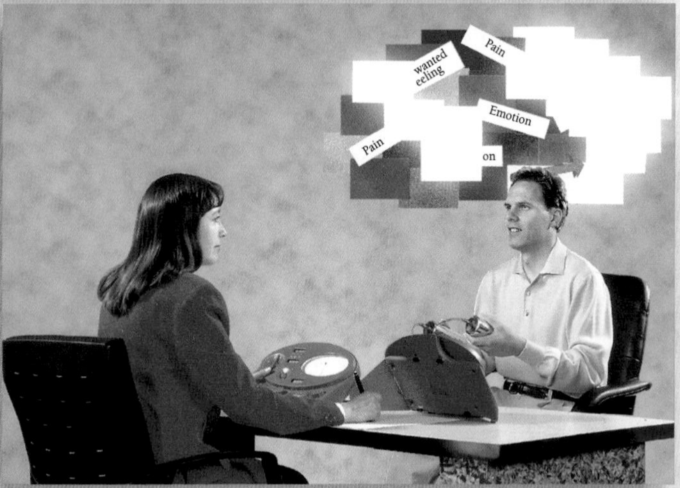

THE ROAD OUT

Only Scientology can fully handle the effects of drugs.

The means to get someone off drugs are now known—nutritional handling and Objective Processes which help the person get through any period of "drying out."

The next action, then, is the Purification program. This program is for any person who has taken drugs or anyone subjected to toxic substances of any kind.

And after a person has successfully finished the Purification program, processing on the Drug Rundown fully completes handling of the mental and spiritual effects of drugs.

Without workable methods to handle the effects of drugs, many people are doomed to live in chemical shackles. While drugs may appear to have short-term benefits, they only mask problems, they don't solve them.

Other drug rehabilitation approaches have failed mainly because of a lack of knowledge. They lack a true understanding of the mind, there is little or no understanding of man's spiritual nature, and the effects of drugs upon the mind and the being are unknown. The result is a materialistic ("man is an animal") approach which ignores these fundamental and crucial factors. All this adds up to proven unworkability.

Scientology, on the other hand, has a workable and extremely effective drug rehabilitation program because it addresses not only the correct problems, but the real sources of those problems.

Through understanding of the true nature of man, the methods to handle the biochemical, mental and spiritual factors of drugs do exist.

Scientology has the answers. ■

TEST YOUR UNDERSTANDING

Answer the following questions about drugs. Refer back to the chapter to check your answers. If you need to, review the chapter. Going over the material several times will increase your certainty and help you better apply the knowledge.

- ❑ *What are drugs?*
- ❑ *Why do people turn to drugs?*
- ❑ *Why does a person who takes drugs "make mistakes"?*
- ❑ *What are the two actions of a pain depressant?*
- ❑ *What are the approaches to withdrawal from drugs?*
- ❑ *Describe what the Cal-Mag Formula consists of and how it works.*
- ❑ *What is the Purification program and how does it help someone who has taken drugs?*
- ❑ *What is the Drug Rundown and why is it needed for a full resolution for someone who has been on drugs?*

PRACTICAL EXERCISES

Here are exercises you can do to help increase your understanding of and ability to apply the data in this chapter.

1 Look around the place where you live or work and find examples of drugs or toxins. For instance, look at the labels of any products that may be in a medicine cabinet, or food labels, etc. Do this until you can easily recognize examples of drugs and toxins in your environment.

2 Look around your environment and note examples of the effects of drug use in society.

3 Obtain the ingredients for Cal-Mag and make a glass of it, following the directions in the chapter.

4 Find a friend or someone you know who has used drugs and process him on one of the Objective Processes given in this chapter until the person has good indicators and has had a cognition as a result of the process. Repeat this with other people you know until you feel confident in your ability to use these processes.

5 Educate someone on the subject of drugs using data from this chapter, with the end result that the person knows what drugs are and their effects, and the only effective solutions for them, as discovered in Scientology.

RESULTS FROM APPLICATION

Government-funded drug rehabilitation programs around the world continue to fail with a lamentable average success rate of 15 percent. This means that eighty-five out of one hundred addicts continue their habits—and is no success at all. But drug rehabilitation programs which use L. Ron Hubbard's technology almost reverse this failing ratio. An independent study in Spain, for instance, showed that 70 percent of graduates from a program based on Mr. Hubbard's work stayed off drugs. In Sweden, another independent study reported that 84 percent of graduates from a similar program were still drug-free two years after completion.

Mr. Hubbard's drug rehabilitation program is delivered in Scientology organizations throughout the world. If you run into any difficulty applying any of the procedures in this chapter, and require assistance, you may contact the nearest church or mission listed at the back of this book.

SCIENTOLOGY PROMOTES DRUG-FREE LIVING

	Use of Alcohol	Use of Street Drugs
High-School Students	89.5%	69.7%
Scientologists	10.2%	0%

A comparison of drug and alcohol use by US teenagers and a cross section of Scientologists indicates the value of Scientology in solving the drug problem.

The effectiveness of using Mr. Hubbard's methods to salvage others from the devastating effects of drug use—and the sense of achievement gained from doing so—is reflected in the following pages:

After starting to use drugs at the age of thirteen, an American man finally admitted to himself nine years later that he was a drug addict. He decided to do something to get off cocaine and other drugs before they destroyed his life totally. Here is his story:

"I joined the US military because I thought the discipline would help me kick my habit and stay away from drugs, but as a gunner paratrooper, I ended up using as much cocaine as I had in civilian life. About a quarter of my division used drugs and we called ourselves the 'flying junkies.' So I left the military after three years because of drug use. I obviously needed something other than military life to help me handle my problem. I began to drift in and out of various drug programs over the next five years. However it wasn't until I used L. Ron Hubbard's technology that I was able to live a drug-free life. Since that time, I have been helping others kick their addictions to everything from heroin to alcohol, using the program."

The Purification program is the only truly effective program of its kind in the world, as a medical doctor in Amsterdam, Holland agrees. After examining drug users before, during and after the Purification program, he said:

"In my opinion, the Purification program which was developed by L. Ron

Hubbard is the only one which has proved to be effective in practice. I speak from experience because I have had contact with addicts before they started the detoxification step of the Purification program. By doing the preparatory steps at the beginning of the program, the person has already changed so much that I sometimes think I have made a mistake and am not sitting opposite a former heroin addict."

Reflections of a father about his son, Robert, over a four-year span:

"Four years ago, Robert came home from Marine training, very quiet and withdrawn, with no interest in work or play; no normal drive to find his way in the world. He seemed to become worse by the week, very listless and depressed; being very naive, I never thought drugs to be the problem.

"After many visits to doctors and clinics, the doctors settled on prescribing the mind-bending drug, Ritalin, to 'improve his way of thinking.' This drug, being federally controlled, was supposed to help him in getting started on a 'normal way of thinking' and doing things other 'normal' people do.

"Robert became addicted to this drug to the extent of hundreds of pills each week. Even though the drug was supposedly controlled, unscrupulous doctors prescribed the medication. He became a legal dope addict. In my state of mind, I called up these doctors and threatened legal action, but Robert would just find another doctor who was anxious to make a fast dollar and get more medication.

"He became so hard to live with and so mean that he would steal from us and lie to and threaten his mother. I finally had him arrested for grand theft just to get him out of the house and in the hope of shocking him into reality. The judge let him out on probation, and he went on taking Ritalin.

"We were at a breaking point and were considering having him sent to prison before he hurt himself or I hurt him (God forbid).

"I was watching television one morning and saw two young men speaking about drug problems and insisting that they could help if one would just call, so I did. Then I talked to my son and we set up a meeting. So Robert went off to a center in Los Angeles that uses Mr. Hubbard's technology. They began to work with him on a twenty-four-hour basis to help him get off drugs.

"Robert began to change for the better—and oh, what a change. No more drugs. He came home on weekends, and was calm and collected and began to talk intelligently and act sanely.

"Four months have passed, and Robert has improved by the week, no longer harassing his mother, no more asking for the impossible or 'twisting' things to suit his way.

"He has really beat the drug and is well on his way to doing something worthwhile.

"Our friends and others now ask how we came to have a son who is so considerate, calm and intelligent-speaking. I just smile and reply that he works with a group of people in Los Angeles that help young people get started on the road of life.

"Good luck, Robert,
from your Dad.

"And thanks to all his friends there, at the center."

SUGGESTIONS FOR FURTHER STUDY

The proliferation and abuse of medical/psychiatric drugs and illegal street drugs is one of society's major concerns. Learning early on that drugs were a barrier to spiritual betterment, L. Ron Hubbard subsequently researched the subject of drugs as part of his development of Scientology. His breakthroughs in this field have not only helped Scientologists, but have revolutionized the entire field of drug rehabilitation and saved thousands of lives. Some of his further writings on the subject are listed here and recommended for additional information about this societal scourge.

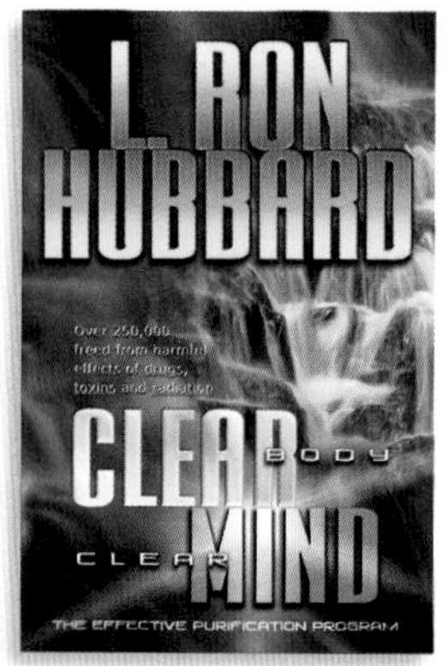

Clear Body, Clear Mind: The Effective Purification Program

The authoritative text on the world's most effective drug rehabilitation program. The Purification program as developed by Mr. Hubbard is not a program for one's body, but is intended to enable an individual to make better and faster spiritual improvement in Scientology processing by getting rid of residual drugs and their effects. This book comprehensively details the program and all its aspects. Explains the discoveries which led to his development of the program and provides an exact description of how and why the program works. Gives all necessary data and technology to enable a person to do the entire program. The truth of the matter is a person is much better off without drugs including psychiatric and medical drugs. This fact is undeniable once one reads this book. But, unlike those who merely decry the problem, Mr. Hubbard provides a uniformly workable solution.

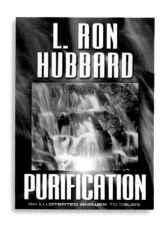

Purification: An Illustrated Answer to Drugs

A fully illustrated, easy-to-understand explanation of drugs and what they do to a person. Shows how the Purification program eliminates drug deposits and other toxins from the body, improving one's well-being, alertness and ability to progress spiritually.

TRs and Objectives Co-audit Course

The combination of communication drills and Objective Processes can have enormous therapeutic value for anyone who has been on drugs, as well as for many people who haven't. On this course, two people pair up and work with each other on drills called Training Routines (TRs) and on an entire series of Objective Processes. They do this on a *co-audit,* meaning *cooperative auditing,* basis. (Auditing is the application of Scientology processes to another for his benefit.) Students study, drill and then audit many different processes on each other, helping another and being helped in return to become more in present time and oriented to the environment, all of which can greatly raise a person's potential for success. (Delivered in Scientology organizations.)

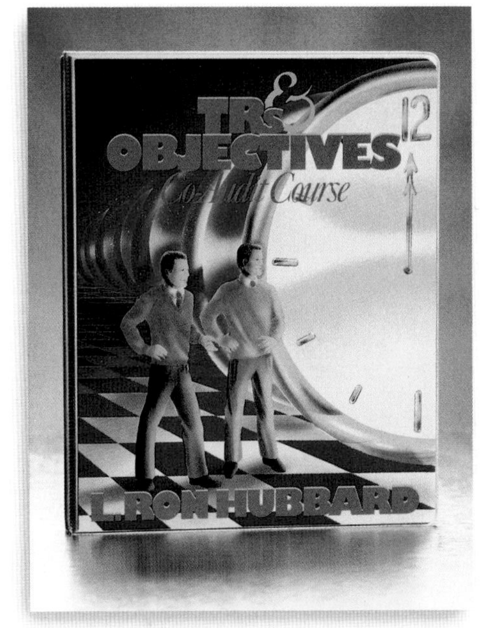

Scientology Drug Rundown Co-audit Course

The mental and spiritual effects of drug use are a vital concern. This is a course done after TRs and Objectives which uses different Scientology processes to address and eradicate the harm that drugs do to the mind and spirit. On a co-audit basis, two people can learn the techniques to accomplish this and bring themselves to greater freedom from the lingering effects of drugs. (Delivered in Scientology organizations.)

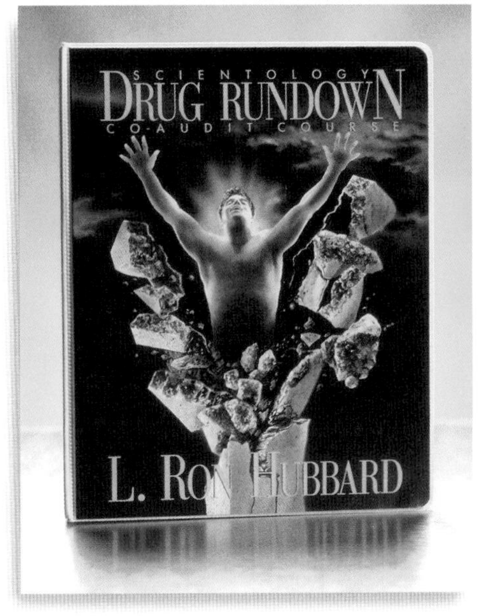

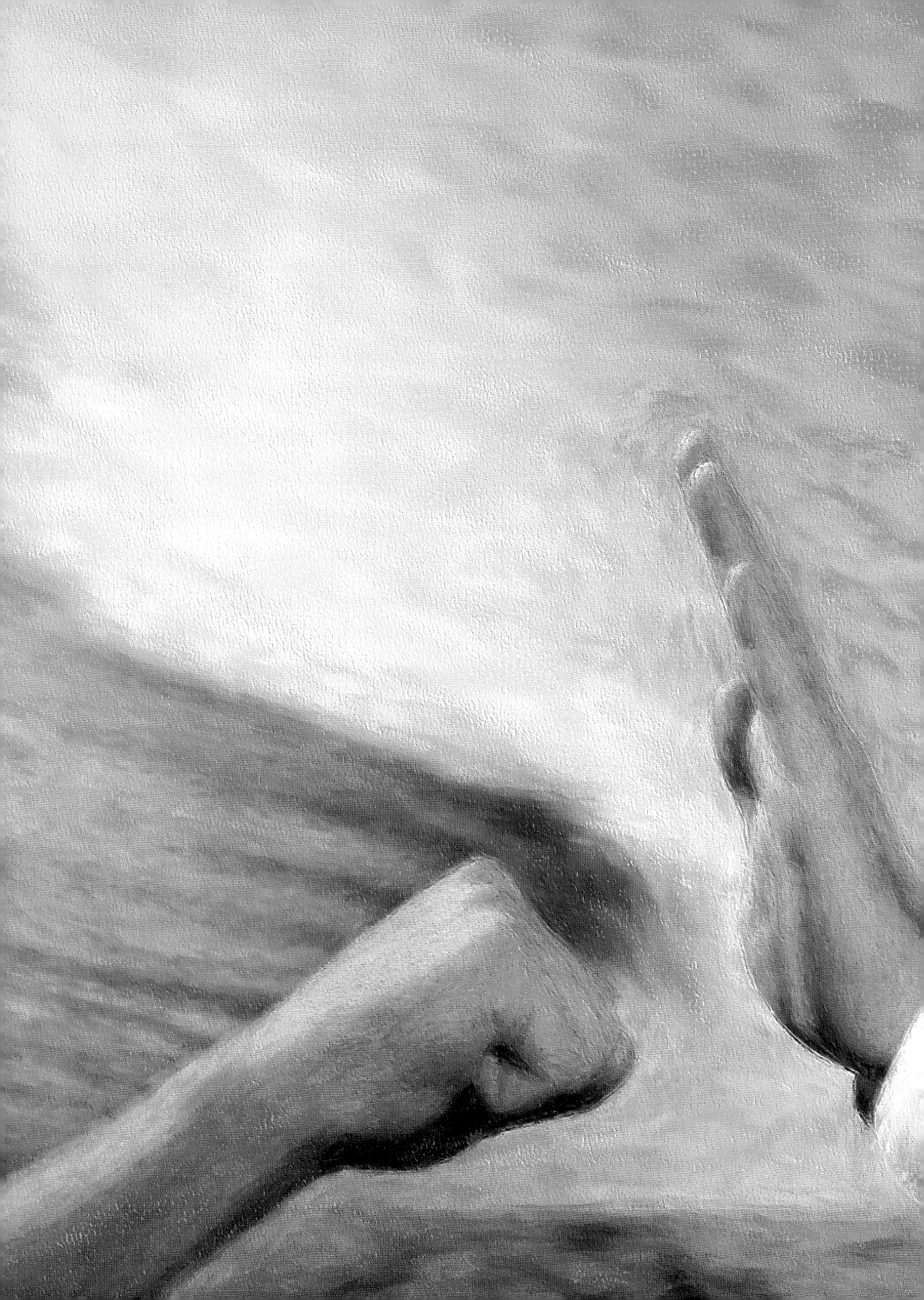

Chapter 8

How to Resolve Conflicts

It seems that people often have trouble getting along together. Families argue, neighbors come to blows, countries lob weapons at each other. Is this the way it has to be?

Anthropologists, sociologists, psychologists and others say it is. Having observed a long history of man's quarrelsome behavior, they claim that man has animal instincts, or that he is antisocial and violent by his very nature.

In truth, man is rather peaceful. But he can be driven, individually and collectively, to hatred and violence.

In researching the causes of violence, L. Ron Hubbard unearthed a fundamental and natural law of human relations which explains why conflicts between people are so often difficult to remedy. And he provided an immensely valuable tool that enables one to resolve any conflict, be it between neighbors, co-workers or even countries.

In this chapter, you will discover how to help others resolve their differences and restore peaceable relations. Peace and harmony between men can be more than just a dream. Widespread application of this law will make it a reality.

The Third Party Law

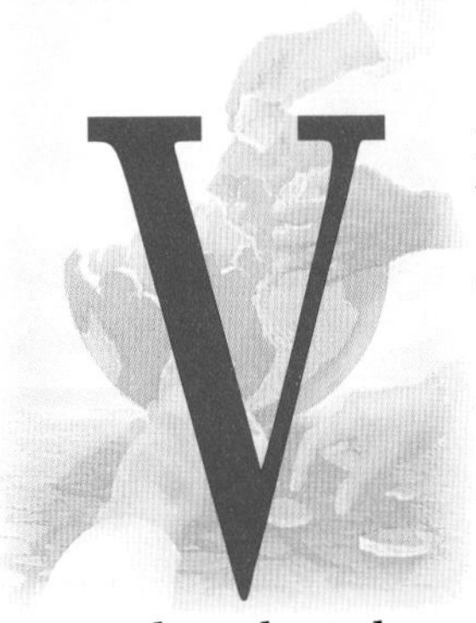

Violence and conflict amongst individuals and nations have been with us for ages and their causes have remained a complete mystery, a mystery finally solved in Scientology.

If Chaldea could vanish, if Babylon turn to dust, if Egypt could become a badlands, if Sicily could have 160 prosperous cities and be a looted ruin before the year zero and a near desert ever since—and all this in *spite* of all the work and wisdom and good wishes and intent of human beings, then it must follow as the dark follows sunset that something must be unknown to man concerning all his works and ways. And that this something must be so deadly and so pervasive as to destroy all his ambitions and his chances long before their time.

Such a thing would have to be some natural law unguessed at by himself.

And there *is* such a law, apparently, that answers these conditions of being deadly, unknown and embracing all activities.

The law would seem to be:

A THIRD PARTY MUST BE PRESENT AND UNKNOWN IN EVERY QUARREL FOR A CONFLICT TO EXIST.

or

FOR A QUARREL TO OCCUR, AN UNKNOWN THIRD PARTY MUST BE ACTIVE IN PRODUCING IT BETWEEN TWO POTENTIAL OPPONENTS.

or

WHILE IT IS COMMONLY BELIEVED TO TAKE TWO TO MAKE A FIGHT, A THIRD PARTY MUST EXIST AND MUST DEVELOP IT FOR ACTUAL CONFLICT TO OCCUR.

It is very easy to see that two in conflict are fighting. They are very visible. What is harder to see or suspect is that a third party existed and actively promoted the quarrel.

The usually unsuspected and "reasonable" third party, the bystander who denies any part of it, *is* the one that brought the conflict into existence in the first place.

The hidden third party, seeming at times to be a supporter of only one side, is to be found as the instigator.

This is a useful law in many areas of life.

It *is* the cause of war.

One sees two fellows shouting bad names at each other, sees them come to blows.

No one else is around. So *they,* of course, "caused the fight." But there *was* a third party.

Tracing these down, one comes upon incredible data. That is the trouble. The incredible is too easily rejected. One way to hide things is to make them incredible.

Clerk A and Messenger B have been arguing. They blaze into direct conflict. Each blames the other. *Neither one is correct and so the quarrel does not resolve since its true cause is not established.*

One looks into such a case *thoroughly*. He finds the incredible. The wife of Clerk A has been sleeping with Messenger B and complaining alike to both about the other.

Farmer J and Rancher K have been tearing each other to pieces for years in continual conflict. There are obvious, logical reasons for the fight. Yet it continues and does not resolve. A close search finds Banker L who, due to their losses in the fighting, is able to loan each side money, while keeping the quarrel going, and who will get their lands completely if both lose.

It goes larger. The revolutionary forces and the Russian government were in conflict in 1917. The reasons are so many the attention easily sticks on them. But only when Germany's official state papers were captured in World War II was it revealed that *Germany* had promoted the revolt and financed Lenin to spark it off, even sending him into Russia in a blacked-out train!

One looks over "personal" quarrels, group conflicts, national battles and one finds, if he searches, the third party, unsuspected by both combatants or, if suspected at all, brushed off as "fantastic." Yet careful documentation finally affirms it.

This datum is fabulously useful.

In marital quarrels the *correct* approach of anyone counseling is to get both parties to carefully search out the *third* party. They may come to many *reasons* at first. These *reasons* are not *beings* (people). One is looking for a third *party,* an actual *being.* When both find the third party and establish proof, that will be the end of the quarrel.

Sometimes two parties, quarreling, suddenly decide to elect a being to blame. This stops the quarrel. Sometimes it is not the right being and more quarrels thereafter occur.

Two nations at each other's throats should each seek conference with the other to sift out and locate the actual third party. They will always find one if they look, and they *can* find the right one. As it will be found to exist in fact.

There are probably many technical approaches one could develop and outline in this matter.

There are many odd phenomena connected with it. An accurately spotted third party is usually not fought at all by either party but only shunned.

Marital conflicts are common. Marriages can be saved by both parties really sorting out *who* caused the conflicts. There may have been, in the whole history of the marriage, several but only one at a time.

Quarrels between an individual and an organization are nearly always caused by an individual third party or a third group. The organization and the individual should get together and isolate the third party by displaying to each other all the data they each have been fed.

Rioters and governments alike could be brought back to agreement could one get representatives of both to give each other what they have been told by *whom.*

Such conferences have tended to deal only in recriminations or conditions or abuses. They must deal in beings only in order to succeed.

This theory might be thought to assert also that there are no bad conditions that cause conflict. There are. But these are usually *remedial by conference unless a third party is promoting conflict.*

In history we have a very foul opinion of the past because it is related by recriminations of two opponents and has not spotted the third party.

"Underlying causes" of war should read "hidden promoters."

There are no conflicts which cannot be resolved unless the true promoters of them remain hidden.

This is the natural law the ancients and moderns alike did not know.

And not knowing it, being led off into "reasons," whole civilizations have died.

It is worth knowing.

It is worth working with in any situation where one is trying to bring peace.

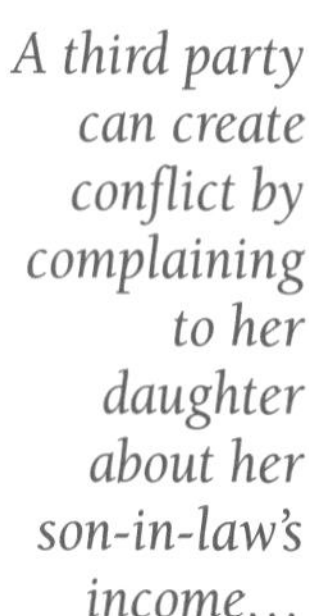

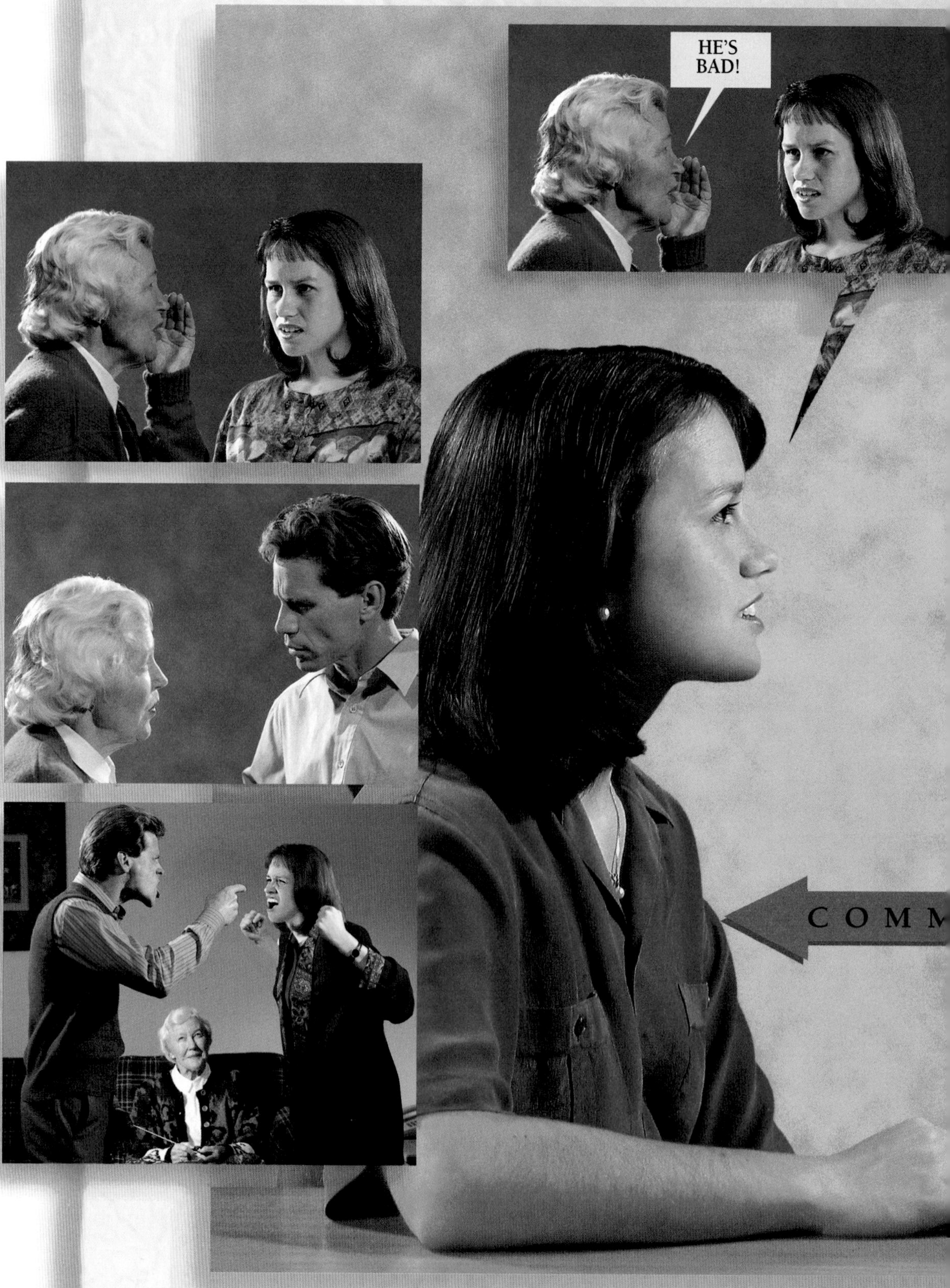

A third party can create conflict by complaining to her daughter about her son-in-law's income…

…and then upsetting the son-in-law by misinterpreting something his wife said.

When the conflict erupts, the third party is often unnoticed and unsuspected.

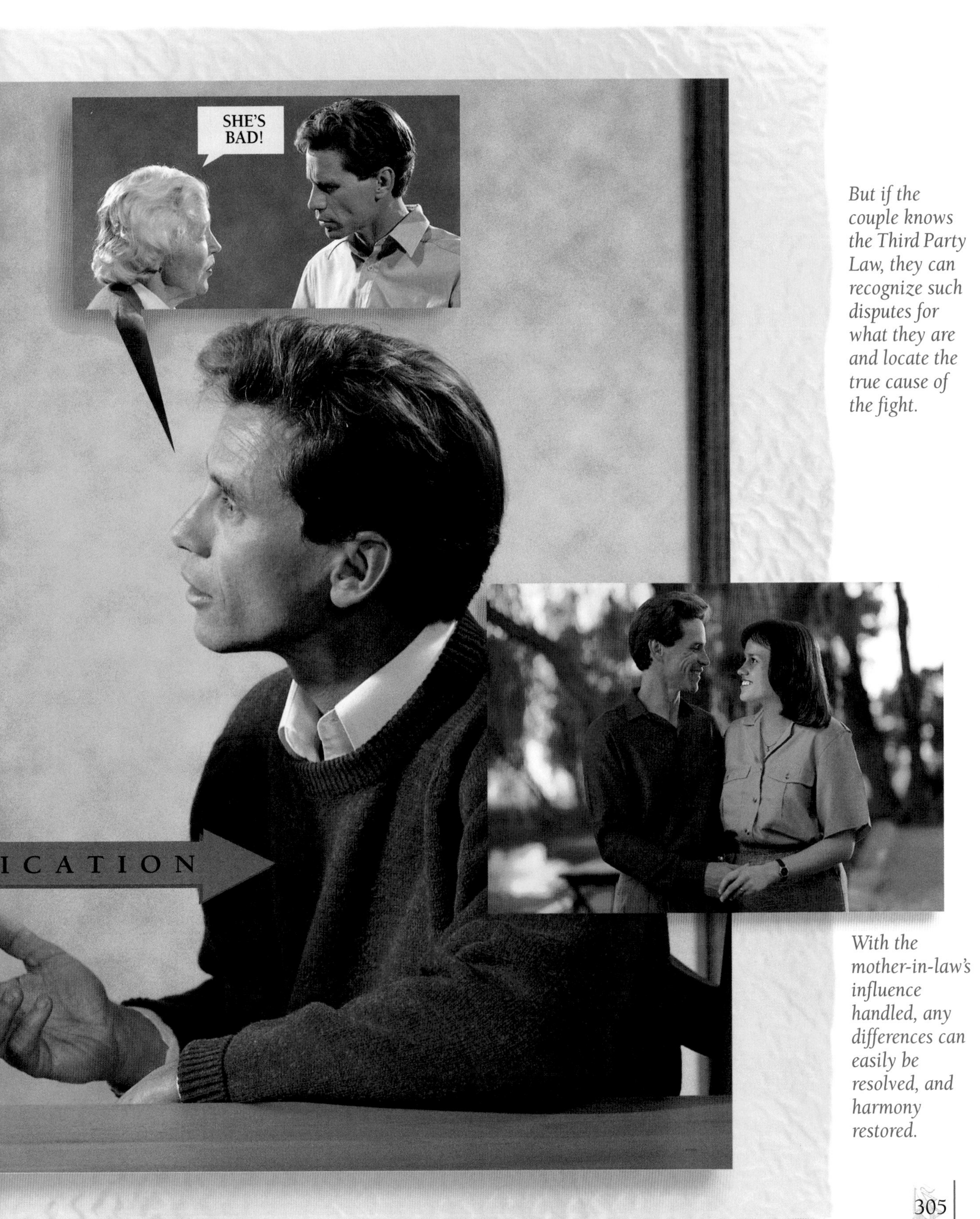

But if the couple knows the Third Party Law, they can recognize such disputes for what they are and locate the true cause of the fight.

With the mother-in-law's influence handled, any differences can easily be resolved, and harmony restored.

Further Discovery

Another very important factor in third party technology is false reports. False reports are written or spoken statements which turn out to be groundless or deceitful or which knowingly contain lies.

We know that a third party is necessary to any quarrel.

In reviewing several organizational upsets, it was found that the third party can go completely overlooked even in intensive investigation.

By giving false reports on others, a third party causes harm and wreaks havoc amongst individuals and groups.

In several cases an organization has lost several guiltless staff members. They were dismissed or disciplined in an effort to solve upsets. Yet the turbulence continued and the area became even more upset by reason of the dismissals.

Running this back further, one finds that the real third party, eventually unearthed, got people shot by *false reports.*

One source of this is as follows:

Staff member X goofs. He is very furious and defensive at being accused. He blames his goof on somebody else. That somebody else gets disciplined. Staff member X diverts attention from himself by various means including falsely accusing others.

This is a third party action which results in a lot of people being blamed and disciplined. And the real third party remaining undetected.

The missing point of justice here is that the disciplined persons *were not faced with their accusers* and were not given the real accusation and so could not confront it.

Another case would be a third party simply spreading tales and making accusations out of malice or some even more vicious motive. This would be a usual third party action. It is ordinarily based on false reports.

Another situation comes about when a person in charge of some area who can't get the area straight starts to investigate, gets third party false reports about it, disciplines people accordingly and totally misses the real third party. This upsets the area even more.

The basis of all really troublesome third party activities is then *false reports.*

There can also be *false perception.* One sees things that don't exist and reports them as "fact."

Therefore we see that we can readily run back an investigation by following a chain of false reports.

In at least one case the third party (discovered only after it was very plain that only he could have wrecked two areas of the organization, one after the other) also had these characteristics:

1. Goofed in his own actions
2. Furiously contested any reports filed on him
3. Obsessively changed everything when taking over an area
4. Falsely reported actions, accusing others
5. Had a high casualty rate of staff in his area

These are not necessarily common to all third parties but give you an idea of what can go on.

From experience in dealing with ethics and justice matters in groups it is apparent that the real source of upset in an area would be *false reports* accepted and acted upon without confronting the accused with all charges and his or her accusers.

A person with any degree of authority in a group should not accept any accusation and act upon it. To do so undermines the security of one and all. One could, as a start, refuse to act on any information unless it were proven by personal investigation not to be the action of some third party.

On being presented with an accusation or "evidence" a person in charge of some activity should conduct an investigation of false reports and false perceptions. In this way one can then verify such reports and arrive at the true source of the trouble and avoid disciplining individuals who may be innocent.

Justice, then, would consist of a refusal to accept any report not substantiated by actual, independent data, seeing that all such reports are investigated and that all investigations include confronting the accused with the accusation and where feasible the accuser, *before* any disciplinary action is undertaken or any penalty assigned.

While this may slow the processes of justice, the personal security of the individual is totally dependent upon establishing the full truth of any accusation before any action is taken.

How to Find a Third Party

The way *not* to find a third party is to compile a questionnaire that asks one and all in various ways, "Have you been a *victim?*" Do not ask questions such as, "Who has been mean to you?" or other questions which would tend to elicit answers that the person has been victimized. This kind of question will not locate the individual stirring up conflicts between people but may only name executives and others in the group who are trying to get people to do their jobs and be productive!

Anyone who uses this approach (1) does not find any third party and (2) causes people to mentally or physically collapse to the extent that they cannot function causatively.

By definition, a third party is *one who by false reports creates trouble between two people, a person and a group or a group and another group.*

The object of the investigation, then, is to find out who has been spreading false reports in order to stir up conflicts between people or groups. To find a third party one has to ask those involved in the dispute questions along the following lines:

1a. Have you been told you were in bad?

b. What was said?

c. *Who* said it?

2a. Have you been told someone was bad?

b. What was said?

c. *Who* said it?

3a. Have you been told someone was doing wrong?

b. What was said?

c. *Who* said it?

4a. Have you been told a group was bad?

b. What was said?

c. *Who* said it?

A questionnaire like this should have a limiter such as "On your job _____?" or "In your marriage _____?" or "In this family _____?"

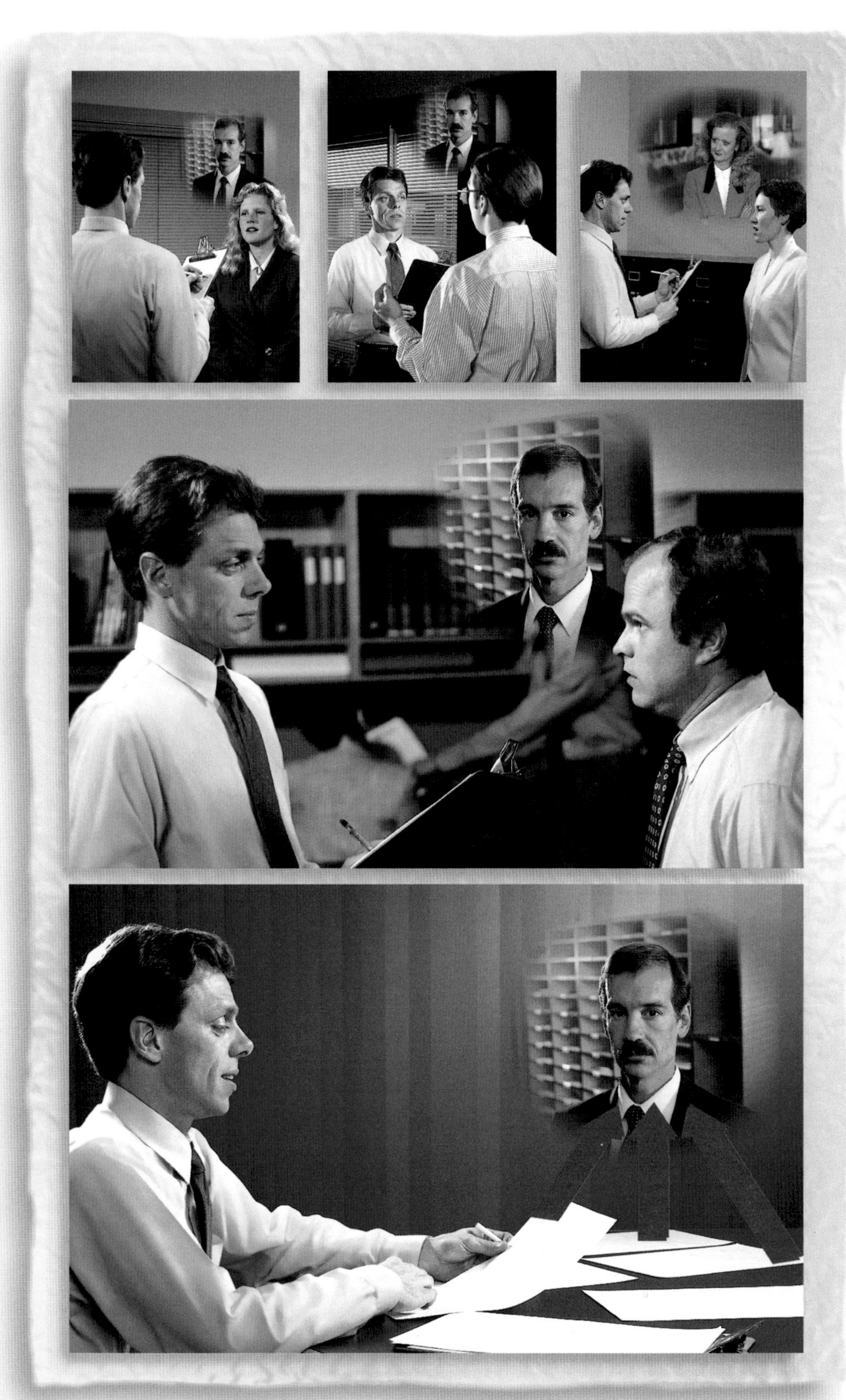

To find a third party, ask who has been telling people that others were bad, doing wrong, etc.

An entire group can be asked such questions, and when the results are viewed…

…one person's name will appear far more often than others. This is the person to investigate for creating disharmony and conflicts.

It may also have a lot of answers so leave ample space for each question.

By then combining names given, you have one name appearing far more often than the rest. This is done by counting names. You then investigate this person.

By following this procedure, you will find out exactly who has been stirring up conflicts and thus open the door to their resolution.

With this tool in your hands you will be able to change conditions between family members, associates and groups you come into contact with and restore harmony.

Such a remedy for previously unresolvable conflicts never existed before Scientology. It is the solution to a host of ills that have worried men for ages. ■

Test Your Understanding

Answer the following questions about handling conflicts. Refer back to the chapter to check your answers. If you need to, review the chapter. Going over the material several times will increase your certainty and help you better succeed in applying it.

- ❑ *What is the Third Party Law?*
- ❑ *Describe an instance of this law in effect.*
- ❑ *Explain what false reports have to do with the Third Party Law.*
- ❑ *How do you find a third party?*

Practical Exercises

Here are exercises you can do to increase your ability to resolve conflicts, whether handling one you may be involved in or helping others resolve conflicts they have.

1 To gain experience in recognizing false reports or false perceptions, find an example of a false report in your environment, such as something a neighbor said, something said at your job, etc.

2 Repeat the above practical assignment several more times until you can confidently recognize false reports.

3 Find two people who are involved in some kind of unresolving quarrel or conflict and resolve it using the Third Party Law.

4 Now find two other people or groups who are involved in a quarrel or conflict and resolve it using the data in this chapter. Repeat this until you are able to resolve conflicts using the Third Party Law.

Results from Application

Using the Third Party Law, people have been able to resolve their differences, upsets have ceased and peaceable relations have been restored.

This is an indispensable tool to handle conflicts that will not otherwise resolve, whether these involve familial situations, interpersonal relationships in the workaday world, or stress between groups or even nations.

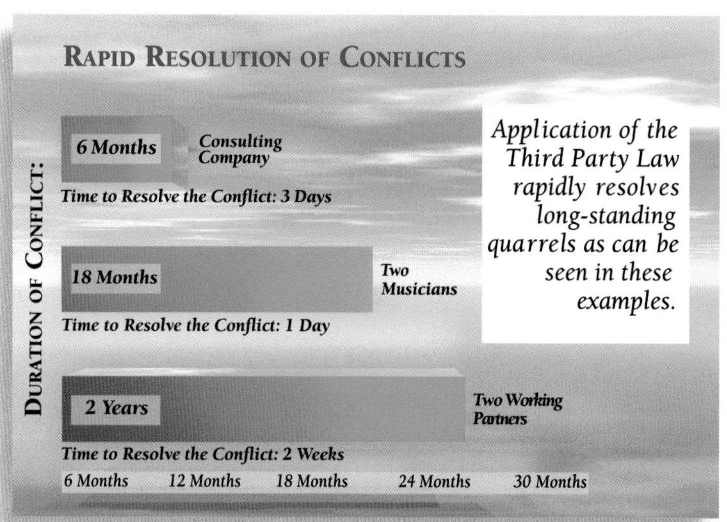

When, for example, the Director General of Justice from an independent state in South Africa first took over his government position, he found numerous conflicts had to be resolved before *any* progress could be made to improve his society. He read Mr. Hubbard's discovery about the Third Party Law and realized he had found the tool he needed to handle these conflicts. When making a special presentation to acknowledge Mr. Hubbard on behalf of the law enforcement officials in his country, the Director General said:

"I use L. Ron Hubbard's Third Party Law almost every day. It is like magic in resolving conflicts and is one of the most effective tools I have ever found to bring about peace and harmony among different groups. L. Ron Hubbard is truly a great man and I say this for a special reason. It is because he has given us wisdom, and not kept it to himself."

While paying a brief visit to a couple in Sydney, Australia, a man noticed the wife was somewhat quarrelsome with her husband. He showed her Mr. Hubbard's Third Party Law and told her to apply it to the situation. She was halfhearted about this as it didn't seem to be much of a troublesome situation to her. However, she did what their visitor suggested and later wrote to him saying:

"That night I sat down with my husband and brought the matter up. To our complete amazement, we found that each of us had been separately told, by the same person, that the other was bad. And each of us considered that person our special friend—in fact, we had separately often gone to her for advice! The more we discussed this, the more realizations we had and our affinity for each other soared and soared. Prior to this, neither of us had thought it was particularly low, but now it

seems it has no bounds. ***Thank you*** *for telling me to do this, I gained* ***complete*** *certainty on the workability of this technology on the Third Party Law."*

Miraculous results were obtained when a man from Burbank, California, used the Third Party Law to resolve a conflict between two business partners which would just not clear up.

"I conducted a hearing on the parties concerned and in the course of this, I determined that a third party investigation was needed, as the communication between the people involved simply would not improve.

"The results were truly miraculous. Not only did the communication go back in with a ***bang,*** *but I watched one of the parties, who had been ill for three years, change before my eyes. She realized that it had been due to this situation and the third partying involved that she had become ill. You would be amazed at how good it feels to be able to give help to others that is* ***real*** *help."*

Some international business partners had been locked in a long-term conflict that showed no signs of resolving. They were advised to get a third party investigation done into the matter. This was done and the results were fantastic. One of the businessmen concerned reported:

"After two days of third party investigation, a conflict which had lasted ten months finally came to an end and we are now friends with our business partners again. This was the most incredible phenomenon we have seen! After the investigation was complete, we were able to reach agreement on issues where none had been possible before. This technology worked like magic. Scientology is the game where everyone wins!"

Suggestions for Further Study

L. Ron Hubbard's discovery and codification of the Third Party Law was a major breakthrough—just one of many made in his extensive research into human relations and administrative technology. The following references are advised for study by anyone interested in these areas.

Scientology: A New Slant on Life

A collection of L. Ron Hubbard's essays on a wide variety of subjects including justice, professionalism, the anatomy of failure, human character and man's search for his soul. Each essay contains invaluable insights and practical knowledge.

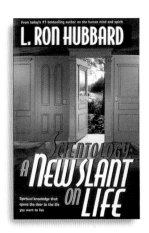

Introduction to Scientology Ethics

Augments knowledge of the Third Party Law with L. Ron Hubbard's development of a workable system of ethics. This book provides a framework for application of third party technology and will assist both in conducting third party investigations and dealing effectively with a third party once found. In addition to its use in discovering and handling the source of conflicts, the technology of ethics is essential if one hopes to lead a happy and successful life.

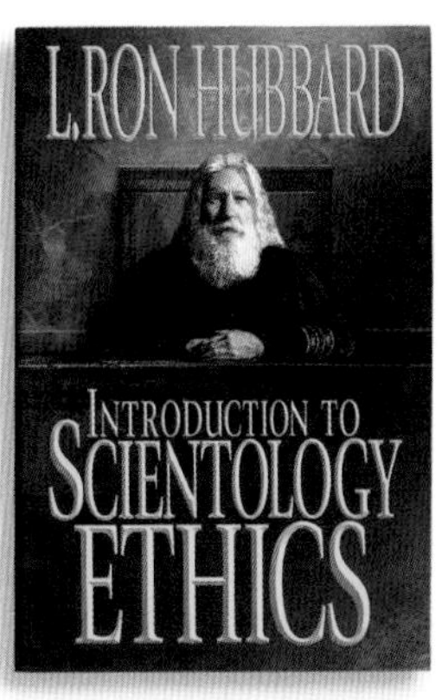

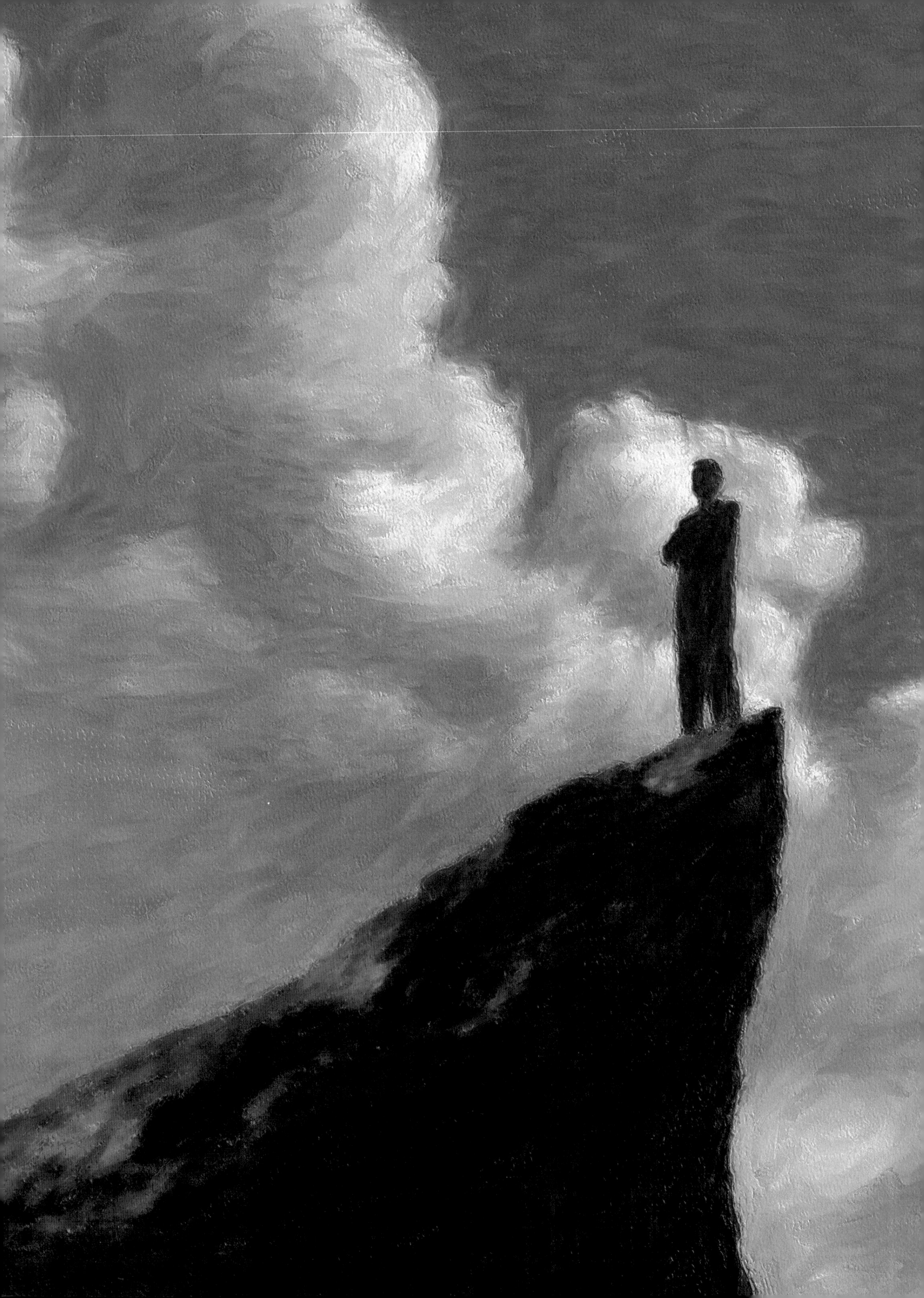

Chapter 9

Integrity and Honesty

What causes people to withdraw from participation in life? A carefree child grows reserved and wary as a teenager. A successful career woman who leaves one personal relationship after the other suffers from lack of self-esteem. A retired man looks back at his life with regret over the choices he made.

There is a reason for these all-too-common scenarios. They don't "just happen," nor are they subject to fate. L. Ron Hubbard amassed a huge body of research which squarely addresses and resolves the underlying reason for withdrawal from others and loss of integrity. And he developed a precise way for you to help individuals regain their feelings of honesty and self-worth. Broken dreams and regret about the past do not have to continue to pull people away from involvement in the present.

There is an actual mechanism which makes people withdraw from relationships, from families, groups and, indeed, their dreams. And such situations can be remedied. In this chapter, you will discover how you can help others regain their integrity—and their zest for life. It is a new view of an old problem, and what it means is that you no longer need to sit on the sidelines and helplessly observe the anguish of others. Instead, you will have in your hands tools which thoroughly resolve such misery.

MORAL CODES

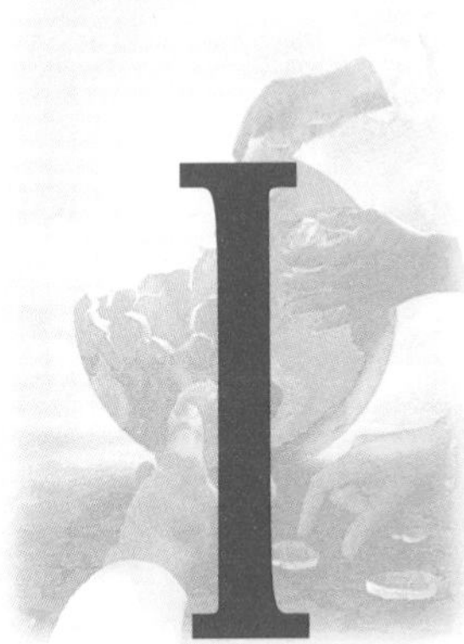

In any activity in which people interact, *moral codes* are developed. This is true of any group of any size—a family, a team, a company, a nation, a race.

What *is* a moral code? It is a series of agreements to which a person has subscribed to guarantee the survival of a group.

Take, for example, the Constitution of the United States. This was an agreement made by the original thirteen states as to how they would conduct their affairs. Wherever that Constitution has been breached, the country is now in trouble. It first stated that there must not be any income tax. Later, that was violated. Then they changed another point in it, and another and another. And each time they have done this, it has caused problems.

Why are they in trouble? Because there are no agreements other than the basic agreement.

Man has learned that where he has agreed upon codes of conduct or what is proper, he survives, and where he has not agreed, he doesn't survive. And so when people get together, they always draw up a long, large series of agreements on what is moral (that is, what will be contributive to survival) and what is immoral (what will be destructive of survival).

Moral, by these definitions, means those things which are considered to be, at any given time, survival characteristics. A survival action is a moral action. And those things are considered immoral which are considered contrasurvival.

When two or more persons have a mutual agreement, they act together—which we call *coaction.* Dancing with someone is a coaction; having a fight with someone is a coaction; working within an organization is coaction.

In naval experience, there is a known datum that a ship's crew is not worth anything until they have braved some tremendous danger or fought together. You could have a ship sailing with a new crew and, even though they are trained for their duties, nothing works: the supplies never seem to get aboard, the fuel never seems to flow freely to the engines, nothing happens except a confusion. Then one day the ship meets a great storm, with huge, raging seas, and with every crew member aboard working together to bail the water out of the engine room and to keep the screws turning. Somehow or another they hold the ship together, and the storm abates (lessens, diminishes). Now, for some peculiar reason, we have a real ship.

Whether you have a group of two men in partnership or an entire nation which is being formed after the conquest of land from another race—it does not matter the size of the group—they enter into certain agreements. The longevity of the agreement does not have much to do with it. It could be an agreement for a day, an agreement for a month or an agreement for the next five hundred years.

People, then, in forming groups, create a series of agreements of what is right and what is wrong, what is moral and what is immoral, what is survival and what is nonsurvival. That is what is created. And then this disintegrates by transgressions (violations of agreements or laws). These transgressions, unspoken but nevertheless transgressions, by each group member gradually mount up to a disintegration.

In Scientology these transgressions and their effects have been examined in great detail. There are two parts which encompass the mechanism at work here.

A harmful act or a transgression against the moral code of a group is called an *overt act*. When a person does something that is contrary to the moral code he has agreed to, or when he omits to do something that he should have done per that moral code, he has committed an overt act. An overt act violates what was agreed upon.

An unspoken, unannounced transgression against a moral code by which the person is bound is called a *withhold*. A withhold is an overt act a person committed that he or she is not talking about. It is something a person believes that, if revealed, will endanger his self-preservation. Any withhold comes *after* an overt act. Thus, an overt act is something *done;* a withhold is an overt act *withheld* from another or others.

The only person who can separate one from a group is himself, and the only mechanism he can do it through is withholding. He withholds transgressions against the moral code of the group from the other members of the group and therefore he individuates (separates) from the group, and the group therefore disintegrates.

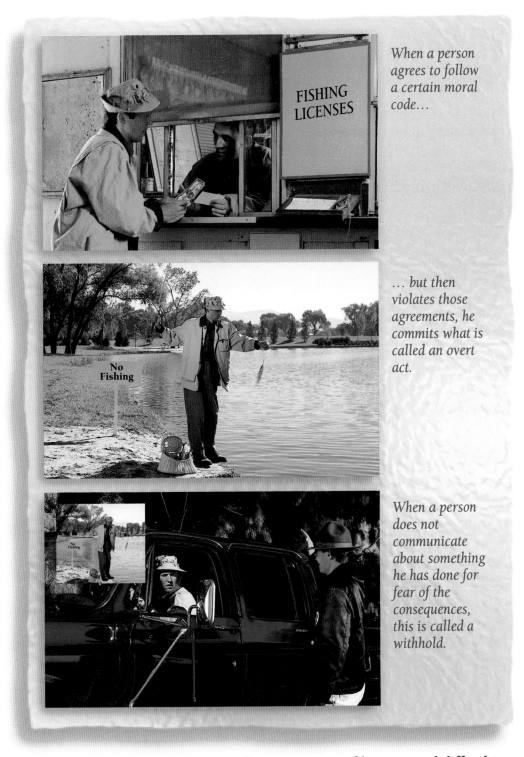

When a person agrees to follow a certain moral code…

… but then violates those agreements, he commits what is called an overt act.

When a person does not communicate about something he has done for fear of the consequences, this is called a withhold.

The social ills of man are chiefly a composite of his personal difficulties. The workable approach is to help the *individual* handle his personal difficulties for the betterment of himself and the society of which he is a part.

Justification

When a person has committed an overt act and then withholds it, he or she usually employs the social mechanism of *justification.* By "justification" we mean explaining how an overt act was not really an overt act.

We have all heard people attempt to justify their actions and all of us have known instinctively that justification amounted to a confession of guilt. But not until now have we understood the exact mechanism behind justification.

Short of applying Scientology procedures, there was no means by which a person could relieve himself of consciousness of having done an overt act, except to try to *lessen the overt.*

Some churches and other groups have used confession in an effort to relieve a person of the pressure of his overt acts. However, lacking a full understanding of all the mechanisms at play, it has had limited workability. For a confession to be truly effective, revelation of one's wrongdoing must be accompanied by a full acceptance of responsibility. All overt acts are the product of irresponsibility in some area or aspect of life.

Withholds are a sort of overt act in themselves but have a different source. Scientology has proven conclusively that man is basically good—a fact which flies in the teeth of older beliefs that man is basically evil. Man is good to such an extent that when he realizes he is being very dangerous and in error he seeks to minimize his power and if that doesn't work and he still finds himself committing overt acts he then seeks to dispose of himself either by leaving or by getting caught and executed. Without this computation, police would be powerless to detect crime—the criminal always assists himself to be caught. Why police punish the caught criminal is the mystery. He wants to be rendered less harmful to the society and wants rehabilitation. Well, if this is true then why does he not unburden himself? The fact is this: unburdening is considered by him to be an overt act.

People withhold overt acts because they conceive that telling them would be another overt act. It is as though people were trying to absorb and hold out of sight all the evil of the world. This is wrongheaded. By withholding overt acts, these are kept afloat and are themselves, as withholds, entirely the cause of continued evil.

In view of these mechanisms, when the burden became too great, man was driven to another mechanism—the effort to lessen the size and pressure of the overt. He or she could only do this by attempting to reduce the size and repute of the person against whom the overt was committed. Hence, when a man or a woman has done an overt act, there usually follows an effort to reduce the goodness or importance of the target of the overt. Hence, the husband who betrays his wife must then state that the wife was no good in some way. Thus, the wife who betrayed her husband had to reduce the husband to reduce the overt. In this light, most criticism is justification of having done an overt.

This does not say that all things are right and that no criticism anywhere is ever merited. Man is not happy. And the overt act mechanism is simply a sordid "game" man has slipped into without knowing where he was going. So there are rightnesses and wrongnesses in conduct and society and life at large, but random, nagging criticism when not borne out in fact is only an effort to reduce the size of the target of the overt so that one can live (he hopes) with the overt. Of course, to criticize unjustly and lower repute is itself an overt act and so this mechanism is not in fact workable.

This is a downward spiral. One commits overt acts unwittingly. He then seeks to justify them by finding fault or displacing blame. This leads him into further overts against the same people which leads to degradation of himself and sometimes those people.

Society is set up to punish most transgressions in one way or another. Punishment is just another worsening of the overt sequence and degrades the punisher. But people who are guilty of overts demand punishment. They use it to help restrain themselves from (they hope) further transgressions. It is the victim who demands punishment and it is a wrongheaded society that awards it. People get right down and beg to be executed. And when you don't oblige, the woman scorned is sweet tempered by comparison.

When you hear scathing and brutal criticism of someone which sounds just a bit strained, know that you have your eye on overts against that criticized person.

We have our hands here on the mechanism that makes this a crazy universe. Knowing the mechanism, it is possible to derive an effective handling to defuse it. There are further ramifications of it, however, which should be understood first.

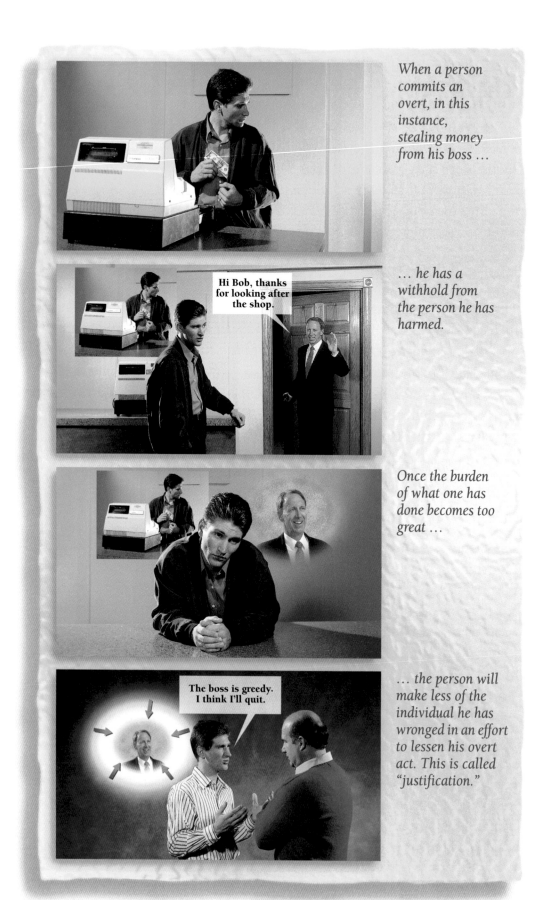
When a person commits an overt, in this instance, stealing money from his boss …
… he has a withhold from the person he has harmed.
Hi Bob, thanks for looking after the shop.
Once the burden of what one has done becomes too great …
… the person will make less of the individual he has wronged in an effort to lessen his overt act. This is called "justification."
The boss is greedy. I think I'll quit.

Blow-Offs

Scientology technology includes the factual explanation of departures, sudden and relatively unexplained, from jobs, families, locations and areas. These departures are called *blow-offs*.

This is one of the things man thought he knew all about and therefore never bothered to investigate. Yet this amongst all other things gave him the most trouble. Man had it all explained to his own satisfaction and yet his explanation did not cut down the amount of trouble which came from the feeling of "having to leave."

For instance, man has been frantic about the high divorce rate, about the high job turnover in plants, about labor unrest and many other items, all stemming from the same source—sudden departures or gradual departures.

We have the view of a person who has a good job, who probably won't get a better one, suddenly deciding to leave and going. We have the view of a wife with a perfectly good husband and family leaving it all. We see a husband with a pretty and attractive wife breaking up the affinity and departing.

Man explained this to himself by saying that things were done to him which he would not tolerate and therefore he had to leave. But if this were the explanation, all man would have to do would be to make working conditions, marital relationships, jobs, training programs and so on all very excellent and the problem would be solved. But on the contrary, a close examination of working conditions and marital relationships demonstrates that improvement of conditions often worsens the amount of blow-off. Probably the finest working conditions in the world were achieved by Mr. Hershey of chocolate bar fame for his plant workers. Yet they revolted and even shot at him. This in its turn led to an industrial philosophy that "the worse workers were treated, the more willing they were to stay," which in itself is as untrue as "the better they are treated, the faster they blow off."

One can treat people so well that they grow ashamed of themselves, knowing they don't deserve it, that a blow-off is precipitated. And, certainly, one can treat people so badly that they have no choice but to leave. But these are extreme conditions and in between these we have the majority of departures: The wife is doing her best to make a marriage and the husband wanders off on the trail of a promiscuous woman. The manager is trying to keep things going and the worker leaves. These, the unexplained, disrupt organizations and lives and it's time we understood them.

People leave because of their own overts and withholds. That is the factual fact and the hard-bound rule. A man with a clean heart can't be hurt. The man or woman who must, must, must become a victim and depart is departing because of his or her own overts and withholds. It doesn't matter whether the person is departing from a town or a job. The cause is the same.

Almost anyone, no matter his position and no matter what is wrong can remedy a situation if he or she really wants to. When the person no longer wants to remedy it, his own overt acts and withholds against the others involved in the situation have lowered his own ability to be responsible for it. Therefore, departure is the only apparent answer. To justify the departure, the person blowing off dreams up things done to him, in an effort to minimize the overt by degrading those it was done to. The mechanics involved are quite simple.

It is an irresponsibility on our part, now that we know this full mechanism, to permit this much irresponsibility. When a person threatens to leave a town, position, job or training program, the only kind thing to do is to get off that person's overt acts and withholds. To do less sends the person off with the feeling of being degraded and having been harmed.

It is amazing what trivial overts will cause a person to blow. One time a staff member was caught just before he blew and the original overt act against the organization was traced down to his failure to defend the organization when a criminal was speaking viciously about it. This failure to defend accumulated to itself more and more overts and withholds, such as failing to relay messages, failure to complete an assignment, until it finally utterly degraded the person into stealing something of no value. This theft caused the person to believe he had better leave.

It is a rather noble commentary on man that *when a person finds himself,* as he believes, *incapable of restraining himself from injuring a benefactor, he will defend the benefactor by leaving.* This is the real source of the blow-off. If we were to better a person's working conditions in this light, we would see that we have simply magnified his overt acts and made it a certain fact that he would leave. If we punish, we can bring the value of the benefactor down a bit and thus lessen the value of the overt. But improvement and punishment are neither one answers. The answer lies in Scientology and using Scientology procedures to move the person up to a high enough responsibility to take a job or a position and carry it out without all this weird hocus-pocus of "I've got to say you are doing things to me so I can leave and protect you from all the bad things I am doing to you." That's the way it is and it doesn't make sense not to do something about it now that we know.

Uneasy lies the head that has a bad conscience. Clean it up and you have a better person.

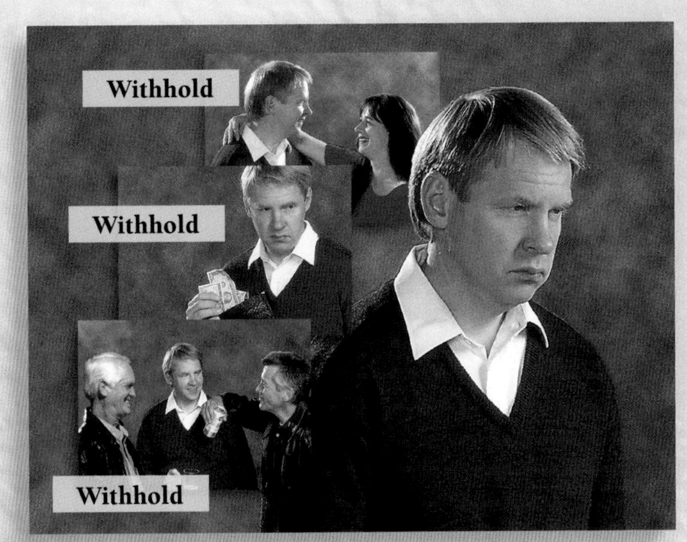

When a person accumulates enough overts and withholds against another or an area, in this case, in a marriage…

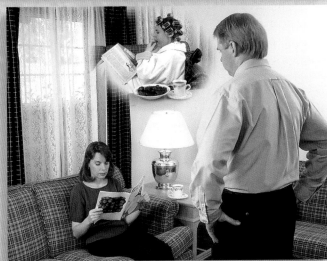

…he will become critical and begin to find fault with that person or area …

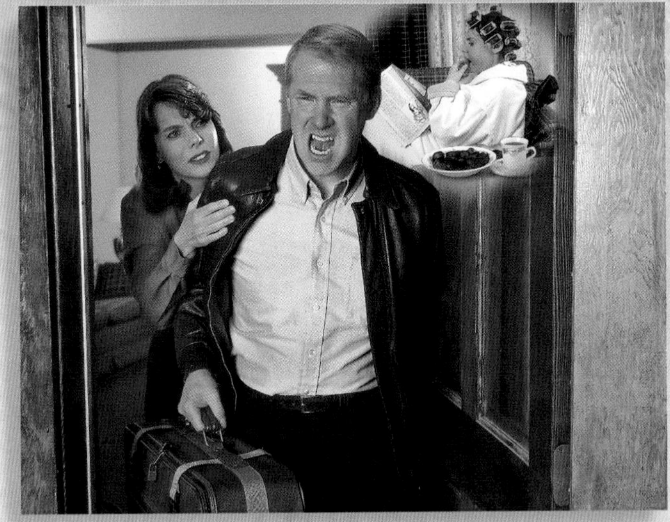

…which to him justifies a departure, a blow-off. People leave because of their own overts and withholds.

THE OVERT-MOTIVATOR SEQUENCE

There is another aspect to the mechanism of overt acts. It is called the *overt–motivator sequence,* and it further explains much of human behavior.

An *overt,* as seen, is a transgression against the moral code of a group and could additionally be described as an aggressive or destructive *act* by the individual against some part of life.

A *motivator* is an aggressive or destructive act received by the person or part of life.

The viewpoint from which the act is viewed resolves whether the act is an overt or a motivator.

The reason it is called a "motivator" is because it tends to prompt that one pays it back—it "motivates" a new overt.

When one has done something bad to someone or something, one tends to believe it must have been "motivated."

When one has received something bad, *he* also may tend to feel *he* must have done something to deserve it.

The above points are true. The actions and reactions of people on the subject are often very falsified.

People go about believing they were in an auto accident when in actual fact they caused one.

Also people may believe they caused an accident when they were only *in* one.

Some people, on hearing of a death, at once believe they must have killed the person even though they were far away.

Police in large cities have people turn up and confess to almost every murder as a routine.

One doesn't have to be crazy to be subject to the overt–motivator sequence.

The overt–motivator sequence is based upon and is in agreement with Newton's law of interaction that for every action there is an equal and contrary reaction.

The plain law of interaction is that if you have two balls, a red one and a yellow one, suspended by strings and you take the red ball and drop it against the yellow ball, the yellow ball is going to come back and hit the red ball.

That is Newton's law of interaction at work. People who have gone down (deteriorated) and are beginning to follow totally the physical universe use this law as their exclusive method of operation.

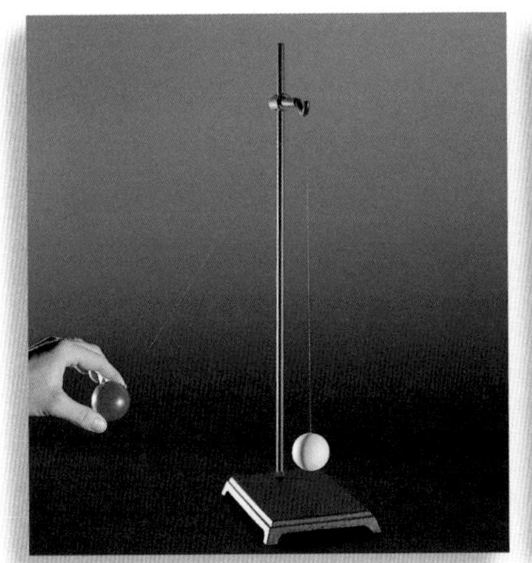

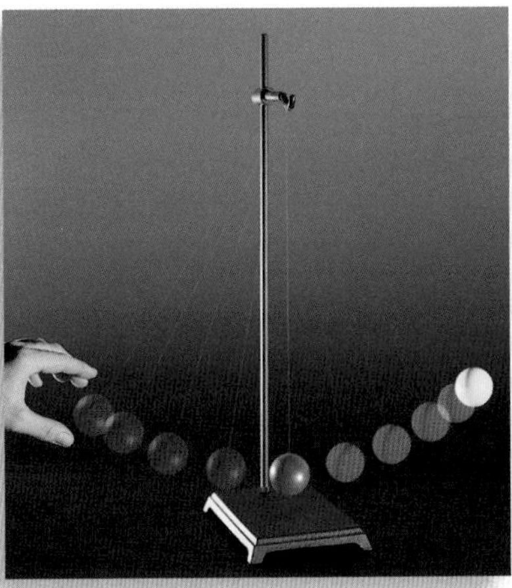

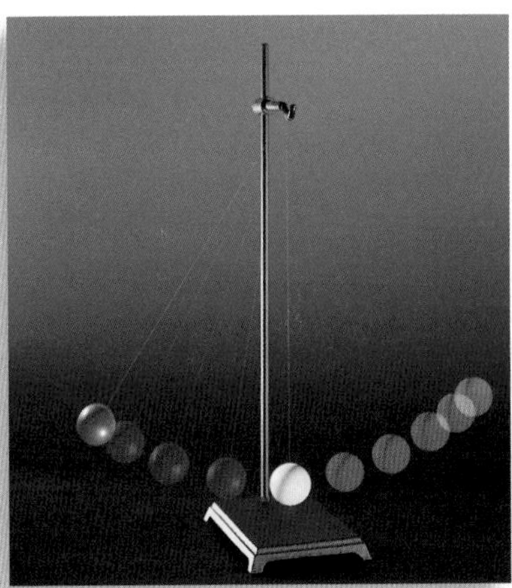

Revenge: "You hit me, I'll hit you."

National defense: "If we get enough atomic weapons, we will of course be able to prevent people from throwing atomic weapons at us."

There is more to the overt–motivator sequence, however, than just Newton's law of interaction.

If Joe hits Bill, he now believes he should be hit by Bill. More importantly, he will actually get a somatic (a physical pain or discomfort) to prove he has been hit by Bill, even though Bill hasn't hit him. He will make this law true

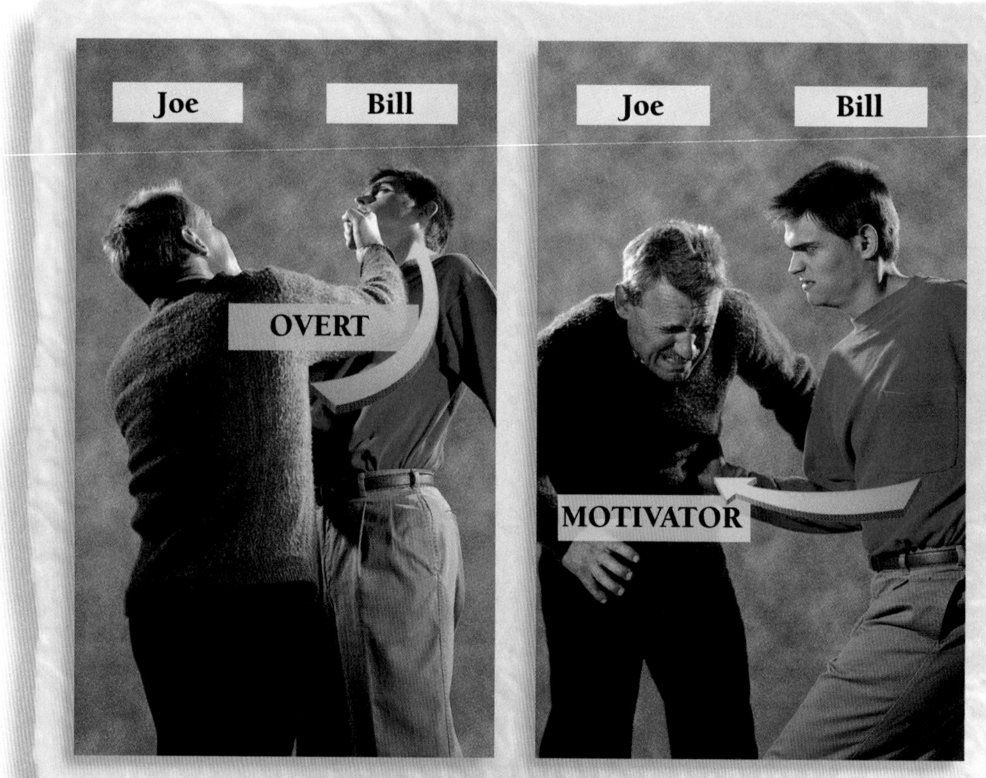

A harmful action is either an overt or a motivator depending on the viewpoint. A motivator tends to prompt another overt (the person who got hit, Bill, is likely to hit back or seek revenge), thus involving the person in many difficulties in areas of his life where he has committed overts.

regardless of the actual circumstances. And people go around all the time justifying, saying how they've been hit by Bill, hit by Bill, hit by Bill.

Even though it hasn't occurred, human beings on a low reactive (irrational) basis will insist that it has occurred. And that is the overt–motivator sequence.

This is a very valuable thing to know.

For example, if you hear a wife saying how the husband beats her every day, look under her pillow for the bat that she uses because sure as the devil, if she is saying that the yellow ball has hit the red ball, notice that the red ball had to hit the yellow ball first.

This mechanism does much to explain certain human activities.

YOU CAN BE RIGHT

Rightness and wrongness form a common source of argument and struggle. These relate closely to overts and withholds and the overt–motivator sequence.

The effort to be right is the last conscious striving of an individual on the way out. "I-am-right-and-they-are-wrong" is the lowest concept that can be formulated by an unaware person.

What *is* right and what *is* wrong are not necessarily definable for everyone. These vary according to existing moral codes and disciplines and, before Scientology, despite their use in law as a test of "sanity," had no basis in fact but only in opinion.

In Scientology a more precise definition arose. And the definition became as well the true definition of an overt act. An overt act is not just injuring someone or something: an overt act is an act of *omission* or *commission* which does the least good for the least number of people or areas of life, or the most harm to the greatest number of people or areas of life. This would include one's family, one's group or team and mankind as a whole.

Thus, a wrong action is wrong to the degree that it harms the greatest number. A right action is right to the degree that it benefits the greatest number.

Many people think that an action is an overt simply because it is destructive. To them all destructive actions or omissions are overt acts. This is not true. For an act of commission or omission to be an overt act it must harm the greater number of people and areas of life. A failure to destroy can be, therefore, an overt act. Assistance to something that would harm a greater number can also be an overt act.

An overt act is something that harms broadly. A beneficial act is something that helps broadly. It can be a beneficial act to harm something that would be harmful to many people and areas of life.

Harming everything and helping everything alike can be overt acts. Helping certain things and harming certain things alike can be beneficial acts.

The idea of not harming anything and helping everything are alike rather mad. It is doubtful if you would think helping enslavers was a beneficial action and equally doubtful if you would consider the destruction of a disease an overt act.

In the matter of being right or being wrong, a lot of muddy thinking can develop. There are no absolute rights or absolute wrongs. And being right does not consist of being unwilling to harm and being wrong does not consist only of not harming.

There is an irrationality about "being right" which not only throws out the validity of the legal test of sanity but also explains why some people do very wrong things and insist they are doing right.

The answer lies in an impulse, inborn in everyone, to *try to be right*. This is an insistence which rapidly becomes divorced from right action. And it is accompanied by an effort to make others wrong, as we see in hypercritical persons. A being who is apparently unconscious is *still* being right and making others wrong. It is the last criticism.

We have seen a "defensive person" explaining away the most flagrant wrongnesses. This is "justification" as well. Most explanations of conduct, no matter how far-fetched, seem perfectly right to the person making them since he or she is only asserting self-rightness and other-wrongness.

Scientists who are irrational cannot seem to get many theories. They do not because they are more interested in insisting on their own odd rightnesses than they are in finding truth. Thus, we get strange "scientific truths" from men who should know better. Truth is built by those who have the breadth and balance to see also where they're wrong.

You have heard some very absurd arguments out among the crowd. Realize that the speaker was more interested in *asserting* his or her own rightness than in *being right.*

A thetan—the spiritual being, the person himself—*tries* to be right and *fights* being wrong. This is without regard to being right *about* something or to do actual right. It is an *insistence* which has no concern with a rightness of conduct.

One tries to be right *always,* right down to the last spark.

How, then, is one ever wrong?

It is this way:

One does a wrong action, accidentally or through oversight. The wrongness of the action or inaction is then in conflict with one's necessity to be right. So one then may continue and repeat the wrong action to prove it is right.

This is a fundamental of aberration (irrational thought or conduct). All wrong actions are the result of an error followed by an insistence on having been right. Instead of righting the error (which would involve being wrong) one insists the error was a right action and so repeats it.

As a being goes downscale, it is harder and harder to admit having been wrong. Nay, such an admission could well be disastrous to any remaining ability or sanity.

For rightness is the stuff of which survival is made. This is the trap from which man has seemingly been unable to extricate himself: overt piling upon overt, fueled by asserted rightness. There is, fortunately, a sure way out of this web, as we shall next see.

The impulse to be right lies within everyone.

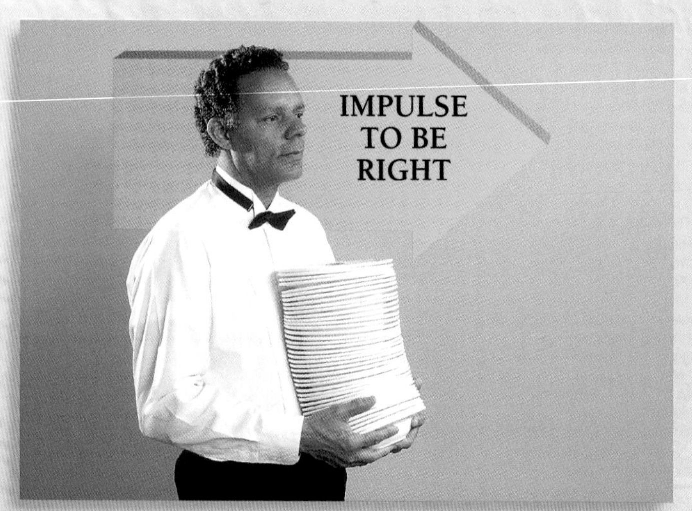

When a wrong action occurs, the person is thrown into conflict between his wrong action and impulse to be right …

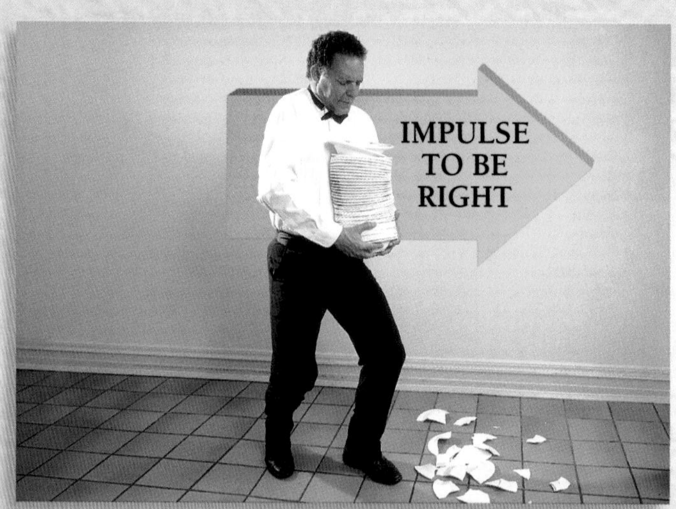

… and he may continue to do the action in an effort to assert his rightness.

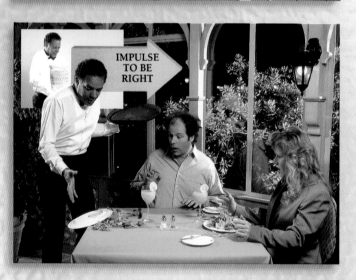

WRITING UP OVERTS AND WITHHOLDS

It has been long-standing knowledge in Scientology that in the presence of overts and withholds, abbreviated "O/Ws," no gains (improvements) occur.

Overts are the biggest reason a person restrains and withholds himself from action.

A person who has overts and withholds becomes less able to influence his own life and the lives of others around him and falls out of communication with those people and things he has committed overts against.

Writing up one's overts and withholds offers a road out. By confronting the truth an individual can experience relief and a return of responsibility.

Basic Theory

The theory behind the action of writing up one's overts and withholds is contained in the Scientology Axioms, published in their entirety in the book *Scientology 0-8: The Book of Basics*. An *axiom* is a statement of natural law on the order of those of the physical sciences.

A portion of Axiom 38 of the Scientology Axioms is particularly applicable:

1: *Stupidity is the unknownness of consideration.*

2: *Mechanical definition: Stupidity is the unknownness of time, place, form and event.*

1: *Truth is the exact consideration.*

2: *Truth is the exact time, place, form and event.*

Thus we see that failure to discover truth brings about stupidity.

Thus we see that the discovery of truth would bring about an as-isness by actual experiment.

As-isness is the condition in which a person views anything exactly as it is, without any distortions or lies, at which moment it vanishes and ceases to exist.

Thus we see that an ultimate truth would have no time, place, form or event.

Thus, then, we perceive that we can achieve a persistence only when we mask a truth.

Lying is an alteration of time, place, event or form.

Lying becomes alter-isness (an altered or changed reality of something), becomes stupidity.

Anything which persists must avoid as-isness.

Thus, anything, to persist, must contain a lie.

Writing up one's overts and withholds can accomplish an as-isness and thereby relieve a person of the burden of his transgressions.

O/W Write-up Format

When people do O/W write-ups, abuses can occur if the specifics of the action are not known and followed.

The first step to be done before one undertakes the action of an O/W write-up is to clear up the procedure of exactly how such write-ups are done.

Experience has proven that people have run into trouble on O/W write-ups when the format (including the key words and terms) was not *word cleared* before embarking on the action. (Word Clearing is that body of Scientology procedures used to locate words a person has misunderstood in subjects he has studied and get the words defined by looking them up in a dictionary.)

Format:

The format for doing an O/W write-up is as follows:

1. Write down the exact overt of commission or omission.

2. Then state explicitly the specifics regarding the action or inaction, including:

a. Time (Definition: the moment of an event, process or condition. A definite moment, hour, day or year as indicated or fixed by a clock or calendar; a precise instant or date; the period during which something [as an action] exists or continues.)

b. Place (Definition: the location of occurrence or action. A specific location; a particular portion of space or the earth's surface of a definite or indefinite size but of definite position.)

c. Form (Definition: the arrangement of things; the way in which parts of a whole are organized. In general, the arrangement of or relationship between the parts of anything as distinguished from the parts themselves. A specific formation or arrangement.)

d. Event (Definition: something that happens or comes to pass; a distinct incident. A more or less important or noteworthy occurrence. The actual outcome or final result.)

One has to get the time, place, form and event, and one has to get a done or a failure in order to get as-isness.

Example:

"1. I hit a friend's car when backing out of my parking space at work and caused about five hundred dollars' worth of damage to his car.

"2. On the 30th of June 1987, when I was leaving work, I was backing out of my parking space and hit the back end of my friend Joe's car. There was no one else around and the parking lot was almost empty. I drove away without leaving a note or telling Joe, knowing that I caused about five hundred dollars damage to his car which he had to pay for."

or, when there is a withhold or withholds to be gotten off:

1. Write down the withhold.

2. Then state explicitly the specifics regarding the action or inaction withheld, including:

a. Time

b. Place

c. Form

d. Event

For example:

"1. I cheated on my wife (Sally) by seeing another woman and never told her about this.

"2. Three years ago, when I was first married to Sally, I cheated on her by seeing another woman. I have never told Sally about this. One morning (in June 1985) I had told Sally I would take her to the movies that night and on my way home from work, when I was at Jones' Department Store, I saw an old girlfriend of mine (Barbara). I asked Barbara to go out to dinner with me that night and she accepted. (She did not know that I was married.) I told her I would pick her up at 8:00 P.M. that night. When I got home from the store I told Sally I had to go back to work to get some things done and would not be able to go to the movies with her.

"I then went out to dinner in another city with Barbara (at the Country Inn) so that I would not risk seeing any of my friends."

Administering O/W Write-ups

The action of writing up one's overts and withholds can be applied to anyone, and the breadth of its application is unlimited.

Examples:

A person is not correctly performing the duties of his job and has to be bypassed by someone senior to him in order to handle (the client or business or work assignment). Such a person is instructed to write up his O/Ws.

A person is brutally critical and leaves a training program he is on. The person in charge of the training activity has him write up his O/Ws.

It could be that a person is being very critical and fault-finding. He could experience relief from writing up his O/Ws.

The following steps are the procedure for getting a person to do an O/W write-up:

1. The first action is for the person administering the O/W write-up to: (a) study and word clear this chapter (by "word clear" is meant define, using a dictionary and the glossary in the back of this book, any words not fully understood), (b) clear the words included in step 4 below, (c) word clear the O/W write-up format.

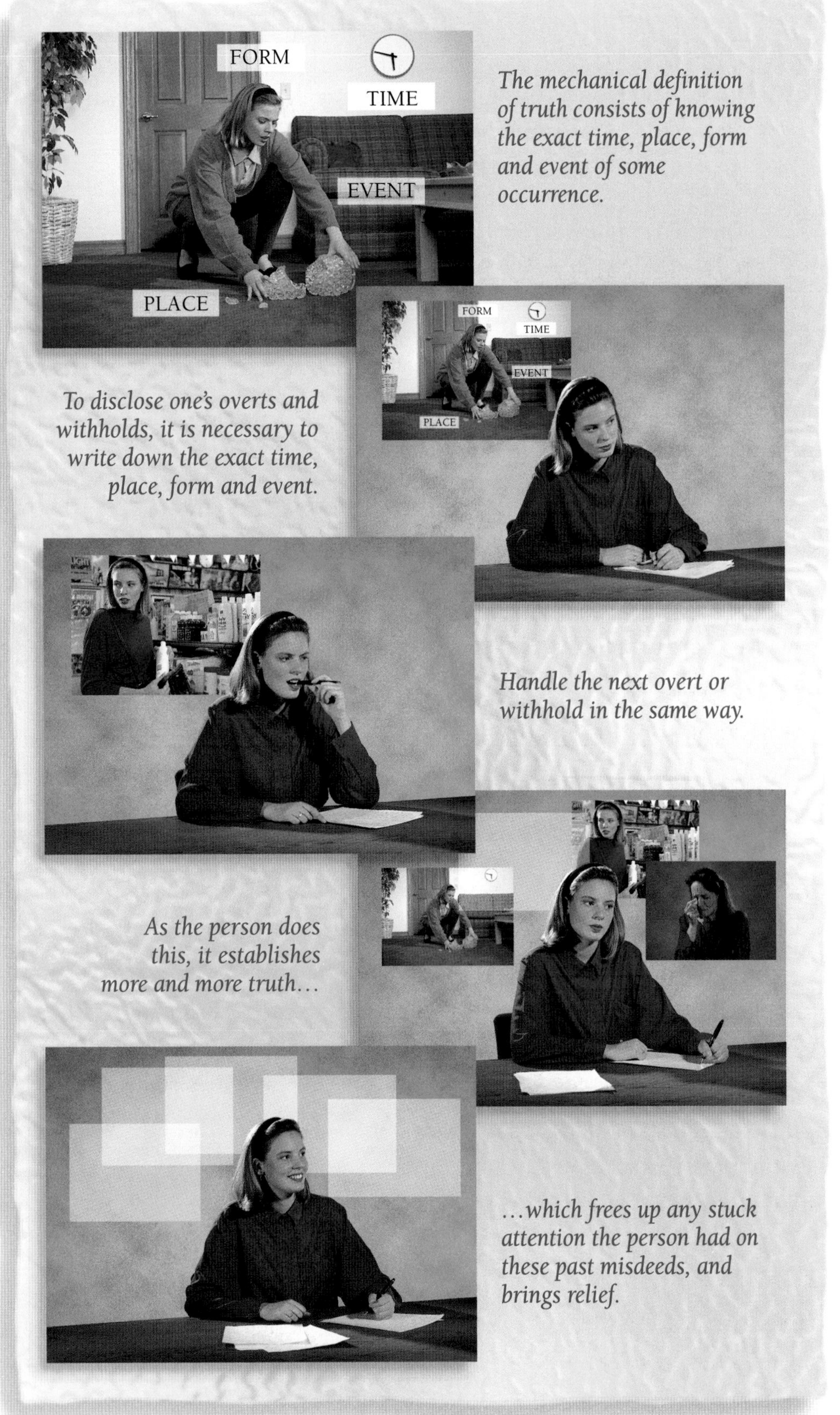

The mechanical definition of truth consists of knowing the exact time, place, form and event of some occurrence.

To disclose one's overts and withholds, it is necessary to write down the exact time, place, form and event.

Handle the next overt or withhold in the same way.

As the person does this, it establishes more and more truth…

…which frees up any stuck attention the person had on these past misdeeds, and brings relief.

2. Ensure that a space is provided where a person can write up his overts and withholds undistracted.

3. Provide paper and pen.

4. Have the person clear the following words, as defined in the text of this chapter: *overt, withhold, motivator, justification, overt–motivator sequence.*

5. Have the person read this chapter and word clear the O/W write-up format as covered above, to full understanding.

6. Have the person write up his O/Ws, exactly per the O/W write-up format above.

In doing an O/W write-up a person writes up his overts and withholds until he is satisfied that they are complete. The person will feel very good about it and experience relief. One would not engage in carrying on an O/W write-up past this point.

When he has finished, have him give the O/W write-up to you. Read the write-up, ensuring the format was used, and thank him for writing these up. This acknowledgment is important as it lets the person know his communication has been received by someone. There should, however, be no comments or opinions expressed about the content of his write-up.

Once acknowledged, you can then give the write-up back to the person.

Writing up one's overts and withholds is a simple procedure with unlimited application. A husband and wife could write up their overts and withholds on their marriage. An employee could write up his O/Ws concerning his job. A rebellious student could write down his transgressions at school.

One can straighten out any area of life by coming to grips once and for all with one's violations against the various moral codes to which he agreed and later transgressed. The relief which can accompany the unburdening of one's misdeeds is often very great. One can again feel a part of a group or relationship and regain respect for oneself, the trust and friendship of others and a great deal of personal happiness.

This is extremely useful technology.

HONEST PEOPLE HAVE RIGHTS, TOO

After you have achieved a high level of ability, you will be the first to insist upon your rights to live with honest people.

When you know the technology of the mind, as a trained Scientologist does, you know that it is a mistake to use "individual rights" and "freedom" as arguments to protect those who would only destroy.

Individual rights were not originated to protect criminals but to bring freedom to honest men. Into this area of protection then dived those who needed "freedom" and "individual liberty" to cover their own questionable activities.

Freedom is for honest people. No man who is not himself honest can be free—he is his own trap. When his own deeds cannot be disclosed, then he is a prisoner; he must withhold himself from his fellows and is a slave to his own conscience. Freedom must be deserved before any freedom is possible.

To protect dishonest people is to condemn them to their own hells. By making "individual rights" a synonym for "protect the criminal," one helps bring about a slave state for all; for where "individual liberty" is abused, an impatience with it arises which at length sweeps us all away. The targets of all disciplinary laws are the few who err. Such laws unfortunately also injure and restrict those who do not err. If all were honest, there would be no disciplinary threats.

There is only one way out for a dishonest person—facing up to his own responsibilities in the society and putting himself back into communication with his fellow man, his family, the world at large. By seeking to invoke his "individual rights" to protect himself from an examination of his deeds, he reduces just that much the future of individual liberty, for he himself is not free. Yet he infects others who are honest by using *their* right to freedom to protect himself.

Uneasy lies the head that wears a guilty conscience. And it will lie no more easily by seeking to protect misdeeds by pleas of "freedom means that you must never look at me." The right of a person to survive is directly related to his honesty.

Freedom for man does not mean freedom to injure man. Freedom of speech does not mean freedom to harm by lies.

Man cannot be free while there are those amongst him who are slaves to their own terrors.

The mission of a techno-space society is to subordinate the individual and control him, by economic and political duress. The only casualty in a machine age is the individual and his freedom.

To preserve that freedom one must not permit men to hide their evil intentions under the protection of that freedom. To be free a man must be honest with himself and with his fellows. If a man uses his own honesty to protest the unmasking of dishonesty, then that man is an enemy of his own freedom.

We can stand in the sun only so long as we do not let the deeds of others bring the darkness.

Freedom is for honest men. Individual liberty exists only for those who have the ability to be free.

Today in Scientology we know the jailer—the person himself. And we can restore the right to stand in the sun by eradicating the evil men do to themselves.

So do not say that an investigation of a person or the past is a step toward slavery. For in Scientology such a step is the first step toward freeing a man from the guilt of self.

Were it the intention of the Scientologist to punish the guilty, then and only then would a look into the past of another be wrong.

But we are not police. Our look is the first step toward unlocking the doors—for they are all barred from *within*.

Who would punish when he could salvage? Only a madman would break a wanted object he could repair—and we are not mad.

The individual must not die in this machine age—rights or no rights. The criminal and madman must not triumph with their newfound tools of destruction.

The least free person is the person who cannot reveal his own acts and who protests the revelation of the improper acts of others. On such people will be built a future political slavery where we all have numbers—and our guilt—unless we act.

It is fascinating that blackmail and punishment are the keynotes of all dark operations. What would happen if these two commodities no longer existed? What would happen if all men were free enough to speak? Then and only then would you have freedom.

On the day when we can fully trust each other, there will be peace on earth.

Don't stand in the road of that freedom. Be free, yourself. ■

Test Your Understanding

Answer the following questions about the information contained in this chapter. Refer back to check your answers. If you need to, review the chapter. Going over the materials several times will increase your certainty and help you obtain better success in applying them.

- ❑ *Give an example of a moral code.*
- ❑ *What is an overt?*
- ❑ *What is a withhold?*
- ❑ *What is meant by "justification"?*
- ❑ *Explain the mechanism behind sudden and relatively unexplained departures from jobs, locations and areas.*
- ❑ *What is the overt–motivator sequence?*

PRACTICAL EXERCISES

The following exercises will help you understand this chapter and increase your ability to apply the knowledge in it.

1 Look through a newspaper or magazine and find several examples of someone employing the social mechanism of justification. Continue doing this, as needed, until you can easily spot examples.

2 Write down an example of an overt or withhold that you have observed. Then figure out a consequence of this overt or withhold on the person himself or the people around him. Repeat this several more times, as needed, until you get a reality on the effects of overts and withholds.

3 Think of at least two examples of the overt–motivator sequence you have seen or experienced.

4 Find someone you know who would benefit from writing up his overts and withholds. This could be a person who is overly critical about someone or something, a person who is heavily justifying his actions in some area or someone who is extremely defensive about something he has done. Administer an O/W write-up to him. Follow the steps given in the section "Administering O/W Write-ups." Show him this chapter so he understands the benefits of writing up his O/Ws. Have him do a write-up exactly per the format until he is satisfied he has written up his overts and withholds completely and feels good about it.

RESULTS FROM APPLICATION

Thousands have used the works of L. Ron Hubbard to squarely address and resolve the contradictions of existence—good and evil, right and wrong. They have discovered that interpersonal relationships no longer rest on the *hope* of improvement, but upon an actual technology that can invariably bring about improvement. Using this body of data, people can regain self-worth and increase their ability to be responsible.

Knowing the mechanism which makes people withdraw from relationships of all types and indeed life itself, enables them to rehabilitate their willingness to assume responsibility. For these people, alienation is no longer a fact of life. They know what is right, and live accordingly. And the society around them benefits, as shown in a study conducted in Spain: of a group of hardened criminals who used Mr. Hubbard's methods to become honest citizens, 100 percent committed no crimes at all following their rehabilitation. In view of the normal 80 percent recidivism (a return to criminal habits) rate, this is an amazing statistic.

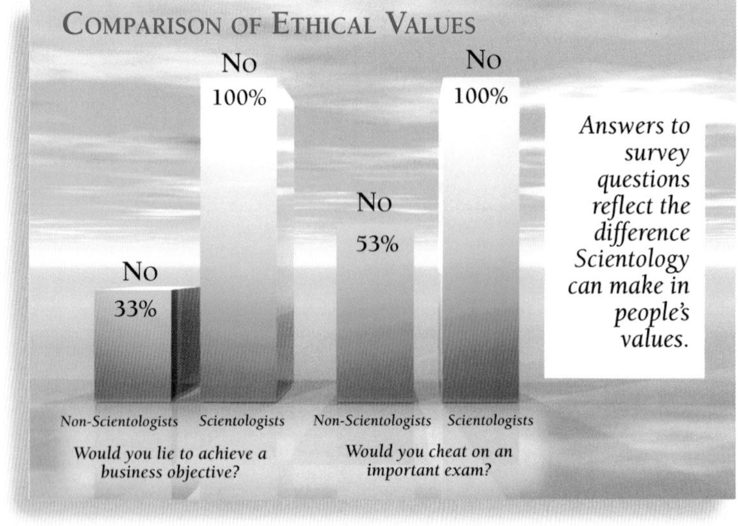

Answers to survey questions reflect the difference Scientology can make in people's values.

In modern society there is no sure way one can alleviate the misery caused by his own transgressions. Mr. Hubbard's technology, however, does provide a means whereby an individual can free himself from the hostilities and sufferings of life. Life-changing results are gained as shown in these stories.

A young man from California discovered that he could take control of his own life using the technology of overts and withholds.

"I was very upset one day as I was driving my car. Things were just not going right: customers had earlier in the day decided not to buy the products I was offering; slow, poor drivers were in front of me, causing me to honk my horn at them; I was mad and unhappy; the day looked grim. All of a sudden, however, I realized that perhaps I should just write up my overts and withholds. I pulled off the road and for whatever reason decided to do it right there in my car. Well, what do you know! I felt much better and realized I could always write up my overts and withholds if things got too out of control for me. I felt so good

and in control of my own destiny. Things went great from there. I was no longer worried the rest of that day and sure enough, my next customer bought everything I had to sell! 'Good' drivers were now in front of me too! I realized **my** *viewpoint made the difference and that I* **could** *do something about it."*

A South African volunteer in charge of a project to get Mr. Hubbard's technology into use in underprivileged black communities said the following after applying the technology of overts and withholds:

"I have two volunteers from the community who are currently writing up overts and withholds. I must say I feel very proud of this. I had perceived one of them as being extremely unfaithful to a number of women and he was stunned when I told him I knew what was happening in his life. It must have shaken him as he stopped being promiscuous instantly, so to speak. He is faithfully writing up detailed overts and withholds and thriving from the relief. He looks absolutely great! His lovely sense of humor and a whole 'new' person is emerging from under all the previous bric-a-brac. The other young man called me to say he has written a whole pad of overts and withholds and is completely exhilarated by the action and what is happening to him as a result. He has just been chosen out of thousands of young men by his country to go overseas to further his education—he cannot believe it!"

Having immigrated to Sweden with his family, a young man was thoroughly upset about how badly life had been treating him. He was miserable and nothing seemed to change this. Eventually, a friend realized that the only way out for this young man would be for him to write up his overts and withholds. He agreed to do this and here is what he said:

"I have been sitting here all day writing overts and withholds, covering my whole life. I have always blamed others for why I was doing so badly—my mother, my father, even my girlfriend, my friends, my new country, the fact that I am a foreigner—but it never occurred to me before that I am the reason I have felt so bad: it was really because of all these things I did that I carried around inside me. No wonder I have been doing so badly and why others do so badly! I feel 100 kilograms lighter!"

In California, a schoolteacher had a chronic liar as a pupil. He would lie even in circumstances where there was no reason to. He was "punished" for doing this—his privileges were taken away, he was made to do work during recesses, etc. Yet no matter what was done, there was no change. Here is what happened when this teacher decided to get him to write up his overts and withholds to handle this:

"I spent five days helping the boy to do an O/W write-up. All of the overts he wrote up had 'lying' as the form of the overt. After the fourth day of writing, he finally told me the first time he had ever lied was when he had hurt his little brother and made him cry. His mom had walked into the room and asked if he'd hurt his brother and he said, 'No.' She accepted his answer and it was then he realized he could 'lie and get away with it.' His face was bright after he told me this. Contentment and relief glowed within him. That was three years ago. This boy is now a pleasure to be around and there has not been one instance of lying since."

A woman in Los Angeles was in very poor physical condition which she had been trying to handle for months and months without result. Her life was a mess, so much so that she hardly knew where to turn for help. Luckily, a chaplain who knew the technology of overts and withholds came on the scene.

"I have been writing up my overts and withholds for the past several days. I have a physical problem that has not improved for the better part of a year. Yesterday my physical therapist told me there was a ***marked*** *improvement in muscle tone and in my overall health. I know it is because I am taking responsibility for my own condition. This technology is saving my life."*

A girl from Florida was writing up her overts and withholds and trying to think of anything else she could possibly write as she didn't feel quite satisfied with her write-up. She suddenly thought of an incident from about a year and a half before when she had carelessly misplaced her purse and had subsequently lost it and at the time made no effort to find it. Here is what occurred as a result:

"As I wrote this up, I realized that I actually had some stuck attention but I didn't really think much about it at the time. The next day, roughly twenty-four hours from the time I had written this up, I went to collect my mail and found that my purse had been sent to me, still containing everything that I had left in it! This was a year and a half after it had gone missing in another city entirely. Now, I am not saying that the purpose of writing up overts and withholds is for getting missing things back, but I realized that it was something that I had not taken responsibility for and had ignored, and as soon as I took some responsibility for it and was no longer being the effect of it, something happened and I was no longer holding it away from myself. I could have my purse again, at which time I got it back."

SUGGESTIONS FOR FURTHER STUDY

Mr. Hubbard's discoveries and developments related to overts and withholds have, for the first time, opened the door to relief from the burden of one's transgressions, full recovery of personal integrity and greatly increased freedom and survival potential. The materials listed below contain much additional data on overts and withholds, and should be studied by anyone who intends to use it to help others.

Introduction to Scientology Ethics

There exist in today's society major confusions on the subjects of ethics, justice and morals. *Introduction to Scientology Ethics* contains the simple and sensible answers to these confusions. Covering the fundamentals of the Scientology ethics and justice systems, the book is invaluable for improving your own life and the lives of others around you.

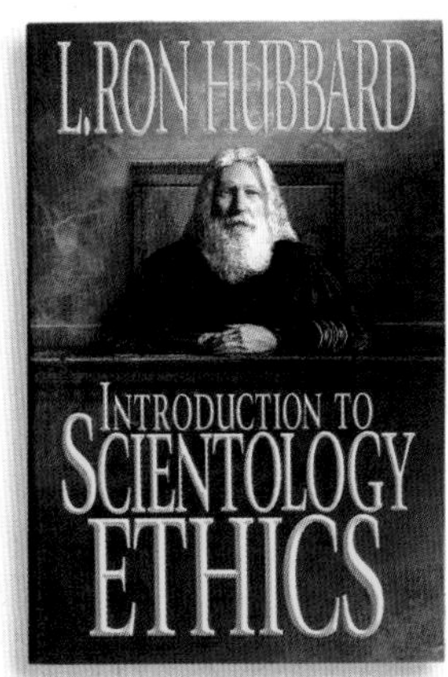

Personal Values and Integrity

Personal integrity plays a key role in living a happy life. Pressures from society can compromise that integrity and deny you real happiness. The Personal Values and Integrity course gives you the straight facts on determining your own values and keeping your personal integrity high despite the stresses of today's world. Here is knowledge to increase your ability to live and be happy while remaining true to yourself. (Delivered in Scientology organizations.)

State of Man Congress

This series of nine lectures by Mr. Hubbard, recorded in 1960, contains his initial breakthroughs on the subject of overts and withholds. He expands upon the materials contained in this chapter, covering the relationship of overts and withholds to survival, responsibility, recovery of one's true identity and the restoration of creative abilities. Other topics discussed include how different forms of governments function and the application of Scientology to society.

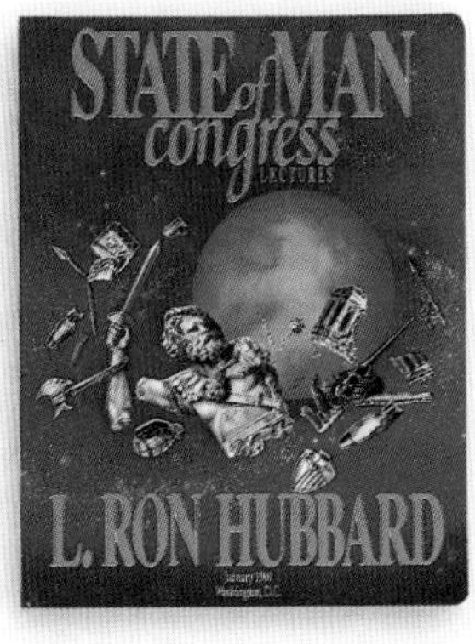

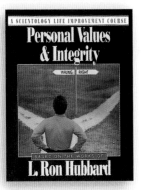

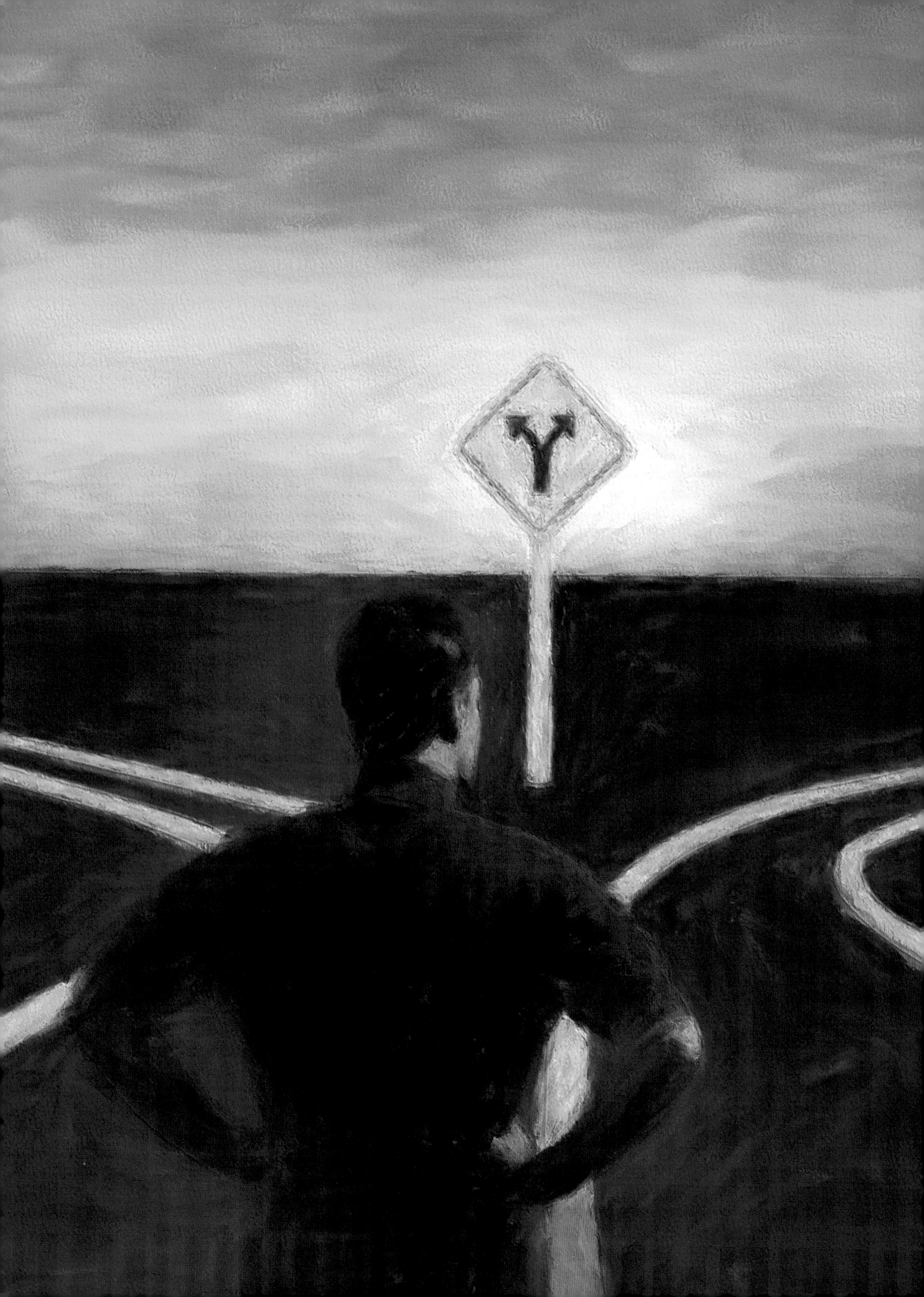

Chapter 10

Ethics and the Conditions

Man has long found ethics to be a confusing subject. In recent decades it has become more so. How does a person know if what he is doing is right or wrong? When he sees dishonest men hold power, criminals go free and traditional values cast aside, maybe he feels he should take the easy way out. "Others cheat on their taxes, why shouldn't I?" "Other kids shoplift, what's the harm?" But, regardless of anything else, a person has to live with himself. With many pressures pushing and pulling at a person, how can he be sure his choices will be best for himself, his family and every aspect of his life and his future?

L. Ron Hubbard achieved a remarkable breakthrough in the field of ethics which included not only simplification and codification of the subject, but development of a workable technology with applicability to our daily lives, one which brings about increased happiness, prosperity and survival.

These fundamentals, taken from Mr. Hubbard's body of work, even when combined with the previous chapter, "Integrity and Honesty," which provides yet more information on the subject, do not present the entirety of ethics technology available in Scientology. However, they do provide an exact means for an individual to gradiently raise his ethics level, increase his survival potential in any area of life and help others do the same. Thus ethics technology is the key tool you need to succeed in **all** *aspects of existence.*

The Basics of Ethics

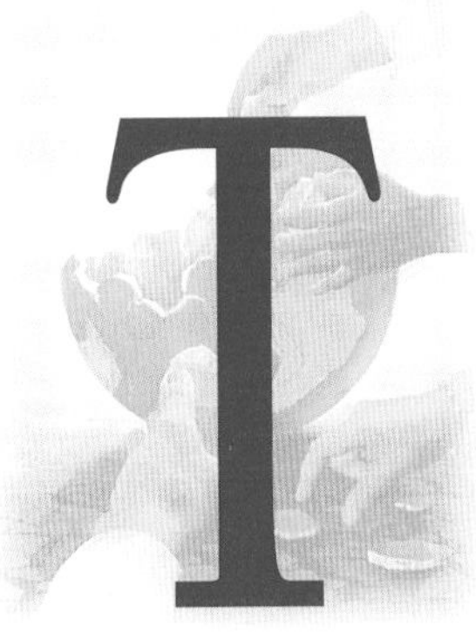

Throughout the ages, man has struggled with the subjects of right and wrong and ethics and justice.

The dictionary defines *ethics* as "the study of the general nature of morals and of the specific moral choices to be made by the individual in his relationship with others."

The same dictionary defines *justice* as "conformity to moral right, or to reason, truth or fact," or "the administration of law."

As you can see, these terms have become confused.

All philosophies from time immemorial have involved themselves with these subjects. And they never solved them.

That they have been solved in Scientology is a breakthrough of magnitude. The solution lay, first, in their *separation*. From there it could go forward to a workable technology for each.

Ethics consists simply of the actions an individual takes on himself. It is a personal thing. When one is ethical or "has his ethics in," it is by his own determinism and is done by himself.

Justice is the action taken on the individual by the group when he fails to take these actions himself.

History

These subjects are, actually, the basis of all philosophy. But in any study of the history of philosophy it is plain that they have puzzled philosophers for a long time.

The early Greek followers of Pythagoras (Greek philosopher of the sixth century B.C.) tried to apply their mathematical theories to the subject of human conduct and ethics. Some time later, Socrates (Greek philosopher and teacher, 470?–399 B.C.) tackled the subject. He demonstrated that all those who were claiming to show people how to live were unable to defend their views or even define the terms they were using. He argued that we must know what courage, and justice, law and government are before we can be brave or good citizens or just or good rulers. This was fine, but he then refused to provide definitions. He said that all sin was ignorance but did not take the necessary actions to rid man of his ignorance.

Socrates' pupil, Plato (Greek philosopher, 427?–347 B.C.) adhered to his master's theories but insisted that these definitions could only be defined by pure reason. This meant that one had to isolate oneself from life in some ivory tower and figure it all out—not very useful to the man in the street.

Aristotle (Greek philosopher, 384–322 B.C.) also got involved with ethics. He explained unethical behavior by saying that man's rationality became overruled by his desire.

This chain continued down the ages. Philosopher after philosopher tried to resolve the subjects of ethics and justice.

Unfortunately, until now, there has been no workable solution, as evidenced by the declining ethical level of society.

So you see it is no small breakthrough that has been made in this subject. We have defined the terms, which Socrates omitted to do, and we have a workable technology that anyone can use to help get himself out of the mud. The natural laws behind this subject have been found and made available for all to use.

Ethics

Ethics is so native to the individual that when it goes off the rails he will always seek to overcome his own lack of ethics.

He knows he has an ethics blind spot the moment he develops it. At that moment he starts trying to put ethics in on himself, and to the degree that he can envision long-term survival concepts, he may be successful, even though lacking the actual tech of ethics.

All too often, however, the bank is triggered by an out-ethics situation; and if the individual has no tech with which to handle it analytically, his "handling" is to mock up motivators. In other words, he tends to believe or pretend that something was done to him that prompted or justified his out-ethics action, and at that point he starts downhill.

It is *not* his attempt to get his ethics in that does him in. It is the automaticity of the bank which kicks in on him and his use of a bank mechanism at this point which sends him down the chute. When that happens, nobody puts him down the chute harder, really, than he does himself.

And, once on the way down, without the basic technology of ethics, he has no way of climbing back up the chute—he just caves himself in directly and deliberately. And even though he has a lot of complexities in his life, and he has other people doing him in, it all starts with his lack of knowledge of the technology of ethics.

This, basically, is one of the primary tools he uses to dig himself out.

Basic Nature of Man

No matter how criminal an individual is, he will be trying, one way or another, to put ethics in on himself.

This explains why Hitler invited the world to destroy Germany. He had the whole war won before September 1939, before he declared war. The Allies were giving him everything he wanted; he had one of the finest intelligence organizations that ever walked; he had Germany well on the way to getting her colonies back and the idiot declared war! And he just caved himself and Germany right in. His brilliance was going at a mad rate in one direction and his native sense of ethics was causing him to cave himself in at a mad rate in the other direction.

The individual who lacks any ethics technology is unable to put in ethics on himself and restrain himself from contrasurvival actions, so he caves himself in. And the individual is not going to come alive unless he gets hold of the basic tech of ethics and applies it to himself and others. He may find it a little unpalatable at first, but when you're dying of malaria you don't usually complain about the taste of the quinine: you may not like it, but you sure drink it.

Justice

When the individual fails to put in his own ethics, the group takes action against him and this is called justice.

I have found that man cannot be trusted with justice. The truth is, man cannot really be trusted with "punishment." With it he does not really seek discipline; he wreaks injustice. He dramatizes his inability to get his own ethics in by trying to get others to get their ethics in: I invite you to examine what laughingly passes for "justice" in our current society. Many governments are so touchy about their divine rightness in judicial matters that you hardly open your mouth before they burst into uncontrolled violence. Getting into police hands is a catastrophe in its own right in many places, even when one is merely the plaintiff, much less the accused. Thus, social disturbance is at maximum in such areas.

When the technology of ethics isn't known, justice becomes an end-all in itself. And that just degenerates into a sadism. Governments, because they don't understand ethics, have "ethics committees," but these are all worded in the framework of justice. They are even violating the derivation of the word *ethics.* They write justice over into ethics continuously with medical ethics committees, psychological ethics committees, congressional committees, etc. These are all on the basis of justice because they don't really know what ethics is. They call it ethics but they initiate justice actions and they punish people and make it harder for them to get their own ethics in.

Proper justice is expected and has definite use. When a state of discipline does not exist, the whole group caves in. It has been noted continually that the failure of a group began with a lack of or loss of discipline. Without it the group and its members die. But you must understand ethics *and* justice.

The individual can be trusted with ethics, and when he is taught to put his own ethics in, justice no longer becomes the all-important subject that it is made out to be.

Breakthrough

The breakthrough in Scientology is that we *do* have the basic technology of ethics. For the first time man *can* learn how to put his own ethics in and climb back up the chute.

This is a brand-new discovery; before Scientology it had never before seen the light of day, anywhere. It marks a turning point in the history of philosophy. The individual can learn this technology, learn to apply it to his life and can then put his own ethics in, change conditions and start heading upwards toward survival under his own steam.

I hope you will learn to use this technology very well for your own sake, for the sake of those around you and for the sake of the future of this culture as a whole.

Conditions: States of Operation

An organization or its parts or an individual passes through various states of existence. These, if not handled properly, bring about shrinkage and misery and worry and death. If handled properly they bring about stability, expansion, influence and well-being.

These, arranged from highest to lowest, are:

Power

Power Change

Affluence

Normal Operation

Emergency

Danger

Non-Existence

Liability

Doubt

Enemy

Treason

Confusion

The formulas for these are apparently monitoring formulas for livingness (the state of living).

The first thing to know about them is that each step in a formula is in exact sequence and must be done in *that* sequence. It is totally fatal to reverse the order of sequence of two or more actions. Example: in Emergency economize before you promote. If the sequence is disordered the final result is a smaller organization or less influential person.

A key datum is that if the formulas are not known or not correctly applied, an organism emerges from each crisis smaller.

A person can exist in different conditions. Ethics is the means by which he can raise himself to a higher condition and improve his survival.

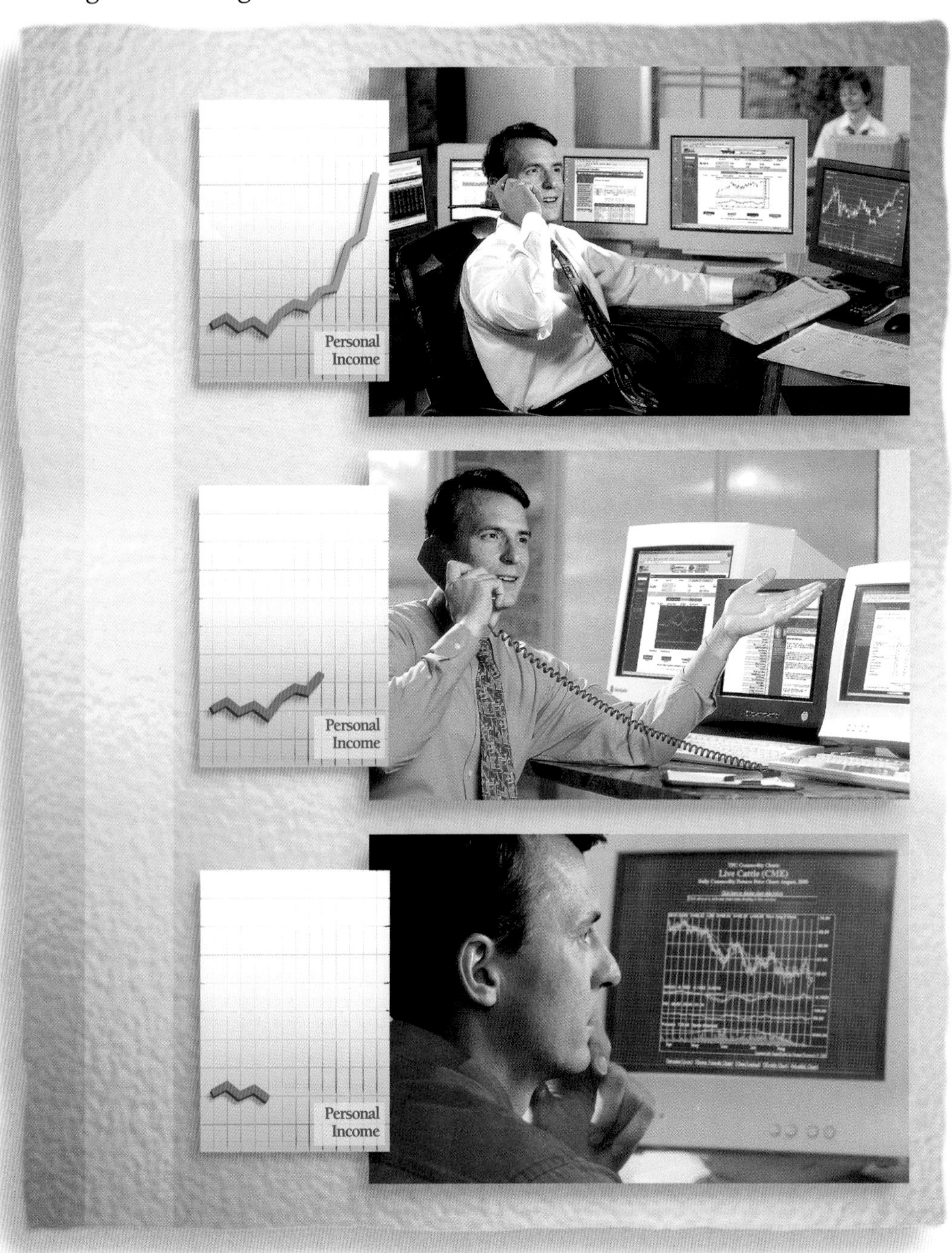

THE MEASUREMENT OF SURVIVAL: STATISTICS

The next thing to know is that one knows what formula to apply only by closely and continually inspecting statistics. By statistics is meant numbers of things, measurement of volume, all relative to time. A statistic not compared to the same type of statistic earlier will not predict any future statistic. A single statistic is meaningless. Statistics are always worse than, the same as or better than they were at an earlier period. Graphing and the reading of graphs is a vital necessity then in monitoring an organization, department or person and applying condition formulas to it.

This is much easier than it appears. If you made $20,000 last year and only $15,000 this year, you obviously are slipping; if you made $30,000 this year you are pretty stable; if you made $50,000 this year you are affluent—as compared to the $20,000 you made last year.

What is the code of conduct you should use to stay healthy under these *conditions?* These are the condition formulas.

The third thing to know is that one can wreck an organization or department or person by applying the wrong condition formula. The person is in an Emergency condition. One applies the condition of Affluence or Power or anything but the Emergency Formula and the person will go bust. The universe is made that way. The right condition must be applied.

STATISTICS—WHAT THEY ARE

What is a statistic? A statistic is a number or amount *compared* to an earlier number or amount of the same thing. Statistics refer to the quantity of work done or the value of it in money.

A down statistic means that the current number is less than it was.

An up statistic means the current number is more than it was.

We operate on statistics. These show whether or not a staff member or group is working or not working, as the work produces the statistic. If he doesn't work effectively, the statistic inevitably goes down. If he works effectively, the statistic goes up.

Negative statistics—some things go up in statistic when they are bad (like car accidents). However, we are not using negative statistics. We only use things that mean good when they go up or mean bad when they go down.

Statistic Graphs

Definition: A graph is a line or diagram showing how one quantity depends on, compares with or changes another. It is any pictorial device used to display numerical relationships.

A graph is not informative if its vertical scale results in graph line changes that are too small. It is not possible to draw the graph at all if the line changes are too large.

If the ups and downs are not plainly visible on a graph, then those interpreting the graph make errors. What is shown as a flat-looking line really should be a mountain range.

By *scale* is meant the number of anything per vertical inch of graph.

The way to do a scale is as follows:

Scale is different for every statistic.

1. Determine the lowest amount one expects a particular statistic to go—this is not always zero.

2. Determine the highest amount one can believe the statistic will go in the next three months.

3. Subtract (1) from (2).

4. Proportion the vertical divisions as per (3).

Your scale will then be quite real and show up its rises and falls.

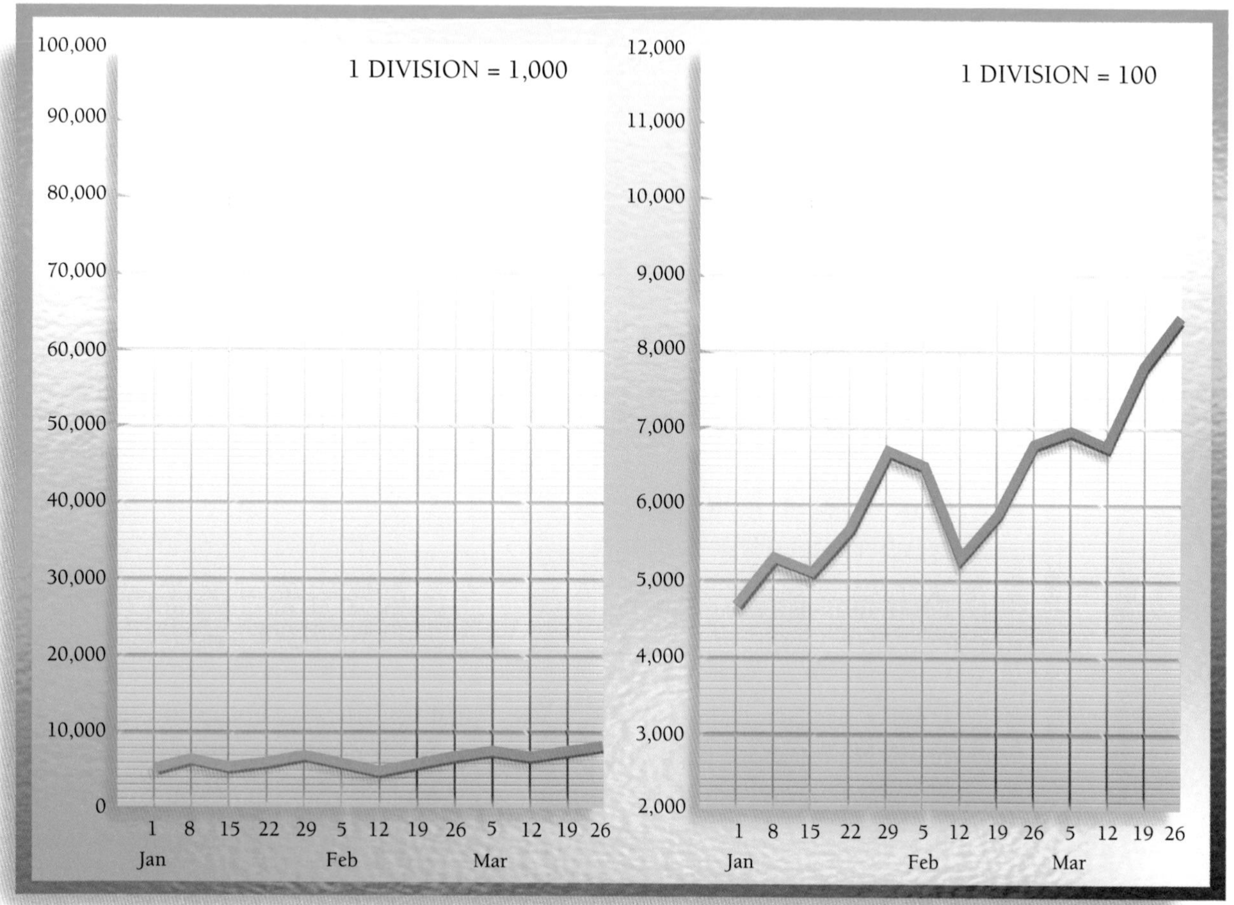

An incorrectly scaled graph does not show changes in a statistic accurately, thus making the graph less useful.

A correctly scaled graph clearly shows changes in a statistic, making it easier to determine which condition to apply.

Here is an *incorrect* example.

We take an organization that runs at $500 per week. We proportion the vertical marks of the graph paper of which there are 100 so each one represents $100. This when graphed will show a low line, quite flat, no matter what the organization income is doing and so draws no attention from executives when it rises and dives.

This is the *correct* way to do it for gross income for an organization averaging $500/week.

1. Looking over the old graphs of the past six months we find it never went under $240. So we take $200 as the lowest point of the graph paper.

2. We estimate this organization should get up to $1,200 on occasion in the next three months, so we take this as the top of the graph paper.

3. We subtract $200 from $1,200 and we have $1,000.

4. We take the 100 blocks of vertical and make each one $10, starting with $200 as the lowest mark.

Now we plot gross income as $10 per graph division.

This will look right, show falls and rises very clearly and so will be of use to executives in interpretation.

Try to use easily computed units like 5, 10, 25, 50, 100, and show the scale itself on the graph (1 div = 25).

The element of hope can enter too strongly into a graph. One need not figure a scale for more than one graph at a time. If you go onto a new piece of graph paper, figure the scale all out again; and as the organization rises in activity, sheet by sheet the scale can be accommodated. For example it took eighteen months to get one organization's statistics up by a factor of 5 (5 times the income, etc.) and that's several pieces of graph paper, so don't let scale do more than represent current expectancy.

On horizontal time scale, try not to exceed three months as one can get that scale too condensed too, and also too spread out where it again looks like a flat line and misinforms.

Correct scaling is the essence of good graphing.

READING STATISTICS

One can determine the condition of a stat by its slant on a graph.

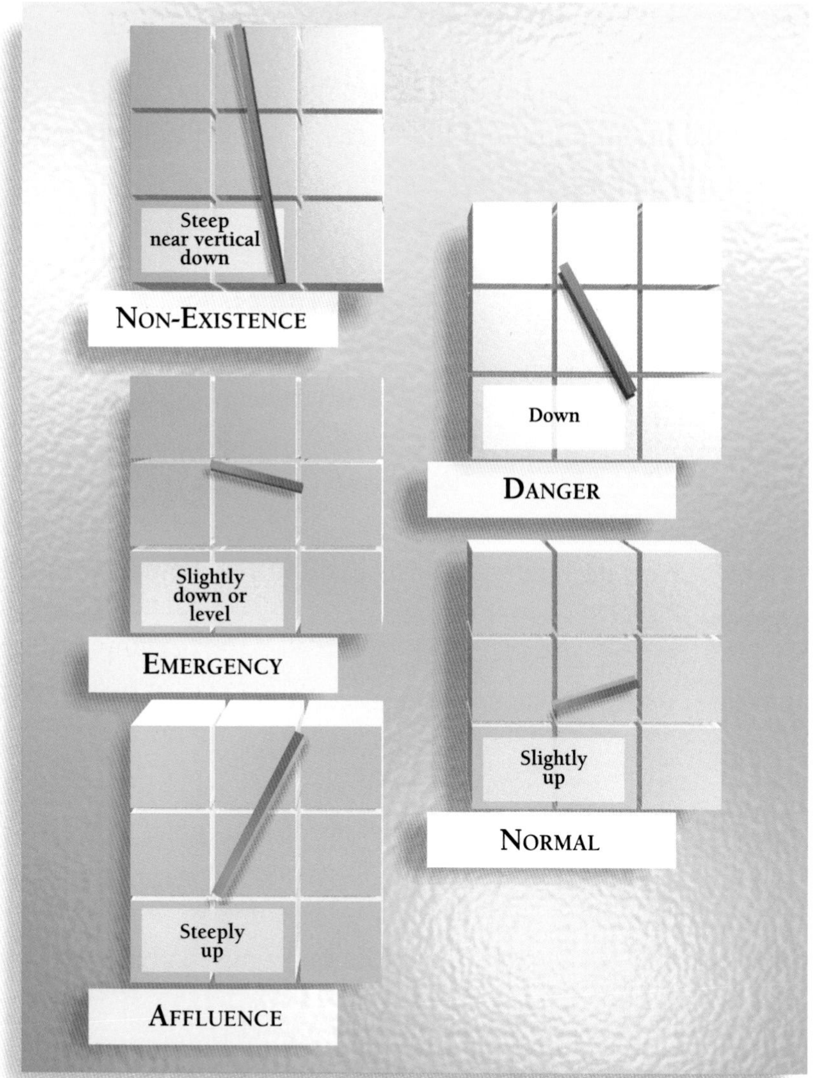

Power is not judged on a one-week basis only nor by a single line on a graph. Power is a Normal *trend* maintained in a high, high range. Trend means the tendency of statistics to average out up, level, or down over several weeks or months. Thus a Power condition must be determined by more than one line on a graph.

Note that these slants for Non-Existence through Affluence are used to determine the stat condition *for the week.*

Statistic Trends Stat Interpretation

The closer one is to the scene of the stat, the more rapidly it can be adjusted and the smaller the amount of time per stat needed to interpret it.

One can interpret one's own personal statistic hour to hour.

A division head can interpret on a basis of day to day.

An Executive Secretary needs a few days' worth of stat.

An Executive Director would use a week's worth of stat.

A more remote governing body would use a TREND (which would be several weeks) of divisional stats to interpret.

In short the closer one is to a statistic the easier it is to interpret it and the easier it is to change it.

One knows he had no stat on Monday—he didn't come to work. So Tuesday he tries to make up for it.

At the other end of the scale, a more remote managing body would have to use a trend of weeks to see what was going on.

A *trend* is an inclination toward a general course or direction.

Trends can be anything from Danger to Power, depending on the slant and its steepness. It is also possible to have a Non-Existence trend.

Plotted by weeks:
A Non-Existence *trend* would look like this:

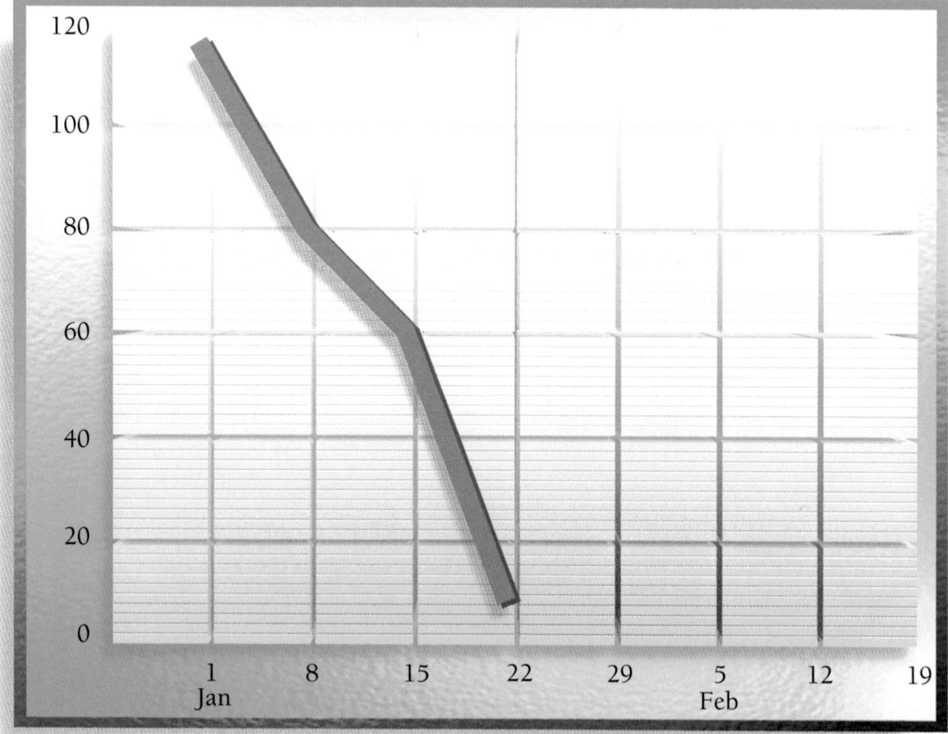

This would also be a Non-Existence *trend:*

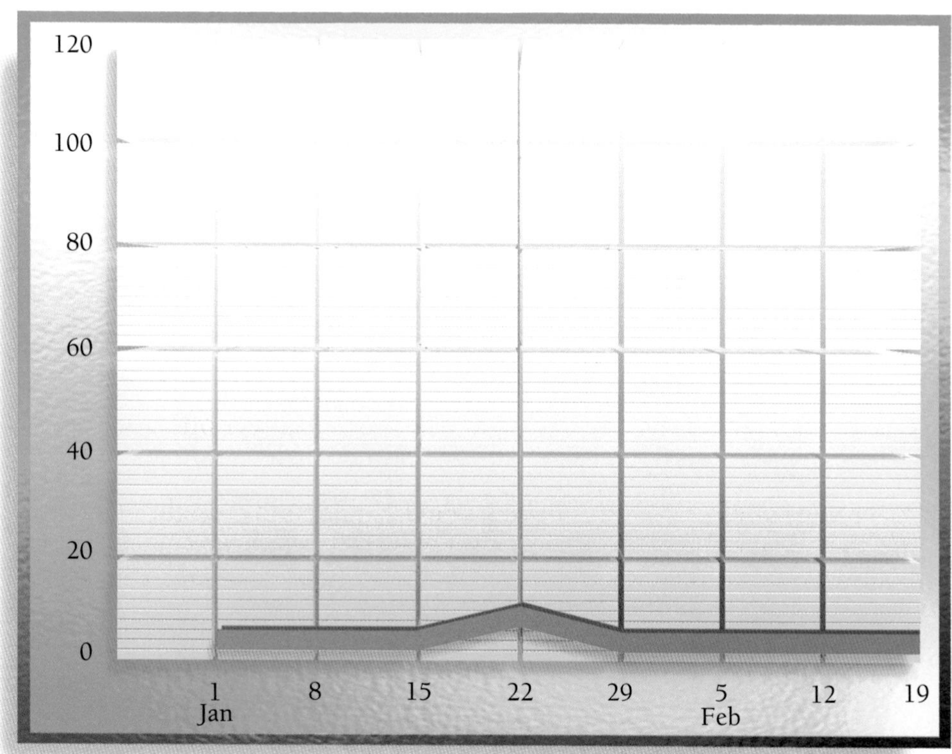

This would be a Danger *trend:*

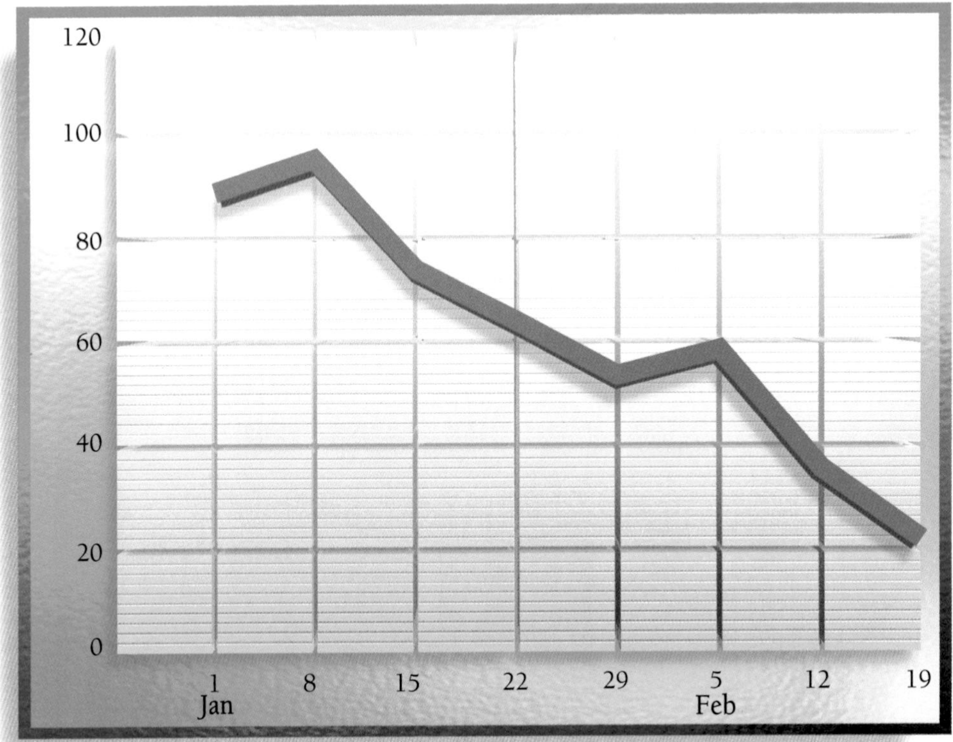

This would be an Emergency *trend:*

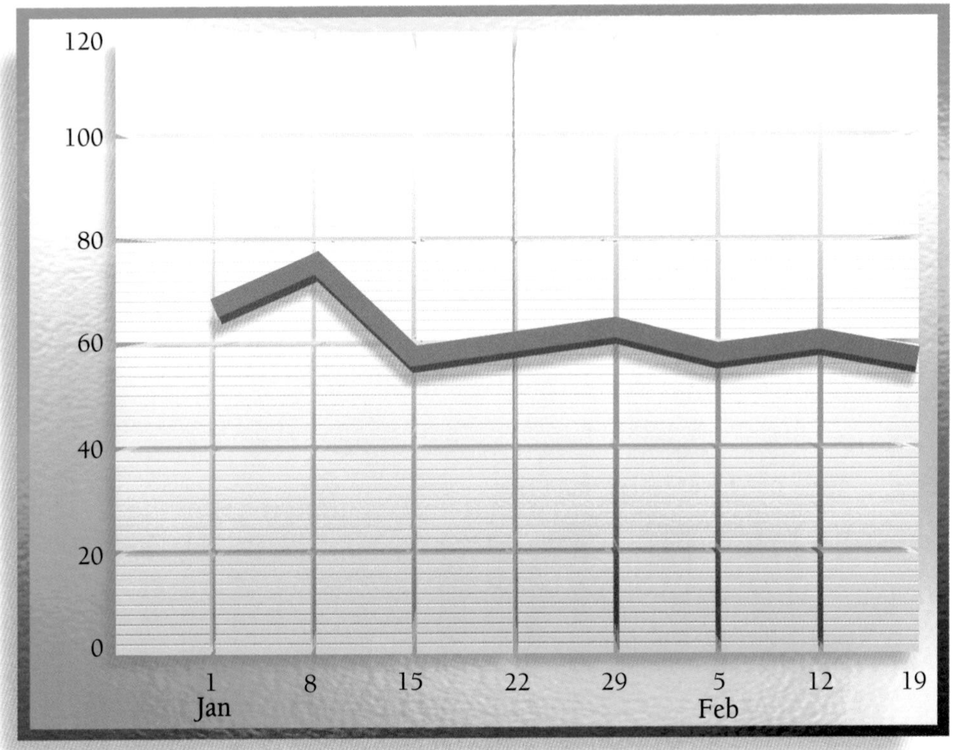

This would be a Normal *trend:*

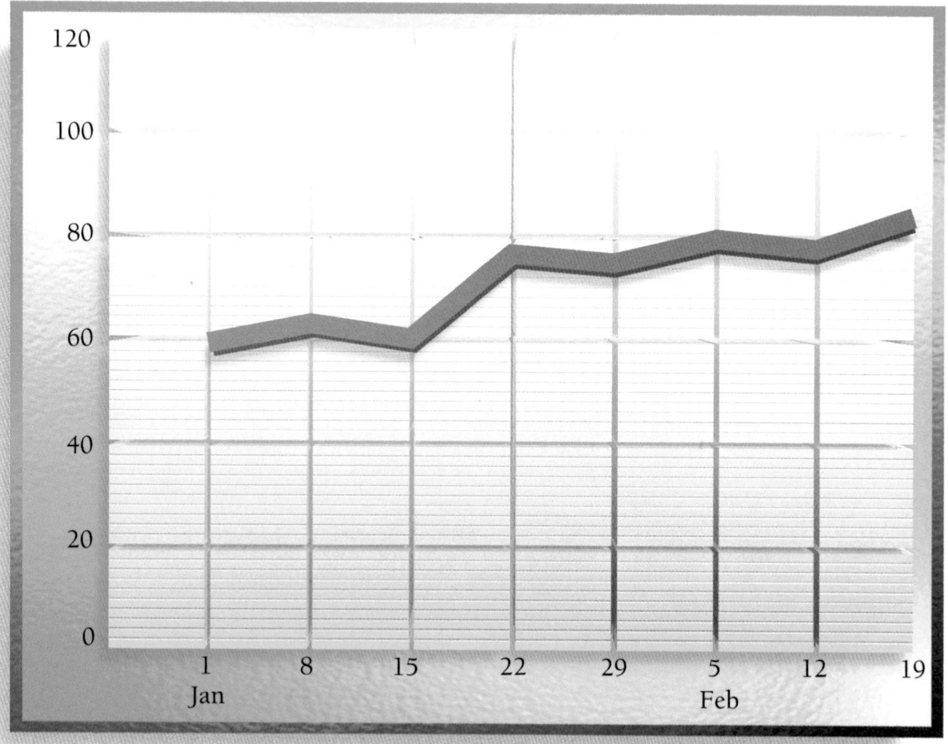

Any slight rise above level is Normal.
This would be an Affluence *trend:*

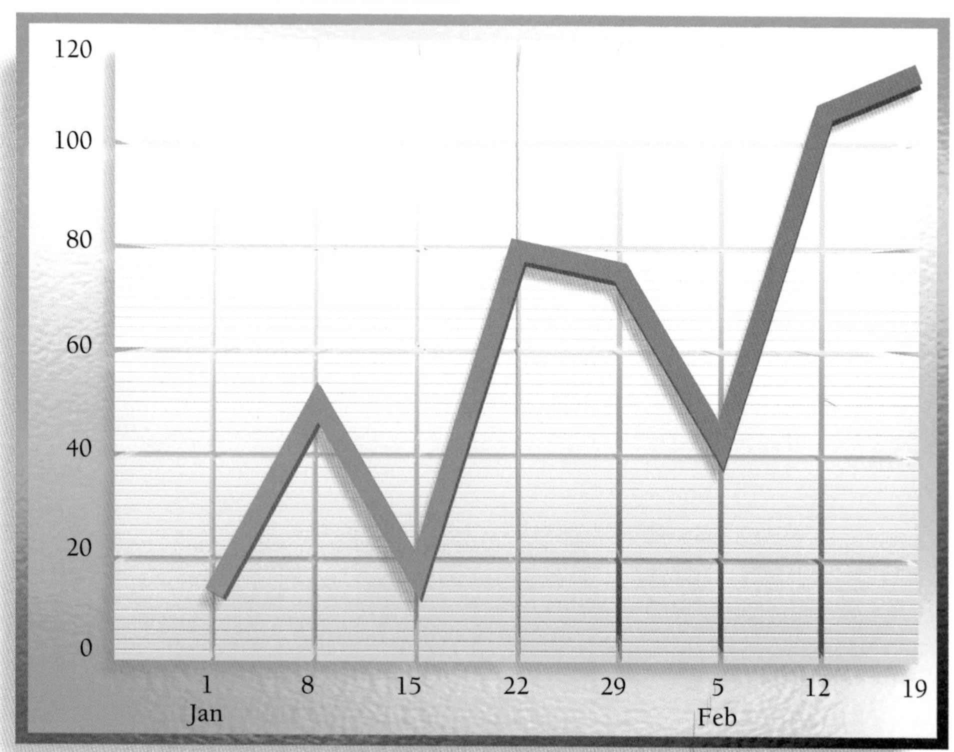

As Power is a *trend* it is not judged by a single line on a graph. Power is a Normal *trend* maintained in a high, high range; thus a Power condition must be determined by more than one week's worth of stats.

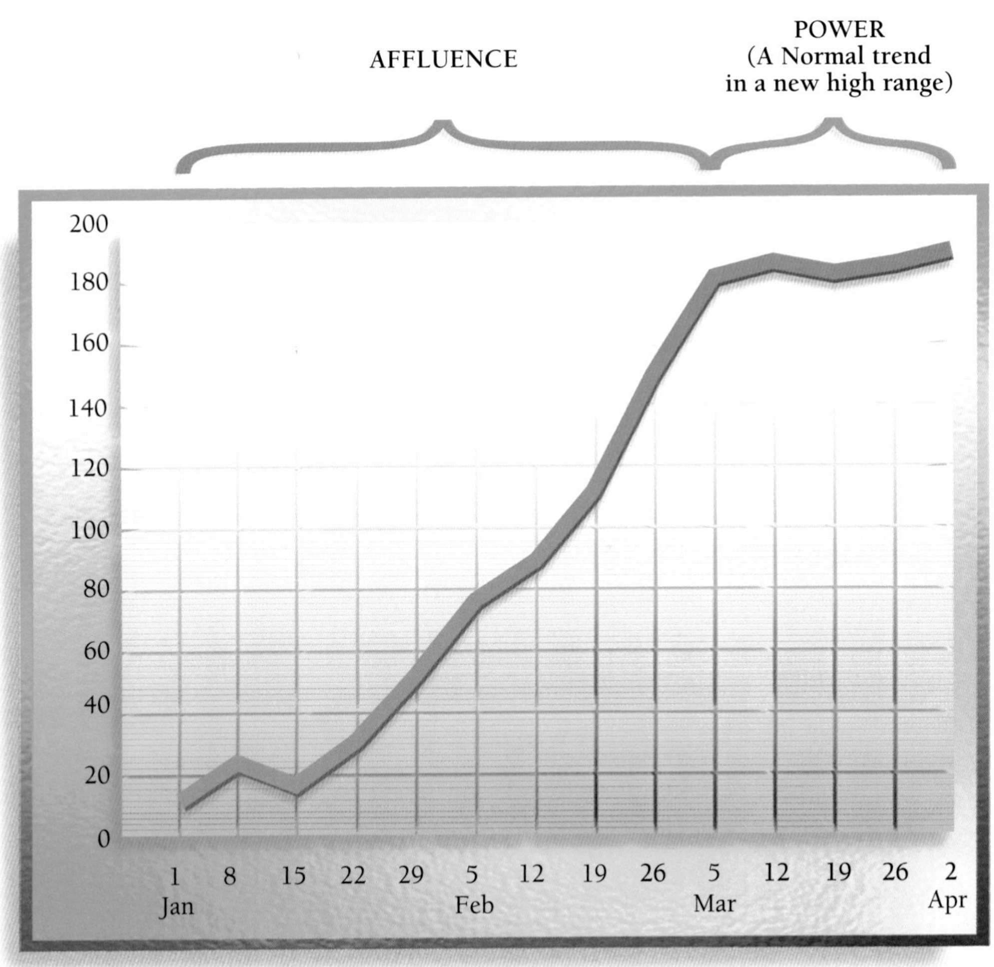

THE CONDITIONS FORMULAS

Here are the conditions and their formulas given in order of advance upward:

The Condition of Non-Existence (New Post Formula)

Every new appointee to a post begins in Non-Existence. Whether obtained by new appointment, promotion or demotion.

He is normally under the delusion that now he is "*THE* ________" (new title). He tries to start off in Power condition as he is usually very aware of his new status or even a former status. But in actual fact *he* is the only one aware of it. All others except perhaps the Personnel Officer are utterly unaware of him as having his new status.

Therefore he begins in a state of Non-Existence. And if he does not begin with the Non-Existence Formula as his guide, he will be using the wrong condition and will have all kinds of trouble.

The Non-Existence Formula is:

1. *Find a communication line.*

2. *Make yourself known.*

3. *Discover what is needed or wanted.*

4. *Do, produce and/or present it.*

A new appointee taking over a going concern often thinks he had better make himself known by changing everything, whereas he (a) is not well enough known to do so and (b) hasn't any idea of what is needed or wanted yet. And so he makes havoc.

Sometimes he assumes he knows what is needed or wanted when it is only a fixed idea with him and is only his idea and not true at all and so he fails at his job.

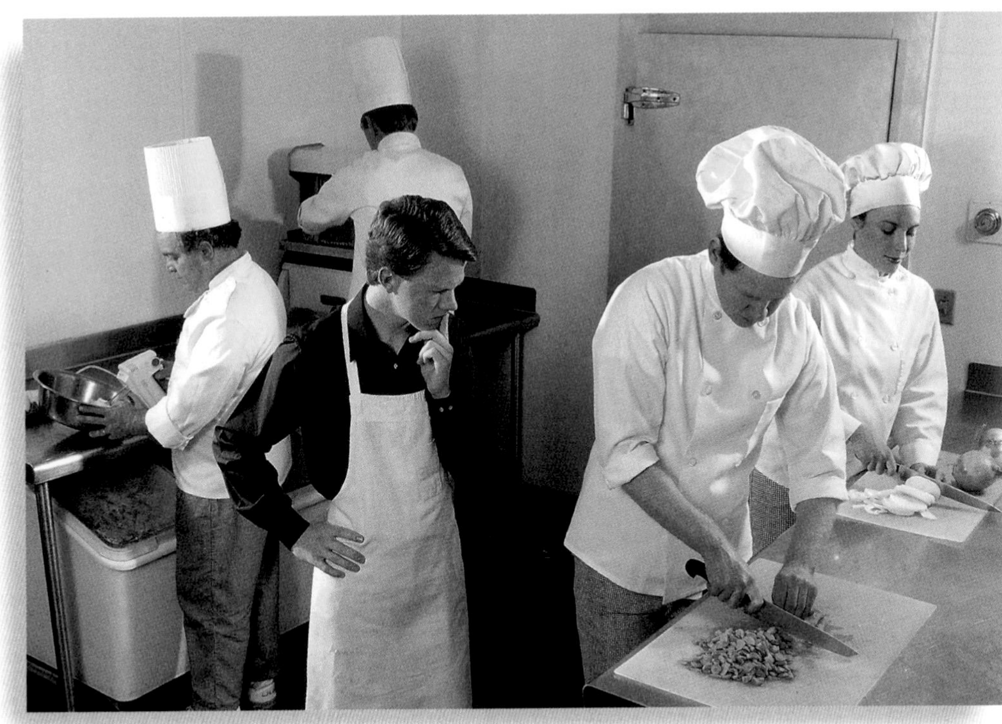

A person begins a new job or activity in a condition of Non-Existence.

Sometimes he doesn't bother to find out what is really needed or wanted and simply assumes it or thinks he knows when he doesn't. He soon becomes "unsuccessful."

Now and then a new appointee is so "status happy" or so insecure or so shy that even when his boss or his staff comes to him and tells him what is needed or wanted he can't or doesn't even acknowledge and really does go into Non-Existence for keeps.

Sometimes he finds that what he is *told* is needed or wanted needs reappraisal or further investigation. So it is always safest for him to make his own survey of it and operate on it when he gets his own firm reality on what is needed or wanted.

If the formula is applied intelligently, the person can expect to get into a zone of bypass where people are still doing his job to fill the hole his predecessor may have left. This is a Danger condition—but it is the next one higher than Non-Existence on the scale. If he defends his job and does his job and applies the Danger Formula, he will come through it.

He can then expect to find himself in an Emergency condition. In this he must follow the Emergency Formula with his post and he will come through *it.*

He can now expect to be in Normal Operation, and if he follows the formula of that, he will come to Affluence. And if he follows *that* formula, he will arrive at Power. And if he applies the Power Formula, he will stay there.

So it is a long way from Power that one starts his new appointment, and if he doesn't go *up* the scale from where he really is at the start, he will of course fail.

This applies to groups, to organizations, to countries as well as individuals.

It also applies when a person fails at his job. He has to start again at Non-Existence and he will build up the same way condition by condition.

Most failures on post are occasioned by failures to follow the conditions and recognize them and apply the formula of the condition one is in when one is in it and cease to apply it when one is out of it and in another.

This is the secret of holding a post and being successful on a job or in life.

Non-Existence Formula Expanded

Many people misapply the Non-Existence Formula and then wonder why they seem to continue in trouble.

Executives sometimes wonder why certain staff personnel never seem to be able to do anything right and out of exasperation wind up handling the whole area themselves.

The answer is a misapplication of and not really doing the Non-Existence Formula on their job.

Experience has shown that even experienced executives and staff members have not in fact ever come out of Non-Existence. And where the organization runs at all, it is carried on the back of one or two key seniors.

The phrase "find a communication line" is shortened down by too many to locating somebody's in-basket and dropping a "needed and wanted" request in it. This is not really finding a communication line.

To handle *any* post you have to have *information* and furnish *information.* Where this is not done, the person finds himself doing projects that get rejected, projects that have to be redone, restraints put on his actions and finds himself sinking down the conditions. He gets in bad with his seniors *because he doesn't acquire and doesn't furnish* the vital information of *what is going on.*

It is the duty of any staff member, new on post or not, *to round up the communication lines that relate to his post, find out who needs vital information from him* and *get those lines in, in, in* as a continuing action.

When a person fails to do just that, he never comes out of Non-Existence. He isn't even up to Danger because nobody knows they are even bypassing him. In other words, when a staff member does not do that, in the eyes of the organization, he is simply a *zero.*

Orders being issued by him usually wind up *cancelled* when discovered by some senior because they are not real. Joe was already handling it. Bill's schedule was thrown out by it. Treasury yells, "How come this wasted expense?"

Pretty soon, when staff hears it's so-and-so's order they just ignore it.

The bright hopes of such a person usually wind up as hopes he will be able to get transferred, the sooner the better. Everybody is against him.

But what really happened?

He never applied the Non-Existence Formula for real and so he stayed in Non-Existence. His actions do not coordinate because he does *not have the lines to give or receive information.*

It is really and factually not up to anyone else to round up his lines for him any more than it is up to others to do his breathing for him. The inhale and exhale of an organization or any activity is the take and give of *vital information and particles.*

Anyone who finds himself in apparent Non-Existence or worse should rush around and find the communication lines that apply to his activity and post and insist that he be put on those lines.

Such a person, staff member or executive has to write down what information he has to have to handle his post and what information others have to have from him to do their jobs.

And then arrange communication lines so that he is an info addressee from secretaries on those lines.

Senior executives such as division heads or heads of an organization do have a responsibility for briefing staff. But they are usually also faced with security problems as well as a wish to look good. And their data is general for the whole division or organization. It does include specifics like "Mrs. Zikes is arriving at 1400 hours" or "the telephone company rep says the bill must be paid by 1200 hours today or we got no phones."

Havoc and overwork for executives occur where the bulk of the staff have omitted to get themselves on important communication lines and keep those lines flowing. Do not send to find why the statistics are down if 90 percent of your staff is in Non-Existence or worse! Simply because they never really found any communication lines.

Therefore the Expanded Non-Existence Formula is:

1. *Find and get yourself on every communication line you will need in order to give and obtain information relating to your duties and materiel.*

2. *Make yourself known, along with your post title and duties, to every person you will need for the obtaining of information and the giving of data.*

3. *Discover from your seniors and fellow staff members and any public your duties may require you to contact, what is needed and wanted from each.*

4. *Do, produce and present what each needs and wants that is in conformation with policy.*

5. *Maintain your communication lines that you have and expand them to obtain other information you now find you need on a routine basis.*

6. *Maintain your origination lines to inform others what you are doing exactly, but only those who actually need the information.*

7. *Streamline what you are doing, producing and presenting so that it is more closely what is really needed and wanted.*

8. *With full information being given and received concerning your products, do, produce and present a greatly improved product routinely on your post.*

I can guarantee that if you do this—and write your information concisely so it is quick to grasp and get your data in a form that doesn't jam your own lines—you will start on up the conditions for actual and in due course arrive in Power.

The Condition of Danger

A Danger condition is normally assigned when:

1. An Emergency condition has continued too long.

2. A statistic plunges downward very steeply.

3. A senior executive suddenly finds himself or herself wearing the hat of the head of the activity because it is in trouble.

To *bypass* someone means to "jump the proper terminal (person or post) in a chain of command."

If you declare a Danger condition, you of course must do the work necessary to handle the situation that is dangerous.

This is also true backwards. If you start doing the work of another on a bypass you will of course unwittingly bring about a Danger condition. Why? Because you unmock the people who should be doing the work.

Further, if you habitually do the work of others on a bypass, you will of course inherit all the work. This is the answer to the overworked executive. He or she bypasses. It's as simple as that. If an executive habitually bypasses, he or she will then become overworked.

Also the condition of Non-Existence will occur.

So the more an executive bypasses, the harder he works. The harder he works on a bypass, the more the section he is working on will disappear.

So purposely or unwittingly working on a bypass, the result is always the same—Danger condition.

If you *have* to do the work on a bypass, you *must* get the condition declared and follow the formula.

If you declare the condition, you must also do the work.

You must get the work being competently done by new appointment or transfer or training of personnel. The condition is over when that portion of the company or organization has visibly, statistically recovered.

So there are great responsibilities in declaring a Danger condition. These are outweighed in burdensomeness by the fact that if you *don't* declare one on functions handled by those under you which go bad, it will very soon catch up with you yourself, willy-nilly, and declared or not, *you* will go into a Danger condition personally.

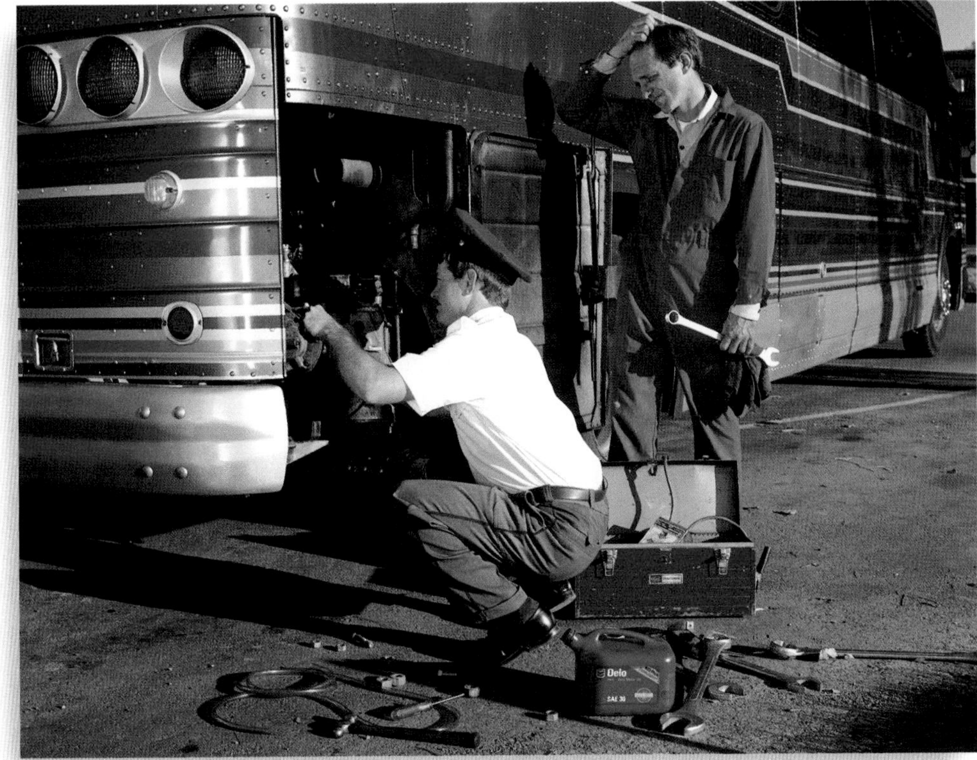

When a person has to be bypassed by another to get his job or activities done, a Danger condition exists.

There's the frying pan—there's the fire. The cheerful note about it is that if the formula is applied, you have a good chance of not only rising again but also of being bigger and better than ever.

And that's the first time *that* ever happened to an executive who started down the long slide. There's hope!

When the formula for handling a Danger condition is not done, an organization or activity or person cannot easily get above that condition thereafter.

A prolonged state of Emergency or threats to viability or survival or a prolonged single-handing will not improve unless the actual Danger Formula is applied.

Danger Formula

<u>**The formula follows:**</u>

1. *Bypass (ignore the junior or juniors normally in charge of the activity and handle it personally).*

2. *Handle the situation and any danger in it.*

3. *Assign the area where it had to be handled a Danger condition.*

4. *Assign each individual connected with the Danger condition a First Dynamic Danger condition and enforce and ensure that they follow the formula completely, and if they do not do so, do a full Ethics investigation and take all actions indicated.*

5. *Reorganize the activity so that the situation does not repeat.*

6. *Recommend any firm policy that will hereafter detect and/or prevent the condition from recurring.*

The senior executive present acts and acts according to the formula above.

First Dynamic Danger Formula

The First Dynamic Danger Formula is:

1. *Bypass habits or normal routines.*

2. *Handle the situation and any danger in it.*

3. *Assign self a Danger condition.*

4. *Get in your own personal ethics by finding what you are doing that is out-ethics and use self-discipline to correct it and get honest and straight.*

5. *Reorganize your life so that the dangerous situation is not continually happening to you.*

6. *Formulate and adopt firm policy that will hereafter detect and prevent the same situation from continuing to occur.*

Here is an example of how the First Dynamic Danger Formula could be applied.

The step "bypass habits or normal routines" means bypass doing all this stuff you have been doing.

Let us say a fellow was accepting money from his uncle and saying he was buying a house with it and he wasn't. He was spending it on a blonde. Now he is in continuous danger. His uncle might find it out at any moment and he expects to inherit his uncle's fortune someday. So he's in a sort of quasi-panic; even though he isn't thinking about it, it's still sitting there.

Now, "handle the situation and any danger in it" could be spotted as the basic reason. Because he has done things he is not telling and he is connected in some way and it's pretty weird and he's liable to be tripped. Well, all right, he'd have to quit doing that—bypass the habits or normal routines of the thing. In other words, quit accepting that money.

But he'd also have to handle the situation and any danger in it. It would be very dangerous to write, "Dear Uncle George: For the last year and a half, all the money you've been sending me to buy a house with, I have been spending on a blonde named Floozie." Well, he'd have to figure out how to handle that so that there wasn't any danger in it. And it might take quite a bit of thinking.

If he just jumped up and said to his uncle, "Well, I've been lying to you, Uncle George. I've been wasting all of your dough," the possibility is that this would come as such a shock to Uncle George that he'd disinherit him, shoot him and so forth—he would really be in danger. So he'd have to figure out how to handle it. It might be as simple as, "Dear Uncle George: I have been getting processed lately with Scientology, and it's making a more honest man out of me. And there are many dishonest things which I have done in my life and one of them is this. Now, you will probably shoot me for having done this, and it is not fair to you but actually I have been using this money to live off of and..."

Then "assign self a Danger condition" is only there because people forget to assign it. And then you "get in your own *personal ethics* by finding what you are doing that is out-ethics and use self-discipline to correct it and get honest and straight." Now, there might be some other "Uncle Georges" (and we've still got to handle this blonde named Floozie). Even though one might have handled the uncle there might be some more.

Then "reorganize your life so that the dangerous situation is not continually happening to you"—well, that's easy, in this hypothetical case of Uncle George. Simply knock it off as far as this Floozie is concerned and instead of being up all night every night and so forth, actually get some sleep and do your job and amount to something. That's a reorganization of it.

And then, "formulate and adopt firm policy that will hereafter detect and prevent the same situation from continuing to occur." In other words, "I'm not going to tell lies so that I can get money," or something like that, is all the guy would have to decide. It's like a New Year's resolution. But people don't keep them because they didn't get in the first five steps. That's why New Year's resolutions aren't kept. You are actually asking the guy at this point to reform.

Junior Danger Formula

Where a Danger condition is assigned to a junior, request that he or she or the entire activity write up his or her overts and withholds and any known out-ethics situation and turn them in at a certain stated time on a basis that the penalty for them will be lessened but if discovered later after the deadline it will be doubled.

A harmful act or a transgression against the moral code of a group is called an *overt act,* or an *overt.* When a person does something that is contrary to the moral code he has agreed to, or when he omits to do something that he should have done per that moral code, he has committed an overt act. An overt act violates what was agreed upon.

An unspoken, unannounced transgression against a moral code by which the person is bound is called a *withhold.* A withhold is an overt act that a person committed that he or she is not talking about. It is something that a person believes that if revealed will endanger his self-preservation. Any withhold comes *after* an overt.

The full procedure for writing up one's overts and withholds is given in Chapter 9, "Integrity and Honesty."

This write-up done, require that the junior and the staff that had to be bypassed and whose work had to be done for them or continually corrected, each one write up and fully execute the First Dynamic Danger Formula for himself personally and turn it in.

When production has again increased, the Danger condition should be formally ended and an Emergency condition assigned and its formula should be followed.

The Condition of Emergency

It is an empirical (observed and proven by observation) fact that nothing remains exactly the same forever. This condition is foreign to this universe. Things grow or they lessen. They cannot apparently maintain the same equilibrium (balance) or stability.

Thus things either expand or they contract. They do not remain level in this universe. Further, when something seeks to remain level and unchanged, it contracts.

Thus we have three actions and only three. First is expansion, second is the effort to remain level or unchanged and third is contraction or lessening.

As nothing in this universe can remain exactly the same, then the second action (level) above will become the third action (lessen) if undisturbed or not acted on by an outside force. Thus actions two and three above (level and lessen) are similar in potential and both will lessen.

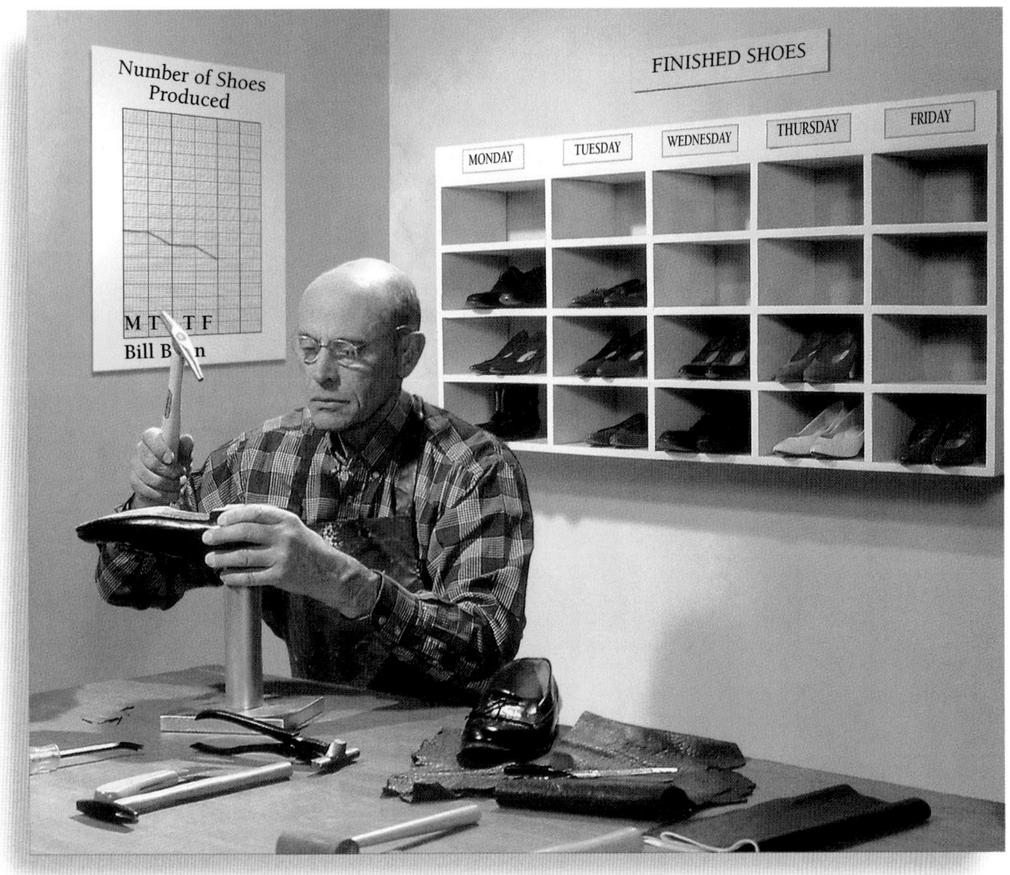

An unchanging or slightly worsening condition requires application of the Emergency Formula.

This leaves expansion as the only positive action which tends to guarantee survival.

To survive, then, one must expand as the only safe condition of operation.

If one remains level, one tends to contract. If one contracts, one's chances of survival diminish.

Therefore, there is only one chance left and that, for an organization or an individual, is expansion.

In order to expand in such a situation, one needs to apply the formula for a condition of Emergency.

One applies the condition of Emergency when:

1. Statistics of an organization, department or portion of an organization or a person are seen to be *declining.*

2. Unchanging statistics of an organization or a portion of an organization or a person.

The formula for the condition of Emergency is:

1. *Promote. That applies to an organization. To an individual you had better say produce. That's the first action regardless of any other action. Regardless of anything else, that is the first thing you have to put attention on. The first broad, big action which you take is promote. Exactly what is promotion? It is making things known; it is getting things out; it is getting oneself known, getting one's products out.*

2. *Change your operating basis. If for instance you went into a condition of Emergency and then you didn't change after you had promoted, you didn't make any changes in your operation, well you just head for another condition of Emergency.*

   So that has to be part of it; you had better change your operating basis; you had better do something to change the operating basis, because that operating basis led you into an emergency so you sure better change it.

3. *Economize.*

4. *Then prepare to deliver.*

5. *Part of the condition of Emergency contains this little line—you have got to stiffen discipline or you have got to stiffen ethics. Organizationally when a State of Emergency is assigned, supposing the activity doesn't come out of that emergency, regardless of what caused the emergency, supposing the activity just doesn't come out of the emergency, in spite of the fact they have been labeled a State of Emergency; they have been directed to follow the formula; they have been told to snap and pop and get that thing straightened out, and they are still found to be goofing; the statistic is going down and continues to go down; what do you do? There is only one thing left to do and that is discipline, because life itself is going to discipline the individual.*

   So the rule of the game is that if a State of Emergency is ignored and the steps are not taken successfully, then you get an announcement after a while that the condition has been continued, and if the condition is continued beyond a specified period of time, why that's it; it has to walk forward into an ethics matter.

The Condition of Normal

You could call Normal a condition of stability and it probably should be called a condition of stability except for this one little factor: This universe does not admit of a static state. It won't admit a no-increase, no-decrease. You cannot have a condition in this universe where there is no increase and no decrease. That's a totally stable condition; there is no such thing in this universe from one end of it to the other. There isn't anything that always remains the same.

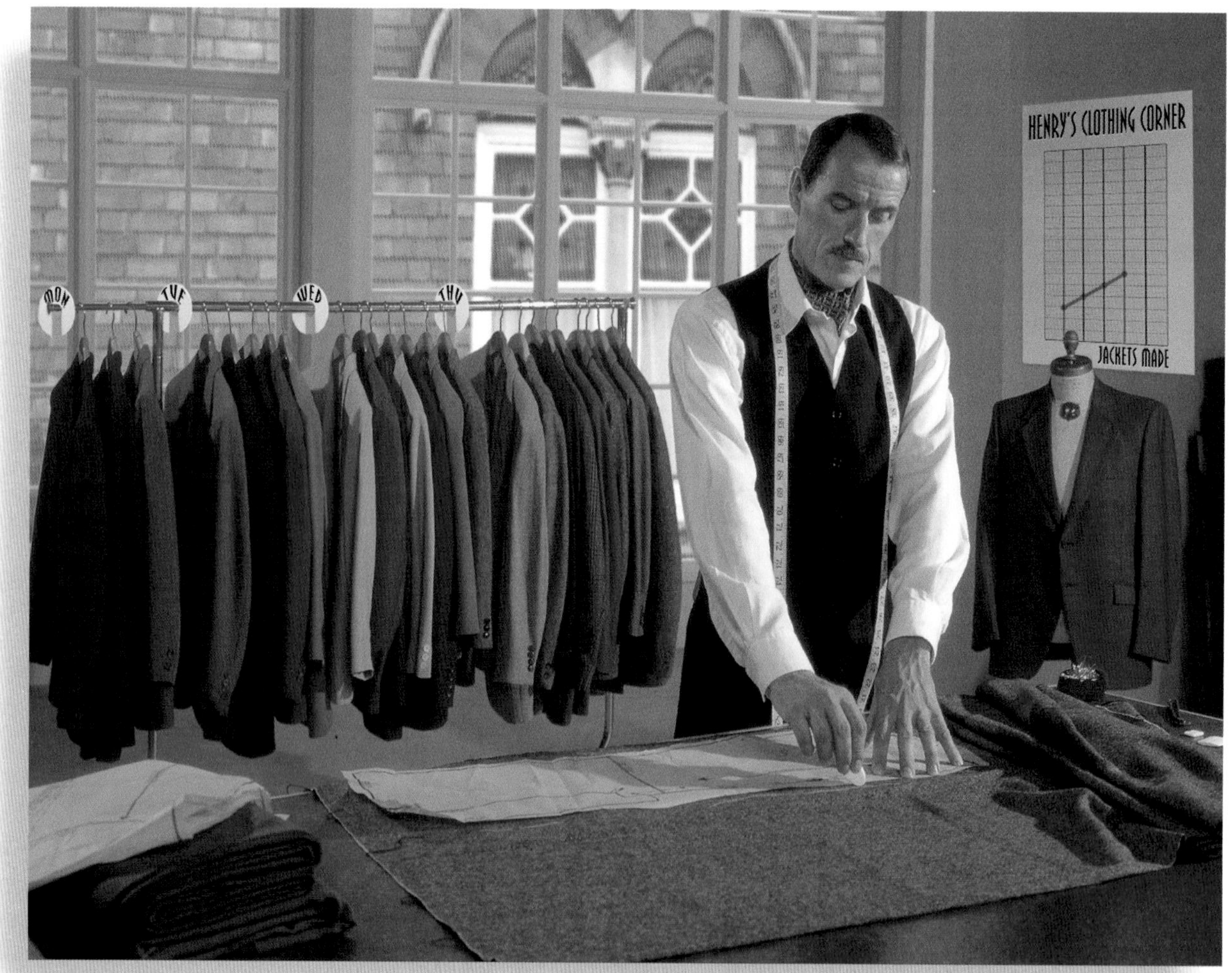

Regular, steady expansion or increase means a condition of Normal Operation exists.

The condition of Normal Operation, then, is not one of "stability"—because it can't be. Normal Operation must be a routine or gradual increase. And there must be a regular, routine, gradual increase. You cannot have a total, even state of existence which does not eventually fall on its head. The second you get this even state in this universe, it starts to deteriorate. So a state of stability would eventually deteriorate.

Well, to prevent a deterioration you must have an increase. That increase doesn't have to be spectacular but it has to be something. There has to be a bit of an increase there.

Normal Formula:

1. *The way you maintain an increase is when you are in a state of Normal Operation you don't change anything.*

2. *Ethics are very mild, the justice factor is quite mild, there are no savage actions taken particularly.*

3. *When a statistic betters then look it over carefully and find out what bettered it, and then do that without abandoning what you were doing before.*

4. *Every time a statistic worsens slightly, quickly find out why and remedy it.*

And you just jockey those two factors, the statistic bettering, the statistic worsening; repair the statistic worsening, and you will find out inevitably some change has been made in that area where a statistic worsens. Some change has been made; you had better get that change off the lines in a hurry.

The Condition of Affluence

When you have a line going steeply up on a graph, that's *Affluence.* Whether it's up steeply for one week or up steeply from its last point week after week after week, it's *Affluence.*

When you've got an Affluence, regardless of how you did it, the Affluence Formula applies.

You *must* apply the Affluence Formula or you will be in trouble. Anyone dealing with Affluence should be aware of the following peculiarities about it.

Affluence is the most touchy condition there is. Misname it or handle it off formula and it can kill you! It is, strangely enough, the most dangerous of all conditions in that if you don't spot it and apply the formula, you spatter all over the street! Spot and handle it right and it's a rocket ride.

The Affluence Formula is:

1. *Economize. Now the first thing you must do in Affluence is economize and then make very, very sure that you don't buy anything that has any future commitment to it; don't buy anything with any future commitments; don't hire anybody with any future commitments—nothing. That is all part of that economy; clamp it down.*

2. *Pay every bill. Get every bill that you can possibly scrape up from anyplace, every penny you owe anywhere under the sun, moon and stars and pay them.*

3. *Invest the remainder in service facilities; make it more possible to deliver.*

4. *Discover what caused the condition of Affluence and strengthen it.*

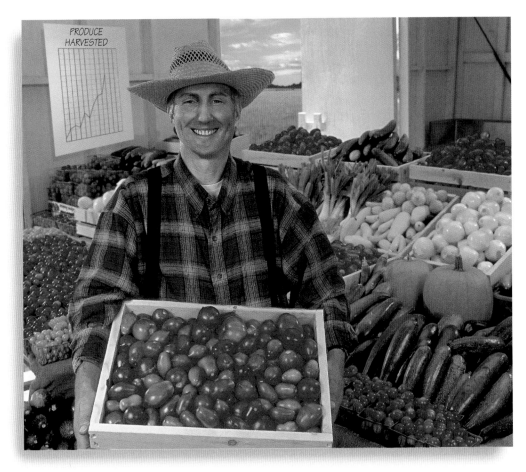

A steep improvement or increased abundance indicates a condition of Affluence.

Action Affluence Formula:

When an Affluence exists based on a statistic measuring one's actions, and disrelated to finance, this is the formula to apply.

1. *Economize on needless or dispersed actions that did not contribute to the present condition. Economize financially by knocking off all waste.*
2. *Make every action count and don't engage in any useless actions. Every new action to contribute and be of the same kind as did contribute.*
3. *Consolidate all gains. Any place we have gotten a gain, we keep it. Don't let things relax or go downhill or roller-coaster. Any advantage or gain we have, keep it, maintain it.*
4. *Discover for yourself what caused the condition of Affluence in your immediate area and strengthen it.*

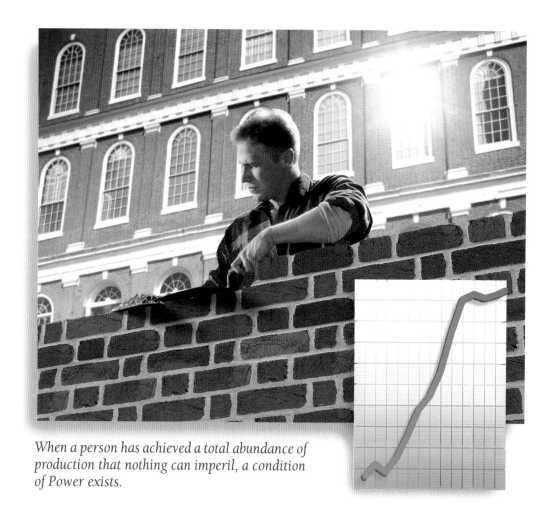

When a person has achieved a total abundance of production that nothing can imperil, a condition of Power exists.

The Condition of Power

A Power stat is a stat in a very high range; a brand-new range in a Normal trend.

A Power stat is not just a stat that is steeply up for a long time. Nor is Power simply a very high stat. Power is not a one-week thing. Power is a *trend.*

Definition: Power is a Normal in a stellar range so high that it is total abundance, no doubt about it.

It is a stat that has gone up into a whole new, steeply high range and maintained that range and now, in that new high range, is on a Normal trend.

Operating in this new range you may get a slight dip in that stat now and then. But it is still Power.

There is another datum that is of importance if one is to correctly recognize and understand this condition:

Why do we call it Power?

Because there is such an abundance of production there that momentary halts or dips can't pull it down or imperil its survival.

And *that* is *Power.*

The question could be asked "How much work can one guy do?" Or "How many bricks can a guy lay in a day?"

Of course, a person can only work so many hours in a day. He can only get so much individual production in a day. But he can get enough production in a day to support himself. He can get his production up into such abundance that he can take some time off. That depends on his efficiency and brightness.

At a certain peak of Affluence he will hit how many bricks he can lay. By increasing practice and efficiency he can keep that level of production going in a Normal.

If he's laying so many bricks that nobody is ever going to think of firing him, why, he's in Power. That's a Power condition for an individual.

Power Formula:

1. *The first law of a condition of Power is don't disconnect. You can't just deny your connections; what you have got to do is take ownership and responsibility for your connections.*
2. *The first thing you have got to do is make a record of all of its lines. And that is the only way you will ever be able to disconnect. So on a condition of Power the first thing you have to do is write up your whole post. You have made it possible for the next fellow in to assume the state of Power Change.*

   If you don't write up your whole post, you are going to be stuck with a piece of that post since time immemorial, and a year or so later somebody will still be coming to you asking you about that post which you occupied.
3. *The responsibility is write the thing up and get it into the hands of the guy who is going to take care of it.*
4. *Do all you can to make the post occupiable.*

When taking over a successful position, a condition of Power Change exists.

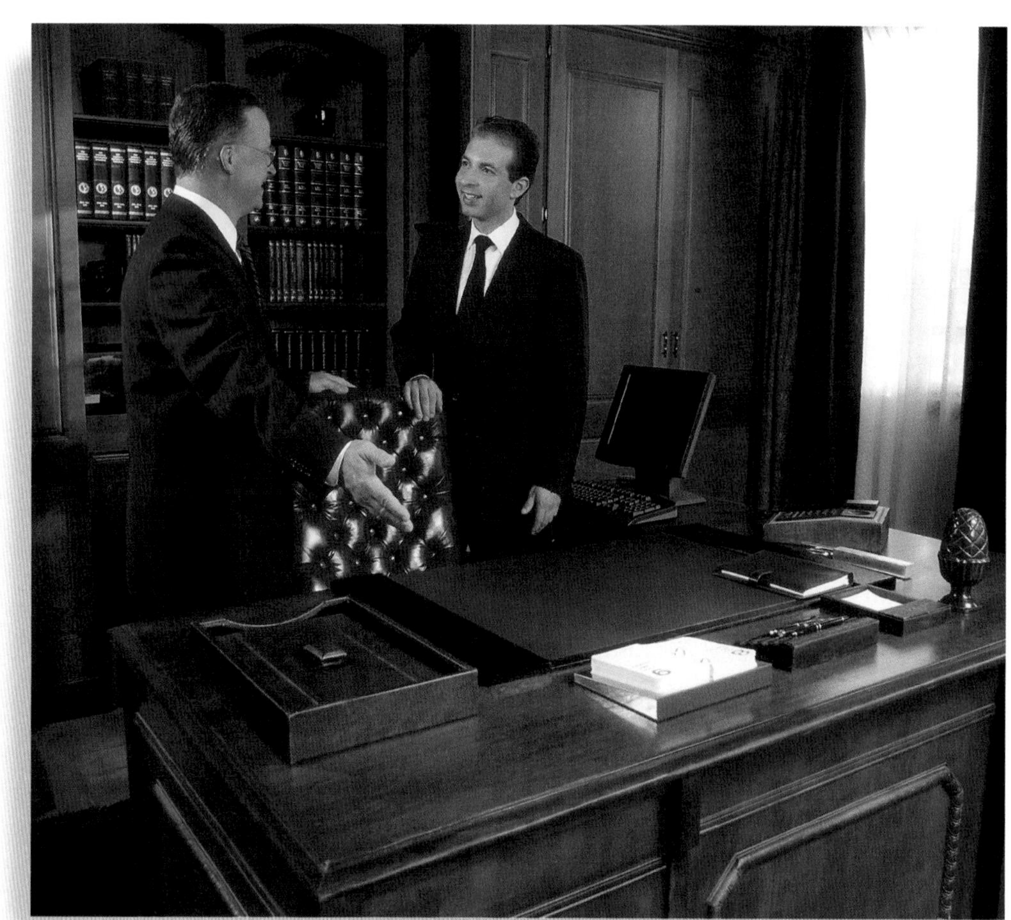

The Condition of Power Change

There are only two circumstances which require replacement, the very successful one or the very unsuccessful one. What a song it is to inherit a successful pair of boots; there is nothing to it; just step in the boots and don't bother to walk. If it was in a normal state of operation, which it normally would have been in for anybody to have been promoted out of it, you just don't change anything.

So, if anybody wants anything signed that your predecessor didn't sign, don't sign it. Keep your eyes open, learn the ropes and, depending on how big the organization is, after a certain time, why, see how it is running and run it as normal operating condition if it's not in anything but a normal operating condition.

Go through the exact same routine of every day that your predecessor went through; sign nothing that he wouldn't sign; don't change a single order;

look through the papers that had been issued at that period of time—these are the orders that are extant—and get as busy as the devil just enforcing those orders and your operation will increase and increase.

Now, the fellow who walks into the boots of somebody who has left in disgrace—the post is in a condition of Emergency, its statistics have crashed causing the boss to be fired—all he has to do when he inherits one in Emergency is just apply the Emergency Formula to it, which is *immediately promote!*

One takes over a *new* post or a collapsed post in Non-Existence. *But* a going concern is taken over by the Power Change Formula.

The keynote of the state of Power Change is study the organization, policy, patterns and activity and *issue no orders* that are not routine—change nothing, innovate nothing. Write up fully the post just left. Mainly observe on the post just taken over. Learn the new post before doing anything.

The formula of the Power Change condition is:

When taking over a new post, change nothing until you are thoroughly familiar with your new zone of power.

Violation of Power Change

A Danger condition can be brought about by a violation of the Power Change condition.

Therefore, those who had a Power Change, must apply the *Power Change Violation Repair Formula:*

1. *Observe, question and draw up a list of what was previously successful in your area or zone of control.*
2. *Observe and draw up a list of all those things that were unsuccessful in your area in the past.*
3. *Get the successful actions IN.*
4. *Throw the unsuccessful actions out.*
5. *Knock off frantically trying to cope or defend.*
6. *Sensibly get back in a working structure.*

COMPLETING CONDITIONS FORMULAS

The ethics conditions formulas flow, one to the next, with the first step of one formula directly following the final step of the previous formula.

But what do you do if your stat graph indicates you've moved up a condition before you even have a chance to finish a formula? Do you just drop that formula and start on the next one? The answer is *"no."* One completes the formula he has begun.

Here's an example. An executive director, in looking over his statistics, sees that they are in Emergency. He immediately sees to it that the *promote* step of the Emergency Formula is begun. Once that is well in hand he begins to *change his operating basis.* He gets on-the-job training actions being done on some of his sales staff and puts three more personnel into one of his major production areas.

But before he has a chance to do each of the remaining steps of the Emergency Formula, the income and delivery statistics move up into Normal Operation.

What does he do? Well, he is now in a condition of Normal by statistics. But the Normal Formula would also cause him to complete the Emergency Formula, because in the Normal Formula you drop out what is unsuccessful and you push what was successful; what was successful here was the Emergency Formula. Thus, this executive director can get continued improvement on the graph by *completing* the Emergency Formula, as the actions on the Emergency Formula are what got him to Normal so quickly. So he would push them until they were completed fully. This doesn't mean he is still in an Emergency condition—the statistics are now rising and the condition *is* Normal. It is a bit of an oddball thing.

As another example, suppose someone is doing a Junior Danger Formula. The person goes step by step through the procedure and writes up his or her overts and withholds and any known out-ethics situation and starts applying the First Dynamic Danger Formula. But before he completes the formula, his stats rise. It would be dangerous indeed for this person to not finish the Danger Formula (e.g., getting done the REORGANIZE YOUR LIFE and FORMULATE AND ADOPT FIRM POLICY steps of the Danger Formula).

That one's stats rise before completing a formula doesn't mean he can't go into the higher condition his statistics now indicate. However, it would be a grave fault not to complete the undone steps of an earlier formula. So, as in the above examples, one has to complete the earlier formula, then complete the next formula and continue on as his graph dictates.

Completing a formula is very vital. One doesn't just name a formula. He gets it *completed.*

CONDITIONS BELOW NON-EXISTENCE

There also exist operating states below Non-Existence.

The Condition of Liability

Below Non-Existence there is the condition of Liability. The being has ceased to be simply nonexistent as a team member and has taken on the color of an enemy.

It is assigned where careless or malicious and knowing damage is caused to projects, organizations or activities. It is adjudicated that it is malicious and knowing because orders have been published against it or because it is contrary to the intentions and actions of the remainder of the team or the purpose of the project or organization.

It is a *liability* to have such a person unwatched as the person may do or continue to do things to stop or impede the forward progress of the project or organization and such a person cannot be trusted. No discipline or the assignment of conditions above it has been of any avail. The person has just kept on messing it up.

The condition is usually assigned when several Dangers and Non-Existences have been assigned or when a long unchanged pattern of conduct has been detected.

When all others are looking for the reason mail is getting lost, such a being would keep on losing the mail covertly.

The condition is assigned for the benefit of others so they won't get tripped up trusting the person in any way.

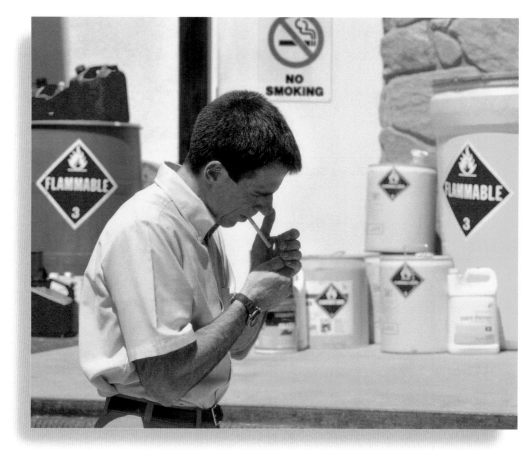

A person is in a condition of Liability when he goes against the orders, intentions and actions of the group and cannot be trusted.

The formula of Liability is:

1. *Decide who are one's friends.*

2. *Deliver an effective blow to the enemies of the group one has been pretending to be part of despite personal danger.*

3. *Make up the damage one has done by personal contribution far beyond the ordinary demands of a group member.*

4. *Apply for reentry to the group by asking the permission of each member of it to rejoin and rejoining only by majority permission, and if refused, repeating (2) and (3) and (4) until one is allowed to be a group member again.*

The Condition of Doubt

When one cannot make up one's mind as to an individual, a group, organization or project, a condition of Doubt exists.

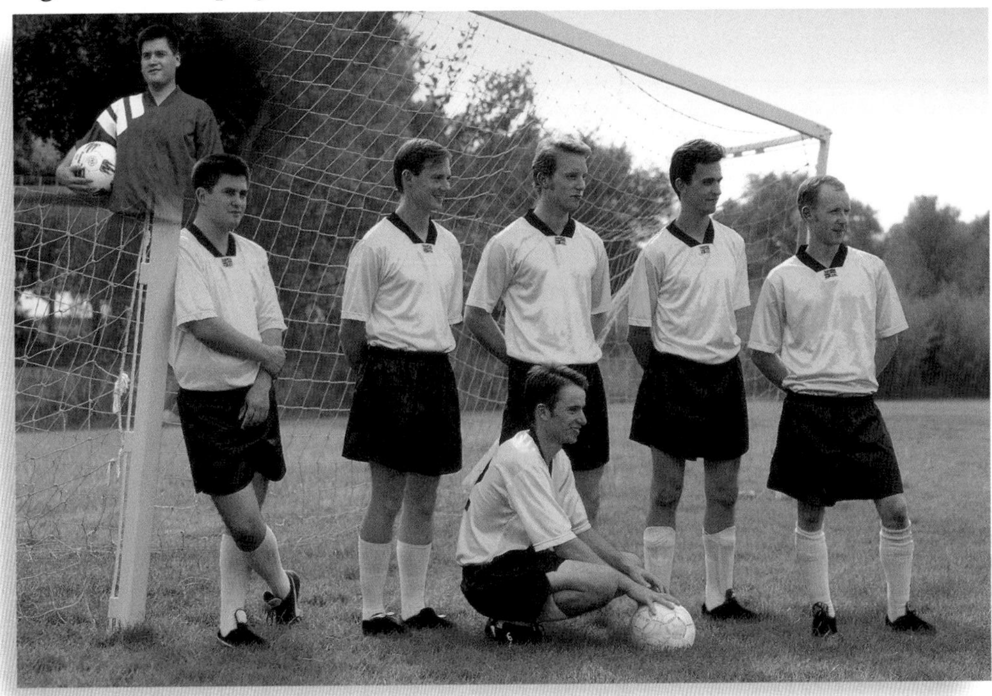

If one cannot come to a decision about a situation, a condition of Doubt exists.

The Doubt Formula is:

1. *Inform oneself honestly of the actual intentions and activities of that group, project or organization, brushing aside all bias and rumor.*
2. *Examine the statistics of the individual, group, project or organization.*
3. *Decide on the basis of "the greatest good for the greatest number of dynamics" whether or not it should be attacked, harmed or suppressed or helped.*
4. *Evaluate oneself or one's own group, project or organization as to intentions and objectives.*
5. *Evaluate one's own or one's group, project or organization's statistics.*
6. *Join or remain in or befriend the one which progresses toward the greatest good for the greatest number of dynamics and announce the fact publicly to both sides.*
7. *Do everything possible to improve the actions and statistics of the person, group, project or organization one has remained in or joined.*
8. *Suffer on up through the conditions in the new group if one has changed sides or the conditions of the group one has remained in if wavering from it has lowered one's status.*

The Condition of Enemy

When a person is an avowed and knowing enemy of an individual, a group, project or organization, a condition of Enemy exists.

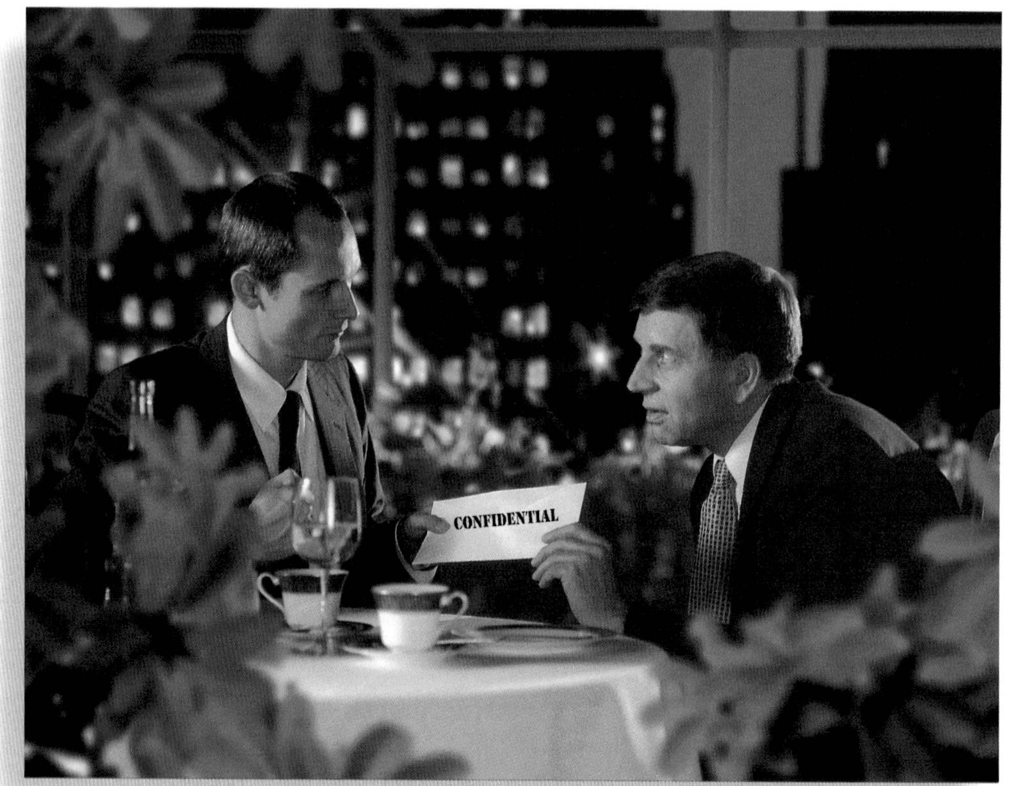

Destructive actions indicate a condition of Enemy.

The formula for the condition of Enemy is just one step:

Find out who you really are.

The Condition of Treason

Treason is defined as betrayal after trust.

The formula for Treason is very correctly and factually "Know *that* you are."

It will be found, gruesomely enough, that a person who accepts a post or position and then doesn't function as it, will inevitably upset or destroy some portion of an organization.

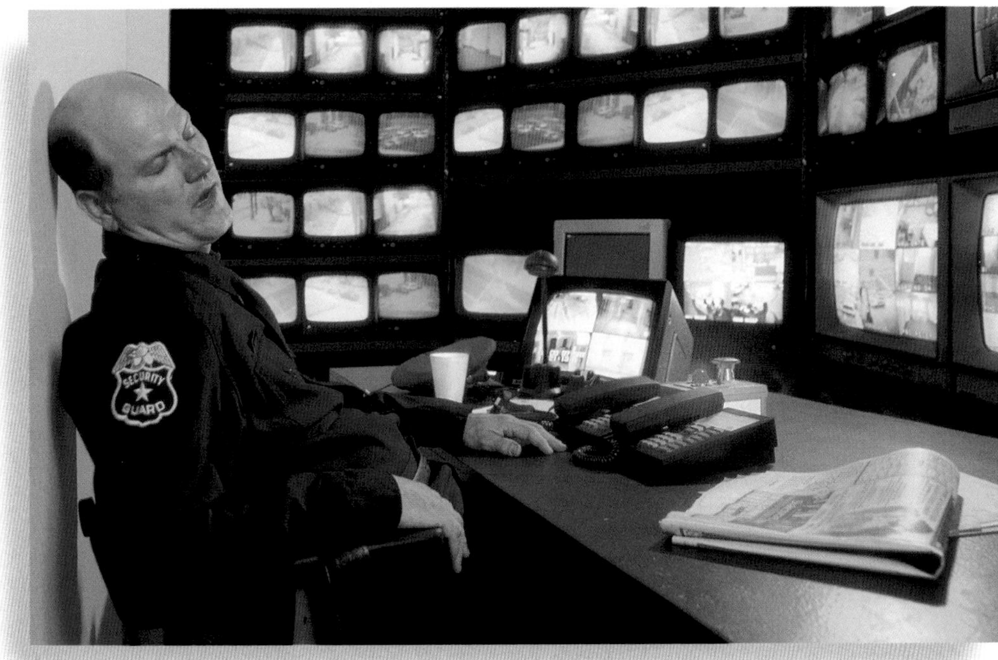

Someone who betrays the duties entrusted to them is in a condition of Treason.

By not knowing that he is the ____________ (post name), he is committing treason in fact.

The results of this can be found in history. A failure to be what one has the post or position name of will result in a betrayal of the functions and purposes of a group.

Almost all organizational upsets stem from this one fact:

A person in a group who, having accepted a post, does not know *that* he is a certain assigned or designated beingness is in *treason* against the group.

<u>The formula for the condition of Treason is:</u>

Find out <u>that</u> you are.

The Condition of Confusion

The lowest condition is a condition of Confusion.

In a condition of Confusion the being or area will be in a state of random motion. There will be no real production, only disorder or confusion.

In order to get out of Confusion one has to find out where he is.

It will be seen that the progress upward would be, in Confusion, find out where you are; in Treason, find out that you are; and for Enemy, find out who you are.

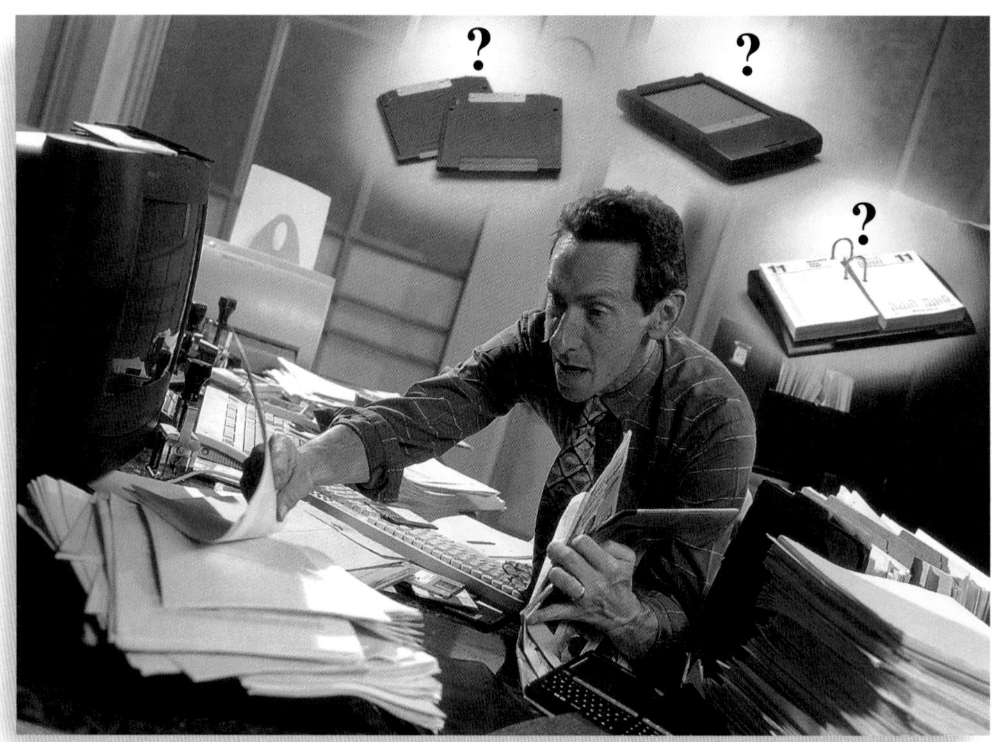

Random, useless activity with no actual production indicates a condition of Confusion.

The formula for Confusion is:

Find out where you are.

Note: It is important that the person who is in Confusion fully understand the definition of Confusion as given below. This is done before the formula itself is started.

Definitions:

1. any set of factors or circumstances which do not seem to have any immediate solution.

More broadly, a confusion in this universe is *random motion*. If you were to stand in heavy traffic you would be likely to feel confused by all the motion whizzing around you. If you were to stand in a heavy storm, with leaves and papers flying by, you would be likely to be confused. A confusion could be called an *uncontrolled randomness*.

Only those who can exert some control over that randomness can handle confusions. Those who cannot exert control actually breed confusions.

A confusion is only a confusion so long as all particles are in motion.

A confusion is only a confusion so long as no factor is clearly defined or understood.

Confusion is the basic cause of stupidity.

2. all a confusion is is unpatterned flow. The particles collide, bounce off each other and stay IN the area. Thus there is no product as to have a *product* something must flow OUT.

The additional formula for the condition of Confusion is:

1. *Locational Processing on the area in which one is.*

Locational Processing is a Scientology technique done to orient and put a person in communication with his environment. This is done by pointing out certain objects and telling the person to "Look at that ________ (indicated object)" and acknowledging the person when he has done so. The objects could include such things as a tree, a building, a street, etc. This is done until the person is happier and has some kind of realization.

The full theory on Locational Processing is given in Chapter 6, "Assists for Illnesses and Injuries."

2. *Comparing where one is to other areas where one was.*

3. *Repeat step 1.*

CONDITIONS APPLICATION

A vital thing to realize is that the formulas of conditions exist. They are part and parcel of any activity in this universe and now that they are known they must be complied with. This takes about 90 percent of chance out of business operation or personal economics. The variables are only how well one estimates the situation and how energetic one is in applying the formulas.

The proper application of the proper formula works. It works no matter how stupidly it is applied only so long as the *right* formula is applied and the exact sequence of steps is taken. Brilliance only shows up in the *speed* of recovery or expansion. Very brilliant applications show up in overnight, sound expansions. Dull applications, given only that they are correct, show up in slower expansions. In other words, nobody has to be a screaming genius to apply them or dream up the necessary ideas in them. One only has to estimate the condition accurately and *act* energetically in applying its steps in exact order. The brighter the ideas, the faster the expansion, that's all. The expansion or gain is itself inevitable. However, if the dullness includes adding needless steps, then one may fail, and if one is so stupid that a wrong estimate is made of conditions and a wrong formula is applied and applied with its steps in wrong sequence, then one jolly well deserves to fail!

Another thing to know is that these conditions apply to a universe, a civilization, an organization, a portion of an organization or a person alike.

The final thing to know is that knowing the formulas carries the responsibility of using them. Otherwise one could be accused of willful suicide! For these *are* the formulas. And they *do* work like magic.

If these formulas are not known or used, expansion is totally a matter of chance or fate, regardless of how good one's ideas are. ■

Test Your Understanding

Answer the following questions about the subject of ethics. Refer back to the chapter to check your answers. If you need to, review the chapter. Going over the material several times will increase your certainty and help you better apply it.

- ❑ *What is the difference between ethics and justice?*
- ❑ *What is a condition?*
- ❑ *What is a condition formula?*
- ❑ *How do statistics measure survival?*
- ❑ *What condition formula do you apply when you begin a new job?*
- ❑ *What do you do if your statistics improve before you have finished all the steps of a condition formula you are applying?*

Practical Exercises

Here are exercises relating to the application of ethics. Doing these will help increase your understanding of the subject.

1 Look around in your environment (your neighborhood, place of work, etc.) and find at least five examples of someone who has his ethics in. Then find five examples of someone who has his ethics out.

2 Look around your environment and locate an individual or activity which is in each of the following conditions: Non-Existence, Danger, Emergency, Normal, Affluence, Power. Do this until you are fully familiar with each condition as a state of existence.

3 Look around your environment and locate an individual or activity which is in a condition below Non-Existence. What condition is the person or activity in?

4 Using a separate sheet of paper, work out the statistic for some area of your life and show this on a graph. Determine what condition should be applied to that statistic.

5 Determine the condition of some aspect of your life, such as your job, your social life, your marriage, family life, anything. Once you have determined the correct condition, write down on a sheet of paper what you would do to apply each step of the formula for that condition.

6 Help someone you know determine the correct condition for a part of his or her life. When the correct condition has been established, show the person the formula for that condition and get the person to work out what he or she would do to apply that formula.

RESULTS FROM APPLICATION

Armed with the technology and tools of ethics developed by Mr. Hubbard, prosperity and a better life can be matters of certainty, not just chance or luck.

The use of ethics technology by the Director of the Juvenile Court in Greensville, Alabama, to deal with the problem of rehabilitating young criminals illustrates its workability. Statistics show that almost one for one, youngsters who embark on a life of crime remain criminals their entire lives. However, through use of Scientology ethics technology in counseling young offenders, this man achieved the unheard-of: 90 percent of the youths he has counseled have not returned to prison after release. More than 500 testimonials have been written by those he has worked with, crediting ethics with having changed their lives forever.

In Greece, a man on trial for car theft was introduced to Scientology ethics. He put the data to use, made a clean breast of his crimes and made many outstanding contributions to the community as amends for his earlier misdeeds. When the man's attorney presented evidence of his reform and new value as a citizen, the judge on the case dismissed all charges.

Visiting her parents for the first time in a number of years, a young California woman was distressed to find that they were having problems with their marriage and were contemplating divorce. Rather than sit by and let that happen, she used what she knew of ethics technology.

"I spent time with my father going over the different conditions and their formulas, as well as basic Scientology data on creating and expanding a marriage. We established

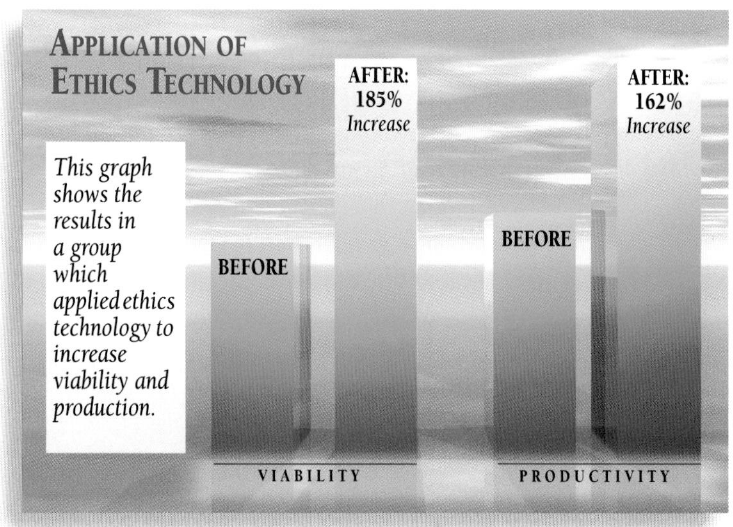

This graph shows the results in a group which applied ethics technology to increase viability and production.

his correct condition with regard to the area and he applied its formula with great success. Next I spent time with my mother, working out how she could apply ethics to the difficulties she faced in the marriage. She realized that she had earlier given up on handling a financial problem with my father, and determined to resolve it. Once they began applying the ethics formulas, my parents' troubles were sorted out and their marriage became happier and more successful than it had been in many years."

Being well versed in Scientology ethics, a community volunteer in South Africa was able to bring calm to an environment that had become turbulent after a series of unsolved thefts.

"I got into communication with the child who was suspected of stealing. Because I made it safe for her, she told me everything she had done. We worked out what she could do for the community to make up for the harm she had done, and she was happy about this. Because there had been so much upset about the thefts, I next assembled all the children (about seventy), and the young girl stood in front of the class and told them what she had done. I told the children that after the meeting there was to be no finger-pointing. They promised there wouldn't be any and officially forgave her. I was a little concerned about how the girl would feel after the meeting, but I found her playing happily with a group of children. I also found out that both the child's parents had been killed a few years earlier, and as she looked quite neglected I took measures to ensure she would be better looked after. The upset in the group was handled and the girl had a chance to become a true member of her group."

A man and his family opened a furniture business in Los Angeles; though they began with nothing, they achieved swift expansion by applying the conditions formulas.

"We studied and applied the data on conditions by Mr. Hubbard and began applying the Non-Existence Formula by the book. It was then that miracles started to happen. We opened up our communication lines and in the second month of operation two large loan companies offered us $50,000 in credit each. We got up into Danger and applied that formula, then Emergency and then Normal. We continued to apply the conditions by the book, achieving more expansion in one year than other businesses normally experience in fifteen years or more. We were even able to open a second store in our first year! Our expansion is stable through the application of the formulas."

The owner of a large restaurant chain uses Mr. Hubbard's data on conditions formulas to help his employees be honest and ethical.

"I had one employee who stole some money and another who allowed a great deal of money to be taken. Both were demoted, assigned the correct ethics condition and allowed to work their way back to executive positions through application of the conditions formulas. Now one of them is a successful franchise owner and the other is a key executive. Had it not been for the conditions formulas, I would have lost two valuable people."

SUGGESTIONS FOR FURTHER STUDY

The materials in this chapter represent only a portion of the complete body of the Ethics Technology Mr. Hubbard developed and codified. The following materials provide a more in-depth coverage of the subject and are highly recommended for a complete grasp of the subject and its application.

Introduction to Scientology Ethics

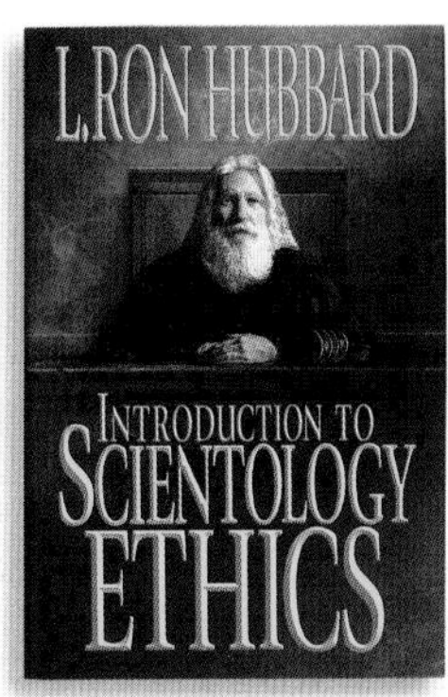

This invaluable reference book contains the complete fundamentals of Scientology Ethics, including the conditions and their formulas, Scientology Ethics and Justice Codes, application of ethics to others and important related information. Everything included in the book is a tool to raise your own condition, to improve the environment and the lives of those around you.

Formulas for Success: The Five Conditions

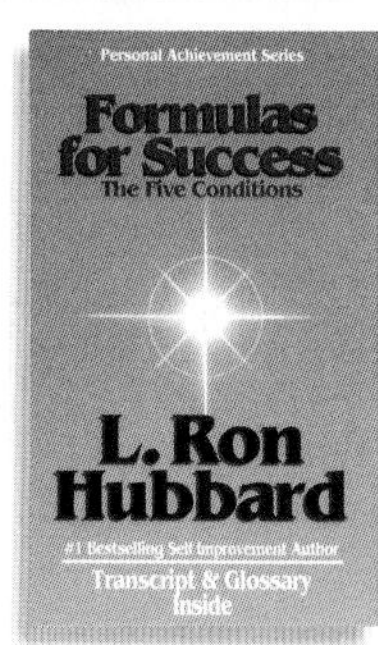

Natural laws govern the conditions of life, with exact steps to take to move *upward.* In this hour-long recorded lecture, Mr. Hubbard describes the ethics conditions and their formulas in detail, illustrating them with captivating examples. An integral part of Scientology Ethics Technology, this material is essential information for any individual to continually achieve higher levels of success.

Personal Values and Integrity

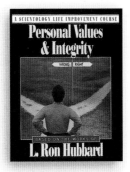

Maintaining one's integrity is a vital part of personal ethics and a happy and prosperous life. This Scientology Life Improvement Course shows you how to maintain (or recover) your integrity in the face of the pressures of day-to-day living. (Delivered in Scientology organizations.)

How to Improve Conditions in Life

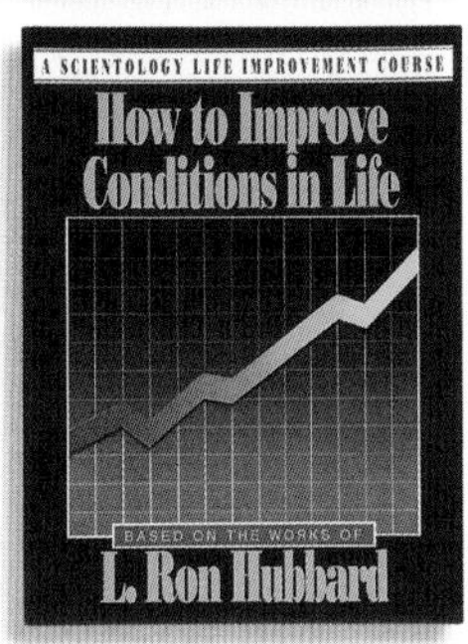

This Scientology Life Improvement Course covers the ethics conditions in detail, with illustrations, demonstrations and practical exercises to help you master their application. The course features data on how to use statistics to accurately determine the correct condition to apply. (Delivered in Scientology organizations.)

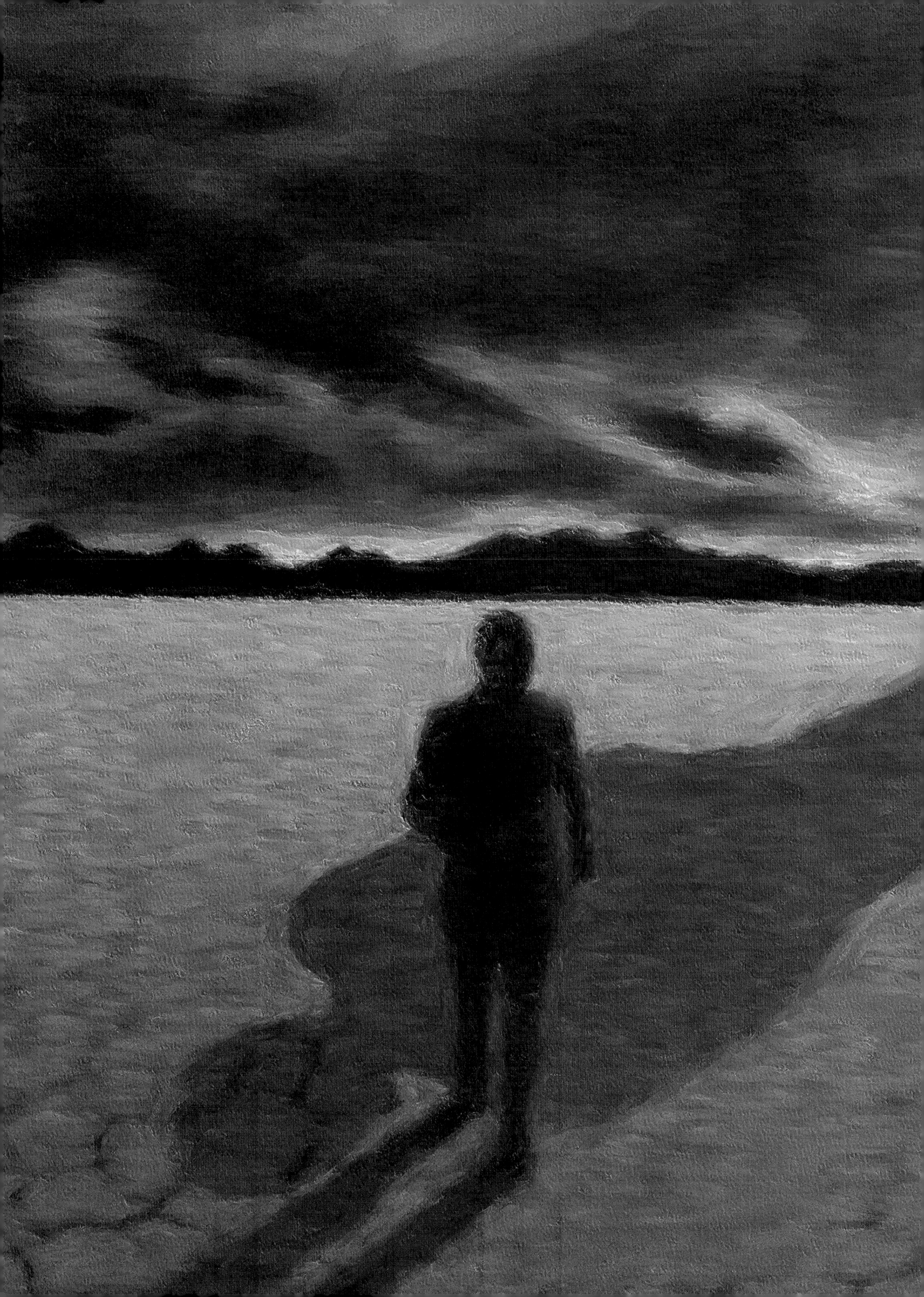

Chapter 11

The Cause of Suppression

Why are some people ill more often than others? Why are some accident-prone? And is there a reason others live their lives on an emotional seesaw, doing well one day and badly the next?

There is an explanation, and it has nothing to do with the gods, fate or the position of the stars. In fact, the actual reason behind these phenomena—and their resolution—has been explained in Scientology.

L. Ron Hubbard was able to see through the complexities of human behavior and discover the underlying factors which explain the phenomenon of **suppression** *in people—for it is suppression by others that causes these seemingly haphazard events. In the excerpts from his writings in this chapter, you will find out how to recognize people who wish you ill and those who should be your friends. You'll discover why some people do poorly in life and how you can help them regain their well-being. You'll learn about the mechanics behind this destructive yet commonplace situation and ways to counteract it. It is data that could actually change your life tangibly and instantly, just as it has changed the lives of others.*

The Antisocial Personality

There are certain characteristics and mental attitudes which cause about 20 percent of a race to oppose violently any betterment activity or group.

Such people are known to have antisocial tendencies.

When the legal or political structure of a country becomes such as to favor such personalities in positions of trust, then all the civilizing organizations of the country become suppressed and a barbarism of criminality and economic duress ensues.

Crime and criminal acts are perpetrated by antisocial personalities. Inmates of institutions commonly trace their state back to contact with such personalities.

Thus, in the fields of government, police activities and mental health, to name a few, we see that it is important to be able to detect and isolate this personality type so as to protect society and individuals from the destructive consequences attendant upon letting such have free rein to injure others.

As they only comprise 20 percent of the population and as only 2½ percent are truly dangerous, we see that with a very small amount of effort we could considerably better the state of society.

Well-known, even stellar, examples of such a personality are, of course, Napoleon and Hitler. Dillinger, Pretty Boy Floyd, Christie and other famous criminals were well-known examples of the antisocial personality. But with such a cast of characters in history we neglect the less stellar examples and do not perceive that such personalities exist in current life, very common, often undetected.

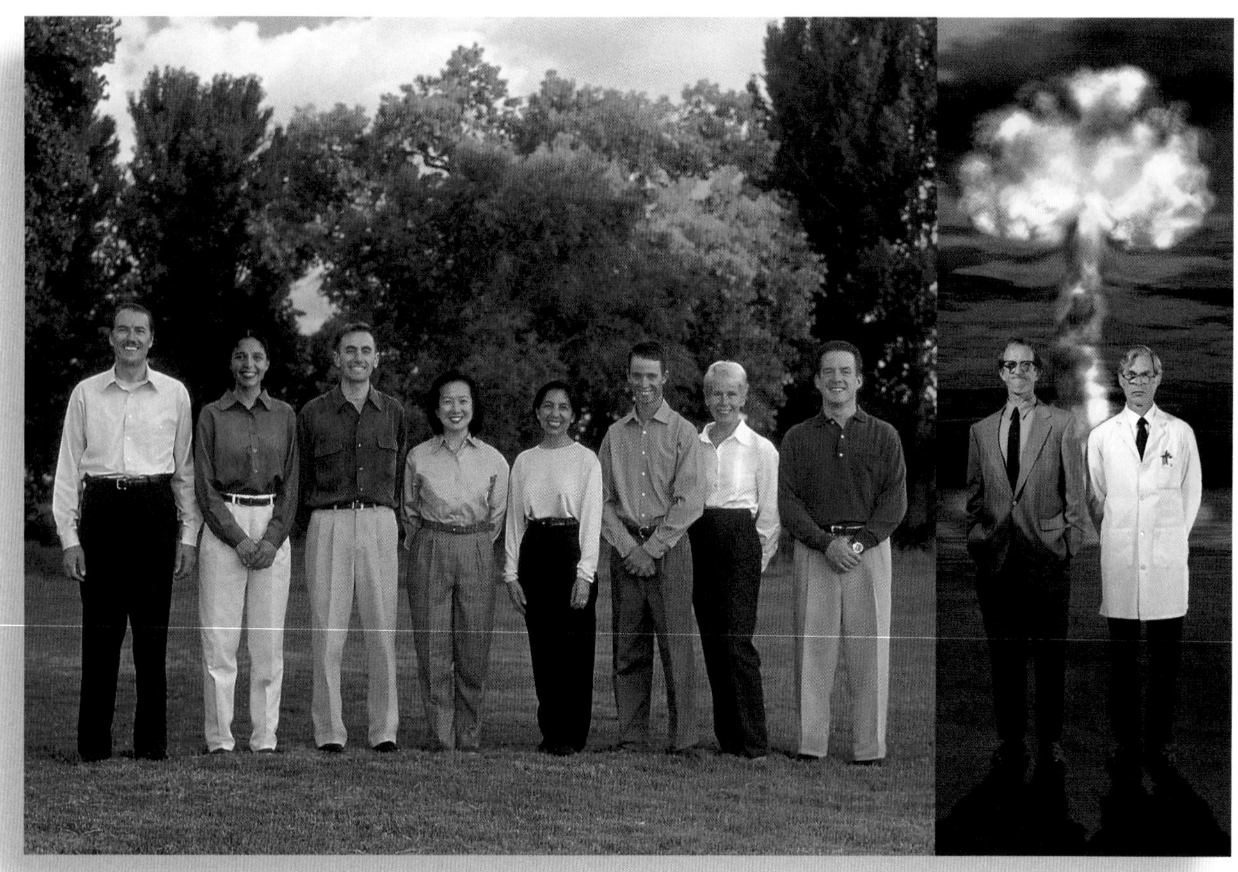

A relatively small proportion of a race, about 20 percent, possess antisocial characteristics. They cause trouble for the remaining 80 percent out of proportion to their number.

When we trace the cause of a failing business, we will inevitably discover somewhere in its ranks the antisocial personality hard at work.

In families which are breaking up, we commonly find one or the other of the persons involved to have such a personality.

Where life has become rough and is failing, a careful review of the area by a trained observer will detect one or more such personalities at work.

As there are 80 percent of us trying to get along and only 20 percent trying to prevent us, our lives would be much easier to live were we well informed as to the exact manifestations of such a personality. Thus, we could detect it and save ourselves much failure and heartbreak.

It is important then to examine and list the attributes of the antisocial personality. Influencing as it does the daily lives of so many, it well behooves decent people to become better informed on this subject.

Attributes

The antisocial personality has the following attributes:

1. He or she speaks only in very broad generalities. "They say..." "Everybody thinks..." "Everyone knows..." and such expressions are in continual use, particularly when imparting rumor. When asked, "*Who* is everybody..." it normally turns out to be one source and from this source the antisocial person has manufactured what he or she pretends is the whole opinion of the whole society.

This is natural to them since to them all society is a large hostile generality, against the antisocial in particular.

2. Such a person deals mainly in bad news, critical or hostile remarks, invalidation and general suppression.

"Gossip" or "bearer of evil tidings" or "rumormonger" once described such persons.

It is notable that there is no good news or complimentary remark passed on by such a person.

3. The antisocial personality alters, to worsen, communication when he or she relays a message or news. Good news is stopped and only bad news, often embellished, is passed along.

Such a person also pretends to pass on "bad news" which is in actual fact invented.

4. A characteristic, and one of the sad things about an antisocial personality, is that it does not respond to treatment or reform.

5. Surrounding such a personality we find cowed or ill associates or friends who, when not driven actually insane, are yet behaving in a crippled manner in life, failing, not succeeding.

Such people make trouble for others.

When treated or educated, the near associate of the antisocial personality has no stability of gain but promptly relapses or loses his advantages of knowledge, being under the suppressive influence of the other.

Physically treated, such associates commonly do not recover in the expected time but worsen and have poor convalescences.

It is quite useless to treat or help or train such persons so long as they remain under the influence of the antisocial connection.

The largest number of insane are insane because of such antisocial connections and do not recover easily for the same reason.

Unjustly we seldom see the antisocial personality actually in an institution. Only his "friends" and family are there.

6. The antisocial personality habitually selects the wrong target.

If a tire is flat from driving over nails, he or she curses a companion or a noncausative source of the trouble. If the radio next door is too loud, he or she kicks the cat.

If A is the obvious cause, the antisocial personality inevitably blames B or C or D.

7. The antisocial cannot finish a cycle of action. Any action goes through a sequence wherein the action is begun, is continued for as long as is required and is completed as planned. In Scientology, this is called a *cycle of action.*

The antisocial becomes surrounded with incomplete projects.

8. Many antisocial persons will freely confess to the most alarming crimes when forced to do so, but will have no faintest sense of responsibility for them.

Their actions have little or nothing to do with their own volition. Things "just happened."

They have no sense of correct causation and particularly cannot feel any sense of remorse or shame therefore.

9. The antisocial personality supports only destructive groups and rages against and attacks any constructive or betterment group.

10. This type of personality approves only of destructive actions and fights against constructive or helpful actions or activities.

The artist in particular is often found as a magnet for persons with antisocial personalities who see in his art something which must be destroyed and covertly, "as a friend," proceed to try.

11. Helping others is an activity which drives the antisocial personality nearly berserk. Activities, however, which destroy in the name of help are closely supported.

12. The antisocial personality has a bad sense of property and conceives that the idea that anyone owns anything is a pretense, made up to fool people. Nothing is ever really owned.

The Basic Reason

The basic reason the antisocial personality behaves as he or she does lies in a hidden terror of others.

To such a person every other being is an enemy, an enemy to be covertly or overtly destroyed.

The fixation is that survival itself depends on "keeping others down" or "keeping people ignorant."

If anyone were to promise to make others stronger or brighter, the antisocial personality suffers the utmost agony of personal danger.

They reason that if they are in this much trouble with people around them weak or stupid, they would perish should anyone become strong or bright.

Such a person has no trust to a point of terror. This is usually masked and unrevealed.

When such a personality goes insane, the world is full of Martians or the FBI and each person met is really a Martian or FBI agent.

But the bulk of such people exhibit no outward signs of insanity. They appear quite rational. They can be *very* convincing.

However, the list given above consists of things which such a personality cannot detect in himself or herself. This is so true that if you thought you found yourself in one of the above, you most certainly are not antisocial. Self-criticism is a luxury the antisocial cannot afford. They must be *right* because they are in continual danger in their own estimation. If you proved one *wrong*, you might even send him or her into a severe illness.

Only the sane, well-balanced person tries to correct his conduct.

Relief

If you were to weed out of your past by proper search and discovery those antisocial persons you have known and if you then disconnected, you might experience great relief.

Similarly, if society were to recognize this personality type as a sick being as they now isolate people with smallpox, both social and economic recoveries could occur.

Things are not likely to get much better so long as 20 percent of the population is permitted to dominate and injure the lives and enterprise of the remaining 80 percent.

As majority rule is the political manner of the day, so should majority sanity express itself in our daily lives without the interference and destruction of the socially unwell.

The pity of it is, they will not permit themselves to be helped and would not respond to treatment if help were attempted.

An understanding and ability to recognize such personalities could bring a major change in society and our lives.

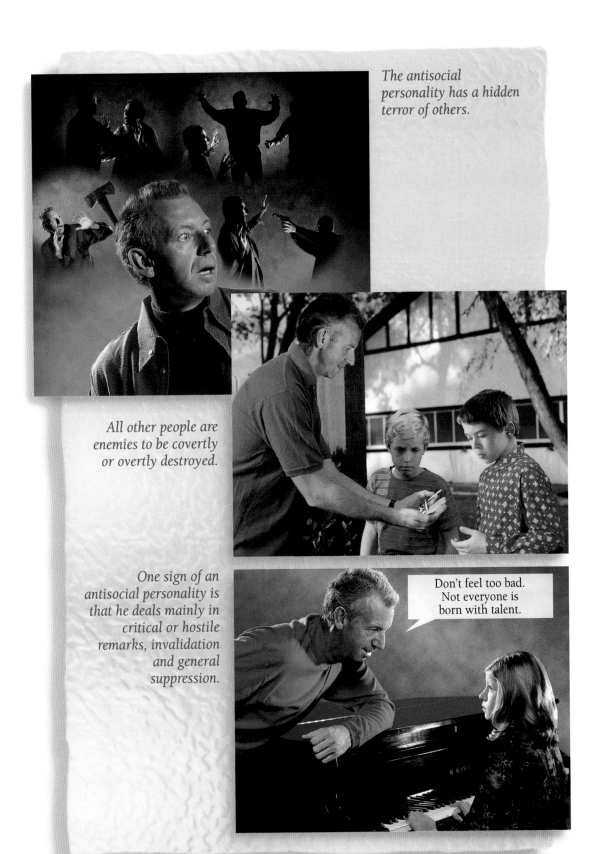

The antisocial personality has a hidden terror of others.

All other people are enemies to be covertly or overtly destroyed.

One sign of an antisocial personality is that he deals mainly in critical or hostile remarks, invalidation and general suppression.

Don't feel too bad.
Not everyone is
born with talent.

THE SOCIAL PERSONALITY

Man in his anxieties is prone to witch hunts.

All one has to do is designate "people wearing black caps" as the villains and one can start a slaughter of people in black caps.

This characteristic makes it very easy for the antisocial personality to bring about a chaotic or dangerous environment.

Man is not naturally brave or calm in his human state. And he is not necessarily villainous.

Even the antisocial personality, in his warped way, is quite certain that he is acting for the best and commonly sees himself as the only good person around, doing all for the good of everyone—the only flaw in his reasoning being that if one kills everyone else, none are left to be protected from the imagined evils. His *conduct* in his environment and toward his fellows is the only method of detecting either the antisocial or the social personalities. Their motives for self are similar—self-preservation and survival. They simply go about achieving these in different ways.

Thus, as man is naturally neither calm nor brave, anyone to some degree tends to be alert to dangerous persons and, hence, witch hunts can begin.

It is therefore even more important to identify the social personality than the antisocial personality. One then avoids shooting the innocent out of mere prejudice or dislike or because of some momentary misconduct.

The social personality can be defined most easily by comparison with his opposite, the antisocial personality.

This differentiation is easily done and no test should ever be constructed which isolates only the antisocial. On the same test must appear the upper as well as lower ranges of man's actions.

A test that declares only antisocial personalities without also being able to identify the social personality would be itself a suppressive test. It would be like answering "Yes" or "No" to the question "Do you still beat your wife?"

Anyone who took it could be found guilty. While this mechanism might have suited the times of the Inquisition, it would not suit modern needs.

As the society runs, prospers and lives *solely* through the efforts of social personalities, one must know them as *they,* not the antisocial, are the worthwhile people. These are the people who must have rights and freedom. Attention is given to the antisocial solely to protect and assist the social personalities in the society.

All majority rules, civilizing intentions and even the human race will fail unless one can identify and thwart the antisocial personalities and help and forward the social personalities in the society. For the very word "society" implies social conduct and without it there is no society at all, only a barbarism with all men, good or bad, at risk.

The frailty of showing how the harmful people can be known is that these then apply the characteristics to decent people to get them hunted down and eradicated.

The swan song of every great civilization is the tune played by arrows, axes or bullets used by the antisocial to slay the last decent men.

Government is only dangerous when it can be employed by and for antisocial personalities. The end result is the eradication of all social personalities and the resultant collapse of Egypt, Babylon, Rome, Russia or the West.

You will note in the characteristics of the antisocial personality that intelligence is not a clue to the antisocial. They are bright or stupid or average. Thus, those who are extremely intelligent can rise to considerable, even head-of-state heights.

Importance and ability or wish to rise above others are likewise not indexes to the antisocial. When they do become important or rise, they are, however, rather visible by the broad consequences of their acts. But they are as likely to be unimportant people or hold very lowly stations and wish for nothing better.

Thus, it is the twelve given characteristics alone which identify the antisocial personality. And these same twelve reversed are the sole criteria of the social personality if one wishes to be truthful about them.

The identification or labeling of an antisocial personality cannot be done honestly and accurately unless one *also,* in the same examination of the person, reviews the positive side of his life.

All persons under stress can react with momentary flashes of antisocial conduct. This does not make them antisocial personalities.

The true antisocial person has a majority of antisocial characteristics.

The social personality has a majority of social characteristics.

Thus, one must examine the good with the bad before one can truly label the antisocial or the social.

In reviewing such matters, very broad testimony and evidence are best. One or two isolated instances determine nothing. One should search all twelve social and all twelve antisocial characteristics and decide on the basis of actual evidence, not opinion.

The twelve primary characteristics of the social personality are as follows:

1. The social personality is specific in relating circumstances. "Joe Jones said..." "*The Star* newspaper reported..." and gives sources of data where important or possible.

He may use the generality of "they" or "people" but seldom in connection with attributing statements or opinions of an alarming nature.

2. The social personality is eager to relay good news and reluctant to relay bad.

He may not even bother to pass along criticism when it doesn't matter.

He is more interested in making another feel liked or wanted than disliked by others and tends to err toward reassurance rather than toward criticism.

3. A social personality passes communication without much alteration and if deleting anything tends to delete injurious matters.

He does not like to hurt people's feelings. He sometimes errs in holding back bad news or orders which seem critical or harsh.

4. Treatment and reform work very well on the social personality.

Whereas antisocial people sometimes promise to reform, they do not. Only the social personality can change or improve easily.

It is often enough to point out unwanted conduct to a social personality to completely alter it for the better.

Criminal codes and violent punishment are not needed to regulate social personalities.

5. The friends and associates of a social personality tend to be well, happy and of good morale.

A truly social personality quite often produces betterment in health or fortune by his mere presence on the scene.

At the very least he does not reduce the existing levels of health or morale in his associates.

When ill, the social personality heals or recovers in an expected manner, and is found open to successful treatment.

6. The social personality tends to select correct targets for correction.

He fixes the tire that is flat rather than attack the windscreen.

In the mechanical arts he can therefore repair things and make them work.

7. Cycles of action begun are ordinarily completed by the social personality, if possible.

8. The social personality is ashamed of his misdeeds and reluctant to confess them. He takes responsibility for his errors.

9. The social personality supports constructive groups and tends to protest or resist destructive groups.

10. Destructive actions are protested by the social personality. He assists constructive or helpful actions.

11. The social personality helps others and actively resists acts which harm others.

12. Property is property of someone to the social personality and its theft or misuse is prevented or frowned upon.

The Basic Motivation

The social personality naturally operates on the basis of the greatest good.

He is not haunted by imagined enemies but he does recognize real enemies when they exist.

The social personality wants to survive and wants others to survive, whereas the antisocial personality really and covertly wants others to succumb.

Basically, the social personality wants others to be happy and do well, whereas the antisocial personality is very clever in making others do very badly indeed.

A basic clue to the social personality is not really his successes but his motivations. The social personality when successful is often a target for the antisocial and by this reason he may fail. But his intentions included others in his success, whereas the antisocial only appreciate the doom of others.

Unless we can detect the social personality and hold him safe from undue restraint and detect also the antisocial and restrain him, our society will go on suffering from insanity, criminality and war, and man and civilization will not endure.

Of all our technical skills in Scientology, such differentiation ranks the highest since, failing, no other skill can continue, as the base on which it operates—civilization—will not be here to continue it.

Do not smash the social personality—and do not fail to render powerless the antisocial in their efforts to harm the rest of us.

Just because a man rises above his fellows or takes an important part does not make him an antisocial personality. Just because a man can control or dominate others does not make him an antisocial personality.

It is his motives in doing so and the consequences of his acts which distinguish the antisocial from the social.

Unless we realize and apply the true characteristics of the two types of personality, we will continue to live in a quandary of who our enemies are and, in doing so, victimize our friends.

All men have committed acts of violence or omission for which they could be censured. In all mankind there is not one single perfect human being.

But there are those who try to do right and those who specialize in wrong and upon these facts and characteristics you can know them.

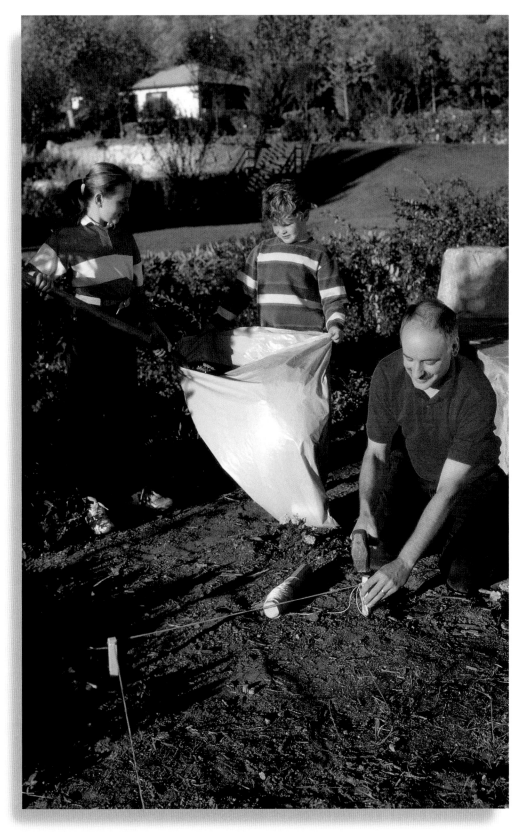

Social personalities are motivated by the desire to help others and do the greatest good for the greatest number. The bulk of humanity is composed of social personalities.

Basic Terms and Definitions

Often a social personality is so mired down in his own difficulties that he cannot *see* improvement is possible. To him, his setbacks and travails are "just life" or "the way things have to be." He has no inkling that such a thing as antisocial personalities exist or that one (or more) were making life miserable for him.

To become aware that such a condition exists requires one understand what the condition is. Following are basic terms and definitions associated with the detection and handling of antisocial personalities and those affected by them. These need to be understood for success in addressing and handling personal suppression.

Suppressive Person: (abbreviated "SP") A person who seeks to *suppress,* or squash, any betterment activity or group. A suppressive person suppresses other people in his vicinity. This is the person whose behavior is calculated to be disastrous. "Suppressive person" or a "suppressive" is another name for the "antisocial personality."

Potential Trouble Source: (abbreviated "PTS") A person who is in some way connected to and being adversely affected by a suppressive person. He is called a *potential* trouble source because he can be a lot of trouble to himself and to others.

An indicator of someone being a potential trouble source is *not* whether that person looks intimidated or not cheerful or is having trouble with his boss. Those are not things that indicate whether someone is a PTS. The indicators are very precise.

The PTS is connected to an SP who is antagonistic to him. The suppressive person keeps the potential trouble source from functioning in life. Therefore, the potential trouble source can do well in life or in some activity and then, when he meets up with or is affected by the suppressive person—who is somehow invalidating or making less of him or his efforts—he gets worse.

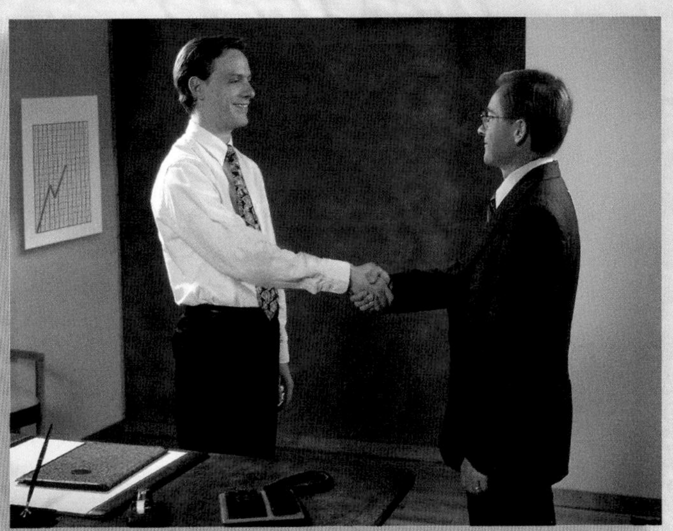

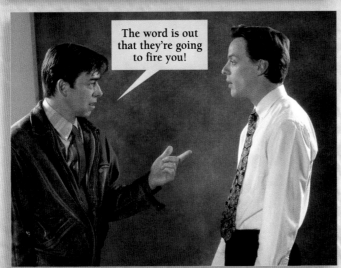

A potential trouble source has periods in life when he does well.

But when he comes under the influence of a suppressive person…

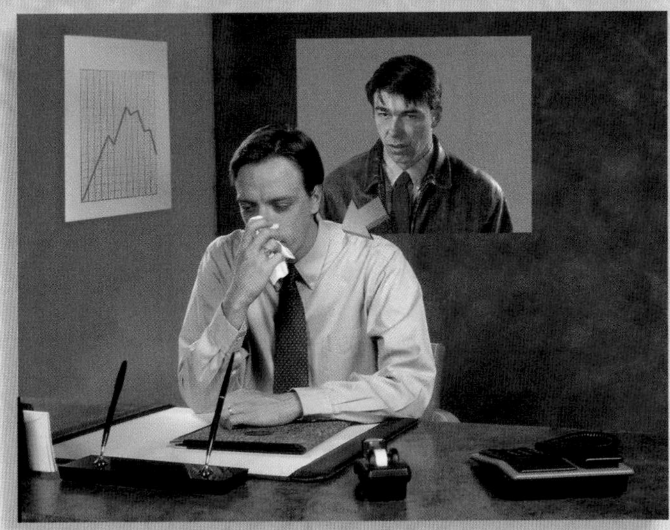

…he begins doing poorly. He may become ill or have accidents and generally do worse in life.

A potential trouble source is doing well and then not doing well, doing well, not doing well. When he is not doing well, he is sometimes ill.

A person in this condition *roller-coasters*. The term *roller-coaster* means to better and worsen—the person gets better, gets worse, gets better, gets worse. Its name was derived from the name of an amusement park ride that rises then plunges steeply.

Another indicator of a potential trouble source is that in the presence of suppression, an individual makes mistakes. When a person makes mistakes or does stupid things, it is evidence that a suppressive person exists in that vicinity.

There are also types of PTS people. The basic ones are as follows.

PTS Type I

The first type of PTS person is one who is associated with or connected to a suppressive person in his present time environment. By "connected to" is meant in the vicinity of, or in communication with in some way, whether a social, familial or business relationship.

An artist may have a "friend" hanging around who is actually a suppressive person, invalidating his work and ambitions. The artist may become ill or give up his work.

A Type I PTS has a suppressive person there in his present time environment trying to squash and invalidate him.

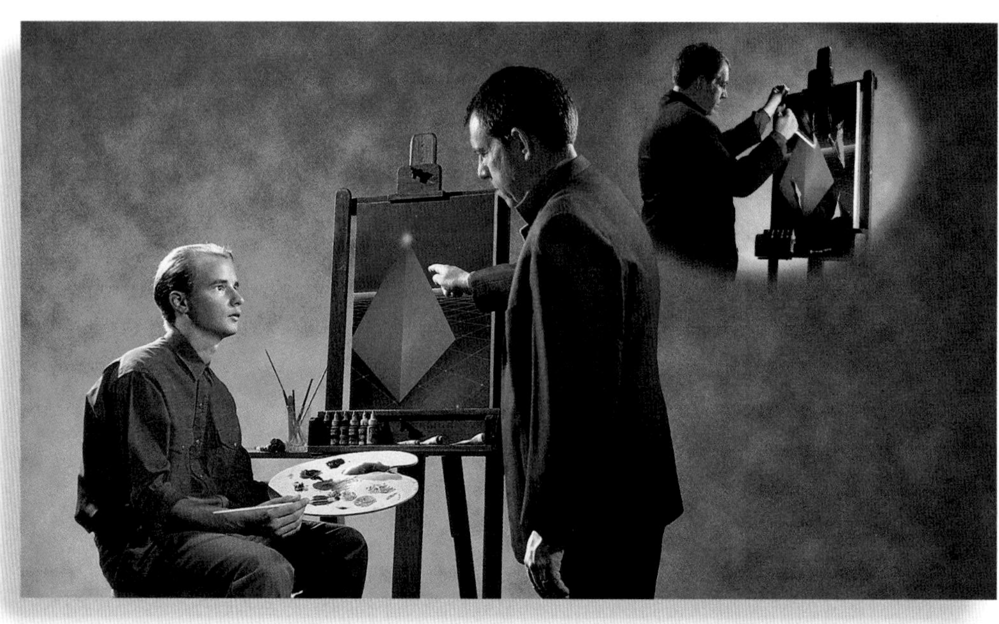

An executive with a suppressive person for a business associate will roller-coaster and may find himself making mistakes in his work, suffering setbacks or becoming sick.

Also, an individual may be involved in betterment activities to increase his abilities and improve his life and the lives of others. Such an individual may be connected to a suppressive person. The SP attacks such betterment activities and the people involved in them, as the suppressive is terrified of anyone becoming stronger or more able.

Thus individuals intimately connected with persons (such as marital or familial ties) of known antagonism to betterment activities are PTS. In practice, these persons have such pressure continually brought to bear upon them by others with undue influence over them, they make poor progress or improvement, and their interest is solely devoted to proving the antagonistic element wrong.

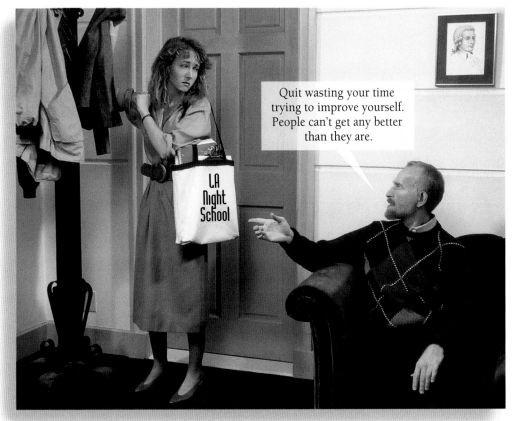

Someone intimately connected to another who opposes their attempts at self-betterment is PTS.

PTS Type II

In the second type of PTS, a *past* suppression is being restimulated by someone or something in the present time environment. When an individual is restimulated, a past bad memory is reactivated due to similar circumstances existing in the present which approximate circumstances of the past, and the person can experience the pain and emotions contained in the past memory. In the case of a PTS Type II, the person wouldn't even have to see the suppressive person to go PTS but can become so just by seeing something that reminds him of the suppressive.

For example, if someone has been suppressed by a postman and sees a letter box when the postman isn't even around, that could be enough to cause him to roller-coaster.

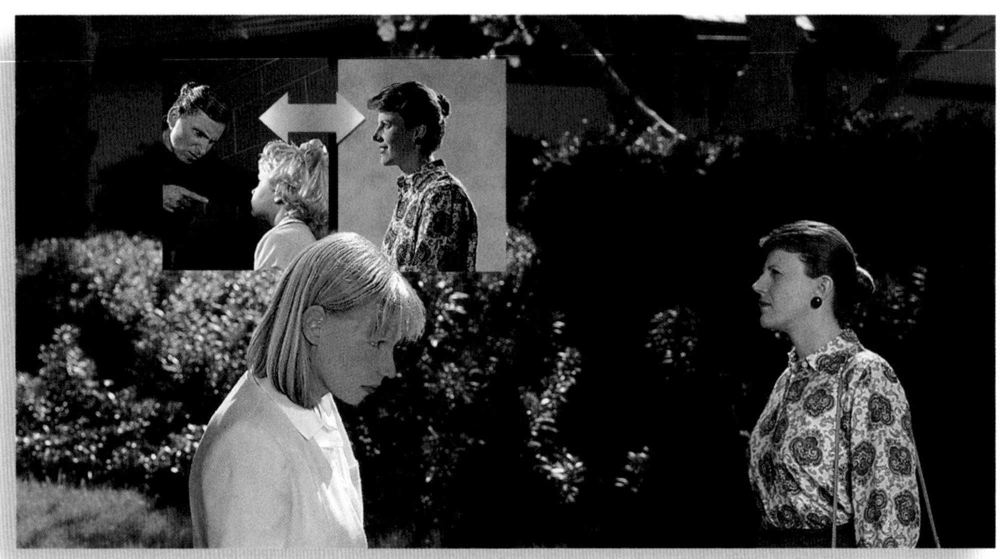

A Type II PTS is reminded of a suppressive person in his past by someone or something in his environment. The actual suppressive is not there in present time but his influence is felt nevertheless.

A PTS Type II always has an *apparent* suppressive who is not *the* suppressive of the PTS person and is confusing the two and is acting PTS only because of restimulation, not because of suppression.

An important thing to know is that *a suppressive is always a person, a being or a group of beings.* A suppressive is *not* a condition, a problem or a conclusion, decision or resolution made by the individual himself.

The Type II PTS is handled by specific Scientology processes. These are exact sets of questions asked or directions given by a trained Scientology practitioner to help a person find out things about himself and improve his condition. Scientology processes received by a Type II PTS help the person locate the suppressive and fully alleviate the undue influences the SP has had on the PTS.

PTS Type III

In this case the Type II's *apparent* SP (suppressive person) is spread all over the world and is often more than all the people there are—for the person sometimes has ghosts about him or demons and they are just more apparent SPs but imaginary as beings as well.

The Type III PTS is mostly found in mental institutions. He is best helped by providing a safe environment and giving him rest and quiet, and no treatment of a mental nature at all. He should receive any medical care needed that is unbrutal in nature.

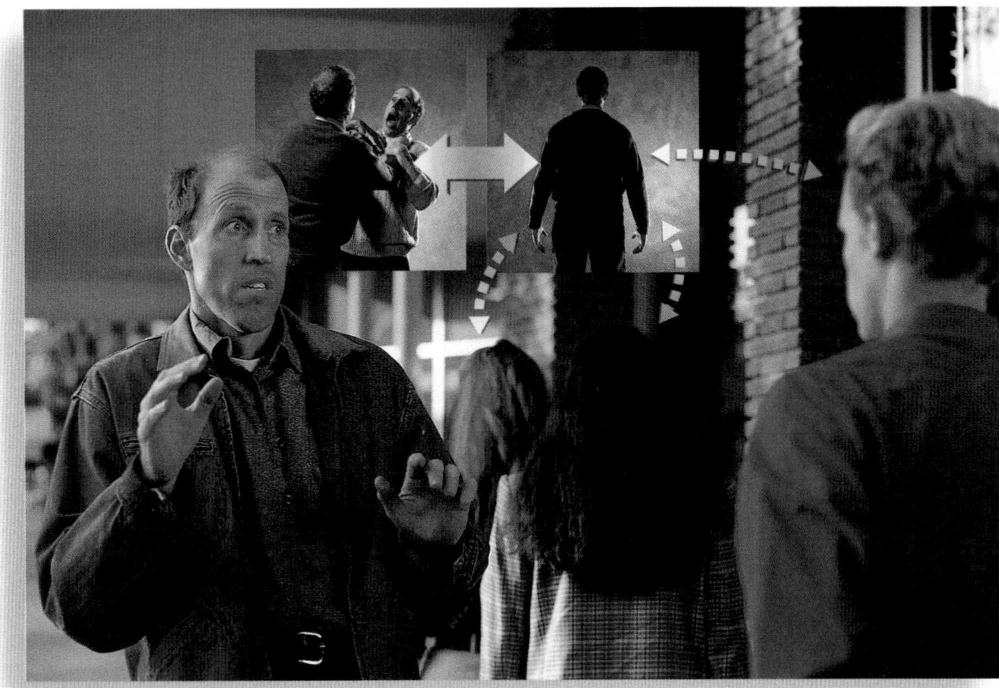

A Type III PTS is also under the influence of a suppressive from his past, but the present time environment is, to him, full of suppressives.

A person who is PTS is often the last person to suspect it. He may have become temporarily or momentarily so. And he may have become so very slightly. Or he may be *very* PTS and have been so for a long time. Therefore, the very first step in handling this condition is to gain an understanding of the fundamentals of the technology concerning potential trouble sources and suppressive persons so that the situation can be handled.

And it *can* be handled.

PTS HANDLING

There are two stable data which anyone has to have, understand and *know are true* in order to obtain results in handling the person connected to suppressives.

These data are:

1. That all illness in greater or lesser degree and all foul-ups stem directly and only from a PTS condition.

2. That getting rid of the condition requires three basic actions: (A) Discover; (B) Handle or (C) Disconnect.

Persons called upon to handle PTS people can do so very easily, far more easily than they believe. Their basic stumbling block is thinking that there are exceptions or that there is other technology or that the two above data have modifiers or are not sweeping. The moment a person who is trying to handle PTSes gets persuaded there are other conditions or reasons or technology, he is at once lost and will lose the game and not obtain results. And this is very too bad because it is not difficult and the results are there to be obtained.

A PTS person is rarely psychotic. But all psychotics are PTS if only to themselves. A PTS person may be in a state of deficiency or pathology (an unhealthy condition caused by a disease) which prevents a ready recovery, but at the same time he will not fully recover unless the PTS condition is also handled. For he became prone to deficiency or pathological illness because he was PTS. And unless the condition is relieved, no matter what medication or nutrition he may be given, he might not recover and certainly will not recover permanently. This seems to indicate that there are "other illnesses or reasons for illness besides being PTS." To be sure, there are deficiencies and illnesses just as there are accidents and injuries. But strangely enough, the person himself precipitates them (causes them to happen) because being PTS predisposes him (makes him susceptible) to them.

In a more garbled way, the medicos and nutritionists are always talking about "stress" causing illness. Lacking full technology on the subject as contained in Scientology, they yet have an inkling that this is so because they see it is somehow true. They cannot handle it. Yet they recognize it, and they state that it is a senior situation to various illnesses and accidents. Well, Scientology has the technology of this in more ways than one.

What is this thing called "stress"? It is more than the medico defines it—he usually says it comes from operational or physical shock and in this he has too limited a view.

A person under stress is actually under a suppression in one or more areas or aspects of his life.

If that suppression is located and the person handles or disconnects, the condition diminishes. If he also receives Scientology processes which address suppression of the individual and if *all* such areas of suppression are thus handled, the person would recover from anything caused by "stress."

Usually, the person has insufficient understanding of life or any area of it to grasp his own situation. He is confused. He believes all his illnesses are true because they occur in such heavy books!

At some time he was predisposed to illness or accidents. When a serious suppression then occurred, he suffered a precipitation or occurrence of the accident or illness, and then with a series of repeated similar suppressions, the illness or tendency to accidents became prolonged or chronic.

To say then that a person is PTS to his current environment would be very limited as a diagnosis. If he continues to do or be something to which the suppressive person or group objected, he may become or continue to be ill or have accidents.

Actually, the problem of PTS is not very complicated. Once you have grasped the two data first given, the rest of it becomes simply an analysis of how they apply to this particular person.

A PTS person can be markedly helped in three ways:

a. Gaining an understanding of the technology of the condition

b. Discovering to what or to whom he is PTS

c. Handling or disconnecting

Someone with the wish or duty to find and handle PTSes has an additional prior step: he must know how to recognize a PTS and how to handle them when recognized. Thus, it is rather a waste of time to engage in this hunt unless one has thoroughly studied the material on suppressives and PTSes and grasps it without misunderstanding the words or terms used. In other words, the first step of the person is to get a grasp of the subject and its technology. This is not difficult to do.

With this step done, a person has no real trouble recognizing PTS people and can have success in handling them which is very gratifying and rewarding.

Let us consider the easiest level of approach:

i. Give the person the simpler materials on the subject and let him study them so that he knows the elements like "PTS" and "suppressive." He may just come to realize the source of his difficulties right there and be much better. It has happened.

ii. Have him discuss the illness or accident or condition, without much prodding or probing, that he thinks now may be the result of suppression.

He will usually tell you it is right here and now or was a short time ago and will be all set to explain it (without any relief) as stemming from his current environment or a recent one. If you let it go at that, he would simply be a bit unhappy and not get well as he is discussing usually a recent disturbing experience that has a lot of earlier similar experiences below it.

iii. Ask when he recalls first having that illness or having such accidents. He will at once begin to roll this back and realize that it has happened before. He will get back to some early this-lifetime point usually.

iv. Now ask him *who* it was. He will usually tell you promptly. And, as you are not trying to do more than release him from the restimulation that occurred, you don't probe any further.

v. You will usually find that he has named a person to whom he is still connected! So you ask him whether he wants to handle or disconnect. Now, as the sparks will really fly in his life if he dramatically disconnects and if he can't see how he can, you persuade him to begin to handle with a gradual approach. This may consist of imposing some slight discipline on him, such as requiring him to actually answer his mail or write the person a pleasant good roads, good weather (calm, warm, friendly) note or to realistically look at how he turned them from being affectionate to being indifferent, disliking or hateful. In short, what is required in the handling is an easy, gradual approach. All you are trying to do is MOVE THE PTS PERSON FROM BEING THE EFFECT OF SUPPRESSION OVER TO BEING IN A POSITION OF SLIGHT GENTLE CAUSE OVER IT.

vi. Check with the person again, if he is handling, and coach him along, always at a gentle good-roads-and-good-weather level.

That is a simple handling. You can get complexities such as a person being PTS to an unknown person in his immediate vicinity that he may have to find before he can handle or disconnect. You can find people who can't remember more than a few years back. But simple handling ends when it looks pretty complex. When you run into such complexity, it can be handled by more advanced procedures in Scientology.

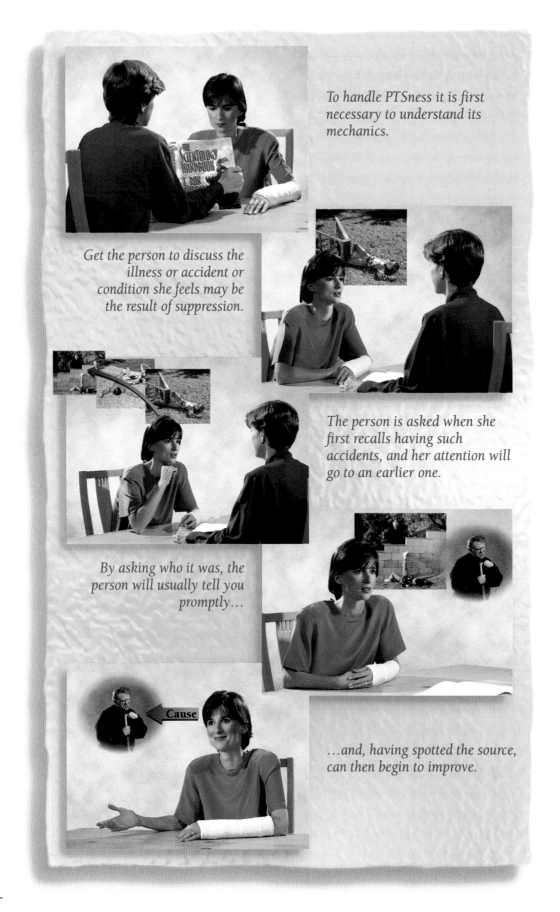

To handle PTSness it is first necessary to understand its mechanics.

Get the person to discuss the illness or accident or condition she feels may be the result of suppression.

The person is asked when she first recalls having such accidents, and her attention will go to an earlier one.

By asking who it was, the person will usually tell you promptly…

…and, having spotted the source, can then begin to improve.

But this simple handling will get you quite a few stars in your crown. You will be amazed to find that while some of them don't instantly recover, medication, vitamins, minerals will now work when before they wouldn't. You may also get some instant recoveries but realize that if they don't, you have not failed.

By doing the PTS handling steps laid out in this section, you have made an entrance and you have stirred things up and gotten the PTS person more aware and just that way you will find he is in a more causative position.

His illness or proneness to accidents may not be slight. You may succeed only to the point where he now has a chance, by nutrition, vitamins, minerals, medication, treatment, and above all, Scientology processing, of getting well. Unless you jogged this condition, he had no chance at all: for becoming PTS is the first thing that happened to him on the subject of illness or accidents.

So do not underestimate what you can do for a PTS. And don't sell PTS technology short or neglect it. And don't push off, or even worse tolerate, PTS conditions in people.

You *can* do something about it.

And so can they.

FURTHER DATA ON PTS HANDLING

A person applying PTS technology to his own life or to another who is roller-coastering can encounter a unique circumstance. The PTS person correctly carries out the standard action to handle a person who is antagonistic to him or his activities, yet the antagonistic source continues to remain antipathetic to the PTS person and/or his activities. In this case, it may require the alternate step to *handle,* which is *disconnect.*

The concept of disconnection relates to the right to communicate.

Perhaps the most fundamental right of any being is the right to communicate. Without this freedom, other rights deteriorate.

Communication, however, is a two-way flow. If one has the right to communicate, then one must also have the right to not receive communication from another. It is this latter concept of the right to not receive communication that gives us our right to privacy.

These rights are so basic that governments have written them into laws—witness the American Bill of Rights.

However, groups have always regulated these rights to one degree or another. For with the freedom to communicate come certain agreements and responsibilities.

An example of this is a marriage: In a monogamous society, the agreement is that one will be married to only one person at one time. That agreement extends to having sexual relations with one's spouse and no one else. Thus, should wife Shirley establish this type of relationship with someone other than her husband Pete, it is a violation of the agreement and resolutions of the marriage. Pete has the right to insist that either this communication cease or that the marriage will cease.

Handle or Disconnect

In this chapter, you have seen the phrase "handle or disconnect." It means simply that.

The term *handle* most commonly means, when used in relation to PTS technology, to smooth out a situation with another person by applying the technology of communication.

The term *disconnection* is defined as a self-determined decision made by an individual that he is not going to be connected to another. It is a severing of a communication line (the route along which a communication travels from one person to another).

The basic principle of handle or disconnect exists in any group.

It is much like trying to deal with a criminal. If he will not handle, the society resorts to the only other solution: It "disconnects" the criminal from the society. In other words, they remove the guy from society and put him in a prison because he won't *handle* his problem or otherwise cease to commit criminal acts against others.

It's the same sort of situation that husband Pete is faced with as mentioned in the first part of this section. The optimum solution is to handle the situation with wife Shirley and her violations of their group (marriage) agreements. But if Pete cannot handle the situation, he is left with no other choice but to disconnect (sever the marriage communication lines if only by separation). To do otherwise would be disastrous, for he is connected to someone antagonistic to the original agreements, decisions, resolutions and responsibilities of the group (the marriage).

A person can become PTS by reason of being connected to someone that is antagonistic to him. In order to resolve the PTS condition, he either *handles* the other person's antagonism (as covered in the materials in this chapter) or, as a last resort when all attempts to handle have failed, he disconnects from the person. He is simply exercising his right to communicate or not to communicate with a particular person.

By applying the technology of handle or disconnect, the person is, in actual fact, doing nothing different than any society or group or marriage down through thousands of years.

The Right to Disconnect

Earlier, the use of disconnection in Scientology had been cancelled. It had been abused by a few individuals who'd failed to handle situations which could have been handled and who lazily or senselessly disconnected, thereby creating situations even worse than the original because it was the wrong action.

Secondly, there were those who could survive only by living on Scientology's lines—they wanted to continue to be connected to Scientologists. Thus, they screamed to high heaven if anyone dared to apply the tech of "handle or disconnect."

This put Scientologists at a disadvantage.

We cannot afford to deny Scientologists that basic freedom that is granted to everyone else: the right to choose whom one wishes to communicate with or not communicate with. It's bad enough that there are governments trying, through the use of force, to prevent people from disconnecting from them.

The bare fact is that disconnection is a vital tool in handling PTSness and can be very effective when used correctly.

Therefore the tool of disconnection was restored to use, in the hands of those persons thoroughly and standardly trained in the technology of handling suppressives and potential trouble sources.

Handling Antagonistic Sources

In the great majority of cases, where a person has some family member or close associate who appears antagonistic to him, it is *not* really a matter of the antagonistic source wanting the PTS to not *get better.* It can more commonly be a lack of correct information about what the PTS person is doing that causes the problem or upset. In such a case, simply having the PTS disconnect would not help matters and would actually show an inability on the part of the PTS to confront the situation. It is quite common that the PTS has a low confront (ability to face without flinching or avoiding) on the person and situation. This isn't hard to understand when one looks at these facts:

a. To be PTS in the first place, the PTS must have committed harmful, contrasurvival acts against the antagonistic source; and

b. When one has committed such acts, his confront and responsibility drop.

When an individual using the data in this chapter to assist another finds that the person is PTS to a family member, he does *not* recommend that the person disconnect from the antagonistic source. The advice to the PTS person is to *handle.*

The handling for such a situation is to educate the PTS person in the technology of PTSness and suppression, and then skillfully and firmly guide the PTS through the steps needed to restore good communication with the antagonistic source. For example, where the PTS person is a Scientologist, these actions eventually dissolve the situation by bringing about an *understanding* on the part of the antagonistic source as to what Scientology is and why the PTS person is interested and involved in it.

When Disconnection Is Used

One can encounter a situation where someone is factually connected to a suppressive person, in present time. This is a person whose normal operating basis is one of making others smaller, less able, less powerful. He does not want anyone to get better, at all.

In truth, an SP is absolutely, completely terrified of anyone becoming more powerful.

In such an instance the PTS isn't going to get anywhere trying to "handle" the person. The answer is to sever the connection.

How a disconnection is done depends on the circumstances.

Example: The person lives next door to, say, a psychiatric clinic and feels PTS due to this environment. The remedy is simple—the person can move to another apartment in another location. He need not write any sort of "disconnection letter" to the psychiatric clinic. He simply changes his environment—which is, in effect, a disconnection from the suppressive environment.

Example: One discovers that an employee at his place of business is an SP—he steals money, drives away customers, wipes out other employees and will not correct no matter what you do. The handling is very simple—the PTS fires him and that's the end of it right there!

The individual's right to communicate (or not) with someone is an inherent freedom. Exercising this right and disconnecting from a suppressive person does not under any circumstances justify any violations of the laws of the land.

The technology of disconnection is essential in the handling of PTSes. It can and has saved lives and untold trouble and upset. It must be preserved and used correctly.

EASE OF HANDLING

In handling the PTS person, the main emphasis has to be on properly doing the steps necessary to handle. If he does so, he will begin to get well, cease to have problems and no longer roller-coaster. One must realize the simplicity of handling the PTS person: it requires no heroic or drastic actions and is done on a very, very gradual approach. It doesn't have to be an explosive handling; it can be very gentle. Handling a PTS condition with a step-by-step approach frees the PTS from the restraints holding him back, brings the person up to a causative position and enables him to achieve a productive and rewarding life.

Detection of antisocial personalities or suppressive persons not only brings relief to the individuals they affect, but recognition of these personalities and an understanding of the havoc they wreak would truly benefit all society. Likewise, knowing the traits of social personalities enables one to wisely choose those individuals for his friends and associates. With this knowledge and its application in everyday life, man can create a sane community and civilization for himself, his family and his fellows. ■

Test Your Understanding

Answer the following questions about suppressive people and overcoming suppression. Refer back to the chapter to check your answers. If you need to, review the chapter. Going over the material several times will increase your certainty and help you better apply it.

- ❑ *How does one determine if a person is social or antisocial?*
- ❑ *What is a suppressive person?*
- ❑ *What is a potential trouble source?*
- ❑ *How can you tell if a person is PTS?*
- ❑ *What are the three basic actions taken to handle a person who is connected to a suppressive?*
- ❑ *Why is it important that a PTS person be educated in the simpler materials of the subject?*
- ❑ *What is a PTS Type I? A PTS Type II? A PTS Type III?*
- ❑ *How does one resolve a PTS condition?*
- ❑ *Under what circumstances would disconnection be a correct action to take in addressing a PTS situation?*

PRACTICAL EXERCISES

These exercises will help you identify and handle suppression. By doing them, your understanding of the subject will increase.

1 Look around your environment and find an example of antisocial behavior in another. Note which antisocial attribute is being demonstrated by the person. Repeat the above nine more times.

2 Look around your environment and find an example of social behavior in another. Note which social attribute is being demonstrated by the person. Repeat the above nine more times.

3 Think of an antisocial characteristic in someone you have known or observed. Then think of a social characteristic in that person or someone else you have known or observed. Do this again and again, spotting examples of antisocial or social characteristics in different people you have known or observed. Keep this up until you feel confident in your ability to recognize antisocial characteristics or social characteristics in people.

4 Find a friend, relative or associate who is ill or roller-coastering. Do a PTS handling on this person, beginning with educating the person on PTSness and continuing all the way through the complete handling: your actions are to include checking with the person again and coaching him along at a good-roads-and-good-weather level until he has moved from being the effect of the suppression to a position of slight, gentle cause over it.

RESULTS FROM APPLICATION

Knowing what causes the precipitation of illnesses and the exact reason why some people do well in life for a time and then do poorly has made a tremendous difference in many lives.

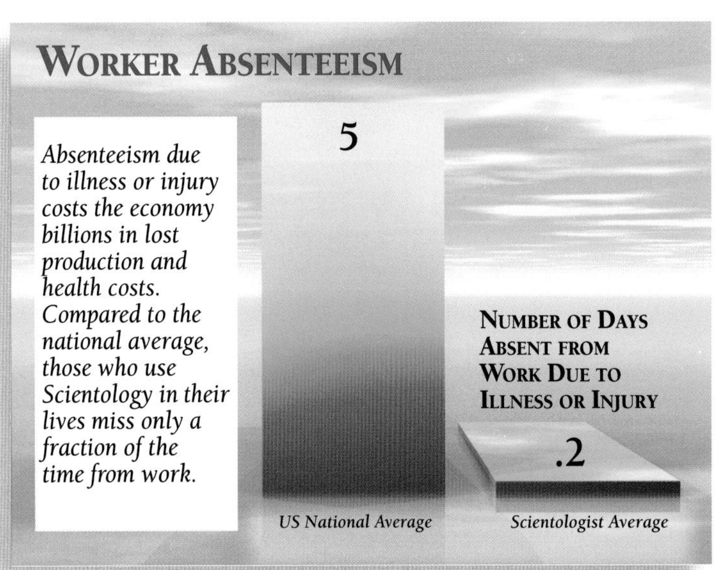

WORKER ABSENTEEISM
Absenteeism due to illness or injury costs the economy billions in lost production and health costs. Compared to the national average, those who use Scientology in their lives miss only a fraction of the time from work.
5
NUMBER OF DAYS ABSENT FROM WORK DUE TO ILLNESS OR INJURY
.2
US National Average
Scientologist Average

People using the discoveries of L. Ron Hubbard do not resort to drugs to relieve stress and anxiety and don't have to mask symptoms with medications. The apathetic advice that one has to learn to live with his condition surrenders to effective action. Illnesses, injuries and goofs of every type are *caused*—and not by an imbalance of chemicals in the brain. Purely physical approaches to resolve nonoptimum conditions which do not involve the individual himself always fall short. More than 80 percent of those who apply Mr. Hubbard's technology on the handling of suppression miss almost no time from work due to illness. None take street drugs. The following are testimonials to the fact that life can be lived free of suppression, illnesses and accidents.

Having spent years trying to handle a physical problem, a legal secretary from St. Louis was finally rescued by a friend who advised him to study Mr. Hubbard's data regarding illness and suppression.

"Boy, what a relief*! I have literally spent thousands of dollars trying to figure out what was going on with my kidney. Well, I now know what kind of effect a person can have on his body when he's in an environment that's holding him down or if he is connected to a person who's constantly telling him how he's not worth much to himself or others. By finding out about this technology I was able to really open my eyes to the fact that I've been living with someone who's been the ruin of my life for years. I was not able to see this before because I was right in the middle of a tornado, you could say, and had become part of that confusion. It's such a relief to no longer feel like I'm on a roller coaster, feeling happy one moment and completely desperate the next. And don't think that you can get bored feeling 'up' most of the time—believe me, it is much more fun than riding a roller coaster that's totally out of control and being monitored by another!"*

A California woman had lost her husband. Although she had been a cheerful person previously, she was now having difficulties in her life and relationships. She wanted another husband and a family, but hadn't been able to achieve this. Instead, she dedicated most of her life to the company she was working for. However, the situation reached the point where she hated her work and had been ill and absent from the job for weeks. Life was passing her by; she had become so depressed that she had considered seeing a psychiatrist. Her sister was concerned when she heard this and decided to apply the technology of handling suppression before the psychiatrist got to her.

"After going through the material about the antisocial personality, my sister realized that the manager of the company where she worked was a suppressive person and was not only the cause of her immediate problems, but also the cause of her late husband's illnesses and problems in life. She saw how the manager had used her and her husband for his own personal gains and was now invalidating her. He had also, with his own unethical behavior, nearly destroyed another couple's marriage.

"My sister was amazed at the relief she experienced when she realized this; she immediately became cause over the situation, talked to the manager and told him exactly what she saw he was doing. She quit the job.

"Shortly after this, I received a letter from my sister saying that she had new friends and a new job and was overjoyed to tell me that she was getting married. Five years later she has a family and is happy and doing very well in life."

The remarriage of her father spelled misfortune for a young girl from Nevada, as she could not get along with her new stepmother. As the years went by, this deteriorated to the point where the girl felt there was no hope for their relationship; she left home at the age of eighteen after a vicious fight with her stepmother. This was upsetting to the rest of the family as the girl and her father had been very close. Some time later she learned about Mr. Hubbard's discoveries on suppressive persons and, using this technology, handled the situation.

"My stepmother had been an alcoholic and had been under treatment by psychologists and psychiatrists for years, trying to handle this condition. Their 'handling' was to give her drugs and tell her what to think and do in life. As a result, her outlook on life had been bleak and very negative. I finally discovered the technology about suppressive persons. I found out who had been suppressing my stepmother and I learned how to help her. Today she doesn't go to psychiatrists anymore, doesn't drink at all, is completely cheerful—we get along great! After all these years, I am ***extremely*** *proud that we have a happy family."*

SUGGESTIONS FOR FURTHER STUDY

The following courses and materials provide additional data on the subjects of suppression and PTSness, and how to detect and handle them. Taken from the extensive body of materials Mr. Hubbard wrote and recorded on these subjects, they can be used to greatly increase one's ability to recognize, confront and shatter suppression, thus enabling an individual to strive for and accomplish his objectives in life.

Overcoming Ups and Downs in Life

Covering the fundamentals of suppression and PTSness and their handling, this Scientology Life Improvement Course includes demonstrations and practical exercises to ensure you know and can apply this important data. The course booklet is illustrated and includes a glossary of terms. (Delivered in Scientology organizations.)

PTS/SP Course Lectures

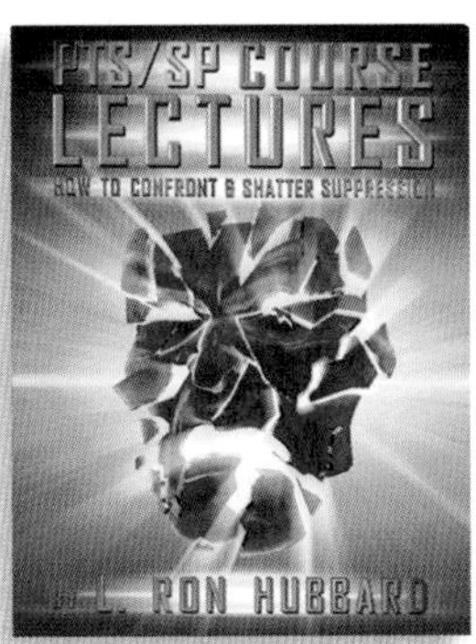

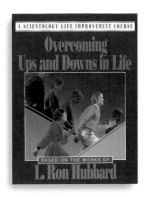

In these recorded lectures, Mr. Hubbard thoroughly covers the subjects of potential trouble sources and suppressive persons and how to effectively handle suppression. Topics discussed include how to recognize the beings behind apparent danger in the environment, exactly how to spot and handle a suppressive person, and how an area that has been subjected to suppression is straightened out.

PTS/SP Course

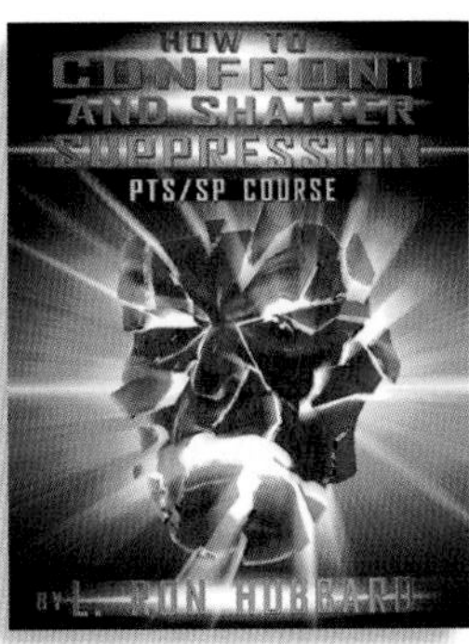

This is an advanced course in the recognition and handling of suppressives and PTS conditions. The course materials include more than sixty technical and administrative issues and articles plus the lectures described above. The end result of this course is someone with a thorough working knowledge of the subject who can apply this technology in his life, to himself and to others. (Delivered in Scientology organizations.)

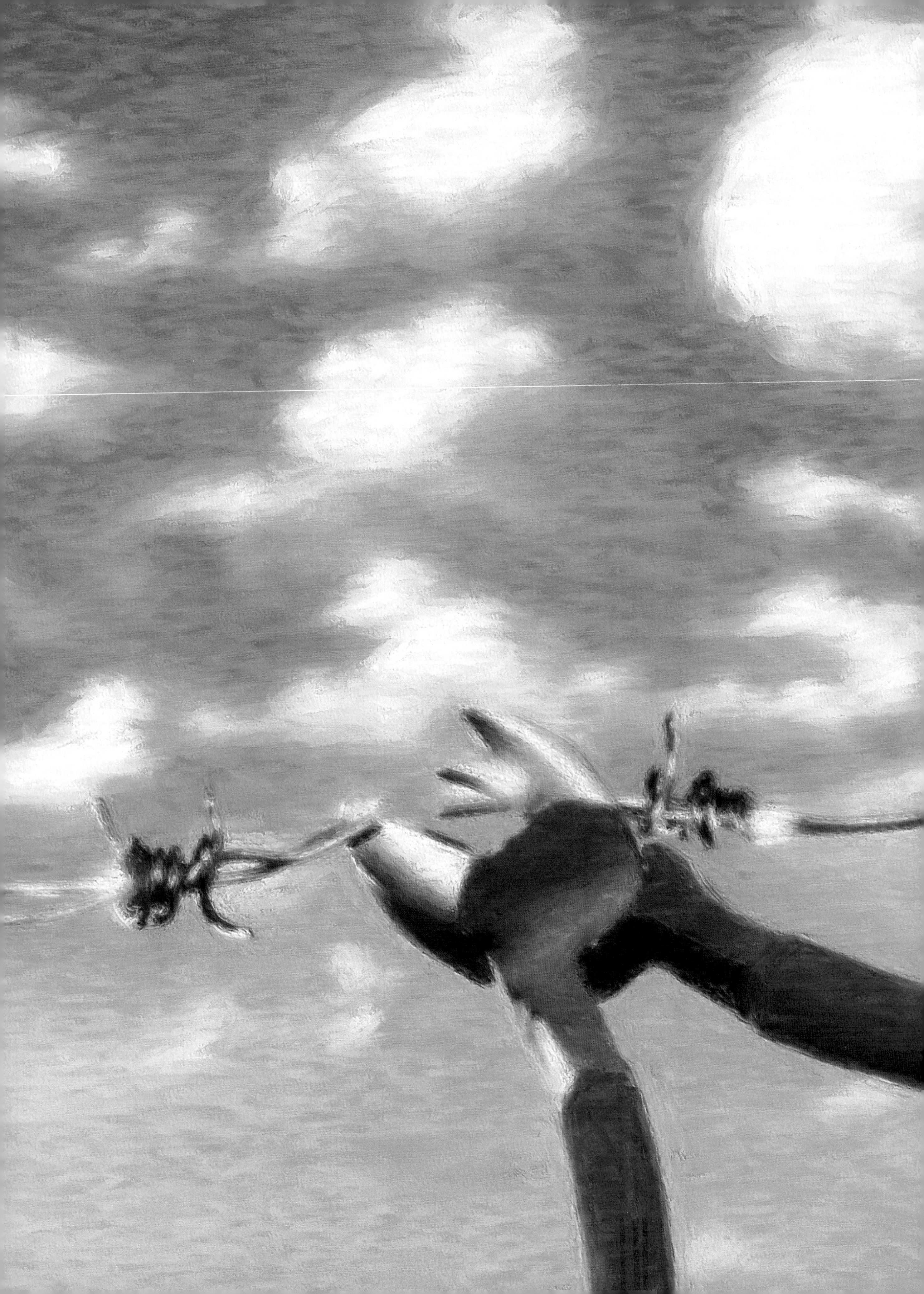

Chapter 12

Solutions for a Dangerous Environment

We live in a perilous world, a dangerous environment. Watch television news or read your daily newspaper and you are subjected to a daily diet of robberies, rapes, riots, murders, fires, earthquakes, floods and famines.

Do you find yourself becoming disturbed by what is happening around you? Do you feel helpless, unable to control these events? Do you even sometimes feel afraid?

In this chapter, L. Ron Hubbard dissects this phenomenon of the dangerous environment, providing methods that will not only help you overcome your fears, but allow you to help others. Applied on a broad scale, this information brings about an enormous calming influence and enables people to lead happier lives. Used on an individual scale—by you—it will enhance the lives of your family, friends and associates.

The Dangerous Environment

Many people are not only convinced that the environment is dangerous, but that it is steadily growing more so. For many, it's more of a challenge than they feel up to.

The fact of the matter is, however, that the environment is *made* to appear much more dangerous than it actually is.

A great number of people are professional dangerous environment *makers*. This includes professions which require a dangerous environment for their existence such as the politician, the policeman, the newspaperman, the undertaker and others. These people sell a dangerous environment. That is their mainstay. They feel that if they did not sell people on the idea the environment is dangerous, they would promptly go broke. So it is in their interest to make the environment far more dangerous than it is.

The environment is dangerous enough.

At one time an idea was put forth that certain societies did not advance because the environment lacked sufficient challenge. One of those advancing the idea was English historian and philosopher Arnold Toynbee (1889–1975) who felt that areas such as Mexico did not progress for that reason. Toynbee's idea on this, however, was born in an ivory tower environment, sitting in libraries reading books, but never going out and talking to any Mexicans.

So Toynbee pronounced with great conclusive exclamation points followed by innumerable university degrees, "The reason the Mexican does not succeed is he has insufficient challenge in his environment. The reason South America isn't an up-and-coming industrial power is insufficient challenge in the environment. The reason the African has not progressed further in civilization is because his environment has insufficient challenge."

What did Toynbee know of it? He spent all his time in the back end of a library, reading books written by men who had spent all of *their* days in libraries! That is no way to learn about life.

In the Philippines, for an added example, a bold, energetic white man arrives and he advises the native Igorots—a tribe which inhabits the northern mountainous region of the Philippines. He says, "If you will just cut a pathway from the village down to the river, then take a bullock cart down to the river in the morning and fill up a water tank and bring it back to the village, your women won't have to be making that long walk to the river. You should engage upon this public works project at once."

He becomes absolutely *outraged* that they don't immediately act on his suggestion and he goes away, thinking, "Aha! Those people have insufficient challenge in the environment. Nothing for them to measure up to. No ambition. Not like us in the West—we have challenge in our environment."

This man had challenge in his environment? Mama spooned Wheaties into his mouth, Papa wrote all the checks as he went through college and his way was paved in all directions with machinery and vehicles. His environment was already licked, so of course he could afford to be bold.

But what really is the environment of the Igorot as he sits by the fire, listening to the white man tell him how he has to cut a path to the river? This Igorot has a little boy, whom he loves very much, but he knows this little boy has only a slim chance of living until he is seven due to disease and bad food. He knows that when the rains come, they won't just be pleasant light rains; they will flood every seed out of the ground and pound the fields to pieces but *if* he can salvage anything out of that, maybe he will live a few more months. He knows all he has to do is walk under the wrong tree and get hit by a poisonous snake, and that will be the end of him. In other words, he already knows he cannot live, so why try?

In other words, the challenge of the environment is absolutely overwhelming for many people.

But does this mean there is no challenge in the environment in the more "civilized" parts of the world? By no means. Consider the situation of a young artist from Terre Haute, Indiana, who moved to New York City. The casual observer might say that he moved because there was no challenge in his environment in Terre Haute. No, here again, the challenge was too much.

This fellow decided to become a painter in the first place because he couldn't face working in the feed store with the same fellow who beat him up during kindergarten, beat him up during grammar school and beat him up in high school. The thought of having to work with this fellow every day was just too much challenge for him. So he became an artist, but nobody in Terre Haute bought paintings and nobody believed in what he was doing. He had no future there; he was facing continual starvation, he was unable to contribute to his community. That was a very hostile environment. So he moved to a friendlier one, Greenwich Village. He would rather starve to death quietly in Greenwich Village than be threatened to death in Terre Haute, Indiana.

We come to the conclusion, then, that any individual—whether white, black, red or yellow—if he has not been able to achieve his own destiny, must be in an environment that he finds overwhelming, and his methods of taking care of that environment must be inadequate to his survival. His existence is as apathetic or as unhappy as his environment seems to him to be overwhelming.

Why then would people go out of their way to actually make the environment appear more dangerous than it already is?

The Merchants of Chaos

There are those who could be called "merchants of chaos." These are people who want an environment to look very, very disturbing. These are people who gain some sort of advantage, they feel, if the environment is made to look more threatening.

An obvious example can be seen in newspapers. There are no good news stories. Newspapermen shove the environment in people's faces and say, "Look! It's dangerous. Look! It's overwhelming. Look! It's threatening." They not only report the most threatening bits of news, but also sensationalize it, making it worse than it is. What more do you want as a proof of their intention? This is the merchant of chaos. He is paid to the degree that he can make the environment threatening. To yearn for good news is foolhardy in a society where the merchants of chaos reign.

The chaos merchant has lots of troops among people with vested interests.

And do not think it an accident that the current justice system will take a dangerous criminal, throw him into prison, make him more antisocial and more dangerous and then release him upon the society. The more crime, the more police are needed.

Ideas of this kind are found in the society to a marked degree. It isn't just the newspaper reporter or the politician; individuals here and there also engage upon this.

A lot of people spend their whole lives as professional chaos merchants; they worry those around them to death. The percentage who do this may be as high as one out of four. For example, a housewife, operating as a merchant of chaos in her sphere of influence, thinks of her husband, "If I can just keep Henry worried enough, he will do what I tell him." She operates on the idea that it is necessary to spread confusion and upset. But along with this goes a concern, "I wonder why Henry doesn't get ahead?" Naturally, she is making him sick.

The truth of the matter, however, is this: the environment is not as dangerous, ever, as it is made to appear. Instead, tremendous numbers of people and vast amounts of money are manufacturing a dangerous environment. In fact, in the 1960s a huge proportion of the national budget of the United States was dedicated to atomic war. But if they hadn't developed the threat, there would not have been one. The money that financed the horror was busy supporting the horror.

It is not to the advantage of those who get their income, appropriations or public interest from the amount of disturbance to make a peaceful environment.

A Calming Influence

Anything that tends to pacify or bring a calmed environment is resisted by the vested interest that backs a disturbed environment.

To the degree Scientology progresses in an area, the environment becomes calmer and calmer. Not less adventurous, but calmer. In other words, the potential hostile, unreachable, untouchable threat in the environment reduces. Somebody who knows more about himself, others and life, and who gets a better grip on situations, has less trouble in his environment. Even though it may only be reduced slightly, it is reduced.

Newspapers can have a depressing effect on a person.

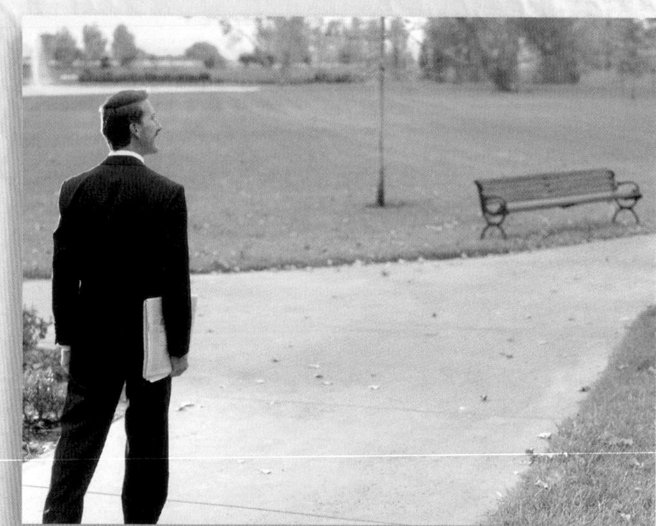

Since they deal largely in bad news, they present a generally bleak picture of the world.

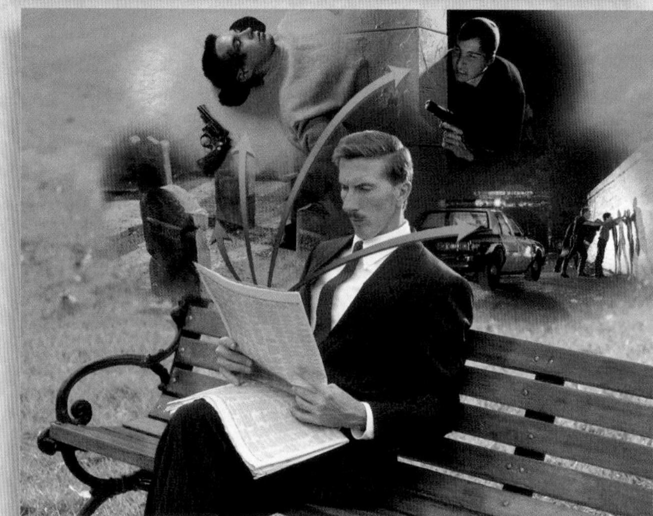

One can carry the bad news around with him and get a negatively distorted idea of his surroundings, which may, in reality, actually be quite calm.

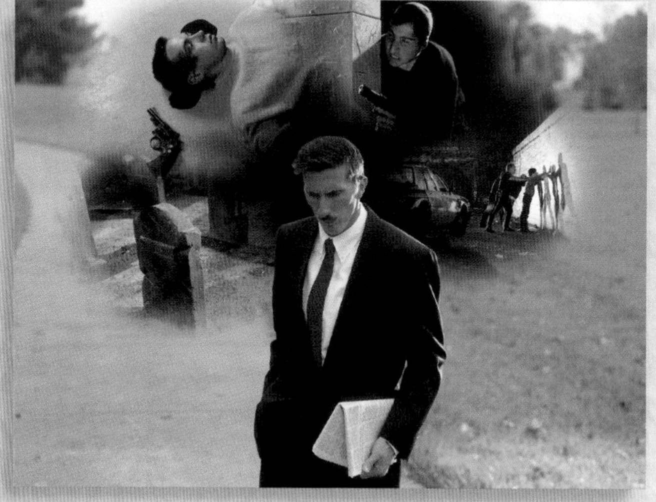

Even somebody who has heard very little of Scientology has less turmoil in his environment. An individual, less threatened by the environment, tends to resurge. He gets less apathetic. He thinks he can do more about life. He can reach outward a little further; therefore he can exert a calming influence upon his immediate environment.

As that progressed forward, more and more individuals would be produced who could bring more and more calm to the environment or handle things better and better. It is only the things which aren't handled which are chaotic. It would result in a situation where the threat of the environment would die out. This overwhelming, overpowering environment would be tamer and tamer. People would be less and less afraid. You would have more and more opportunity of handling the actual problems that exist instead of people dreaming up problems in order to make some money off of it. It would be a different society.

The merchant of chaos does not like calming influences, however. He will fight anything which lessens disturbance in the environment.

For example, a wife has her husband completely under her thumb. She keeps him worried and upset morning, noon and night.

If the husband now engages in some activity which brings more calmness to the environment, there will be repercussions from the wife. If he is less disturbed, he is less under her control. She would naturally fight the thing that was making her husband more calm.

Yet disturbance and chaos fold up in the face of truth. It is lies which keep the universe continuously disturbed. The introduction of truth into a society would produce a calmer environment with less disturbance and therefore less that could be swindled out of that society by merchants of chaos.

Ways to Lessen the Threat

People are looking for a less threatening environment, or at least for a way to better endure the environment they live in.

The concept of the dangerous environment will be understandable to the individual no matter how crudely it is put to him. Just the concept that he considers the environment dangerous and overwhelming and he doesn't quite know where that danger or overwhelm is coming from is an enormous piece of wisdom.

Shrinking back from a very threatening environment that may overwhelm him at any moment, unable to progress forward into greater endurance or power to handle that threatening environment—this is his life.

An individual's health level, sanity level, activity level and ambition level are all monitored by *his* concept of the dangerousness of the environment.

There *are* real areas of danger in the environment, but there are also areas being made to *seem* more dangerous than they really are.

Thus, if a person is marched forward into these sectors of his environment and gotten to inspect them, he can perceive for himself that the environment is not as dangerous as it is being made to seem. And with increased confidence in his ability to handle at least *those* sectors of his environment, his health, well-being, sanity and activity levels will rise as well.

A number of simple procedures can help a person increase his command over his environment. The master question of all these techniques is "What part of the environment isn't threatening?" If one can get him to differentiate and find out there are some parts of the environment that *aren't* threatening, he will make considerable gain.

What is the individual's expectancy at this level? It may be this low—that he just won't be so frightened when the doorbell rings. This sounds like a tiny improvement; nevertheless, it would be quite real to him.

He might just want to handle it so that when he wakes up in the morning he doesn't have an agonizing feeling that something horrible is going to happen if he gets out of bed—and maybe he doesn't even expect that feeling to completely disappear, but hopes it will diminish.

These would be real gains to him, and he would be very happy with them. The funny thing is, the gains he will actually experience will, in most cases, greatly exceed expectations.

Here are the procedures you can use to accomplish this:

1. Find Something That Isn't Being a Threat

When a person gets too upset or confused, one can have him look around his environment and find something that isn't being a threat to him. Carry on doing this until the person is very happy or relieved and has had a realization about himself, the environment or life in general.

A person can also use this technique directly on himself. For example, an individual can be in his office and very worried about something. He may be sitting at his desk with papers piling up. Everything seems to be in a high uproar, and he feels completely overwhelmed. The person himself ought to be able to look at the papers on his desk (the source of the threat) and find something about them that is not a threat. By making such a discovery, the threat will balance out.

2. Don't Read the Newspaper

This is very simple. Tell the person, "**Don't read the newspapers for two weeks and see if you don't feel better.**"

If he doesn't read the newspapers for two weeks, of course he will feel better.

Then tell him, "**Now read the newspaper for a week, and at the end of that week you will find you feel worse. Then make up your mind whether or not you ought to pay any attention to the newspapers.**"

This could be proposed to the person as a simple experiment. It isn't even an expensive experiment—as a matter of fact, it is cheaper *not* to buy newspapers than to buy them.

This is a simple action, but a very effective one which can markedly change a person's outlook on life.

3. Take a Walk

Another way of having a person look at the environment and discover that it isn't so threatening is a technique called "**Take a Walk.**" If a person feels bad, have him take a walk and look at things as he walks.

The effort here is just to get the individual to inspect the environment and find out that there is some slightly greater security in it. One just wants the person to look and find out if the environment is as threatening as it appears to be.

"Take a walk and look at things" is the mildest advice that you could possibly give anybody, and is almost certain to produce a result if the person will do it. It is quite effective.

4. Find Something That Isn't Hostile to You

There are people who feel as if everybody in the environment is hostile to them.

For a person like this, there is another technique that will lessen his fears.

One could ask any of several different questions, depending upon the situation. Examples of these are:

"Find something people say or do around here that isn't hostile to you."

"Is there one person in the company who isn't actively hostile to you?"

"Is there anything said today that wasn't directly and immediately hostile to you?"

Ask the person one of the above questions (or a similar question with a wording more appropriate to the person's situation). For example, ask him, **"Is there one person in the company who isn't actively hostile to you?"**

Continue this until the person feels better, is happier and has had a realization about himself, the environment or life in general.

5. Handling a Loss

A fellow who has just lost his girl, or a woman who has lost her man, feels the horrible sadness and loss it imparts to everything. Actually, everything in the environment will "talk" to him or her about the lost love. For some period of time, it will be impossible for him to look around and not be reminded of this person.

When one's concentration has been heavily on an individual, it is sometimes almost heroically difficult to not associate everything with that person. The trick is to find something that isn't reminding the person of the one he or she lost. One might have to search a long way to find something.

This is the way to recover from a love affair. The situation is in actual fact a simple one: the individual has identified everything in the environment with his unrest. By directing the person's attention to things in the environment which are not so connected and making him find things which are not actively reminding him, one gets a *differentiation* where an *identification* existed before. And where differentiation exists, intelligence and judgment can return.

Do the following:

Tell the person you are going to help them. Tell him or her, "**Find something that isn't reminding you of ________ (name of person he or she lost).**"

Repeat the command, getting the person to find something else that is not reminding him or her of the person until he or she has a realization and feels better about the situation.

This simple procedure can help the person recover from his or her lost love and begin to live again.

6. Arranging One's Life

By having an individual plan a life by which he could live calmly and unthreatened, the life he is living becomes less threatening.

Let us take, for example, the poor fellow who is on a complete treadmill: he has to keep his job, even though it doesn't pay enough and there's no opportunity of advancement, because if he loses it, he feels he won't be able to get another one or he won't be able to survive. This man is in a box of his own making, and he finds that environment very hostile.

Get him to plan a life which would not be so threatening, no matter how imaginative or seemingly unattainable his plan, and he will be able to go on working at his job much more happily and feeling much calmer.

7. Knocking Off Things That Upset One

There is another action which consists of simply having the person stop doing things or associating with people that upset him.

One could say, "**Knock off some of those things in your life that make you upset.**"

"**Who upsets you? Well, don't talk to them for a while.**"

"**What activities leave you feeling worse? Well, just don't do them for a while.**"

"**What things in the environment *aren't* really a threat to you? All right, have you got some of those? Fine. Associate with those. Pay more attention to them.**"

This will benefit the person more than one might imagine.

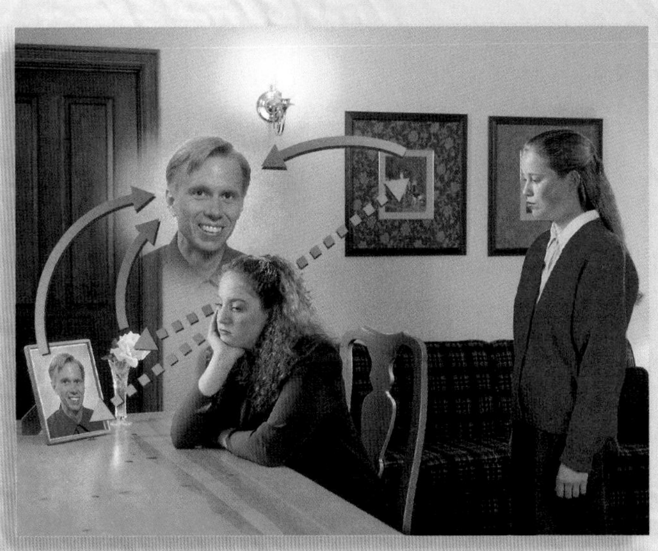

A broken love affair can result in the person being in a state of mind where everything in the environment is a reminder of the loss.

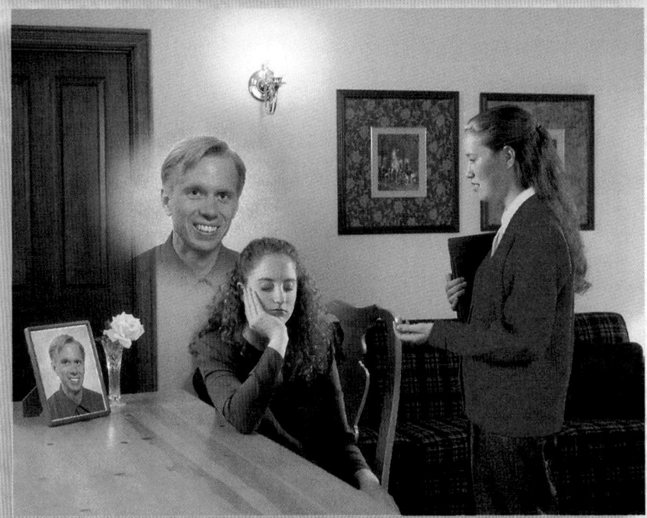

But a person can be helped to recover. If one can find something in the surroundings which does not bring to mind the lost love …

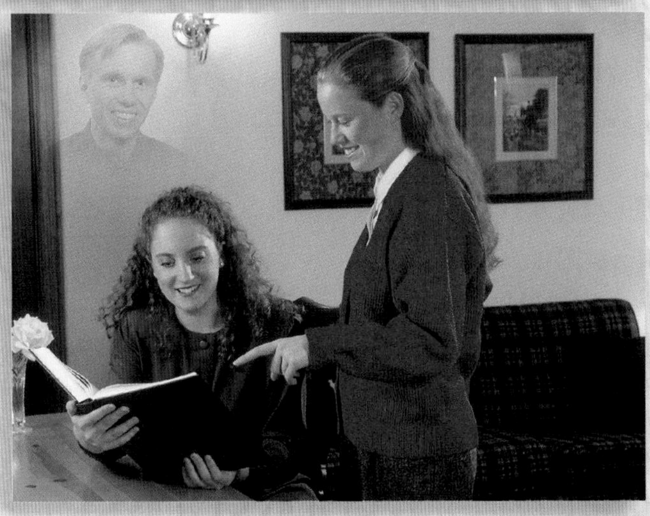

… the person's attention can become unstuck, which allows her to feel better.

CONFRONT

One can safely assume that there is always *something* about a situation the person can confront—by which we mean easily face without flinching.

This is a principle which forms the basis of a solution for many who are overwhelmed by their environments.

For example, a social worker is visiting Mrs. O'Leary in her tenement. Mrs. O'Leary has an awful lot of problems and she is telling them to the social worker: her husband gets drunk all the time and never brings home any pay and the furniture is all broken and the children have no clothes and it's impossible to keep the place clean and so forth.

The social worker can really get somewhere if he can find something that can be confronted by the person he is trying to help and get him to actually do it. Although this sounds very simple and innocuous, it has fantastic workability.

People working in the field of social work usually fail to simply adjudicate the problems involved in the situation and then do something about those problems that *can* have something done about them and that somebody *can* confront to do something about them. So as a net result, a social worker doesn't succeed because he never gives anybody anything they can do.

The well-meaning social worker says, "What you want to do, Mrs. O'Leary, is clean this whole place up, scrub it down from top to bottom—after all, we've given you soap. And get your children cleaned up and put in those nice new dresses we sent you. Now, I'll have a talk with your husband concerning his drinking."

At this point, even if Mrs. O'Leary *would* have cleaned up the whole place and put the children in the clean clothes, she and the social worker part company violently. The social worker has just told Mrs. O'Leary something that she *knows* by experience *cannot be done*. Nobody can talk to her husband about his drinking. She doesn't think that even a full-scale attack by the United States Army could do anything about Mr. O'Leary's drinking. Nothing the social worker does or says from this point on is going to have any effect on Mrs. O'Leary.

Suppose, however, that the social worker listened carefully to Mrs. O'Leary and then applied the principle of giving her something she could actually confront handling. He might have noticed that during their conversation, Mrs. O'Leary had emptied an ashtray for his cigarette. So he says to her, "I'll tell you what I would do. I would start in on this thing a little bit at a time, and I would get the place cleaned up. Now, why don't you keep the ashtrays emptied?" She might even get angry with him, but when the social worker leaves, Mrs. O'Leary will go around and empty the ashtrays.

Finding something that the person can confront handling is essential to getting his or her agreement to handle it. The first level of help is "There is something to be done about it," and the second level contains the element, *"that you can do."* Giving a person something he or she can confront and actually get done starts to give him the idea that the situation can be handled. The next thing you know, Mrs. O'Leary is liable to start getting ideas that she can even do something to make her husband stop drinking.

This principle of giving a person something they can confront doing is fabulously useful in many areas.

People often don't know how to get any further along in life. They *know* they cannot make any improvement in life, that it is impossible to be any better at all. But using this datum, one could easily demonstrate, even to a whole group, that it *is* possible to get better. It would be done in the following manner:

Start by advising the person you want to help, "**Write down on a piece of paper a short list of the problems you have in your life.**"

When he has done that, ask, "**Which one of those is the easiest for you to confront? Now write that down.**"

A person may be in a situation which seems overwhelming to him, so he does not do anything about it.

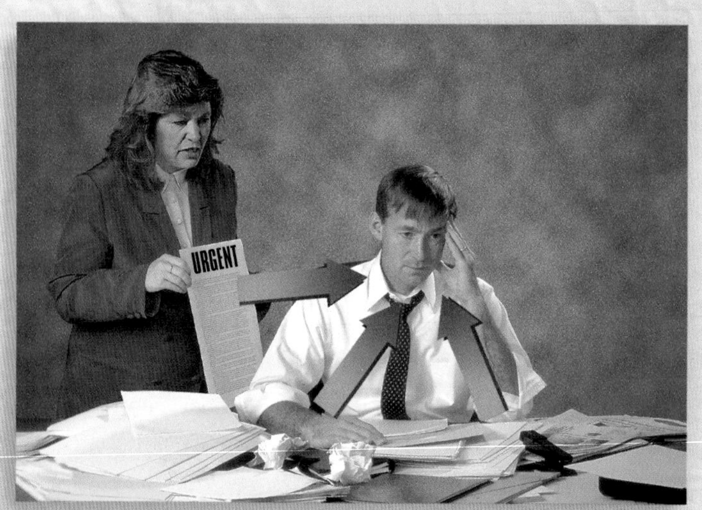

But he can be helped by finding something about the circumstances he can confront handling.

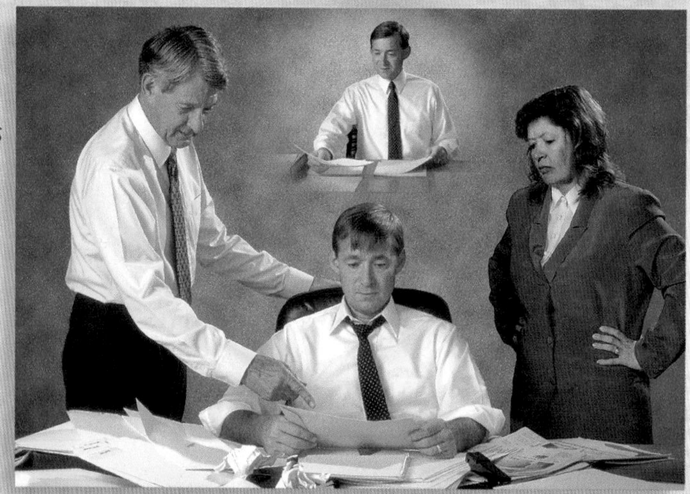

If he can handle one aspect of the situation, his outlook about it can be markedly improved, and he will be able to handle it fully.

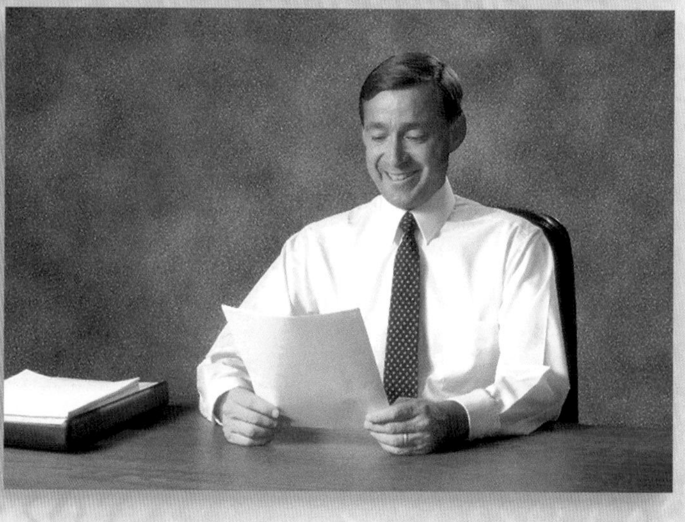

Then tell him, "**Write down what you absolutely know for sure you could do about that last thing you wrote down.**"

And finally, tell him, "**Now, you see what you've written down at the bottom of this page? Do it!**"

Use of this principle can be of enormous assistance to people—in social work, in leading groups, in teaching and lecturing and many other areas.

Don't tell people about problems that they know they cannot do anything about and expect them to be enthusiastic about accomplishing anything.

Neither the problem being pointed out nor the suggested solution must exceed the ability to confront on the part of the person to whom it is being addressed. The easiest thing to relay is an idea, but the idea must not violate the potential to confront of the individual who is expected to execute it.

The sequence is: What is the situation? What part of the situation is potentially confrontable? And what part of that situation will somebody do something about?

Most people stop giving advice because the advice they give is never followed. But if one followed the rules laid out here, he would be a very successful adviser.

Since what the people are being asked to do is confrontable to them, they will be able to handle their problems and succeed at it. As a result, they will be able to see and confront more of their difficulties, and the above sequence can be repeated. A new review of the general situation will find that they have an improved idea of what is potentially confrontable amongst their problems.

The only difficulty one can encounter is that people sometimes start moving with too great a confidence and, like a baby who has just learned how to walk, go tearing across the room at a high run. Unfortunately, they usually fall on their faces on about the third step. They can get overly ambitious. That has to be taken into consideration, and the person warned with, "Don't do any more than this right now."

If you make it your business to (1) rapidly get an estimation of what a person thinks is wrong; then (2) find out which one of these points he can confront; then (3) find out what he is going to do about that point that he thinks he can do; and then (4) get him to do it, and at that point you become terribly insistent on the subject of *getting that point done,* you will have agreement with a capital "A" every time.

THE REAL WORLD

The world simply must not be a better place, according to the chaos merchant. And so long as politicians move upward on scandal, the military establishment gets fatter on more war, and the media profits from the spread of bad news, there will continue to be those who thrive on chaos.

But this is the created world, not the real world. Behind all this upset and disturbance there exists a calmer environment. It is one in which man can live and feel better, a world where people do heroic deeds and neighbors help each other and people overcome vast odds to excel.

The differences between a competent person and an incompetent person are demonstrated in his environment (surroundings). A person is either the effect of his environment or is able to have an effect upon his environment.

The nineteenth-century psychologist preached that man had to "adjust to his environment." This false datum helped begin a racial degeneration.

The truth is that man is as successful as he adjusts the environment to him.

Being competent means the ability to control and operate the things in the environment and the environment itself.

By recognizing the work of the chaos merchant, people can begin to better control their environments. ■

Test Your Understanding

Answer the following questions about handling the dangerous environment. Refer back to the chapter to check your answers. If you need to, review the chapter. Going over the material several times will increase your certainty and help you better apply it.

- ❑ *How is the environment being made to appear more dangerous than it really is?*
- ❑ *What happens when a person has too much challenge in his environment?*
- ❑ *What is a merchant of chaos?*
- ❑ *What does a person's ability to confront have to do with what he can improve in his life?*

Practical Exercises

Here are exercises relating to handling the dangerous environment. Doing these exercises will increase your understanding of how to help people deal with the problems and difficulties in their lives.

1 Look around and find examples where the environment is made to look more dangerous than it really is. Do this until you are certain that the environment is being made to look more dangerous than it really is.

2 Take a walk around the block, looking at things as you walk. After taking the walk, compare how threatening the environment seemed before and how it seems now.

3 Find a friend or family member who is feeling overwhelmed by the environment and help them, using one of the seven techniques given in the section "Ways to Lessen the Threat."

4 Help a person by getting him to write down a short list of the problems he has in his life. Then get him to find which one of those is easiest for him to confront. Get him to write that down. Then get him to write down what he absolutely knows for sure he could do about the last thing he wrote down. Now, get him to take the last thing he wrote down and do it.

Results from Application

L. Ron Hubbard has provided simple actions one can take to help others who are overwhelmed by life. People who use these find that they have in their hands very basic but highly effective weapons against the cynical generality or hopeless attitude that "everything is bad everywhere" and there is no hope for man or anything else.

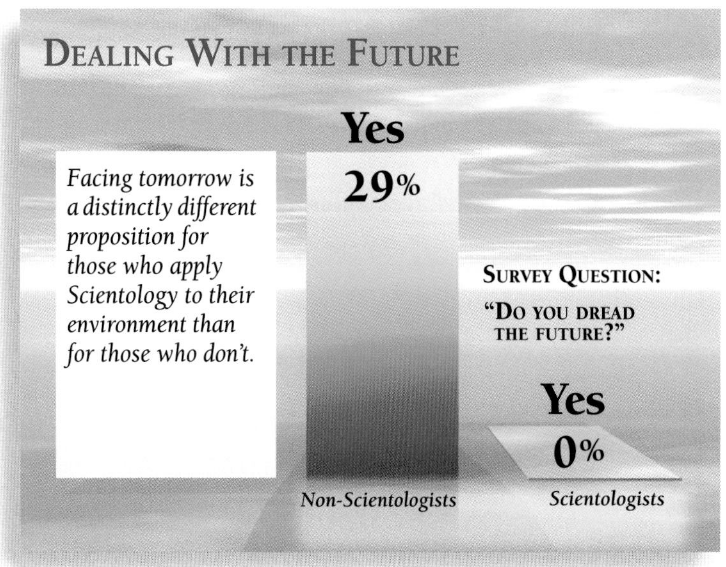
Dealing With the Future
Facing tomorrow is a distinctly different proposition for those who apply Scientology to their environment than for those who don't.
Yes
29%
Non-Scientologists
Survey Question:
"Do you dread the future?"
Yes
0%
Scientologists

Perhaps the most commented-upon aspect of this activity—helping another become more causative over a dangerous environment—is that it really takes very little to help one's fellow man and give him some hope. This fact is reflected in the stories below.

A woman who had studied Mr. Hubbard's discoveries about how to help someone confront and handle a dangerous environment said this about the technology's effectiveness:

"My friend came to see me the night after I finished studying this data and she was full of problems that she had no solutions for. Applying L. Ron Hubbard's technology, I asked her to write down a list of things that were problems in her life, then note which one she thought was the easiest to confront. Then I asked her to write down what she knew for ***sure*** *she could do about that one. The effect of these questions was amazing. She immediately got very bright, whereas she had been very depressed when she first walked in. She dashed out to handle the problem at once, though I had never before seen this woman actually attempt to* ***handle*** *anything in her life—prior to this she had only complained! I saw once again how, with Scientology, a little goes a long way!"*

Continuously getting overwhelmed in her work was a "normal" part of life for a woman from Omaha, Nebraska, until she received some help from a friend.

"I would habitually build up more and more things to do and never finish any of them. Then after a few weeks I would end up in tears, feeling overwhelmed from 'overwork.' The world would look pretty awful and the people in it would all seem pretty mean to me. A friend told me how to write down a list of my problems, pick out the one I could face, then do something about that. From that point on I gained control over situations just by taking one problem at a time, creatively solving that one and then going on to the next, instead of drowning

in how 'impossible' it all seemed. The world did not look so mean after that because I was in charge. This was the first piece of Scientology data anyone had ever applied to me and I have used this in my life ever since. Now I am able to enjoy my work much more."

Unable to tolerate seeing another in distress without doing something about it, a California woman used Mr. Hubbard's technology to help others in trying circumstances. She had many successes with these simple solutions.

"I helped a man and his wife whom I met on the bus one day. The wife was in tears for some reason. I got her to look at those things in the environment which she felt were not hostile to her. She became bright and started working out how she could solve her own problems. Another time I helped a man, who had been very upset and hysterical in his environment, to move to a new place and to take daily walks. He became much saner and started to reach out and help others from his position as a schoolteacher. I have also helped my own family members through a time of upset over the death of my grandmother, using simple processes. Surprisingly, this brought stability and a sense of calmness, even during this trying time. This is simple technology to use that just makes life easier and much more pleasant for others."

Prior to reading any of Mr. Hubbard's technology, a woman in Hawaii thought the world was full of people who couldn't be trusted. Here is what happened when she learned the true source of the dangers in the environment:

"I realized that I had been looking at everything from someone else's point of view. By changing my point of view, it was a whole different world. It was **not** *the world I had previously been taught about at all! This changed so many things for me—I actually started living.*

"I was able to observe better, just by looking at what was really there. The environment wasn't so dangerous anymore, not so frightening. I had been taught at a very young age that you must keep your mouth shut and do what you're told and be **very** *careful because you can't trust anybody. When I actually* **looked,** *I found there were a lot of people around me who were good. This opened up my communication because I could say, 'That's not true—look at this, this and that.'*

"I used this Scientology data on a radio show. People would call in and ask questions. I got one fellow to realize that he **could** *actually make it in life just by observing that others around him were surviving and that he had been fed false information. He is now succeeding in life. His world, like mine, changed from dull gray to a place full of bright colors and enjoyment."*

Suggestions for Further Study

Dealing with the threatening aspect of the environment represents only one facet of L. Ron Hubbard's technology for viewing and handling everyday life. Many fundamental discoveries exist in Scientology which shed new light on our society and provide tools to improve one's survival in it. Studying the materials listed here can help you understand the environment better and handle it more effectively.

Scientology: A New Slant on Life

Contains thirty essays by L. Ron Hubbard which can expand one's understanding of his relationship to his environment and the factors involved in living well and successfully. In a direct, easily understood style, Mr. Hubbard discourses on subjects such as bringing order to life, the race against man's savage instincts, justice, greatness and over twenty other important topics. The knowledge available in this book provides a clearer, more secure view of the world and life.

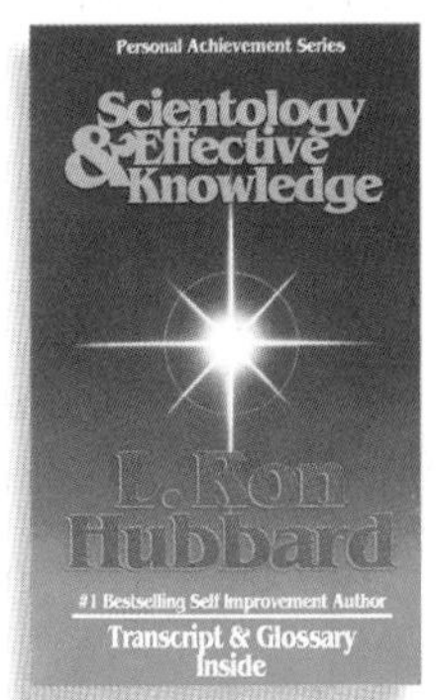

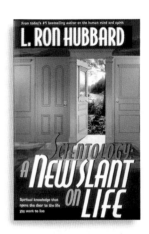

Scientology and Effective Knowledge

In this hour-long recorded lecture, Mr. Hubbard explains why man has remained so long at a loss for workable answers to existence. He explains that there is a level below blindness, which is *imagining* that one can see, and stresses the importance of actually observing the world and the environment to gain true understanding and increase one's effectiveness in dealing with life.

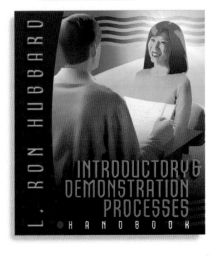

Introductory and Demonstration Processes Handbook

Containing numerous procedures (called "processes") by which specific situations in life can be alleviated, this book is a tool which no one who has an interest in helping others should be without. Contains more than two hundred processes to help people deal with and improve many different parts of their lives. Using these, you can help others to communicate better, resolve problems, become more aware of the environment, confront life and situations more ably and overcome many of the obstacles they might encounter. The handbook is fully indexed, with exact instructions for each process. Provides a complete array of tools for helping others. A course based on this book is available in Scientology organizations.

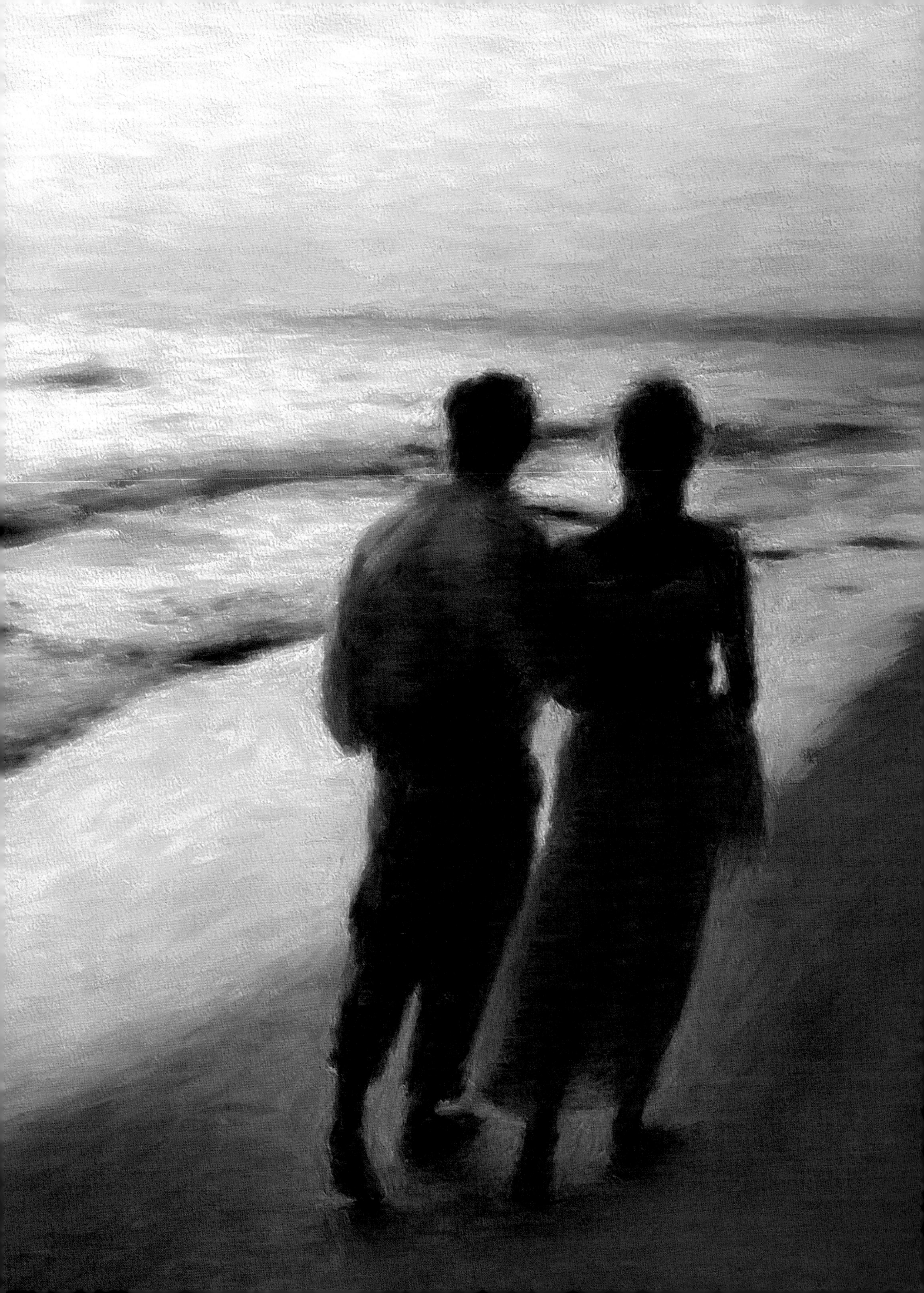

Chapter 13

Marriage

Where once the family was the stable foundation upon which all else was built, today its shattered remnants are the source of much of what troubles society. And while marriages still outnumber divorces, the gap is rapidly closing. Marriage is well on the way to becoming a failed institution.

L. Ron Hubbard wrote extensively on interpersonal relationships and much of it is applicable to this most personal of relationships. In this chapter you will discover methods to make a marriage work, why many marriages fail, how to discover if partners are well suited to each other, and how to save a failing marriage.

While our magazines are filled with the advice of "pop" psychologists, the trend has only worsened. Here are real solutions—workable solutions—that can be applied to improve any intimate relationship.

WHAT IS MARRIAGE?

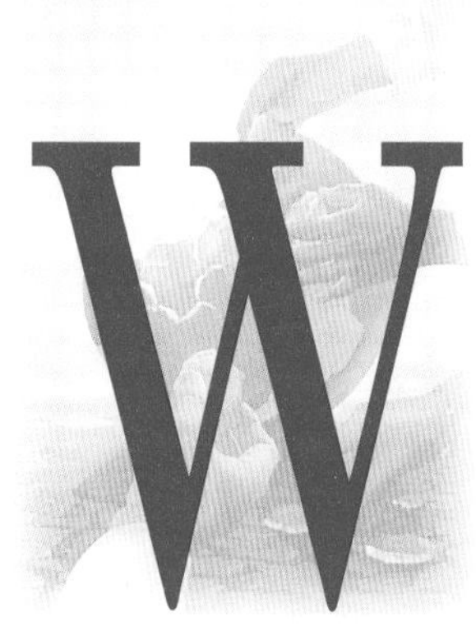

When someone begins on that arrangement called marriage, he is getting into something which is, to say the least, adventurous. When a couple get married, they are doing something they know nothing about. And, from all indications, when they have tried it more than once, they know no more about it the second time than they did the first.

Marriage is the foundation of the family unit. In this society and time, the family is the closest knit, self-perpetuating, self-protecting unit. It is necessary economically and otherwise to the society the way it is set up in present time. A culture will go by the boards if its basic building block, the family, is removed as a valid building block. So one can be fairly sure that he who destroys marriage destroys the civilization.

The marriage relationship, basically, is a *postulated* relationship. A *postulate* is a conclusion, decision or resolution about something. When people stop postulating a marriage, it ceases to exist. That is what happens to most marriages. It isn't the other way around. It isn't that all men are evil, so therefore, contracts such as marriage dissolve usually in infidelity and go all to pieces. That is not true. The reverse is true. When you have a purely postulated relationship, you have to continue to create it. And a family which doesn't continue to create itself as a family will cease to exist as a family. That's about all you need to know about it.

A marriage is something which exists primarily because each partner has postulated its existence and its continued existence. Only with this foundation in place are marriages successful.

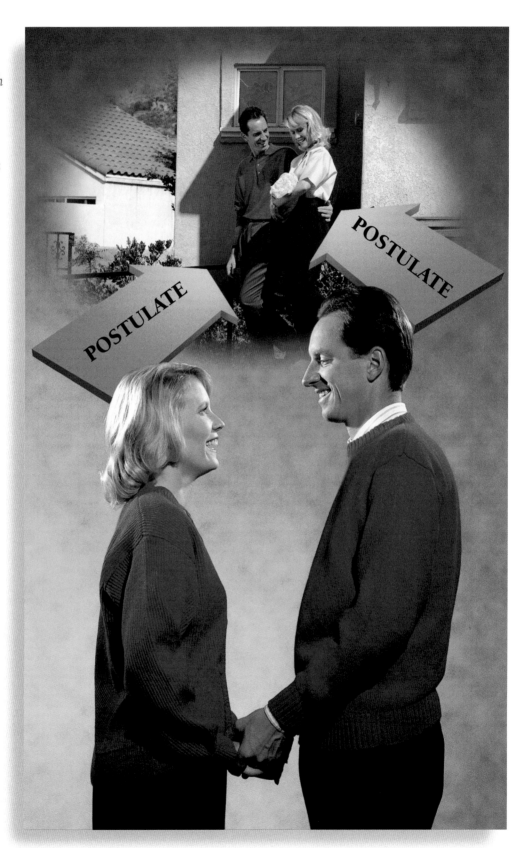

Where people are having trouble with marriage, it is because they are expecting it to run on automatic. They think it will hang together through no effort of their own; unfortunately, it won't. It has to be created.

Perhaps someone whose parents weren't making too good a go of it, looked at this and decided, "Now, look at that! This institution which is inherent in nature, which nothing will ever change, doesn't perpetuate itself and is not much good because it isn't hanging together."

He had a failure. He probably tried to postulate the family into a unit when he was very young. He was working at it, trying to get a Papa-loves-Mama thing going one way or the other, trying to show them that they had something to live for and so forth.

As a matter of fact, one of the reasons a child gets himself injured is to make his parents realize they have responsibilities for the family. Childhood illness and all this sort of thing occur directly after familial upsets.

Nonetheless, whether an individual had in his own parents a good example of a stable marriage or not, it has nothing to do with whether or not he can make a successful marriage.

If you think that everything else is rigged to perpetuate a marriage while you're not trying to keep it going, of course it will end up in destruction. But if you approach this with the realization that a marriage is something you have to postulate into existence and keep there, and when you stop working at it, it will cease, and if you know the technology contained in the remaining part of this chapter, you can make any marriage stick or you can recover any facet of any marriage, or plaster one back together again any way you want to. But it takes a little doing and it takes a little guts and that is an understatement.

Morals and Transgressions

Whenever people get together and operate as groups, they make agreements, whether actually stated or not, regarding what is right and what is wrong, what is moral and what is immoral—in other words, what will be contributive to survival and what will be destructive of survival. This is a moral code—a series of agreements to which a person has subscribed to guarantee the survival of the group. It doesn't matter what the size of the group is—whether it is a group of two people forming a marriage or a whole nation being formed—they enter into certain agreements.

When one or the other of the partners in a relationship or a marriage transgresses against the agreed-upon moral code, he or she often feels that he cannot tell the other about it. But these transgressions, unspoken but nevertheless transgressions, can gradually mount up and cause a disintegration of the relationship.

In Scientology, a harmful act or a transgression against the mores of the group is called an *overt act* or *overt.* When a person does something that is contrary to the moral code he has agreed to, or when he omits to do something that he *should* have done per that moral code, he has committed an overt act. An overt act violates what was agreed upon.

An unspoken, unannounced transgression against a moral code by which the person is bound is called a *withhold.* A withhold is, then, an overt act that a person committed that he or she is not talking about. Any withhold comes *after* an overt act.

These transgressions are the degree that a person has separated himself from free communication with the remainder of the group. If, for example, a man gambles away the money needed to pay the family bills, he has committed an overt act. And if he then hides this fact and never mentions it to his wife or family, he would be *pretending* to be part of the group while no longer being part of it, as he has broken the agreements that the group is based on. It is this factor which causes the disintegration of a group or a family or a marriage.

A marriage which has broken down into a super-separateness of overt acts and withholds is almost impossible to put back together by just postulating it into existence. After people have separated themselves out from each other, they have to "un-separate" themselves again.

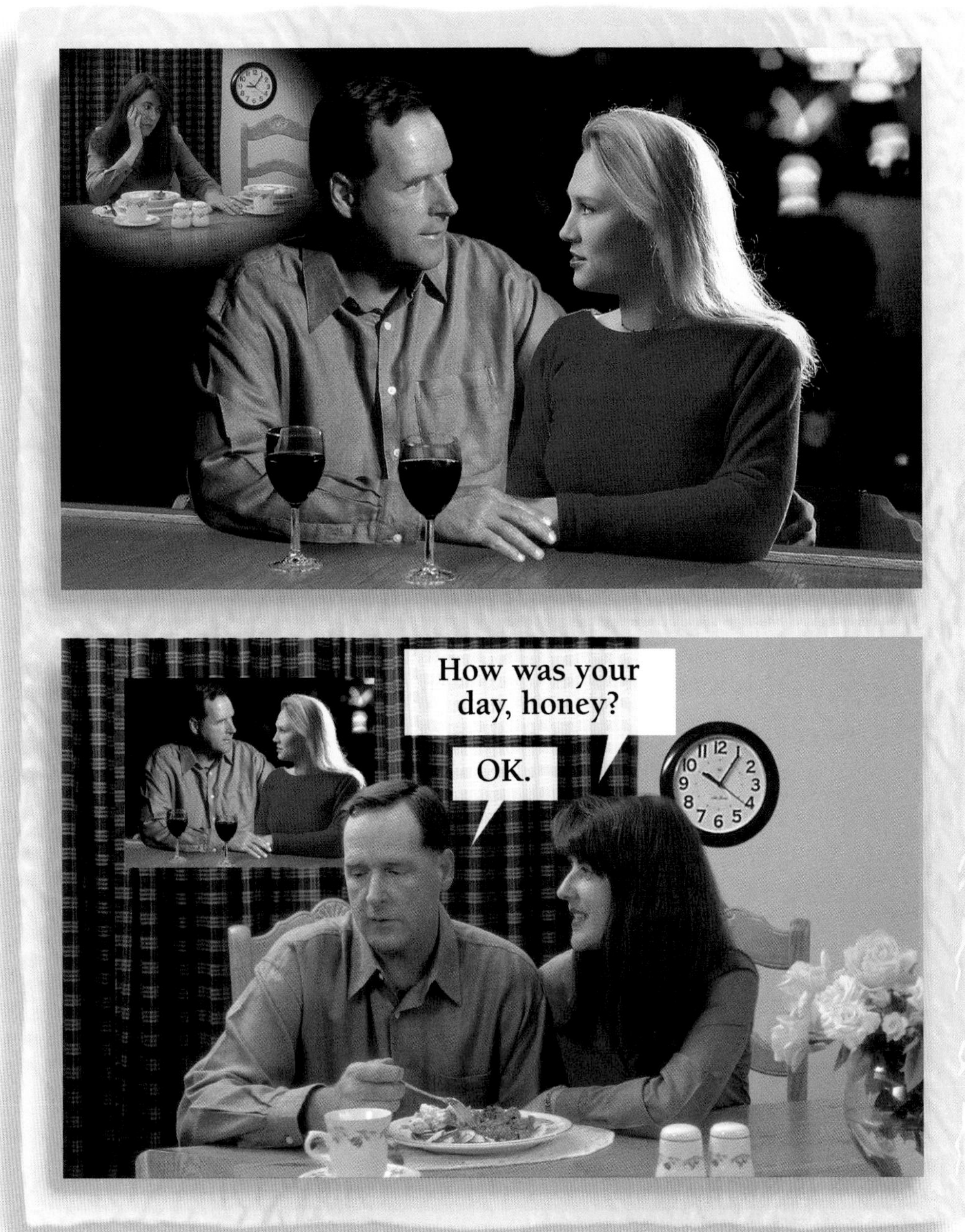

This action is a violation of the agreements of the marriage and is classified as an overt act.

The man is reluctant to communicate to his wife what he did. This is an example of a withhold.

Some who get married may think the way this is supposed to go is: on some bright June day this handsome brute (or not so handsome), and this beautiful girl (or not so beautiful), come together, and they say, "I do, till death do us part…" And they think they have now made a marriage. They haven't even started yet.

They have to find out how they look before breakfast. This arrangement has more to do with cosmetics and razor blades than anything else. They have to learn to live with each other if they can. And to some degree, they have wiped out, more or less by the act of getting married, what they were doing before that and they start from there.

What happens from there on out is what counts. But sometimes things they have done before, which they are violently withholding from each other, don't even let the marriage get started and forty-eight hours later their marriage is on the rocks because there is just too much overt and withhold before they even knew each other.

But even that one can be salvaged.

In a marriage which has ground on for years and years, overt acts and withholds can mount up until the partners "grow apart." It's considered to be traditional that at the end of three years, husbands and wives don't get any "kick" out of each other. This is sort of textbook and "all the psychologists know it," but they don't know *why.* It's the overt acts and withholds.

If at the end of three years this is the case, how about at the end of ten? By that time, many couples have just learned to endure. They are both in propitiation—a state of trying to appease each other or reduce the anger of each other. They are getting along somehow and they would rather have it that way than some other way; they would rather be married than not and they think they're making it okay. They don't think too much about the girl or the guy they should have married instead anymore. It's going along somehow.

Now into that relationship we can introduce one of the most startling assaults: we can clear up the marriage!

All a divorce is, or all an inclination or withdrawal is, is simply too many overts and withholds against the marital partner. It's as uncomplicated as that.

When a marital partner is straining and wanting to leave and saying, "I ought to go" or "I ought not to stay" or "I ought to do something else" or "We ought to split up" or "I'd be much better off if we hadn't," all of those rationales stem immediately from the overt acts and withholds of the partner making those rationales against the other partner.

Actually, the basic reason a person does this is that he's trying to protect the other partner from his own viciousness. So he says, "Well, I'd better leave," "We'd better break it up" or "We should cool it off." And that's usually the gradual approach of a marriage breakup—"Cool it off," "I ought to leave," "We should part." But we can take these things now and "uncool" them off.

Probably while you're trying to clean up a marriage between a couple, they will undoubtedly decide that it's all over and there's no reason to go on with it because one couldn't possibly... The thing that saves the day each time is to get each to remember what *he* himself or *she* herself did. If they just keep that thought firmly in mind, it will come through to a perfect completion.

Remedies

One way to alleviate this condition is to have the husband and wife write up their overts on and withholds from their marital partner. Each spouse writes down his overts and withholds on paper, giving the details of the specific time and place the overt/withhold was done, and what was done and/or withheld. When this is fully done, the person can experience relief and a return of responsibility. (This procedure of writing up one's overts and withholds is covered in full in Chapter 9, "Integrity and Honesty.")

There can be instances where writing up overts and withholds do not fully relieve the discord between the marriage partners. Where this occurs, one should contact a Scientology auditor to help rectify the matter. An auditor is someone who is trained and qualified to apply Scientology processing to individuals for their benefit. Processing is a special form of personal counseling, unique in Scientology, which helps someone view his own existence and which improves his abilities.

Another answer to restore a high level of communication between marital partners is Scientology Marriage Counseling. This is also provided by a Scientology auditor.

A husband and wife can utilize good, honest communication between themselves to create and continue a happy, fulfilling marriage. If both of the people involved work at keeping the agreements they have made and abide by the moral codes, and if the couple keeps the communication free and open between them, they will strengthen their relationship.

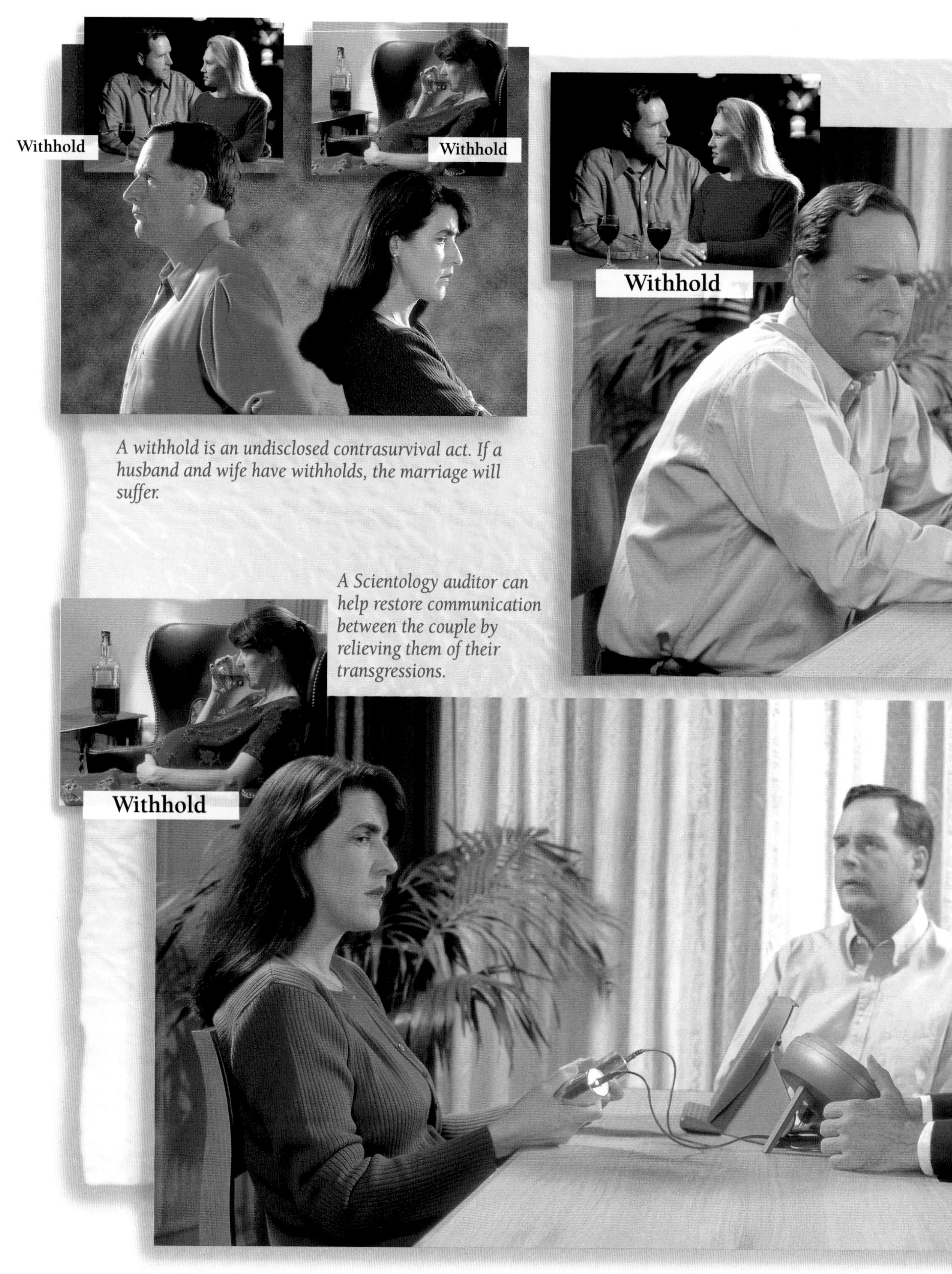

A withhold is an undisclosed contrasurvival act. If a husband and wife have withholds, the marriage will suffer.

A Scientology auditor can help restore communication between the couple by relieving them of their transgressions.

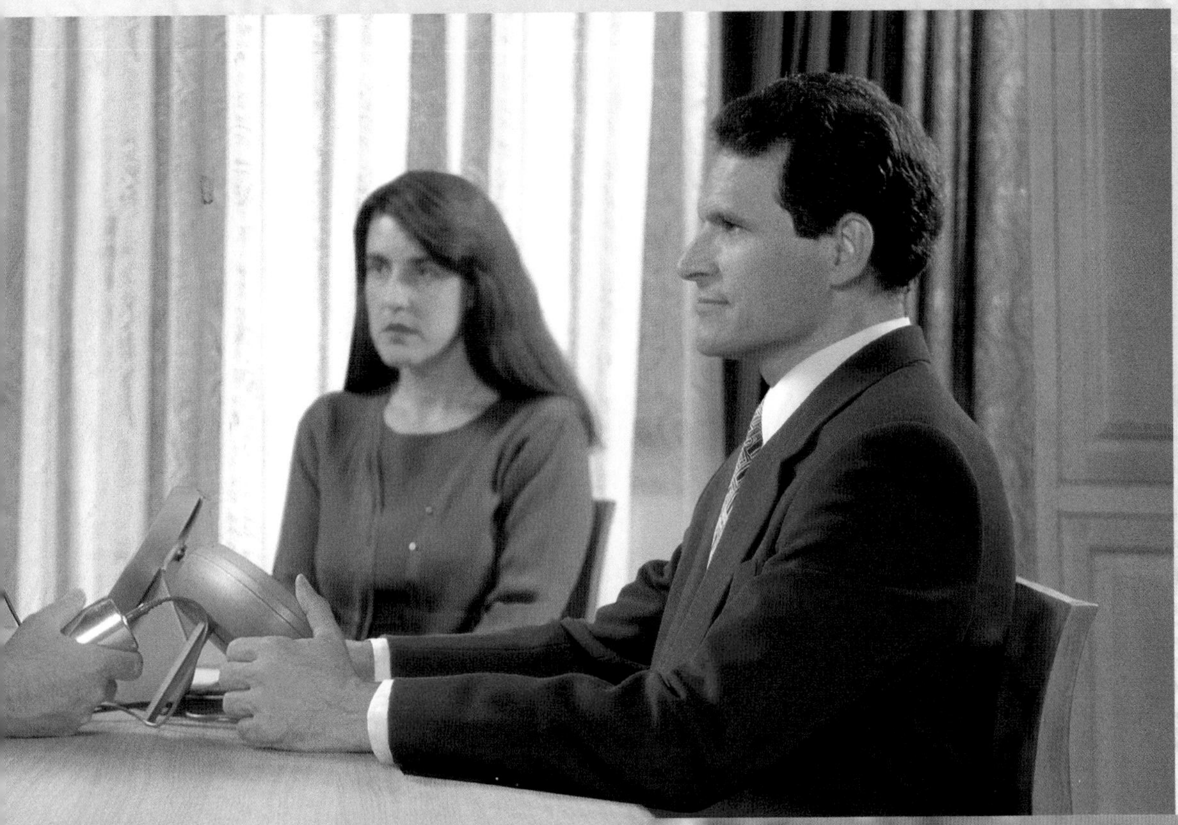

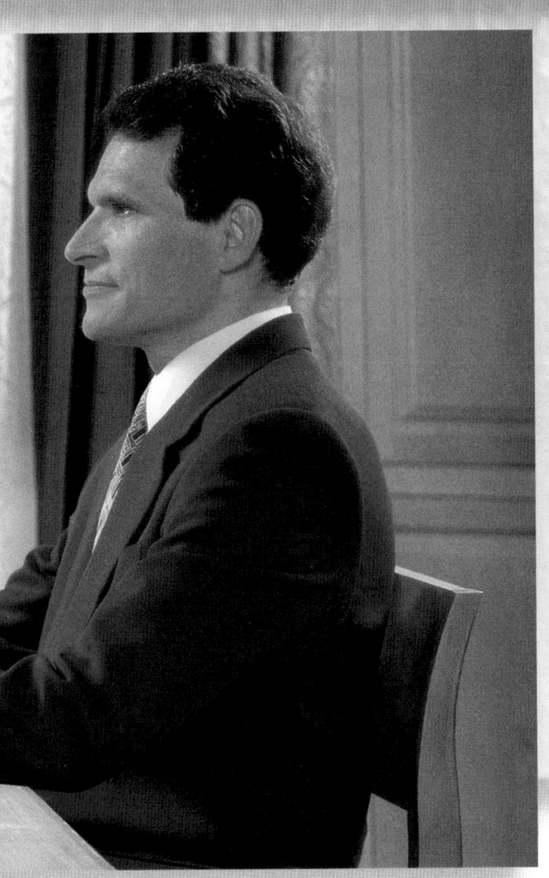

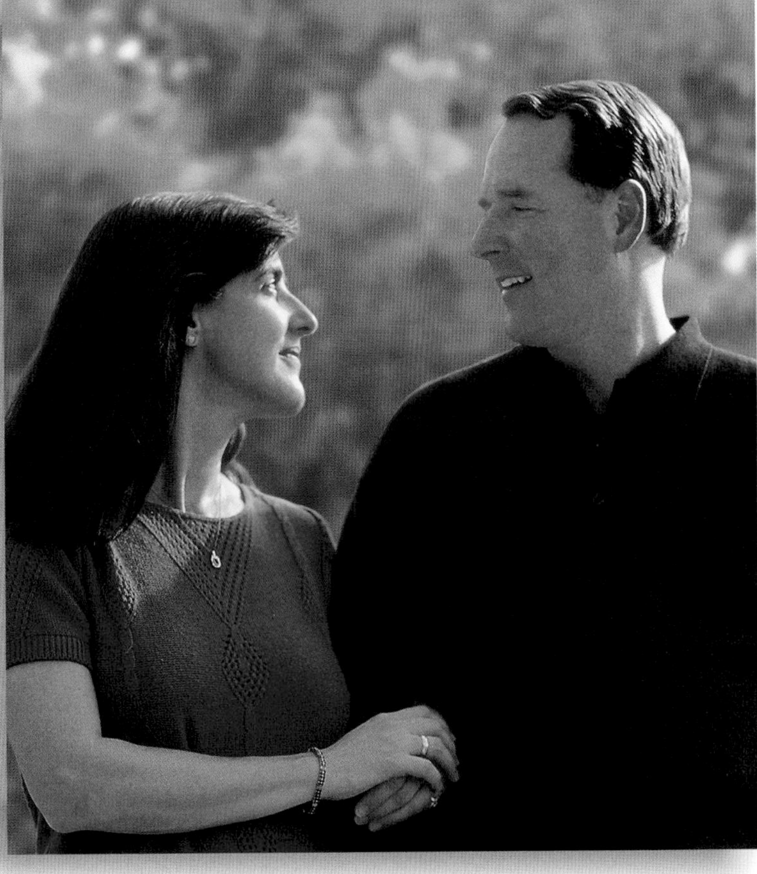

Communication that is free and open is vital to any lasting and fulfilling relationship.

COMMUNICATION IN MARRIAGE

There is another key factor in creating a successful marriage, or repairing one that has deteriorated. This also involves communication—the interchange of ideas between two individuals.

Communication is, in fact, the root of marital success from which a strong union can grow. Noncommunication is the rock on which the ship will bash out her keel.

In the first place, men and women aren't too careful "on whom they up and marry." In the absence of any basic training about neurosis, psychosis, or how to judge a good cook or a good wage earner, that tricky, treacherous and not always easy-to-identify thing called "love" is the sole guiding factor in the selection of mates. It is too much to expect of a society above the level of ants to be entirely practical about an institution as basically impractical as marriage. Thus, it is not amazing that the misselection of partners goes on with such abandon.

There are ways, however, not only to select a marriage partner, but also to guarantee the continuation of that marriage; and these ways are simple. They depend uniformly upon communication.

There should be some parity (equality) of intellect and sanity between a husband and wife for them to have a successful marriage. In Western culture, it is expected that the women shall have some command of the humanities (cultural studies such as language, literature, philosophy and art) and sciences. It is easy to establish the educational background of a potential marriage partner; it is not so easy to gauge their capability on the second dynamic or their sanity. (A dynamic is an urge toward existence in an area of life. The second dynamic is the urge toward existence as a future generation. It has two compartments: sex, and the family unit. Chapter 2 of this book covers the subject of the dynamics.)

In the past, efforts were made to establish sanity with inkblots, square blocks and tests with marbles to find out if anybody had lost any. The resulting figures had to be personally interpreted with a crystal ball and then reinterpreted for application.

In Scientology, there is a test for sanity and comparative sanity which is so simple that anyone can apply it. What is the "communication lag" of the individual? "Lag" means an interval between events. When asked a question, how long does it take him to answer? When a remark is addressed to him, how long does it take for him to register and return? The elapsed time is what is called the communication lag. The fast answer tells of the fast mind and the sane mind, providing the answer is a sequitur—something following logically; the slow answer tells of less ability and sanity. Marital partners who have the same communication lag will get along; where one partner is fast and one is slow, the situation will become unbearable to the fast partner and miserable to the slow one. Further, Scientology when applied will be more swiftly active in the case of the fast partner and so the imparity under processing will grow beyond either's ability to cope with the matter.

How to process a marriage and keep it a marriage is a problem a large number of auditors would like to have answered. It is not too difficult a problem. One simply takes the slow communication lag member of the team and processes that one first, for this will be the harder, longer case. By speeding up the slow one, parity is neared with the fast communication lag partner, and no objection will be offered. If the fast one is chosen for processing, or if both of them enter processing at the same time, the ratio will not be neared but widened and a marital breach will ensue.

The repair of a marriage which is going on the rocks does not always require the processing of the marriage partners. It may be that another family factor is in the scene. This may be in the person of a relative, such as the mother-in-law. How does one solve this factor? This, again, is simple. The mother-in-law, if there is trouble in the family, may be responsible for cutting communication channels or diverting communication. One or the other of the partners, then, is cut off the communication channel on which he belongs. He senses this and objects strenuously to it.

There is another way of cutting communication which happens when jealousy is involved. It is the largest factor in breaking up marriages. Jealousy comes about because of the insecurity of the jealous person and the jealousy may or may not have foundation. This person is afraid of hidden communication lines and will do anything to try to uncover them. This acts upon the other partner to make him feel that his communication lines are being cut; for he thinks himself entitled to have open communication lines, whereas his marital partner insists that he shut many of them. The resultant rows are violent, as represented by the fact that where jealousy exists in a profession such as acting, insurance companies will not issue policies—the suicide rate is too high.

A person who is jealous has something wrong on the subject of communications and, in selecting the partner to be processed first, the auditor should select the jealous person.

The subject of the application of Scientology to marriage could not be covered in many chapters, but here are given the basic clues to a successful marriage—Communicate!

ASSIST FOR A FIGHT WITH A SPOUSE

An "assist" is an action which can be done to alleviate a present time discomfort and help a person recover more rapidly from an accident, illness or upset.

When marital tensions have been left unaddressed and unhandled for some time, they can break out with violence. Severe fights can cause quite an emotional upset for either or both partners, and the threat of loss occasioned by such quarrels can be profound.

Where a fight has occurred between marital partners, the following assist can be used to help handle any resultant emotional trauma of husband and/or wife.

This assist may be done by marital partners on each other after a fight or may be used by another person to help one or both partners.

Procedure

1. Tell the person you are going to help them get over any adverse emotional reaction to the fight.

2. Have the person sit down in a comfortable chair across from you.

3. Say to the person, "Give me places where an angry (husband/wife) would be safe." For example, if you were doing this on a wife, you would say, "Give me places where an angry husband would be safe."

4. Get an answer from the person and acknowledge their answer, with a "Thank you," or "Good," etc.

5. Then say to the person, "Give me places where an angry (husband/wife) would find you safe."

6. Get an answer and acknowledge it.

7. Repeat steps 3–6 over and over again until the person is happy again and has had a realization of some kind—about himself, his spouse, the situation or just life in general.

When this occurs, tell the person "End of assist."

Be certain not to evaluate the person's answers for him or tell him how he should answer or what he should think about the situation. Do not berate the person for his answers. This is destructive and can halt all potential gain from the assist.

This assist is not a handling for the situation which *caused* the conflict or discord. Once the immediate upset is under control, the reasons for the fight should be ascertained. For instance, another party such as a relative or associate of a spouse may be creating friction between the marital partners. When this third party, usually hidden, is exposed as the source of the conflict, it resolves. This would be looked into and handled with the techniques covered in Chapter 8, "How to Resolve Conflicts." Whatever the cause of the difficulty, a full handling for it should be worked out and implemented.

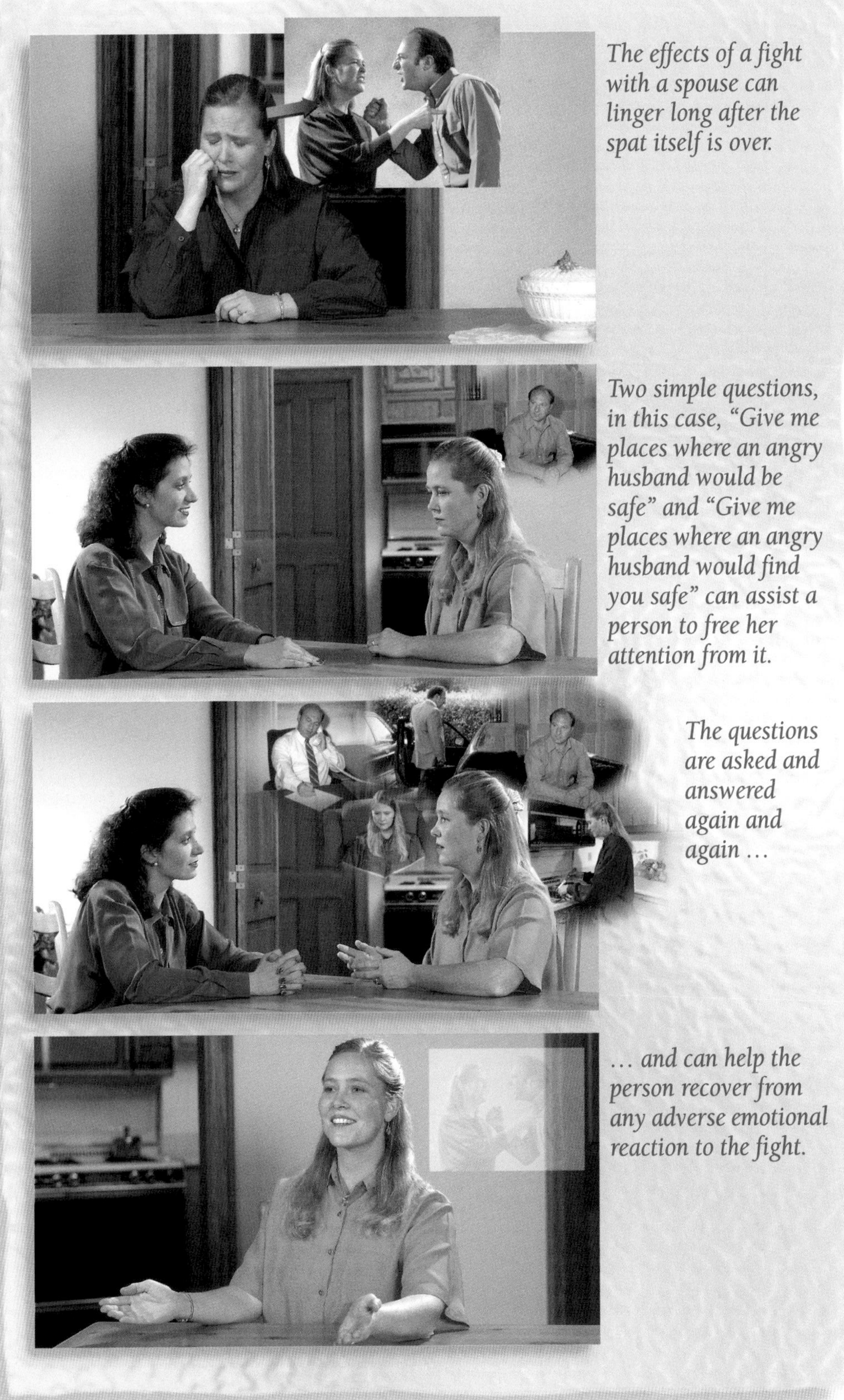

The effects of a fight with a spouse can linger long after the spat itself is over.

Two simple questions, in this case, "Give me places where an angry husband would be safe" and "Give me places where an angry husband would find you safe" can assist a person to free her attention from it.

The questions are asked and answered again and again …

… and can help the person recover from any adverse emotional reaction to the fight.

MAINTAINING A MARRIAGE

A fulfilling marriage has, as an essential ingredient, a high level of communication between the marital partners. When the relationship becomes strained, if they get the overts and withholds off on the marriage, it will be put back together again.

One shouldn't believe that it will go together without a few flying frying pans—you would be a perfectionist if you believed that was going to happen. And don't believe you can all put it together again in one night because the number of overts and withholds can take a little longer to detail.

A marriage can exist but not without two-way communication. And it cannot exist unless it continues to be postulated into existence by the parties involved. If we do these things, we have a marriage.

Marriage, then, would consist of putting together an association between people without overt acts and withholds, postulated into existence and continued for the mutual perpetuation and protection of the members and the group.

It is a very simple arrangement, actually, and a highly satisfactory arrangement if it continues to be simple, but a very complex arrangement if it doesn't continue to be.

It isn't that mothers-in-law are the people who always wreck marriages. You could say offhand that mothers-in-law should all be shot and so forth, and then we would have free marriages and it'd be nice. Or we could have woman's suffrage (their right to vote) and then marriage would be okay, or that we could have complete emancipation, instantaneous divorce, and marriage could be okay.

All of these social, sticky-plaster pieces of nonsense are just efforts to have a marriage without ever really having a marriage. None of these things ever made a marriage—quick divorce or preventing this or that.

The Chinese go the opposite—a marriage occurs but it really doesn't occur because the oldest man of the husband's family is still the head of the family, and the wife still serves the husband's mother, and it all gets very complicated.

We get surrounded by bunches of rules and that sort of thing. We don't care what rules they're surrounded by as long as there is free communication amongst the members of that family—that group. And if there's free communication amongst the members of that group, their affinity is sufficiently high to take the shocks and hammers and pounds of life, and life does hand out a few hammers and pounds and shocks now and again.

If the individuals connected with a family are not self-supportive, then these shocks can be rough one way or the other. The person does something and apparently thinks things are done to him, and he's trying to make it and can't. But on a self-supportive, mutually co-supportive basis, people have a better chance of making it than alone. And that's one of the basic philosophies on which marriage is based.

Of course, a little kid wouldn't make it at all, and none of us would have made it at all, if it hadn't have been for a marriage. The biological pattern of familial relationships and growth is the thing which will carry mankind on.

But a marriage can exist. A marriage, no matter how strained, can be put back together again. ■

TEST YOUR UNDERSTANDING

Answer the following questions about marriage. Refer back to the chapter to check your answers. If you need to, review the chapter. Going over the material several times will increase your certainty and help you better apply it.

- ❑ *Why does a marriage have to continue to be created?*
- ❑ *What is meant by "marriage is a postulated relationship"?*
- ❑ *What is a moral code?*
- ❑ *What causes the withdrawal of a marital partner from his spouse?*
- ❑ *What is communication lag?*

PRACTICAL EXERCISES

Here are exercises relating to marriage. Doing these exercises will help increase your understanding of what marriage is made up of and how a marriage can be improved.

1 Think of a married couple you know and determine what they are doing to create their marriage. Are they both working to keep the marriage created, or is one or the other or both doing less than they should? Think of or directly observe other married couples you know, and estimate how much the partners are doing to create the marriage, until it is very real to you that a marriage is something that is created.

2 Think of some situation you have seen or experienced where someone continued to create something and later ceased to create it.

3 Find someone who is having some kind of marital difficulty and help him or her by having the person read at least some of the data contained in this chapter.

4 Determine the communication lag of someone. Approach another person and ask him a simple question such as, "How many doors are there in this room?" or "What is the date?" Note how long it takes the person to answer the question you asked. From this determine whether the person has a long or short communication lag.

RESULTS FROM APPLICATION

People recognize that a happy marriage and family form a stable building block of society, despite invitations to follow the "modern" philosophy that divorces and single-parent families are inevitable, and marriage "doesn't work." The technology of Scientology is used by thousands to create and maintain successful marriages or to salvage them where they have gone off the rails. In a broad survey of Scientologists, none (0 percent) thought marriage as a state was undesirable and 91.2 percent thought it vital or desirable. Scientology marriages are not only successful, they are productive of stable family units. Only 2.8 percent of all Scientology married couples have no children, whereas in the United States, for example, 49 percent of all married couples have no children. Yet if you were to question an even apparently cynical person about the workability or desirability of marriage, you would probably find that the person does desire a happy marriage and that past failures, either experienced or observed, have buried the desire. Certainly, the following testimonies would seem to bear this out:

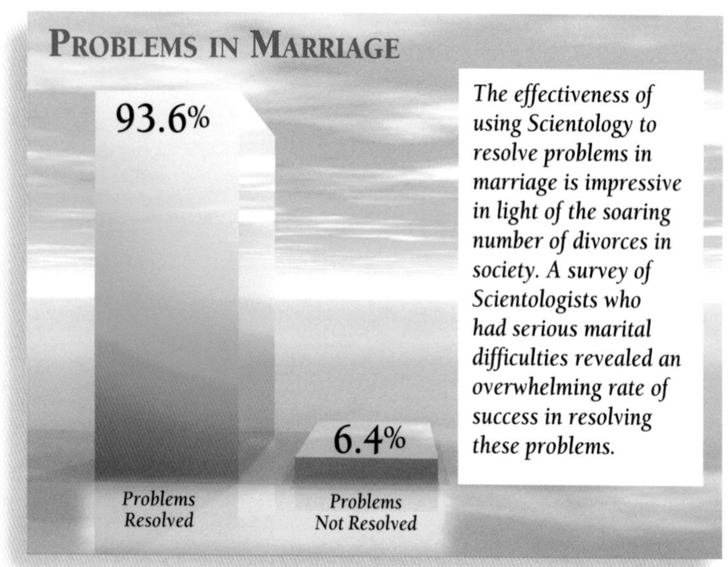

The effectiveness of using Scientology to resolve problems in marriage is impressive in light of the soaring number of divorces in society. A survey of Scientologists who had serious marital difficulties revealed an overwhelming rate of success in resolving these problems.

Two people were having extreme marital difficulties. The husband had absolutely decided to end the marriage and was already in the process of dividing their belongings. A Scientologist was asked by the wife to counsel them. This was the result:

"The wife really wanted to salvage their marriage but her husband didn't, although he did grudgingly agree to go through the counseling. When I first started counseling them, he was doing this as a mere 'formality.' But after a number of hours of counseling, this situation did a 180-degree turnaround and their marriage was salvaged. They were both very much in love again and were spared the trauma that accompanies divorce."

Nothing had worked for a couple from New York who were trying to save their marriage, so they agreed to separate. A friend sent them to a chaplain in a Scientology church for counseling and when that was complete the wife was overjoyed.

"Well, what can I say! I feel wonderful about myself and about my husband. Two weeks ago I couldn't see how we could stay together. Step by step, each of

us took responsibility for ourselves. Then we began to take responsibility for each other. We used to be in very good communication before we drifted apart, but since we completed this counseling, we finish each other's sentences and the same thing comes out of our mouths at the same time! We are both now new people. I owe my life 1,000 times over to the chaplain."

Study of some of Mr. Hubbard's writings on the subject of marriage helped a couple in Los Angeles improve their marriage.

"Each time we learned something new, one or the other of us would apply it. We found that we became a lot more positive in our communication with each other. As we learned more, it was like an adventure—every day of our marriage was something to look forward to, something very exciting, something we created each day. Frankly it had never been that good before. This was just from reading about it. We found each other again—and ourselves."

Through applying the technology of overts and withholds, a young woman from Santa Barbara, California, was able to salvage the marriage of her parents.

"My mother and stepfather were upset with one another and each was telling me bad things about the other. Although I was relatively new to Scientology at that time, one of the things I had learned from Scientology courses was the subject of harmful actions and what causes these and that man, as a being, was basically good.

"Having seen my mother leave one marriage and her second marriage, which started out brilliantly, begin to crumble, I decided to do something about it. I went over a few basics of communication with my parents, and the fact that the basic personality is basically good. I showed them what happens to a person when they commit harmful actions and the results and what makes a person critical about someone as well. They both listened in silence and then I went over the fact that in the beginning of their marriage they had told each other everything and were in very good communication—and how to restore that. When I was sure they fully understood I said that they could apply that to their marriage.

"After that, neither have said a critical thing about the other in the last thirteen years and they are still very much in love. Now they both communicate their love to me and each other and we have a very strong respect for each other."

Disclosing each other's overts and withholds was a matter of course to a Los Angeles married couple who are Scientologists. Talking about this, the husband said:

"Since we get off overts and withholds to each other as a basic action of keeping our marriage going well, we listen to each other. This is such a simple thing, but because of it, our marriage continues to flourish."

A couple in Orange County, California, who had not been getting along at all well together, applied the data in this chapter. The woman said:

"This is the best thing that ever happened in our marriage. I have so much love for my husband—more than ever before. It's the first time that I have been able to tell anyone anything and feel it's okay. There is so much more trust. There was so much unfinished communication that is now finished. Now I know that if anything comes up, our communication can handle it."

In Melbourne, Australia, a married couple were fighting chronically, so much so that even their children couldn't escape the unhappiness of their marriage. They were able to handle this situation using Mr. Hubbard's technology of handling overts and withholds.

"I feel greatly relieved of past upsets and am in **very** *good communication with my husband. The ridding of overts and withholds, no matter how big or small, brings back so much affinity, reality and communication. I can talk to my husband about anything and find that I have a lot more to say and have even broadened my communication to new topics not talked about before. The blow-ups are no longer there; if there is an issue, it is discussed calmly. The children no longer have their ears dunned and their communication has really come up too.* **Anyone** *who is having marriage trouble and can't communicate* **must must** *apply the technology of handling overts and withholds. I feel quite 'new' again spiritually, and heaps more happy."*

Despite a sincere wish to have a marriage that would last a lifetime, a young woman had already been divorced twice.

"I have been married three times. Before I found Mr. Hubbard's discoveries on marriage, I thought I was destined to go from marriage to marriage looking for the 'perfect' man. Boy, was I wrong about this! I have been married to my husband for seven years and because I now know **why** *I 'could never be happy with' my earlier husbands, and because I have the tools now to be* **really** *happy, I know this marriage is for the rest of our lives."*

Suggestions for Further Study

This chapter covers only a portion of the technology L. Ron Hubbard developed to help someone choose a marriage partner, improve an already successful marriage or repair one which is in trouble. Your understanding of and capability in this crucial area of life can be advanced through study of the following materials.

Starting a Successful Marriage

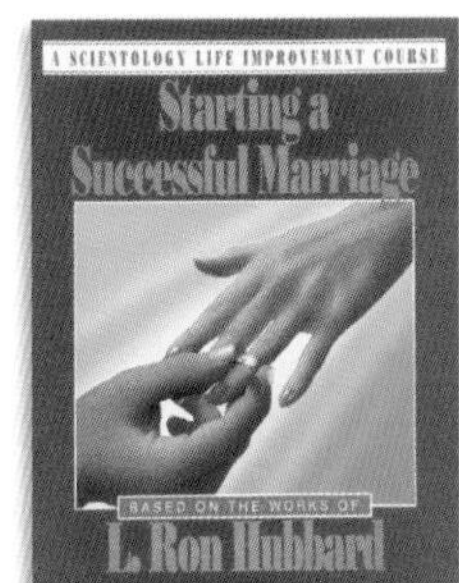

Finding a compatible partner is necessary to having a lasting, happy marriage. This course not only provides one with the technology to understand people, thus enabling one to more intelligently choose a partner, but also gives tools which can get a marriage off on the right foot and keep it moving in the proper direction. (Delivered in Scientology organizations.)

How to Maintain a Successful Marriage

Many people start well in marriage, but don't have the knowledge they need to actually expand and improve the relationship. Knowing how to communicate well, how to increase affinity and how to resolve disputes is vital for the success of a marriage. This course can prepare a couple against the pitfalls they might encounter, and teach them how to build a happy, stable relationship. (Delivered in Scientology organizations.)

How to Improve Your Marriage

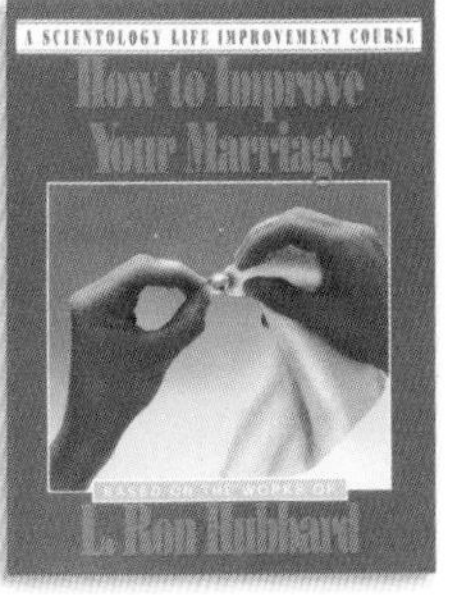

Couples sometimes encounter seemingly unresolvable situations in marriage. The only options, they feel, are to endure it somehow or else break it up. But there *are* ways to improve and even solve such situations. This course explains why couples become dissatisfied with each other, and gives practical handlings to restore love and mutual support in a marriage. (Delivered in Scientology organizations.)

Creating the Second Dynamic Lectures

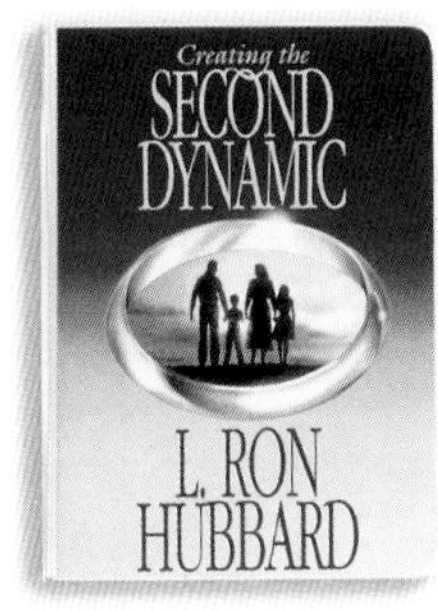

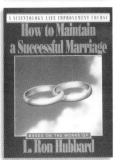

A dynamic is an urge toward existence in an area of life. The second dynamic is the urge toward existence as a future generation. It has two compartments: sex, and the family unit. In this series of lectures, Mr. Hubbard reveals how to straighten out second dynamic problems, including data that is vital to know in selecting a marriage partner in the first place, how to repair a failing marriage and how to live with and raise children. These lectures can help you achieve a much greater understanding of the second dynamic.

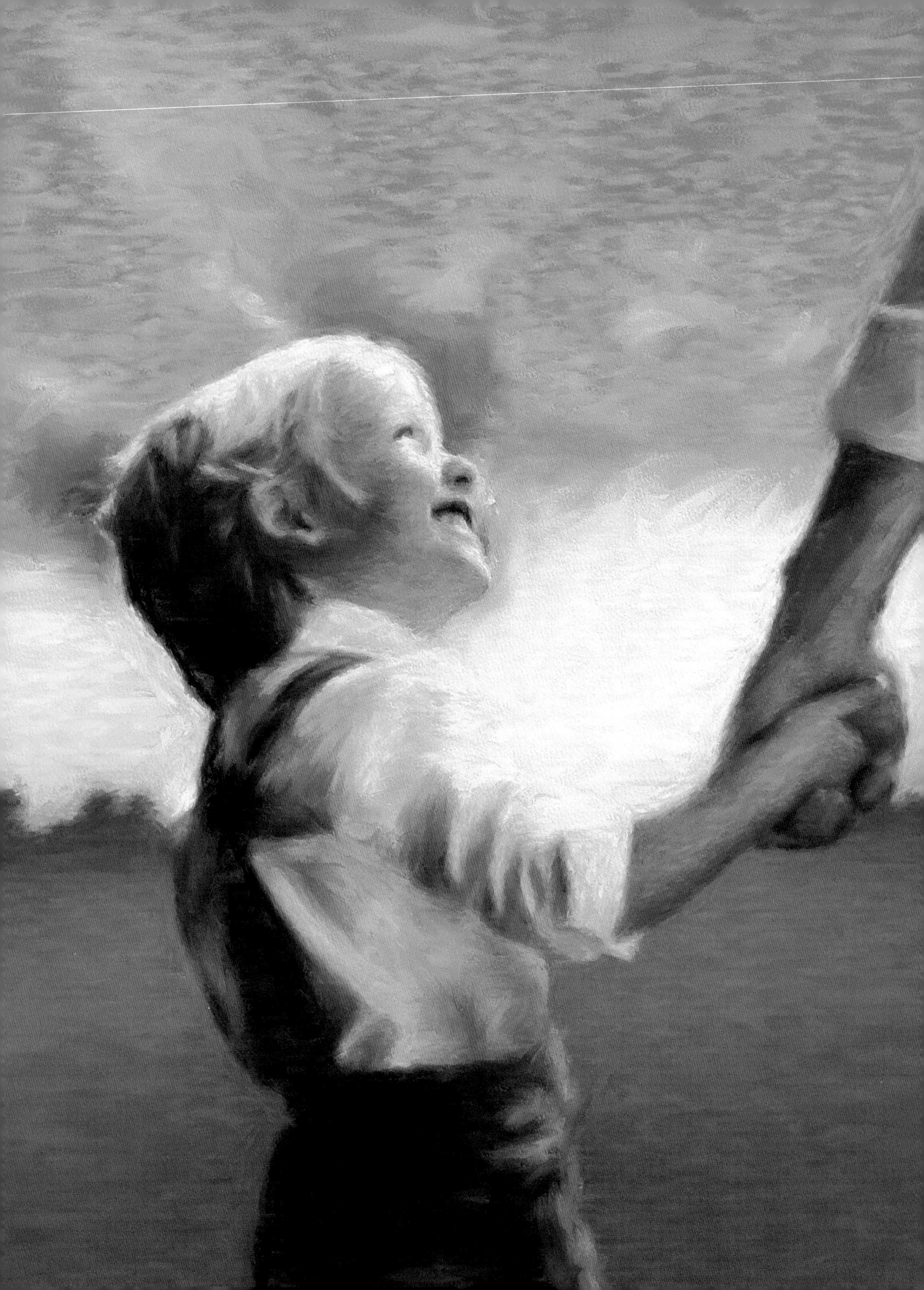

Chapter 14

CHILDREN

How to raise a happy, healthy child is not something most parents are taught. In fact, many just stumble through the entire process, albeit with the best intentions. Consequently, it is all too common to find an unhappy state of affairs in families, with constant friction between parents and children.

It is not a natural state of affairs. In fact, it can be avoided entirely. L. Ron Hubbard developed many methods to bring out the best in a child—and its parents. In this chapter, you will read about some of these methods and discover how to raise a child without breaking his spirit, how to have a child who is willing to contribute to the family, and how to help a child quickly get over the daily upsets and tribulations of life.

Raising children should be a joy. And can be. In fact, it can be one of the most rewarding of all human experiences. The application of Scientology principles to the bringing up of children can ensure that they are happy, loving and productive, and that they become valued members of the societies in which they live.

HOW TO LIVE WITH CHILDREN

The main problem with children is how to live with them. The adult is the problem in child raising, not the child. A good, stable adult with love and tolerance in his heart is about the best therapy a child can have.

The main consideration in raising children is the problem of training them without breaking them. You want to raise your child in such a way that you don't have to control him, so that he will be in full possession of himself at all times. Upon that depends his good behavior, his health, his sanity.

Children are not dogs. They can't be trained like dogs are trained. They are not controllable items. They are, and let's not overlook the point, men and women. A *child* is not a special species of animal distinct from man. A child is a man or a woman who has not attained full growth.

Any law which applies to the behavior of men and women applies to children.

How would you like to be pulled and hauled and ordered about and restrained from doing whatever you wanted to do? You'd resent it. The only reason a child "doesn't" resent it is because he's small. You'd half murder somebody who treated you, an adult, with the orders, contradiction and disrespect given to the average child. The child doesn't strike back because he isn't big enough. He gets your floor muddy, interrupts your nap, destroys the peace of the home instead. If he had equality with you in the matter of rights, he'd not ask for this "revenge." This "revenge" is standard child behavior.

Self-determinism is that state of being wherein the individual can or cannot be controlled by his environment according to his own choice. In that state the individual has self-confidence in his control of the material universe and other people.

A child has a right to his self-determinism. You say that if he is not restrained from pulling things down on himself, running into the road, etc., etc., he'll be hurt. What are you as an adult doing to make that child live in rooms or an environment where he *can* be hurt? The fault is yours, not his, if he breaks things.

The sweetness and love of a child is preserved only so long as he can exert his own self-determinism. You interrupt that and to a degree you interrupt his life.

There are only two reasons why a child's right to decide for himself has to be interrupted—the fragility and danger of his environment and *you*. For you work out on him the things that were done to you, regardless of what you think.

There are two courses you can take. Give the child leeway in an environment he can't hurt and which can't badly hurt him and which doesn't greatly restrict his own space and time. And through Scientology services, you can clean up your own aberrations (departures from rational thought or behavior) to a point where your tolerance equals or surpasses his lack of education in how to please you.

When you give a child something, it's *his*. It's not still yours. Clothes, toys, quarters, what he has been given, *must remain under his exclusive control*. So he tears up his shirt, wrecks his bed, breaks his fire engine. It's *none of your business*. How would you like to have somebody give you a Christmas present and then tell you, day after day thereafter, what you are to do with it and even punish you if you failed to care for it the way the donor thinks you should? You'd wreck that donor and ruin that present. You know you would. The child wrecks your nerves when you do it to him. That's revenge. He cries. He pesters you. He breaks your things. He "accidentally" spills his milk. And he wrecks the possession *on purpose* about which he is so often cautioned. Why? Because he is fighting for his own self-determinism, his own right to own and make his weight felt on his environment. This "possession" is another channel by which he can be controlled. So he has to fight the possession and the controller.

Doubtless, some people were so poorly raised they think *control* is the ne plus ultra (highest point) of child raising. If you want to control your child, simply break him into complete apathy and he'll be as obedient as any hypnotized half-wit. If you want to know how to control him, get a book on dog training, name the child Rex and teach him first to "fetch" and then to "sit up" and then to bark for his food. You can train a child that way. Sure you can. But it's your hard luck if he turns out to be a bloodletter (a person who causes bloodshed).

Of course, you'll have a hard time of it. This is a *human being*. It will be tough because man became king of the beasts only because he couldn't as a species be licked. He doesn't easily go into an obedient apathy like dogs do. *Men* own *dogs* because men are self-determined and dogs aren't.

The reason people started to confuse children with dogs and started training children with force lies in the field of psychology. The psychologist worked on "principles" as follows:

"Man is evil."

"Man must be trained into being a social animal."

"Man must adapt to his environment."

As these postulates aren't true, psychology doesn't work. And if you ever saw a wreck, it's the child of a professional psychologist. Attention to the world around us instead of to texts somebody thought up after reading somebody's texts, shows us the fallacy of these postulates.

The actuality is quite opposite the previous beliefs.

The truth lies in this direction:

Man is basically good.

Only by severe aberration can man be made evil. Severe training drives him into nonsociability.

Man must retain his personal ability to adapt his environment to him to remain sane.

A man is as sane and safe as he is self-determined.

In raising your child, you must avoid "training" him into a social animal. Your child begins by being more sociable, more dignified than you are. In a relatively short time the treatment he gets so checks him that he revolts. This revolt can be intensified until he is a terror to have around. He will be noisy, thoughtless, careless of possessions, unclean—anything, in short, which will annoy you. Train him, control him and you'll lose his love. You've lost the child forever that you seek to control and own.

Permit a child to sit on your lap. He'll sit there, contented. Now put your arms around him and constrain him to sit there. Do this even though he wasn't even trying to leave. Instantly, he'll squirm. He'll fight to get away from you. He'll get angry. He'll cry. Recall now, he was happy before you started to hold him.

Your efforts to mold, train, control this child in general react on him exactly like trying to hold him on your lap.

Of course you will have difficulty if this child of yours has already been trained, controlled, ordered about, denied his own possessions. In mid-flight, you change your tactics. You try to give him his freedom. He's so suspicious of you he will have a terrible time trying to adjust. The transition period will be terrible. But at the end of it you'll have a well-ordered, well-trained, social child, thoughtful of you and, very important to you, a child who loves you.

The child who is under constraint, shepherded, handled, controlled, has a very bad anxiety postulated. His parents are survival entities. They mean food, clothing, shelter, affection. This means he wants to be near them. He wants to love them, naturally, being their child.

But on the other hand his parents are nonsurvival entities. *His whole being and life depend upon his rights to use his own decision about his movements and his possessions and his body.* Parents seek to interrupt this out of the mistaken idea that a child is an idiot who won't learn unless "controlled." So he has to fight shy, to fight against, to annoy and harass an enemy.

Here is anxiety. "I love them dearly. I also need them. But they mean an interruption of my ability, my mind, my potential life. What am I going to do

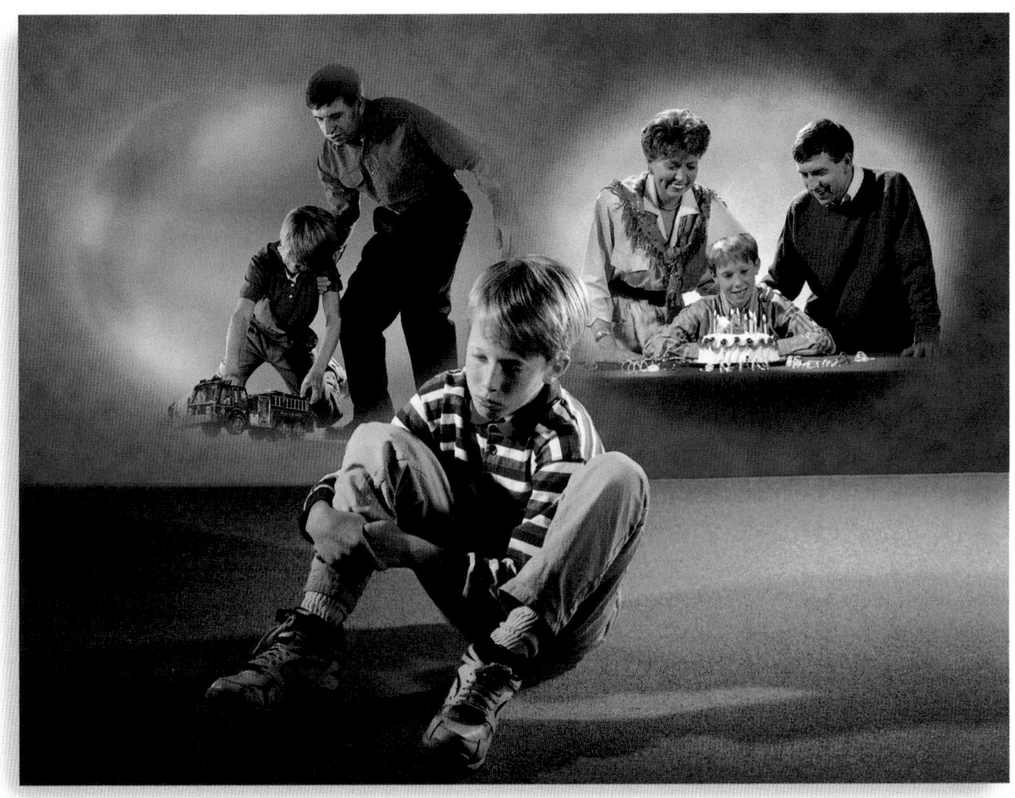

A child needs his parents' support for many aspects of his survival. But if they also severely interrupt his decisions of his life he is given a huge problem which can cause him much worry.

about my parents? I can't live with them. I can't live without them. Oh, dear, oh, dear!" There he sits running this problem through his head. That problem, that anxiety, will be with him for eighteen years, more or less. And it will half wreck his life.

Freedom for the child means freedom for you. Abandoning the possessions of the child to their fate means eventual safety for the child's possessions.

What terrible willpower is demanded of a parent not to give constant streams of directions to a child! What agony to watch his possessions going to ruin! What upset to refuse to order his time and space!

But it has to be done if you want a well, a happy, a careful, a beautiful, an intelligent child!

A Child's Right to Contribute

You have no right to deny your child the right to contribute.

A human being feels able and competent only so long as he is permitted to contribute as much or more than he has contributed to him.

A man can over-contribute and feel secure in an environment. He feels insecure the moment he under-contributes, which is to say, gives less than he receives. If you don't believe this, recall a time when everyone else brought something to the party but you didn't. How did you feel?

A human being will revolt against and distrust any source which contributes to him more than he contributes to it.

Parents, naturally, contribute more to a child than the child contributes back. As soon as the child sees this he becomes unhappy. He seeks to raise his contribution level; failing, he gets angry at the contributing source. He begins to detest his parents. They try to override this revolt by contributing more. The child revolts more. It is a bad dwindling spiral because the end of it is that the child will go into apathy.

You *must* let the child contribute to you. You can't order him to contribute. You can't command him to mow the grass and then think that is contribution. He has to figure out what his contribution is and then give it. If he hasn't selected it, it isn't his, but only more control.

A baby contributes by trying to make you smile. The baby will show off. A little older he will dance for you, bring you sticks, try to repeat your work motions to help you. If you don't accept those smiles, those dances, those sticks, those work motions in the spirit they are given, you have begun to interrupt the child's contribution. Now he will start to get anxious. He will do unthinking and strange things to your possessions in an effort to make them "better" for you. You scold him. That finishes him.

Something else enters in here. And that is *data.* How can a child possibly know what to contribute to you or his family or home *if* he hasn't any idea of the working principles on which it runs?

A family is a group with the common goal of group survival and advancement. The child not allowed to contribute or failing to understand the goals and working principles of family life is cast adrift from the family. He is shown he is not part of the family because he can't contribute. So he becomes antifamily—the first step on the road to being antisocial. He spills milk, annoys your guests and yells outside your window in "play." He'll even get sick just to make you work. He is shown to be nothing by being shown that he isn't powerful enough to contribute.

You can do nothing more than accept the smiles, the dances, the sticks of the very young. But as soon as a child can understand, he should be given the whole story of the family operation.

What is the source of his allowance? How come there is food? Clothes? A clean house? A car?

Daddy works. He expends hours and brains and brawn and for this he gets money. The money, handed over at a store, buys food. A car is cared for because of money scarcity. A calm house and care of Daddy means Daddy works better and that means food and clothes and cars.

Education is necessary because one earns better after he has learned.

Play is necessary in order to give a reason for hard work.

Give him the whole picture. If he's been revolting, he may keep right on revolting. But he'll eventually come around.

First of all a child needs *security.* Part of that security is understanding. Part of it is a code of conduct which is invariable. What is against the law today can't be ignored tomorrow.

You can actually handle a child physically to defend your rights, so long as he owns what he owns and can contribute to you and work for you.

Adults have rights. He ought to know this. A child has as his goal, growing up. If an adult doesn't have more rights, why grow up? Who the devil would be an adult these days anyway?

The child has a duty toward you. He has to be able to take care of you; not an illusion that he is, but actually. And you have to have patience to allow yourself to be cared for sloppily until by sheer experience itself—not by your directions—he learns how to do it well. Care for the child? Nonsense! He's probably got a better grasp of immediate situations than you have, you beaten-up adult. Only when he's almost psychotic with aberration will a child be an accident-prone.

You're well and enjoy life because you aren't *owned*. You *couldn't* enjoy life if you were shepherded and owned. You'd revolt. And if your revolt was quenched, you'd turn into a subversive. That's what you make out of your child when you own, manage and control him.

Potentially, parent, he's saner than you are and the world is a lot brighter. His sense of values and reality are sharper. Don't dull them. And your child will be a fine, tall, successful human being. Own, control, manage and reject and you'll get the treatment you deserve—subversive revolt.

WORKING WITH A CHILD'S WILLINGNESS

How then, without using force, do you get a child to do things?

If you take an individual and *make* him play a musical instrument (as parents and schools do), his ability to play that instrument will not improve. We would first have to consult with him as to what his ambitions are. He would eventually at least have to agree with the fact that it is a good thing to play an instrument.

Take, for example, a "bad boy." He cannot be put in school and has to be sent to a military school. They are going to force him in order to change him. Occasionally this bad boy is sent to a school which simply thinks the best way to handle such cases is to find something in which he is interested and to allow him to do it. Such a school once existed in California and consecutively produced geniuses. The roster of World War II's scientists practically marched from that particular school. They figured that it must have been the example set by the professor, his purity in not smoking cigars or something like that.

What actually happened was this: They took a boy with whom nobody got any results and said, "Isn't there anything you would like to do?" The boy said "No," and they answered, "Well, fuss around in the lab or grounds or something and someday you may make up your mind." The boy thought this over and decided that he wanted to be a chemist. Nobody ever sent him to a class and told him to crack a book, and nobody ever complained very much when he blew up something in the laboratory, and the next thing you knew the boy was an excellent chemist. Nobody interrupted his desire to be a chemist. It existed then, and from that point on he was not himself interrupting his willingness to be a chemist. Educationally, this is a very interesting point.

Consulting Willingness

People will permit you to take things away from them if you do it gracefully and don't upset their willingness too much. The way you make a greedy or a selfish child is to *make* him, against his will, give up things to other children. You will eventually drive him into the "only-one" category—feeling he is the only person who really matters at all. Parents usually never consult the child's willingness. They consult his havingness, his ability to own or possess, then handle it and they have a spoiled child.

It is interesting to watch a child that has been around somebody who always consulted him but didn't take very good care of him as opposed to a child who had the best of care but who never was consulted.

A little boy is sitting on the floor playing with blocks and balls and is having a good time. Along comes the nurse who picks him up and takes him into the other room and changes his diapers, and he screams bloody murder the whole way. He doesn't like it. She keeps on doing this to him, placing him around, never consulting his power of choice and he will eventually grow up obsessed with the power of choice. He has to have his way. He becomes very didactic—assertive of his own rightness. He is trying to hold down the last rungs of it, and his ability will be correspondingly poor, particularly in the handling of people.

Now, this is quite different. You know the child is hungry, and you know he ought to eat. The child will eat if he is kept on some sort of routine. If supper is served routinely at 6:00, he will get used to eating at 6:00, and his willingness will never quite be overwhelmed. He finds out that food is there at 6:00 and so he makes up his mind to eat at 6:00. You provide the food and he provides the willingness. If you don't override that, he will never have any trouble about food.

Then somebody comes along and talks to him and says, "Wouldn't you like to go into the other room and change your clothes?" and the answer is "No." You are making a horrible mistake if you proceed from that point on the basis of "Well, I'll give you a piece of candy," persuade, seduce, coax, etc. That is psychology, the way psychologists handle situations, and it doesn't really work.

You take one of two courses. Either you use excellent control with lots of communication, or you just let him grow. There is no other choice. Kids don't like to be mauled and pulled around and not consulted. You can talk to a child and if your degree of affection, agreement and communication with him are good, you can make him do all sorts of things. He will touch the floor, his head, point you out and find the table. He will fool around for a while and after that you can just say do so-and-so and "Let's go and eat," and he will do it. He has found out that your commands are not necessarily going to override the totality of his willingness. So your commands are therefore not dangerous. You have confronted him and he can confront you. Therefore you and he can do something.

A child sometimes says "I want to stay up with you" and they insist on doing so, exerting their power of choice. Just letting children do what they are doing and not interfering with them and not exerting any control on them is psychology. They are never going to be in communication with anybody; they won't grow or get experience in life for they didn't change their havingness. They didn't have to change their mind, work, exercise or do anything. But they respond very readily to good control and communication, but it certainly takes good communication to override this—not persuasion but good communication.

People think that persuasion works with children. It doesn't. It's communication that does the trick. You say, "Well, it's time for you to go to bed now," and he says, "No." Don't stay on the subject. Leave it alone and just talk about something else, "What did you do today?" "Where?" "How?" "Oh, did you? Is that a fact?" "Well, how about going to bed?" and the answer will be "Okay."

One doesn't have to use force. Go into communication with the child, and control follows this as an inevitability. Omit control from the beginning when bringing up a child and he who looks to you for a lot of his direction and control is gypped. He thinks you don't care about him.

However, as in the case with the playing of musical instruments, learning of languages or the arts and abilities, consult the child's *willingness.*

ALLOWING CHILDREN TO WORK

The basic difficulty with all juvenile delinquency is the one-time apparently humane program of forbidding children to labor in any way.

Doubtless it was once a fact that child labor was abused, that children were worked too hard, that their growths were stunted and that they were, in general, used. It is highly doubtful if the infamous Mr. Marx ever saw in America young boys being pulled off machines dead from work and thrown onto dump heaps.

Where there was an abuse of this matter, there was a public outcry against it, and legislation was enacted to prevent children from working. This legislation with all the good intention of the world is, however, directly responsible for juvenile delinquency.

Forbidding children to work, and particularly forbidding teenagers to make their own way in the world and earn their own money, creates a family difficulty so that it becomes almost impossible to raise a family, and creates as well, and particularly, a state of mind in the teenager that the world does not want him, and he has already lost his game before he has begun it. Then with something like universal military training staring him in the face so that he dare not start a career, he is of course thrust into a deep subapathy (state of disinterest below apathy) on the subject of work, and when he at length is faced with the necessity of making his own way in the world, he rises into an apathy and does nothing about it at all.

It is highly supportive of this fact that our greatest citizens worked, usually when they were quite young. In the Anglo-American civilization the highest level of endeavor was achieved by boys who, from the age of twelve, on farms, had their own duties and had a definite place in the world.

Children, in the main, are quite willing to work. A two-, three-, four-year-old child is usually found haunting his father or her mother trying to help out either with tools or dust rags; and the kind parent who is really fond of the children responds in the reasonable and long-ago-normal manner of being patient enough to let the child actually assist. A child so permitted then develops the idea that his presence and activity is desired and he quite calmly sets about a career of accomplishment.

The child who is warped or pressed into some career, but is not permitted to assist in those early years, is convinced that he is not wanted, that the world has no part of him. And later on he will come into very definite difficulties regarding work. However, the child who at three or four wants to work in this modern society is discouraged and is actually prevented from working, and after he is made to be idle until seven, eight or nine, is suddenly saddled with certain chores.

Now, this child is already educated into the fact that he must not work and so the idea of work is a sphere where he "knows he does not belong," and so he always feels uncomfortable in performing various activities.

Later on in his teens, he is actively prevented from getting the sort of a job which will permit him to buy the clothes and treats for his friends which he feels are demanded of him, and so he begins to feel he is not a part of the society. Not being part of the society, he is then against the society and desires nothing but destructive activities.

HANDLING A CHILD'S UPSETS AND MISHAPS

This section provides many techniques for a parent or anyone to use to help a child recover rapidly from the bumps, bruises, scrapes, scares and upsets that are often part of growing up.

For the most part, the techniques which follow utilize communication between oneself and the child as their main therapeutic agent. Communication is vitally important in dealing with children, as it is in any aspect of Scientology.

The actions described below all classify as assists. An assist is an action undertaken to help an individual obtain relief from an immediate troublesome difficulty. These assists should be used in addition to those in Chapter 6, "Assists for Illnesses and Injuries" whenever circumstances require. The benefits for the child and the family can be considerable.

Childhood Injuries

There are many things one can do to aid a child who suffers a minor fall, cut or the like. In young children, often just letting them cry out seems to be enough. When a child is hurt, most people find themselves speaking comforting and consoling words almost before they know it. And what they say is usually what they have said a hundred times before when the child was hurt. This can remind the child of the whole chain of earlier injuries.

Parents can help a child most by saying nothing. It may take a short while to train themselves not to speak when the child is hurt, but it is not difficult to form the habit of remaining silent. Silence need not inhibit affection. One may hold the child, if he wants to be held, or put an arm around him. Often, if nothing is said, a young child will cry hard for a minute or so, and then suddenly stop, smile, and run back to what he was doing. Allowing him to cry seems to release the tension resulting from the injury and no assist is needed if this occurs. In fact, it is often very difficult to make the child return to the moment of injury if he has released the tension this way.

"Tell Me About It"

If the child does not spontaneously recover after a moment or two of crying, then wait until he has recovered from the short period of lowered awareness that accompanies an injury. It is usually not difficult to tell when a child is dazed and when he is not. If he still cries after the dazed period, it is usually because other previous injuries have been restimulated (reactivated due to similar circumstances in the present approximating circumstances of the past). In this case, an assist is valuable. On older children (age five and up) an assist is usually necessary.

When the child is no longer dazed, ask him, "What happened? How did you get hurt? Tell me about it."

As he begins to tell about it, switch him to the present tense if he doesn't tell the story in the present tense spontaneously. Try it this way:

"Well—I was standing on a big rock and I slipped and fell, and..." (crying)

"Does it hurt when you are standing on the rock?"

"No."

"What happens when you are standing on the rock?"

"I slip..." (crying)

"Then what happens?"

"I fall on the ground."

"Is there grass on the ground?"

"No—it's all sandy."

"Tell me about it again."

You can take the child through it several times until he gets bored or laughs. There is nothing difficult about it. After a child has had a few assists this way, he will, upon being injured, run to the person who can administer this painless help and reassurance, demanding to "tell about it."

A child who has hurt herself can be markedly assisted by communication.

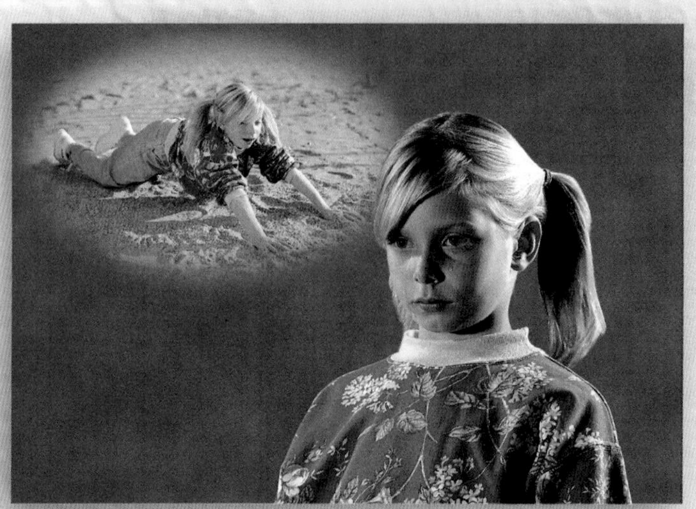

Getting her to explain what happened can be therapeutic.

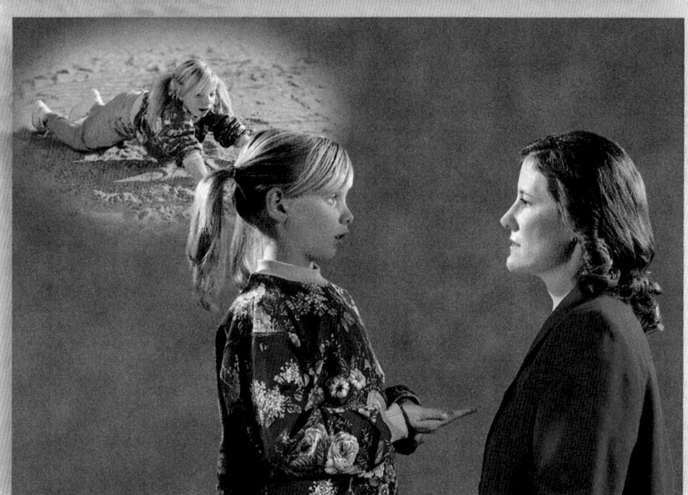

Telling it to someone who's interested will dissipate any upset and enable the child to feel better.

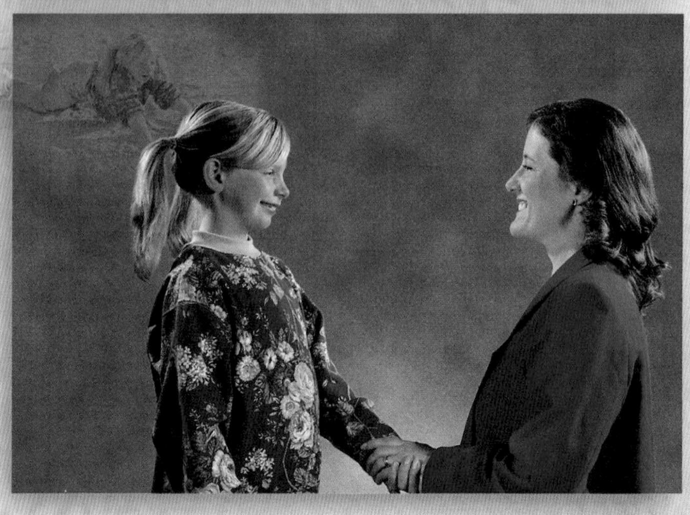

Directing a Child's Attention

Many people habitually tell a child, "Don't do that or you'll get sick," "My goodness, you're certainly getting a bad cold," "You'll get sick if you keep on with that," "I just know Johnny's going to get measles if he goes to school," and countless other such pessimistic suggestions. They also use thousands of "Don'ts," "Can'ts," and "Control yourself" phrases. Parents may watch themselves for these phrases, and avoid their use as much as possible. With a little imagination and practice, it is not difficult to find ways of keeping children safe without using constant verbal restraints. As much as possible, suggestions made to a child should be positive. Graphically illustrating what happens to a glass bottle when it drops will get the idea across better than a thousand screams of "Get away from that!" or "Put that down!"

Smooth, gentle motions and a quiet voice will go far toward averting restimulation when children are being handled. Anyone who wishes to work successfully with children will cultivate these attributes. They are particularly valuable in emergencies.

If a child's attention must be obtained quickly because of a potentially dangerous situation developing too far away to enable the guardian to reach the child in a hurry, calling his name loud enough to be heard will do the trick harmlessly. It is much better than screamed injunctions to "Stop!" "Stay there!" "Don't do that!" and so on. It is not nearly so likely to restimulate him.

Remembering

Asking the child to remember may be used in hundreds of situations that arise from day to day: whenever the child is fretful, unhappy and crying over something; when he is feeling slightly sick; when he is obviously restimulated by something; when he has overheard a dramatization (a replay in the present of something that happened in the past) or someone has punished him severely or uncorked a dramatization directed toward him; when he feels rejected—in fact, every time a child is unhappy or nervous for any reason or when you know that he has had a highly restimulative experience.

The principle here is to get at the specific phrases and situations causing the restimulations. Of course this technique can be used only after the child has learned to talk enough to give a coherent account of what he is thinking and feeling.

If the child is feeling upset (not seriously ill) you may begin by asking him when he felt this way before. Usually a child will remember. As you ask further questions about what was happening, what he was doing at the time, who was talking, what was said, how he felt, he will describe the scene graphically. When he does so, simply have him go through it again a few times. When you come to the end say, "Tell me about it again. Where were you when Daddy was talking?" "Tell it again." Or, simply, "Let's see now, you were sitting on the couch when Daddy says—what does he say?" Any simple phrase which will return the child to the beginning of the scene may be used.

There is no need to make this action complex. Children understand "Tell it again." They love to hear stories over and over again, themselves, and they love to tell their stories to an interested audience. But don't be overly sympathetic. Show affection and interest, yes. But don't croon or moan, "Poor baby, poor little thing!" or similar phrases. To do so may tend to prompt the child to consider the injury or upset *valuable* in that it got him special attention and sympathy.

The more you can enter a child's reality, the better you will be able to help him. Imitate his voice tones, his "Yeah!" "You did!" "And then what?"—adapt yourself to his graphic mimicry, widened eyes, breathless interest or whatever his mood and tone may be—but not to the extent of parroting, of course. If you cannot do it well, then just be simple, natural and interested.

Often, when he is restimulated, a child will use one or two phrases over and over again. In that case you can start with, "Who says that?" or "Who's saying that to you?" or "When did you hear that?"

Sometimes he will insist, "I say it, 'Shut up, you old fool!'" or whatever the phrase is. Then ask, "Who else says it?" or "See if you can remember when you heard somebody else say it," and he will usually start telling you about an incident.

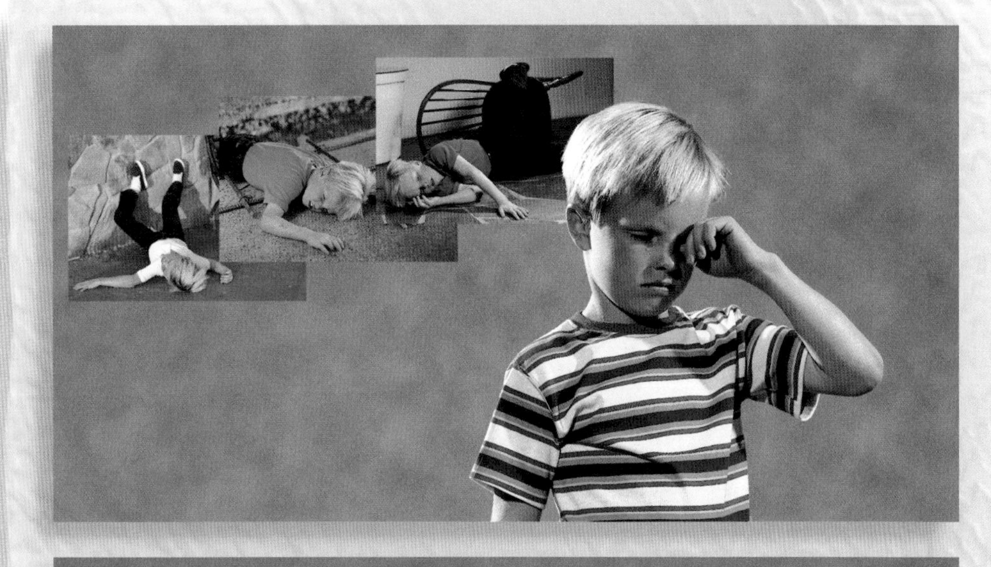

When a child experiences something upsetting or traumatic, similar incidents can reactivate in his mind.

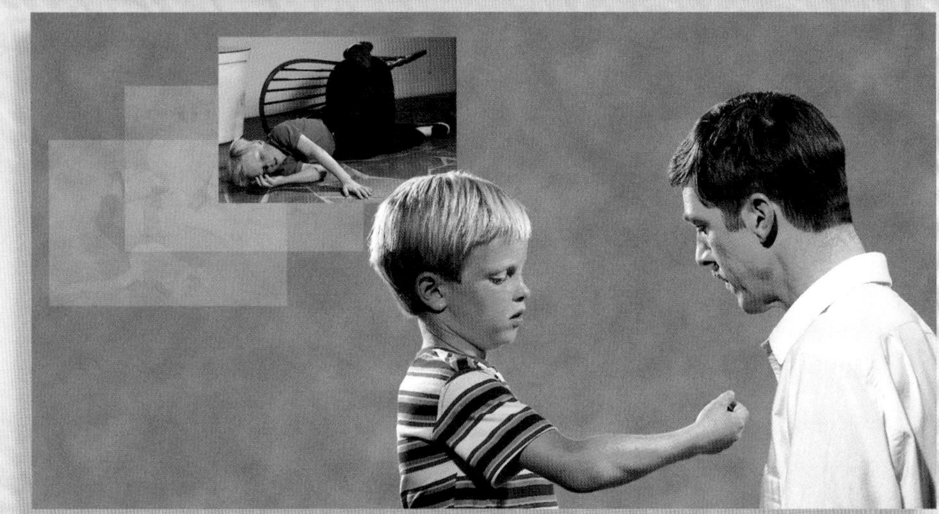

These fall away when the child is gotten to talk about the current upset.

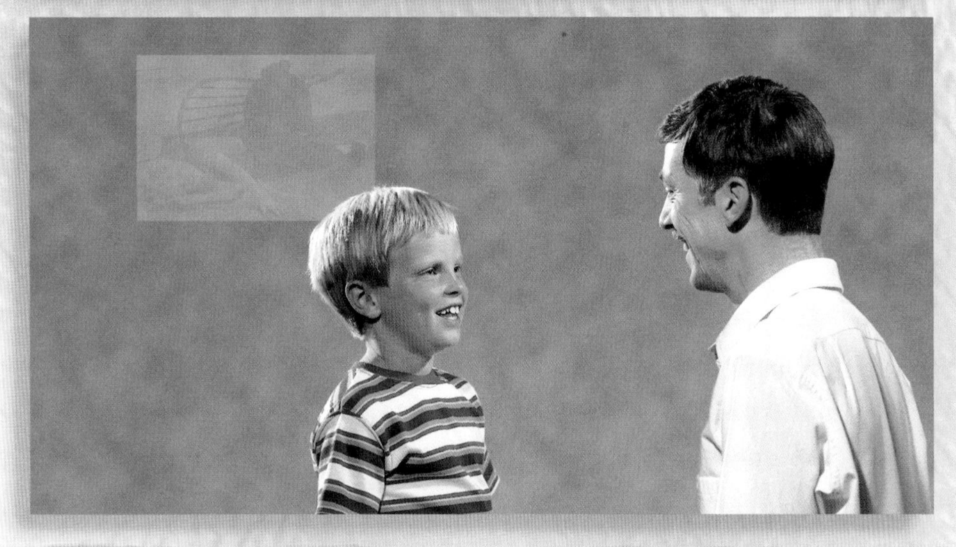

The child should be guided into relating what happened as though it were occurring in the present. This will discharge any trauma connected with it.

One woman, working with her daughter, was astounded when the child said, "You said it, Mummy, a long time ago." "Where were you when I said it?" "Oh, I was only a little thing—in your tummy." This probably won't happen often. But as the child gets the idea, it may happen sooner or later. Whatever the incident, just go on with questioning to build up the incident. "What were you doing? Where were you? Where was I? What was Daddy saying? What did it look like? What did you feel like?" and so on. Have the child recall the incident a few times until he laughs. This will release him from the restimulation.

Use of Dolls or Stuffed Animals

If the father knows that the child has overheard a dramatization or has been severely punished or scolded, he may handle this a few hours after the event by asking about it. "Do you remember when I shouted at Mother last night?" If the child is not used to expressing his anger to his parents, or if he has been severely repressed in the past, it may take some coaxing to get him to tell about it. While doing so, try to assure him by your manner that it is perfectly all right for him to talk about it. If he simply cannot, you might try to get him to play it out. If the child plays with dolls or toy animals you may, in play with him, get him to make the dolls or toys act out the dramatization.

"This is the mama doll. And this is the papa doll. What does the mama doll say when she is mad?" Very often this will take the child right into the scene, and if you let him really open up and describe the scene without condemnation, listening in a sympathetic, interested way, and encouraging him with a well-placed, "Yes...and then what?" he will soon drop the pretense and begin to tell you directly what he overheard. Even if he does not do this and, as children often do, he runs over the scene a couple of times with his dolls or toys, it will lessen in intensity to a large extent.

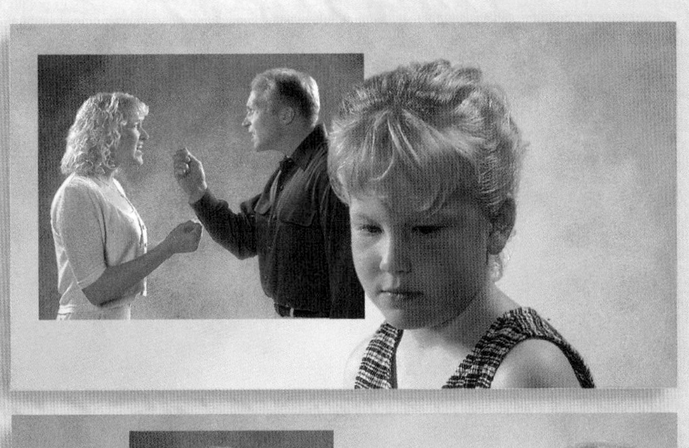

Overhearing an upset or fight between parents can be extremely disturbing.

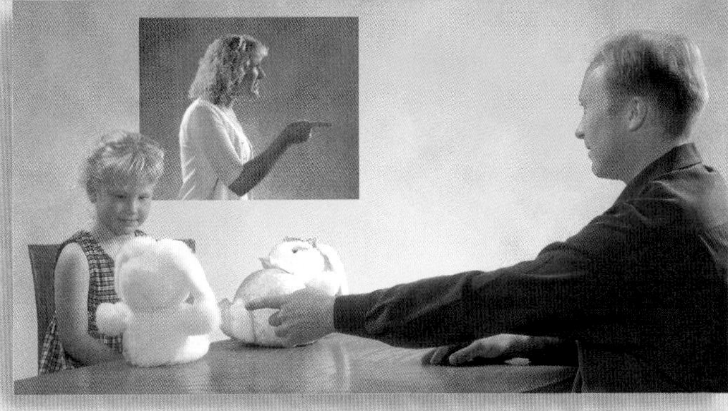

A parent can help dissipate the child's concern by getting her to use dolls to demonstrate what happened.

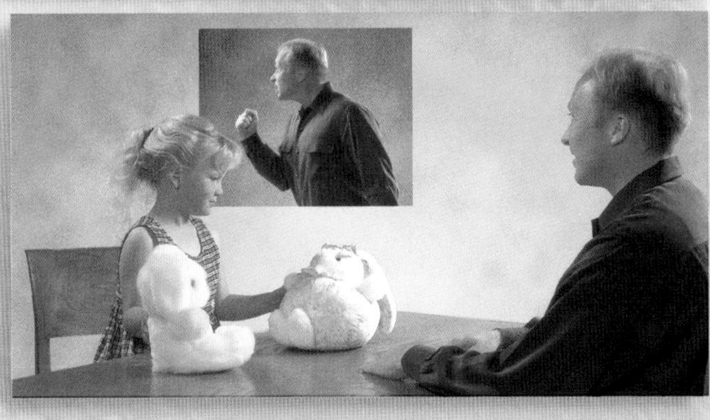

The child re-creates the experience with the dolls…

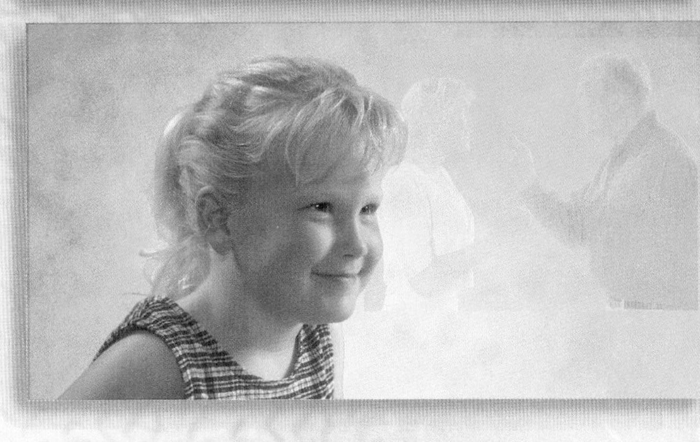

… and any lingering upset on the child's part can quickly fade away.

Drawing Pictures

Instead of dolls or toys, you may have the child draw pictures. "Draw me a picture of a woman and a man.... What are they doing? Draw me a picture of a woman crying," and so on. The emphasis should always be on the adult who was dramatizing, and not on the child who was bad, if that happened. Drawing pictures, playing house with a child: "And then you say...?" "And then I say...?" or simply getting the child to make up a story about it will help.

Anger

With children who have not been inhibited in their expressions of anger against parents, these subterfuges (deceptions) are not usually necessary. They will tell freely and dramatize scenes they overheard or scoldings they got, if you act as an interested audience and encourage them to build up the scene. If you watch children playing, you will often see them doing exactly that, mimicking their parents and other adults in their dramatizations.

Sometimes just asking a child, "What happened to make you feel bad?" or "What did I say to make you feel that way?" will bring out and alleviate the restimulative elements in the present situation.

Everyone is familiar with the violent threats children can think up when they are frustrated: "I'll tear him to pieces and throw him in the river; I'll make them all go in a closet and lock it up and throw away the key and then they'll be sorry," and so on. If you encourage them by "Yes? And then what will you do?" or "Gee, that would be something!" they will keep on for a while and then they often will suddenly pop right out of the upset and go on with what they were doing.

If a child is angry, let him be angry, even if you are the victim. Let him act out his anger, and usually it will disappear quickly. But if you try to suppress it, it will grow worse and last longer. Letting a child react to a frustrating situation without further suppression seems to release the energy of the frustration and will bring him out of it more quickly than almost anything else.

Fear

If a child is in fear, let him tell you about it, giving him all the encouragement you can. This is particularly effective in nightmares. Wake the child, hold him quietly until his crying calms a little, and ask him about the nightmare, taking him through it several times until he is no longer frightened. Then ask him about a pleasant memory, and have him tell you that before leaving him. If he doesn't want to sleep alone after that, do not make him face his fear. Stay with him and encourage him to talk about it until he is no longer afraid, even if this takes some time. In asking about fears, you can use the phrase "the same as." If the child is afraid of the dark, ask him, "What is the same as dark?" If he is afraid of animals, a similar question will cause him to analyze his fear. Perhaps you will not always be successful on the first questioning, but if you continue patiently you'll soon get an answer that will tell you an incident he has his attention on and you can help the child handle this by talking about what occurred.

Grief

If the child is in grief, a good way to begin is, "What are you crying about?" After a child has told what he is crying about a few times, each time being helped by questioning about the incident, and when his crying has abated (become less), you may ask, "What else are you crying about?"

Actually, just letting him cry until he gets out of it will often be enough. This is especially true if you are in close contact with him and he knows he can count on you for support and assistance.

Don't try to stop a child from crying by simply telling him not to cry. Either handle the incident that caused the crying by asking what happened and getting him to tell about it until he is laughing, or let him cry it out while you caress or hold him. No words in this case; just affection.

Irritableness

If the child is simply fretful and "unmanageable," you can often get him out of it by diverting his attention, by introducing a new and fascinating story or picture book or a toy or, in the case of a very young child, something which glitters. This is an old technique, but it is valid. If the child is fretful, the chances are that he is in boredom, which means that the particular activity he was interested in has been suppressed somehow. He is looking for something new but is unable to find it. If you can give him something to interest him, he will become more cheerful quickly. Do not, however, make frantic efforts to attract his attention, plaguing him with jerky movements and such attention diverters as, "See, baby, see the pretty watch!" and if that fails to have an instantaneous effect, jumping to some other object. This will often only confuse him. Move smoothly and quietly, keep your voice soft and calm, and direct his attention to one new thing. That should be enough.

If none of these work, you can sometimes free him from the dramatization by bringing him up to present time with intense physical stimulation, like playful wrestling or some other vigorous exercise.

If you can get the child's attention long enough, you can ask him to tell you about some nice thing that happened. He may do it reluctantly at first, but as you encourage it he will often go right into the pleasurable memory, and pretty soon he will be cheerful again.

Making a new game of remembering provides a constructive and pleasant way to keep a child occupied during long trips, periods of waiting, periods of convalescence, and so on.

Children naturally have a good ability to recall. They love to talk about past moments of pleasure. A good deal of a child's conversation is filled with the wonderful things he has done or hopes to do, and he often talks spontaneously about times where he has been frightened or unhappy.

Teach a child to relate all pleasure moments by asking him what happened when he went to the zoo or went swimming. When he begins to tell you, switch him subtly to present tense, as suggested, if he fails to do so himself. Tell him to feel the water, feel himself moving, see what is going on, hear what people are saying and the sounds around him. This will help build his recall of the various things he perceived. But don't insist on a full account of the perceptions if the child is swiftly and surely recalling the incident, telling about it fluently. It doesn't take much to get a child to do this.

You can introduce the game by saying, "Let's play remembering," or "Tell me about when you went to…" or "Let's pretend we're going to the zoo again," or any other such casual phrase. Enter into the tale as much as you can, adopting the child's tone and manner if you can do it easily, and always being interested and eagerly awaiting the next detail.

Whenever a child comes to tell you about an accident he had or something that frightened him or made him unhappy, listen to it and have him go over it several times. As children learn how to "play remembering" and learn what it does for them, they will begin to ask for this when they want or need it.

There are many more assists that can be used to help children. Consult the Suggestions for Further Study section at the end of this chapter to find a book containing these.

Again, the main points in dealing with a child's upsets or injuries are:

1. Give assists for minor injuries, if necessary, or let the child cry it out if that seems to be enough.

2. Get the child to remember the last time it happened or get him to tell you in full what happened that made him unhappy.

3. Teach a child to remember by having him tell you past pleasure moments.

4. Use recall of pleasure moments or other techniques for bringing the child out of moments of upset up to present time.

Such care will keep the child healthier and happier.

Healthy Babies

An incorrectly fed baby is not only unhappy, he is unhealthy, a matter of concern to any new parent. Proper nourishment is, of course, a necessary ingredient to good health. Based on personal experience, here is something that worked; it is being offered as a helpful tip to parents who seek better ways to raise healthy children.

Some hospitals and medicos have adopted, apparently, the slogan, "A Fat Baby Today Means a Patient Tomorrow."

Some prepared food issued at hospitals and by baby doctors has been found to upset a baby. It is a powdered mess one is supposed to dissolve in water and feed to the baby.

If you ever tasted it, you would agree with the baby. It's terrible.

More than that, it is total carbohydrate and does not contain the protein necessary to make tissue and bone. It only makes fat. When you see one of these bloated, modern babies, know that it is being fed exactly on a diet of mixed milk powder, glucose and water, total carbohydrate.

The largest cause of upset in a baby's early life is just rations. The baby might be fed, yes. But with what? Terrible tasting, high-carbohydrate powdered milk solutions, or skim breast milk from an overworked mother. A ration *must* contain a heavy percentage of *protein*. Protein is the building block for nerves and bones. A soldier, wounded, will not heal without heavy protein intake. Ulcers will not get well without a heavy protein diet being given.

To make brain, bone and tissue, the baby *must* be given protein. And from two days old to at least three years. That makes strong, pretty, alert babies that sleep well and do well.

This problem was first tackled as a personal matter. As a father with a little boy who was not going to live, fast action had to be taken to save him. He had to be (1) gotten *out* of the hospital and (2) the trouble discovered and (3) remedied. The total time available was less than twenty-four hours. He was dying.

So (1) he was gotten out of the hospital. And (2) it was found he wouldn't or couldn't eat. And (3) a formula that provided him the nutrition he needed was developed and given to him.

The formula utilized barley. Roman troops had marched while living on a diet of barley, the cereal with the highest protein content. This formula is the nearest approach to human milk that can be assembled easily. It is an old Roman formula, no less, from around 2,200 years ago.

It's a bit of trouble, of course. You have to sacrifice a pot or a small kettle to cook the barley in (it really wrecks a pot, so you just have a barley pot and use only it). And you have to cook barley for a long time to get barley water, and you may forget and it burns. But even so, it's worth it in terms of a calmer house and a healthy baby.

You mix up a full twenty-four-hour batch of this barley recipe every day, bottle it in sterilized bottles and put it where it will remain cold. And you heat a bottle up to 98.6° F or thereabouts (test it by squirting some on the back of the hand to see if it's too warm or too cool) before you give it to the baby.

And, although you *try* to keep the baby on a schedule, you are foolish not to feed him or her when the baby is hungry.

A baby, having eaten a full ration, usually sleeps for hours anyway. If they don't, there is always a reason, such as a pin or a piece of coal in the bed, wet diapers, something. When a baby who shouldn't be crying, does, hunt until you find out why. Don't follow the schools of (1) the baby is just willful or (2) it's a serious illness that requires an immediate operation. Somewhere between we find the real reason.

Barley Formula for Babies

The foremost reason a baby doesn't do well is poor rations. And to remedy that, here is a formula one can use:

15 ounces of barley water

10 ounces of homogenized milk

3 ounces of corn syrup

The amount of syrup should be varied—depending on the baby—some like it weak—some take it stronger.

This formula can be multiplied by any number according to the number of bottles desired but the ratio remains the same.

To make the barley water, put about half a cup of *whole barley* in a piece of muslin, tie loosely to allow for expansion. It is *slowly* boiled in a covered, vented pot not made of aluminum for 6½ hours in about 4 pints of water. (In venting the pot, one allows steam to escape either through a vent built in the lid [if there is one] or by placing the cover slightly askew so there is an opening between the cover and pot.) Barley water will turn very, very pink. This gives about the right consistency of barley water for making the formula as above.

You don't feed the baby the actual barley, only the water mixed with the milk and corn syrup, in the ratio as given in the formula above.

Do not add anything else to this formula, such as vitamins or cream "to make the formula more nutritious." The formula is as laid out above.

Use this formula and have healthier babies!

HOW TO PREPARE THE BARLEY FORMULA

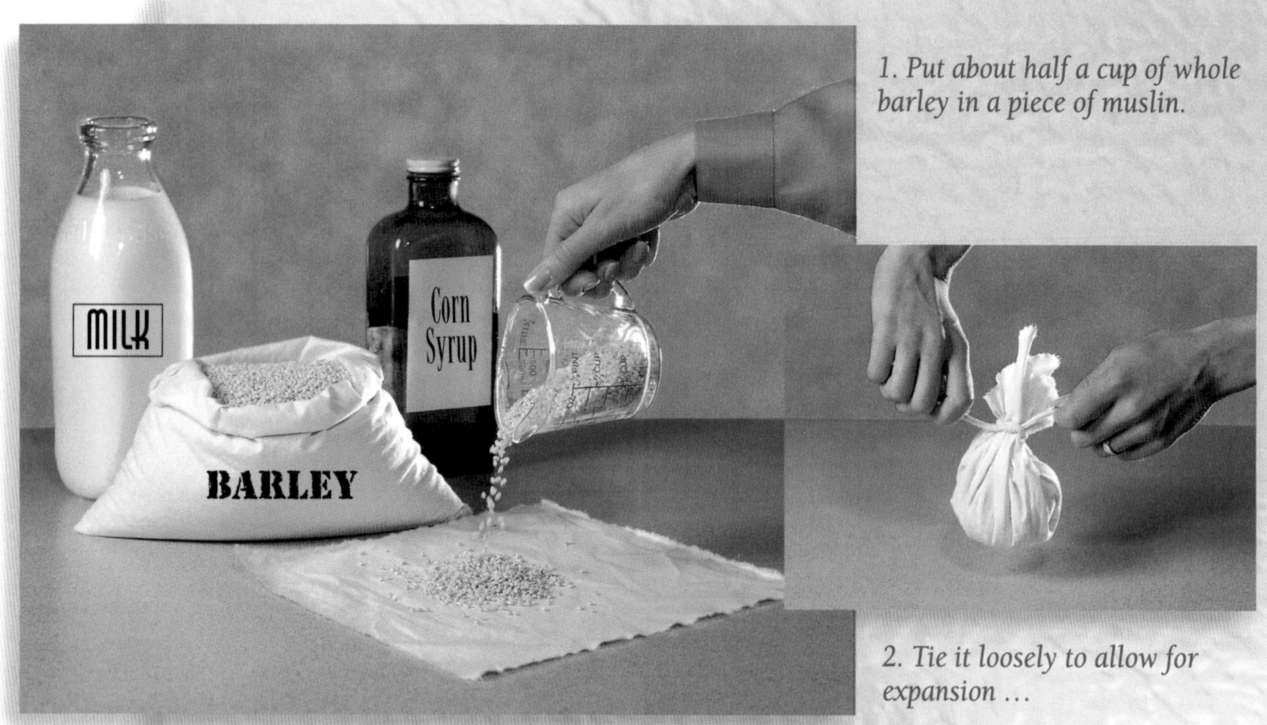

1. Put about half a cup of whole barley in a piece of muslin.

2. Tie it loosely to allow for expansion …

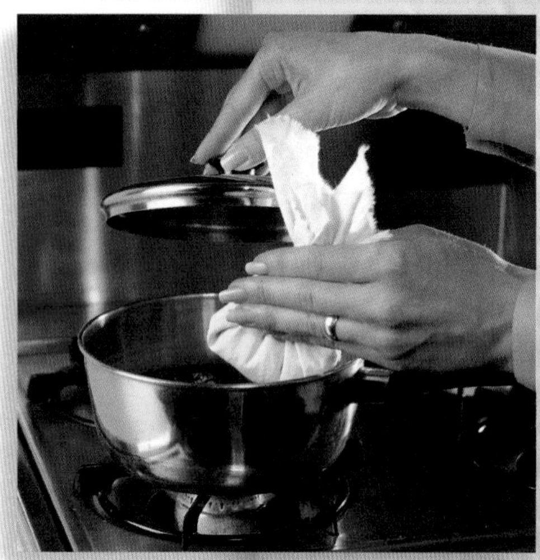

3. … and place it in the pot containing 4 pints of water.

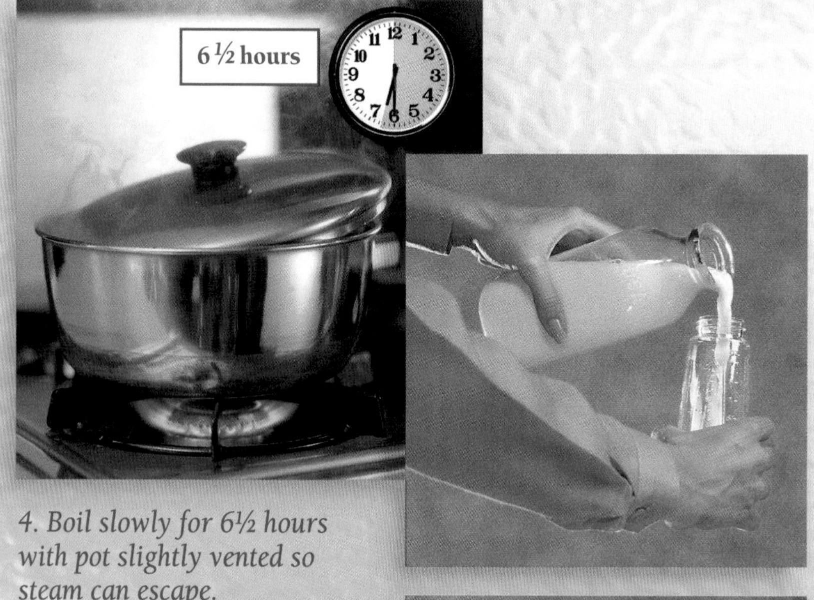

4. Boil slowly for 6½ hours with pot slightly vented so steam can escape.

5. Mix the formula using a ratio of: 15 ounces of barley water, 10 ounces of homogenized milk, 3 ounces of corn syrup.

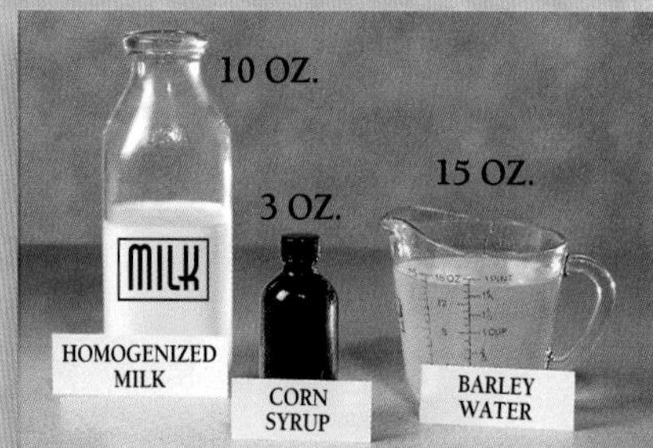

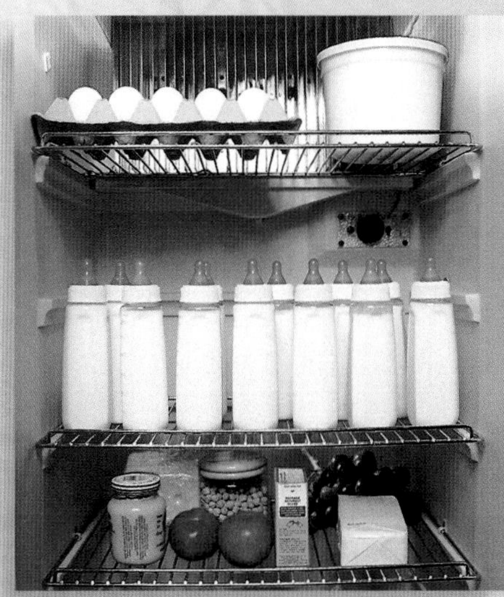

6. Keep the formula cold until feeding time.

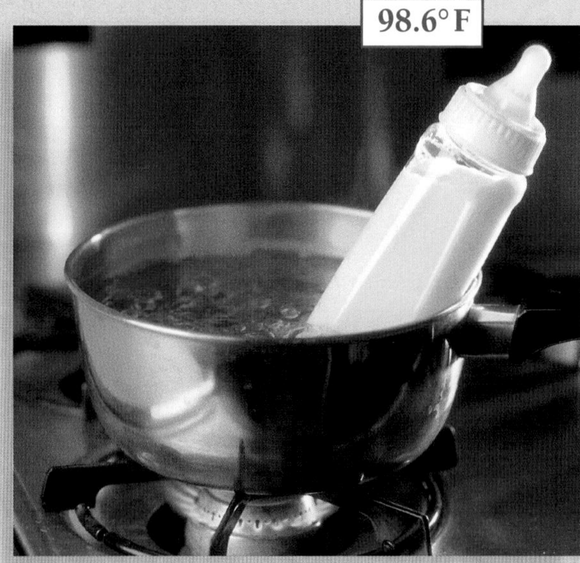

7. Heat a bottle to 98.6° F (body temperature).

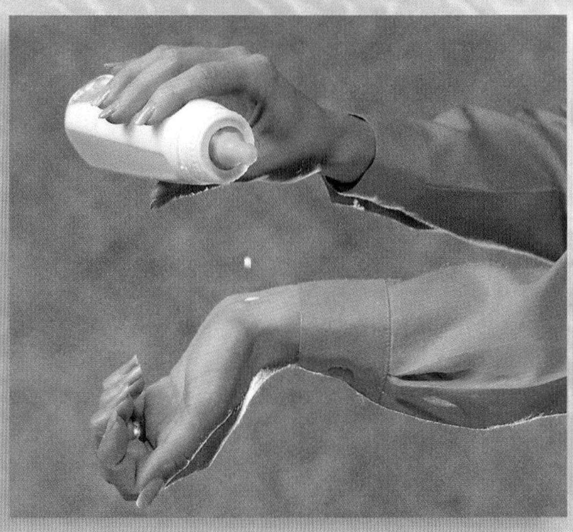

8. Squirt a few drops on your hand to ensure neither too hot nor too cold. Then give it to the baby.

BARLEY FORMULA

Put about half a cup of whole barley in a piece of muslin.

Tie loosely.

Boil slowly for 6½ hours in about 4 pints of water.

Mix the formula in a ratio of:

15 ounces of barley water

10 ounces of homogenized milk

3 ounces of corn syrup

CREATING TOMORROW'S SOCIETY

Working with children can be a fascinating adventure. The person who applies insight and patience along with his skill in applying the knowledge and techniques laid out in this chapter will be rewarded by seeing children progress to become cooperative, healthy members of the society. The task may seem impossible and heartbreaking at times, but in the end there will be an unequaled sense of accomplishment, of having done something really worthwhile for the advancement of future generations. ■

TEST YOUR UNDERSTANDING

Answer the following questions about the handling of children. If you need to, review the chapter. Going over the material several times will increase your certainty and help you better apply it.

- ❑ *How do you train a child without breaking him?*
- ❑ *How does self-determinism relate to a child's behavior?*
- ❑ *What happens to a child when you deny his right to contribute?*
- ❑ *Why is consulting a child's willingness important?*
- ❑ *How do you handle an angry child?*
- ❑ *Why is protein considered a must for babies?*

PRACTICAL EXERCISES

The following exercises will help you understand this chapter and increase your ability to deal with children better.

1 Observe someone handling a child. Notice if the person tries persuasion or force to get a child to do something against his will. If so, what were the results and how would the materials of this chapter have been applied instead? Then observe someone else handling a child and do the same as you did in the first example.

2 Write down an example of how a child can contribute to you. Describe the circumstances you would encounter and what you would do to allow the child to contribute in that circumstance. Then, do this again—thinking of another example of how a child could contribute to you and how you would handle the circumstance.

3 Applying the material in this chapter, consult a child's willingness and get him to do something you need or want him to do.

4 Using the data you read in this chapter, locate and handle a child who has hurt himself and does not spontaneously recover. Ensure you apply the data about saying nothing when the child is hurt. Carry out the steps to handle the child until he gets bored or laughs.

5 Handle a child who is crying until he stops crying. Apply the data in the section, "Tell Me About It," having the child relay his story in present time if he doesn't do this spontaneously. Carry out the steps to handle the crying child until he gets bored or laughs.

6 Write down five examples of actions a parent could do or things he could say which would direct a child's attention and keep him safe without using constant verbal restraints.

7 Improve a child's memory by having him tell you past pleasure moments. Use the techniques found in the chapter section, "Handling a Child's Upsets and Mishaps" to accomplish this result.

RESULTS FROM APPLICATION

It isn't easy to raise children well in today's busy and pressured society. The demands of work and finances, the high divorce rate, the availability of drugs in our schools, the failing educational system all contribute to an unstable family environment. It isn't easy for parents or for their children.

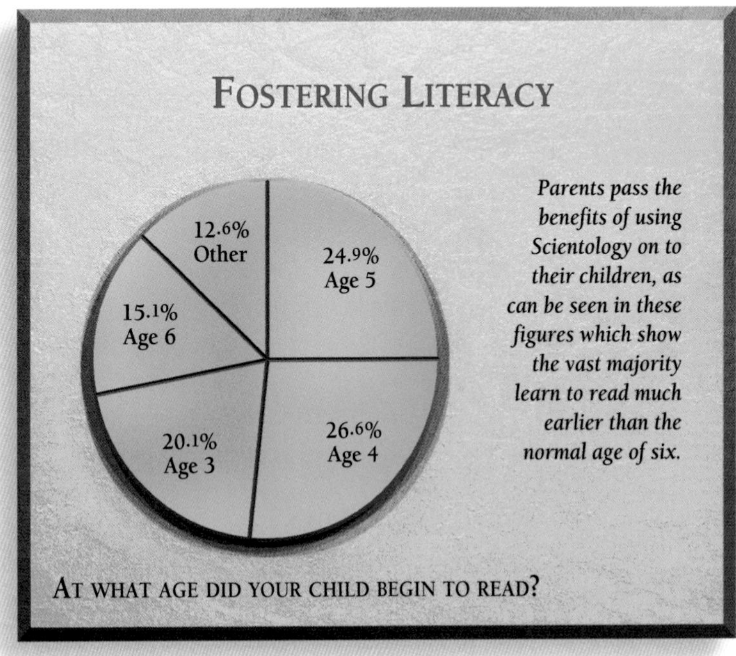

FOSTERING LITERACY
12.6% Other
24.9% Age 5
15.1% Age 6
20.1% Age 3
26.6% Age 4
Parents pass the benefits of using Scientology on to their children, as can be seen in these figures which show the vast majority learn to read much earlier than the normal age of six.
AT WHAT AGE DID YOUR CHILD BEGIN TO READ?

Yet the technology of how to raise happy children does exist. And it has been used by thousands of parents and others to change lives.

All of the Scientology principles which apply to adults also apply to children, but there is also an entire body of work that specifically addresses these men and women who have not "attained full growth." By using this wisdom, raising children can be a joyful and rewarding experience.

The examples below demonstrate that people can indeed bring up children who are able to survive and be happy in this sometimes confusing world.

A woman married a man who had three children. Her sister saw that she was mishandling these children in much the same way as she had been mishandled as a child.

"I had just learned some of Mr. Hubbard's discoveries of how the mind works and how mishandling children can be handed down from one generation to the next. So with these basics, I sat my sister down and went over with her how she had been ignored and mistreated as a child, to which she agreed. I also got her to see that she was very able and naturally wanted to do the correct thing, even when she was a small child. I asked her how she would have responded if someone had actually communicated with her when she was a child and also got her to look at how she could do this with her stepchildren and she brightened up a lot. After that my sister, who had previously not liked or wanted children, changed dramatically. She started enjoying the children and also decided to have one of her own. Since this time she allows her children to communicate to her and be the individuals they are. She loves being a mother now and I believe that this has made her life much happier, not to mention the lives of her children."

Applying L. Ron Hubbard's data about handling small children to the life of a young boy, a nanny brought about a remarkable change:

"The little boy loved being at school, but on the way home each day would fight with his brothers in the car, yelling and fussing about where to sit and so forth. This would continue at the dinner table, where he was really unpleasant to be around and would upset the rest of the family. His parents didn't know what to do to handle him except to send him to his room. This only resulted in the yelling coming from the room until he tired out. I applied the datum that in such circumstances there is a specific thing wrong and one must hunt to find out what it is. I found out that since he had started school, he had no longer been taking naps in the afternoon and he was exhausted at the end of the day. So I moved his bedtime to earlier and in a matter of days he was a most charming, lovable five-year-old boy who eagerly talked about what he did at school and said, 'Please pass the salt' with a smile at the dinner table. To his parents this was a miracle. I made a good impression, but really it was just applying L. Ron Hubbard's technology."

A mother living in Auckland, New Zealand, was quite frantic about her first baby as he cried every few hours, day and night. The family doctor said the child was in good health and could not account for the crying.

"One day I was in our local Scientology church and picked up an article by L. Ron Hubbard about how to have healthy babies. One of his recommendations was to feed a baby with a barley formula which was given in the article. I went home determined to try it out. The results were very worthwhile. In two days my son had settled down to sleeping between feeding times. At the end of a week he began sleeping through his night feeding time. I was so thankful for the extra rest! I later discovered he was cutting teeth—he cut all of them without crying. Diaper rash and upset stomachs were unknowns in our home and he grew so strong that he began walking at seven months. I can honestly say that the barley formula not only had a calming effect on our son but upon the whole household, as I went on to feed our other two children the same way."

Having studied what L. Ron Hubbard wrote about raising children, a father in Los Angeles decided to use this data in the raising of his son. He said:

"I felt I owed my child a parent who didn't pass on the 'family traditions'—bad habits of child raising. I knew I would fall into the rut of a parent with not enough understanding if I didn't do something about it. So I studied L. Ron Hubbard's data so that I could give my son a proper upbringing. The difference that it made, which is observable not only to me but to other parents, is that my son has a real interest in keeping his possessions in order and cared for and he often comments on other people (adults as well) who don't. My wife and I have never required that he be concerned about these things. The secret of accomplishing this lies in applying the data and is actually what you don't understand, not what your child doesn't understand. You would be remiss in your duties as a parent if you didn't read and use this technology."

SUGGESTIONS FOR FURTHER STUDY

This chapter contains some fundamental applications of Dianetics and Scientology to the raising of children. The materials listed below provide more of Mr. Hubbard's breakthroughs related to giving a child a happy and fulfilling life, and are recommended study for parents, couples planning a family or anyone who works with children.

How to Be a Successful Parent

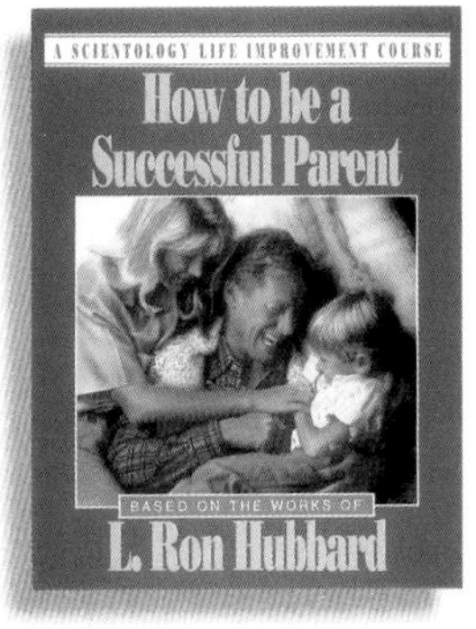

Raising an independent and responsible child is not a hit-or-miss activity. This course contains vital knowledge on the role of love and affection, how to create an understanding relationship with a child, the exact use of discipline without reducing self-determinism, and more.

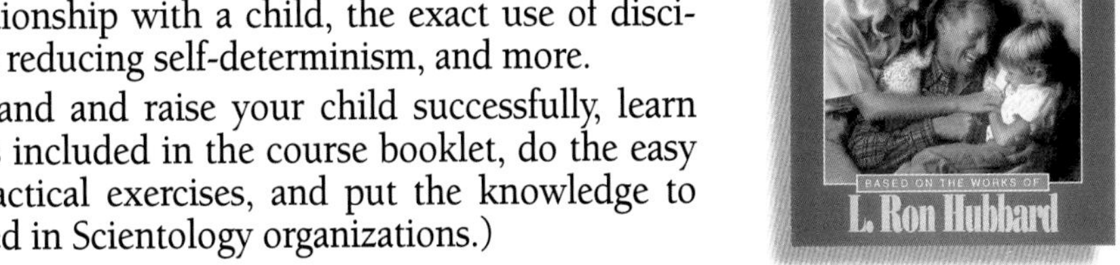

To understand and raise your child successfully, learn the principles included in the course booklet, do the easy drills and practical exercises, and put the knowledge to use. (Delivered in Scientology organizations.)

Child Dianetics

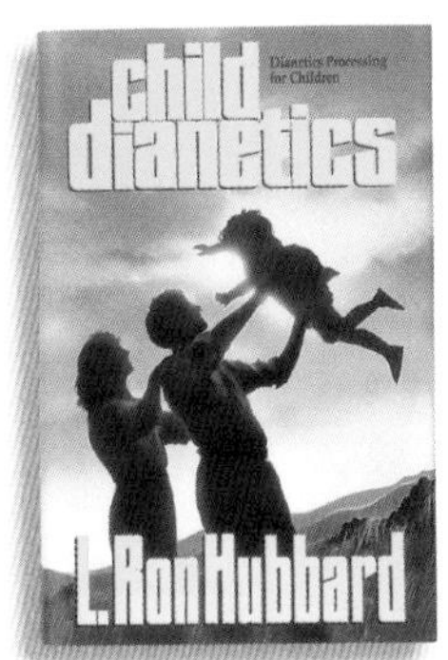

A new approach to rearing children utilizing the principles of Dianetics. Greatly expands on the material in this chapter, giving a full understanding of how to apply the techniques presented plus much further data. Includes case histories of children on whom the techniques covered in the book were applied.

With this view of children and the practical measures in Mr. Hubbard's book, one can engender a child's love and respect, and help him grow to lead a happy and successful adult life.

Children's Communication Course

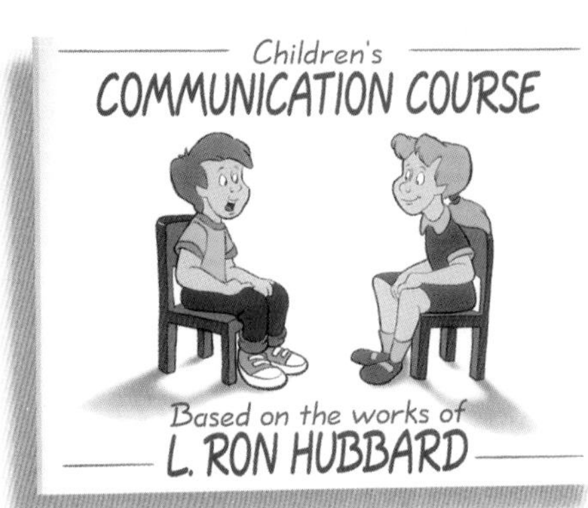

This is a course specifically designed *for* children, not about children.

Mr. Hubbard isolated that communication is a vital part of life and is key to happiness and success. His breakthrough discoveries in this field make it possible for anyone to communicate easily and be really understood.

This course gives a child simple practical exercises to learn basic communication skills which enable him or her to communicate freely with anyone, overcome shyness, get a question answered, handle others with understanding, make himself or herself fully understood, get a point across, and more. Includes an easy-to-read, fully illustrated text and is suitable for children between the ages of 8 and 12. Any child can learn how to communicate well and feel confident in life. (Delivered in Scientology organizations.)

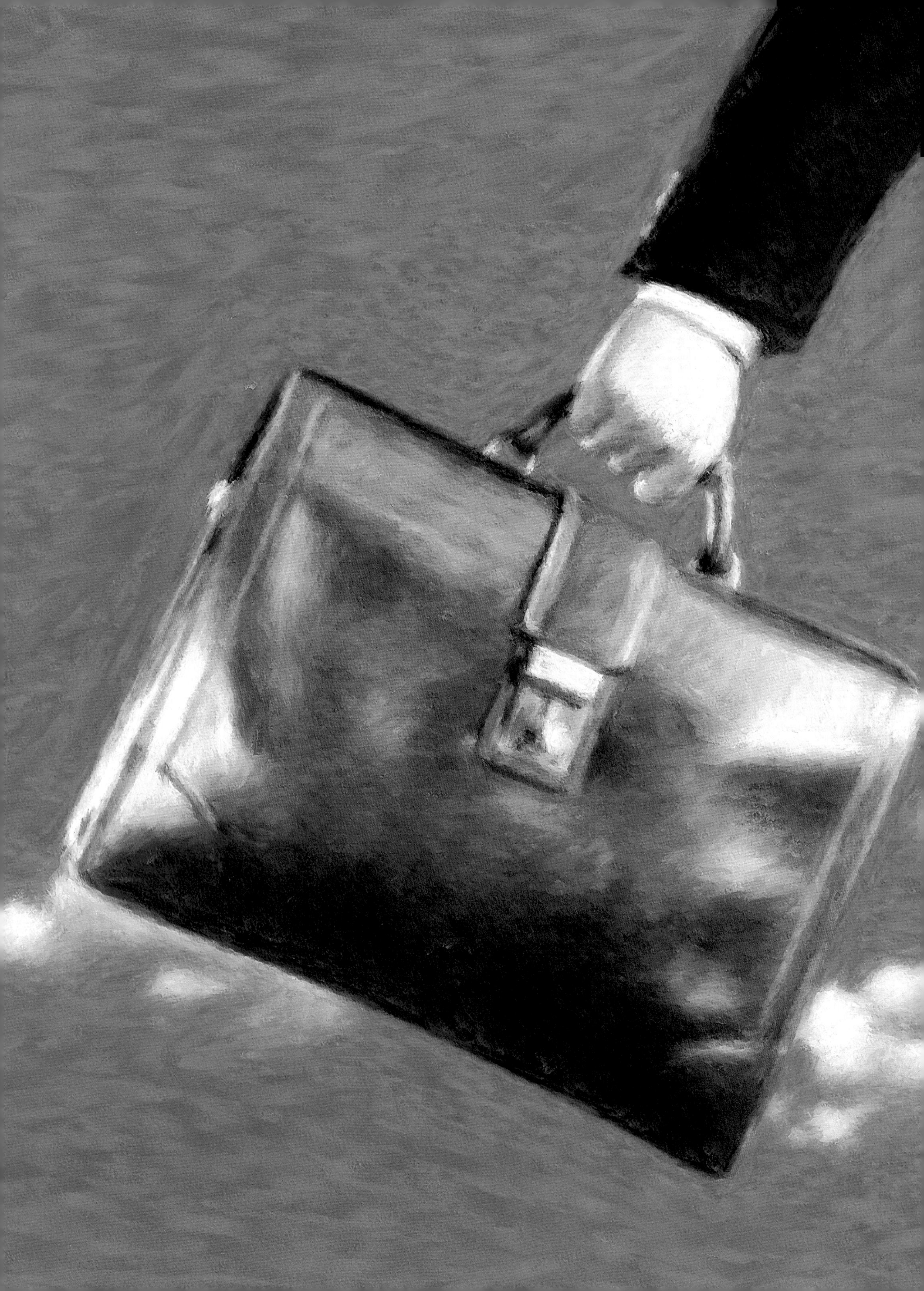

Chapter 15

TOOLS FOR THE WORKPLACE

Plummeting productivity, massive layoffs, sour relations between management and labor, executive incompetence and dishonest business dealings all plague the workplace. It is small wonder that the act of work is a source of stress and anxiety for millions.

How to increase job efficiency and productivity, how to handle upsets and confusion in the workplace and how to overcome exhaustion are all matters that concern both the laborer and the manager. Their resolution would bring about not only greater security but greater satisfaction.

This chapter contains some of the wide array of principles and techniques L. Ron Hubbard developed for application in the workplace. Work not only **can** *be both rewarding and fulfilling, but as the major activity in most of our lives, it* **should** *be. Utilization of this information will help you make it just that.*

Handling Confusion in the Workplace

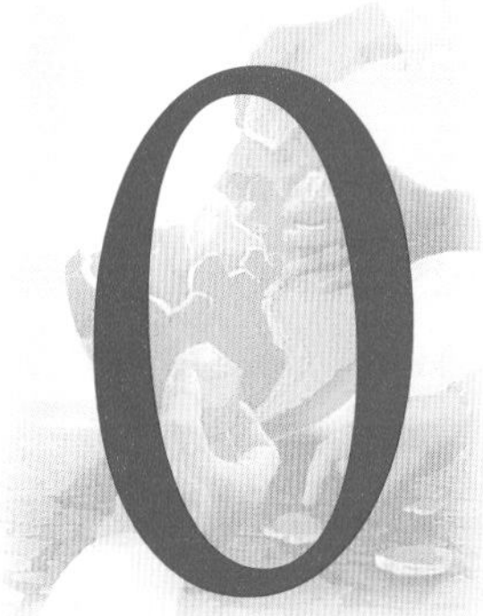

One might be led to believe there was something confusing about navigating one's career in the world of work. And confusion there is, to one who is not equipped with guides and maps.

As one looks at the many factors which might derange his life and undermine his security, the impression is, confusion seems well founded and it can be said with truth that all difficulties are fundamentally confusions. Given enough menace, enough unknown, a man ducks his head and tries to swing through it blindly. He has been overcome by confusions.

Enough unsolved problems add up to a huge confusion. Every now and then, on his job, enough conflicting orders bring the worker into a state of confusion. A modern plant can be so poorly managed that the entire thing appears to be a vast confusion to which no answer is possible.

Luck is the usual answer one resorts to in a confusion. If the forces about one seem too great, one can always "rely on his luck." By luck we mean "destiny not personally guided." When one turns loose of an automobile wheel and hopes the car will stay on the road by luck, he is often disappointed. And so it is in life. Those things left to chance become less likely to work themselves out. One has seen a friend shutting his eyes to the bill collectors and gritting his teeth while he hopes that he will win at the races and solve all his problems. One has known people who handled their lives this way for years. Indeed, one of English novelist Charles Dickens' great characters had the entire philosophy of "waiting for something to turn up." But luck, while we grant that it *is* a potent element, is only necessary amid a strong current of confusing factors. If one has to have *luck* to see him through, then it follows that one isn't any longer at his own automobile wheel and it follows, too, that one is dealing with a confusion.

It would be wise, then, to understand exactly what a confusion is and how it could be resolved.

Confusion and the Stable Datum

A confusion can be defined as any set of factors or circumstances which do not seem to have any immediate solution. More broadly, a confusion is *random motion.*

If you were to stand in heavy traffic you would be likely to feel confused by all the motion whizzing around you. If you were to stand in a heavy storm, with leaves and papers flying by, you would be likely to be confused.

Is it possible to actually understand a confusion? Is there any such thing as an "anatomy of confusion"? Yes, there is.

If, as a switchboard operator, you had ten calls hitting your board at once, you might feel confused. But is there any answer to the situation? If, as a shop foreman, you have three emergencies and an accident all at the same time, you might feel confused. But is there any answer to that?

A confusion is only a confusion so long as *all* particles are in motion. A confusion is only a confusion so long as no factor is clearly defined or understood.

Confusion is the basic cause of stupidity. To the stupid all things except the very simple ones are confused. Thus if one knew the anatomy of confusion, no matter how bright one might be, he would be brighter.

If you have ever had to teach some ambitious young person who was not too bright, you will understand this well. You attempt to explain how such and so works. You go over it and over it and over it. And then you turn him loose and he promptly makes a complete botch of it. He "didn't understand," he "didn't grasp it." You can simplify your understanding of his misunderstanding by saying, very rightly, "He was confused."

Ninety-nine percent of all education fails, when it fails, on the grounds that the student was confused.

And not only in the realm of the job, but in life itself, when failure approaches, it is born, one way or another, from confusion. To learn of machinery or to live life, one has to be able either to stand up to confusion or to take it apart.

We have in Scientology a certain doctrine (principle) about confusion. It is called the *Doctrine of the Stable Datum.*

If you saw a great many pieces of paper whirling about a room they would look confused until you picked out *one* piece of paper to be the piece of paper by which everything else was in motion. In other words, a confusing motion can be understood by conceiving one thing to be motionless.

In a stream of traffic all would be confusion unless you were to conceive one car to be motionless in relation to the other cars and so to see others in relation to the one.

The switchboard operator receiving ten calls at once solves the confusion by labeling, correctly or incorrectly, one call as the first call to receive her attention. The confusion of ten calls all at once becomes less confusing the moment she singles out one call to be answered. The shop foreman confronted by three emergencies and an accident needs only to elect his *first* target of attention to start the cycle of bringing about order again.

Until one selects *one* datum, *one* factor, *one* particular in a confusion of particles, the confusion continues. The *one* thing selected and used becomes the *stable datum* for the remainder.

Any body of knowledge, more particularly and exactly, is built from *one datum.* That is its *stable datum.* Invalidate it and the entire body of knowledge falls apart. A stable datum does not have to be the correct one. It is simply the one that keeps things from being in a confusion and on which others are aligned.

Now, in teaching an ambitious young man to use a machine, he failed to grasp your directions, if he did, because he lacked a stable datum. *One fact* had to be brought home to him first. Grasping that, he could grasp others. One is

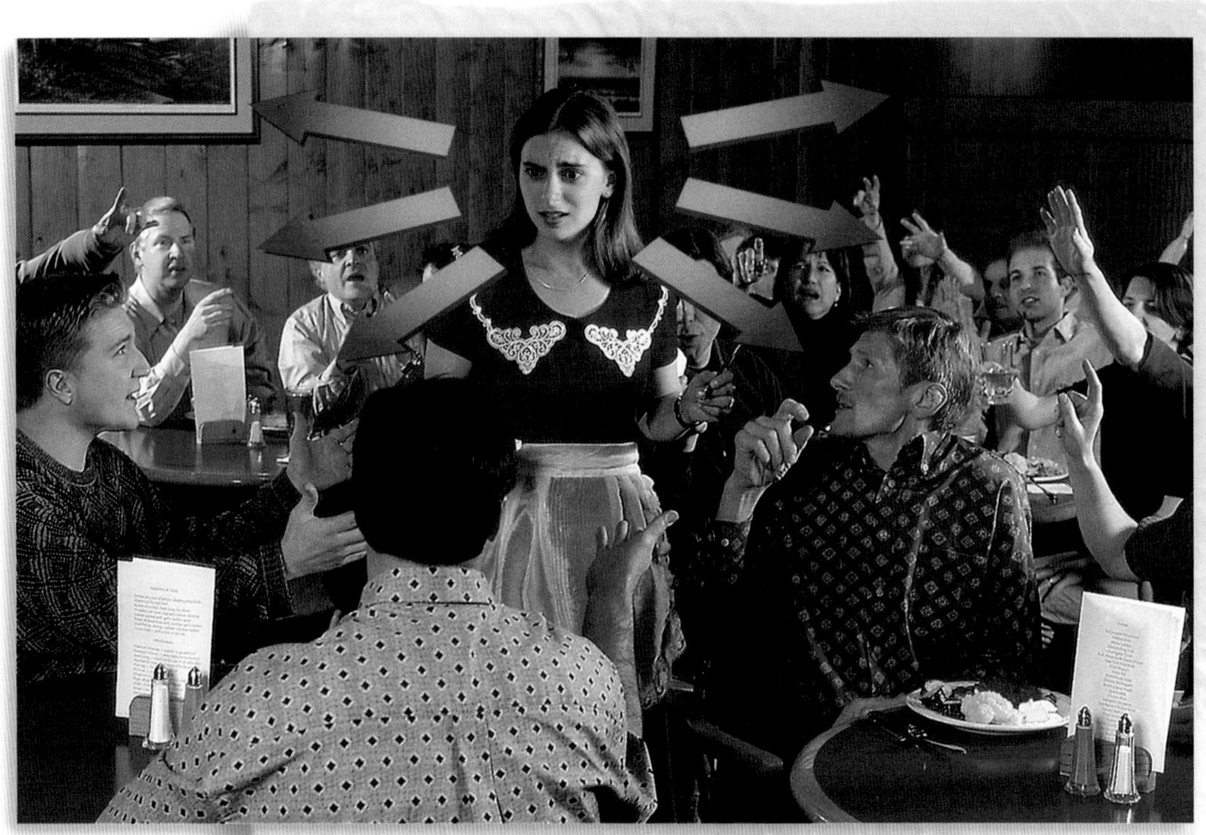

A confusion exists when all particles are in motion.

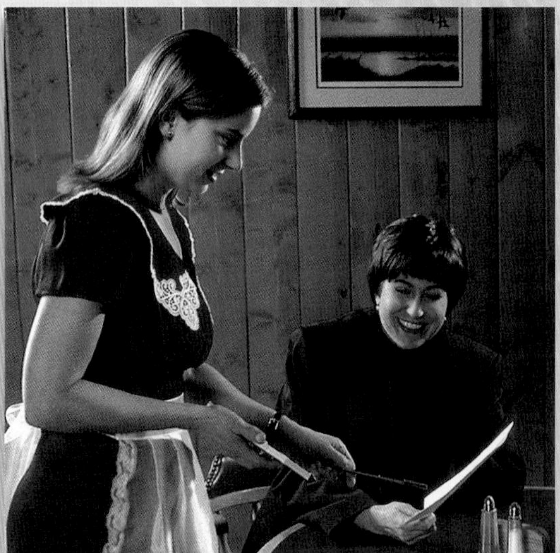

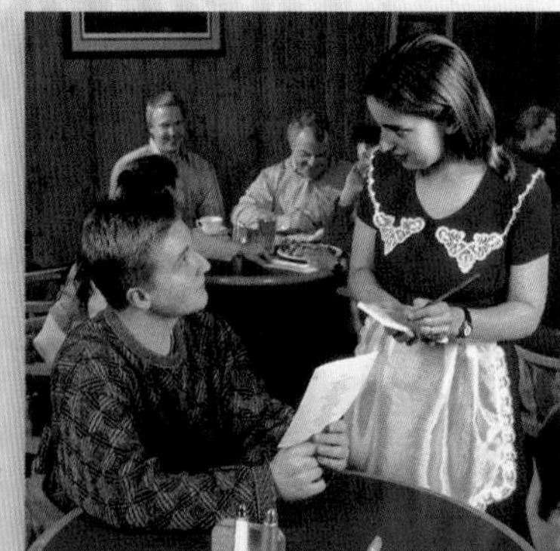

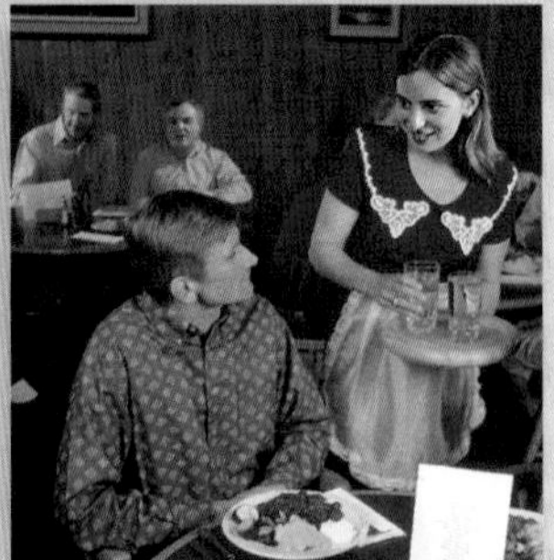

It becomes less confusing when one item is singled out and becomes the stable datum for the remainder.

stupid, then, or confused in any confusing situation until he has fully grasped *one fact* or one item.

Confusions, no matter how big and hard to overcome they may seem, are composed of data or factors or particles. They have pieces. Grasp one piece and locate it thoroughly. Then see how the others function in relation to it and you have steadied the confusion and, relating other things to what you have grasped, you will soon have mastered the confusion in its entirety.

In teaching a boy to run a machine, don't throw a torrent of data at him and then point out his errors: that's confusion to him, that makes him respond stupidly. Find some entrance point to his confusion, *one datum*. Tell him, "This is a machine." It may be that all the directions were flung at someone who had no real certainty, no real order of existence. "This is a machine," you say. Then make him sure of it. Make him feel it, fiddle with it, push at it. "This is a machine," tell him. And you'd be surprised how long it may take, but you'd be surprised as well how his certainty increases. Out of all the complexities he must learn to operate it, he must know *one datum* first. It is not even important *which* datum he first learns well, beyond that it is better to teach him a *simple basic datum*. You can show him what it does, you can explain to him the final product, you can tell him why *he* has been selected to run this machine. *But* you *must* make one basic datum clear to him or else he will be lost in confusion.

Confusion is uncertainty. Confusion is stupidity. Confusion is insecurity. When you think of uncertainty, stupidity and insecurity, think of confusion and you'll have it down pat.

What, then, is certainty? Lack of confusion. What then is intelligence? Ability to handle confusion. What then is security? The ability to go through or around or to bring order to confusion. Certainty, intelligence and security are lack of, or ability to handle, confusion.

How does luck fit into confusion? Luck is the hope that some uncontrolled chance will get one through. Counting on luck is an abandonment of control. That's apathy.

Control and Confusion

There is *good* control and *bad* control. The difference between them is certainty and uncertainty. Good control is certain, positive, predictable. Bad control is uncertain, variable and unpredictable. With good control one can be certain, with bad control one is never certain. A foreman who makes a rule effective today but not tomorrow, who makes George obey but not James, is exercising bad control; in that foreman's wake will come uncertainty and insecurity, no matter what his personal attributes may be.

Because there can be so much uncertain, stupid control, some of us begin to believe that all control is bad. But this is very far from true. Control is necessary if one would bring any order into confusions. One must be able to control things, his body, his thoughts, at least to some degree, to do anything whatever.

A confusion could be called an *uncontrolled randomness.* Only those who can exert some control over that randomness can handle confusions. Those who cannot exert control actually breed confusions.

The difference between good and bad control then becomes more obvious. The difference between good and bad here is *degree.* A thorough, positive control can be predicted by others. Therefore it is good control. A nonpositive, sloppy control cannot be predicted; therefore it is a bad control. Intention also has something to do with control. Control can be used for constructive purposes or destructive purposes; but you will discover that when destructive purposes are *intended,* bad control is used.

Thus there is a great deal to this entire subject of *confusion.* You may find it rather odd for confusion itself to be used here as a target. But you will find that it is an excellent common denominator to all that we consider evil in life. And if one can become master of confusions, his attention is freed for constructive activity. So long as one is being confused by confusions, all he can think about are destructive things—what he wants to do most is to destroy the confusion.

So let us then learn first how to destroy confusions. And this, we find, is a rather simple thing. When *all* particles seem to be in motion, halt one and see how the others move according to it and then you will find less confusion present. With one adopted as a *stable datum* others can be made to fall in line. Thus an emergency, a machine, a job or life itself can be viewed and understood and one can be free.

Let us take a glance at how this works. There are a number of things which might influence obtaining, holding and improving a job. One can handle this entire problem, as people most often do, by entering into the problem the single datum, "I can get and hold a job." By clutching to this as a single belief, the confusions and insecurities of life become less effective, less confusing.

But suppose one has done this: Suppose that without further investigating the problem, one, when young, gritted his teeth and shut his eyes and said, "I can get and hold a job, come what may. Therefore I am not going to worry about the economics of existence anymore." Well, that was fine.

Later on, without warning, one got fired. One was out of work for ten weeks. He felt then, even when he did get a new job, less secure, less confident. And let us say that some accident occurred and one was out of a job again. When once more unemployed, he was once more even less confident, less secure. Why?

Let us take a look at the opposite side of this Doctrine of the Stable Datum. If we do, we learn that confusions are held ineffective by stable data and that, when the stable datum is shaken, the confusion comes into being again.

Let us envision a confusion as stopped. It is still scattered but it is stopped. What stopped it? The adoption of a stable datum. Let us say that one was bothered badly in the home by a mother-in-law. One day, after a quarrel, one stalked out and by inspiration said to himself, "All mothers-in-law are evil." That was a decision. That, rightly or wrongly, was a stable datum adopted in a confusion. At once one felt better. He could deal with or live with the problem now. He knew that "all mothers-in-law" were evil. It wasn't true, but it was a stable datum. Then one day, when he was in trouble, his mother-in-law stepped forward, unwaveringly loyal, and paid not only the rent but the other debt, too. At once he felt very confused. This act of kindness should not have been a thing to bring in confusion. After all, hadn't she solved the problem? Then why does one feel upset about it? *Because the stable datum has been shaken.* The entire confusion of the past problem came into action again by reason of the demonstrated falsity of the stable datum.

To make anyone confused, all you have to do is locate their stable data and invalidate them. By criticism or proof it is only necessary to shake these few stable data to get all a person's confusions back into action.

You see, stable data do not have to be true. They are simply adopted. When adopted, then one looks at other data in relation to them. Thus the adoption of *any* stable datum will tend to nullify the confusion addressed. *But* if that stable datum is shaken, invalidated, disproven, then one is left again with the confusion. Of course, all one has to do is adopt a new stable datum or put the old stable datum back in place, but he'd have to know Scientology in order to accomplish this smoothly.

Let us say one has no fears of national economy because of a heroic political figure who is trying his best. That man is the stable datum to all one's confusions about national economy. Thus one "isn't worried." But one day circumstances or his political enemies shake him as a datum. They "prove" he was really dishonest. One then becomes worried all over again about national economy. Maybe you adopted some philosophy because the speaker seemed such a pleasant chap. Then some person carefully proves to you that the speaker was actually a thief or worse. One adopted the philosophy because one needed some peace from his thoughts. Invalidating the speaker would then at once bring back the confusion one faced originally.

All right. We looked at the confusion of the workaday world when we were young and we held it all back by stating grimly, "I can get and keep a job." That was the stable datum. We did get a job. But we got fired. The confusion of the workaday world then became very confusing. If we have only the one stable datum, "I can get and keep a job," then, assuredly, one is going to spend some confusing periods in his working life. A far, far better stable datum would be, "I understand about life and jobs. Therefore I can get, hold and improve them."

Confusion need not be an unavoidable and persistent part of one's working life. By employing the Doctrine of the Stable Datum one can gradually bring order and understanding to any situation.

REACH AND WITHDRAW

With an understanding of confusion and the need for good control to bring order, one can easily observe workers and executives who breed confusions with bad control. There is a very simple but extremely powerful method to get a person familiarized and in communication with things so that he can be more in control of them. This is called Reach and Withdraw.

One would not expect a person to have much control or understanding of or skill in something with which he was not familiar.

The keynote of familiarity is communication.

A person is out of communication with something because he is withdrawing from it and is not about to reach out to or contact any part of it.

If a person cannot reach and withdraw from a thing, he will be the effect of that thing.

If a person can reach for something and withdraw from it, he could be said to be in communication with that thing.

To be in communication with something is to be in a more causative position in relation to it.

By REACH we mean touching or taking hold of. It is defined as "to get to," "come to" and/or "arrive at."

By WITHDRAW we mean move back from, let go.

The Reach and Withdraw procedure brings a person into communication with and into a more causative position in relation to objects, people, spaces, boundaries and situations.

In the physical universe, communication with objects, forms, spaces and boundaries is best established by actual physical contact.

Reach and Withdraw is a valuable tool to use to get a person into good communication with his work environment, especially the tools and objects he uses.

A pilot would do Reach and Withdraw on all the objects and spaces of his airplane, his hangar, the earth; a secretary would do Reach and Withdraw on her typewriter, her chair, walls, spaces, her desk, etc.

Feeling comfortable with the tools of one's trade is a very important step in getting out products. One can increase the amount of production tremendously with this action.

For example, a flight surgeon who was trained in this procedure used Reach and Withdraw on his squadron and for one whole year there was not one single accident, not even so much as the touch of a wing tip to a wing tip. It is probably the only squadron in history that went a whole year without even a minor accident.

Procedure

Reach and Withdraw procedure is easily learned. It can be done on any object or area. It can be done on an individual's job environment, on a new piece of equipment, a machine, anything. It is done until the person is in good communication with his general environment or specific area being addressed.

1. Take the person to the area where you will be doing Reach and Withdraw. Explain to him you are going to do Reach and Withdraw and explain the procedure.

2. Tell him the commands to be used and ensure he understands these. The commands are:

A. "Reach that _________." (naming and pointing to an object or person or area)

B. "Withdraw from that _________." (naming and pointing to the same object or person or area)

A thing or part of something (e.g., "the big red button on the front of the machine") or a space or a person is named in the blank.

3. Give him the first command. For example, "Reach that big red button on the front of the machine."

Always point to the object (or person, space, etc.) each time you give a command so there will be no mistake made by the person doing it.

4. When the person has carried out the command, acknowledge him by saying "Thank you," or "Good," etc.

5. Now give the second command, "Withdraw from that big red button on the front of the machine." Acknowledge him when he has done so.

6. Continue to alternate the commands A, B, A, B and so on, with an acknowledgment after the execution of each command, having the person touch different parts of the object or area.

7. Reach and withdraw from that one thing, space or person until the individual either has a minor win, or until three consecutive sets of commands have been executed with no change in the person's motions or attitude. By "minor win" is meant a small improvement for the person, such as his feeling a bit better about the object or area, or simply experiencing an increased feeling of well-being.

8. Next, another object, space or person is chosen and the commands are taken to a win on that item.

Don't keep the person reaching and withdrawing endlessly from the same *part* of anything that is being used but go to different points and parts of an object being touched.

Walk around with the person doing the action, ensuring that he actually does get in physical contact with the points or areas of objects, spaces or people.

Choose objects in such a way as to progress from smaller objects to the larger objects available, touching different parts of each one in turn to a minor win of some sort on that object or three sets of commands with no change. Also include walls and floors and other parts of the environment in doing this procedure.

When doing the action on a space or a room rather than an object, have the person walk into the room and walk out of the room over and over.

9. Continue until the person has a major win or a good realization and is very happy about the whole area being addressed. A major win would be a large improvement for the person such as a new awareness of his work area or a certainty about his job. Reach and Withdraw would not be continued past such a point.

Reach and Withdraw on the objects, people, situations, spaces and boundaries of a person's job will greatly assist his control, familiarity and understanding of it.

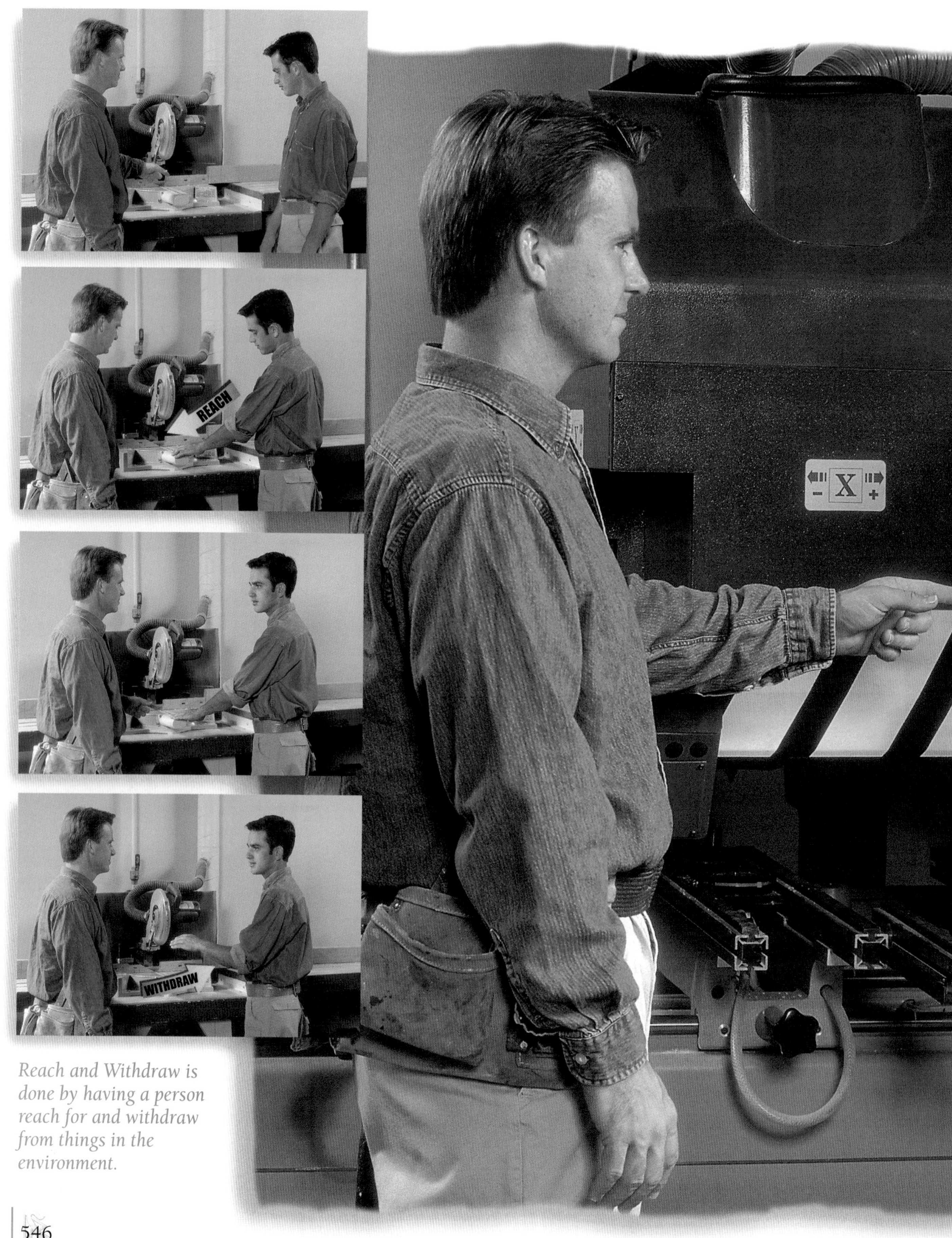

Reach and Withdraw is done by having a person reach for and withdraw from things in the environment.

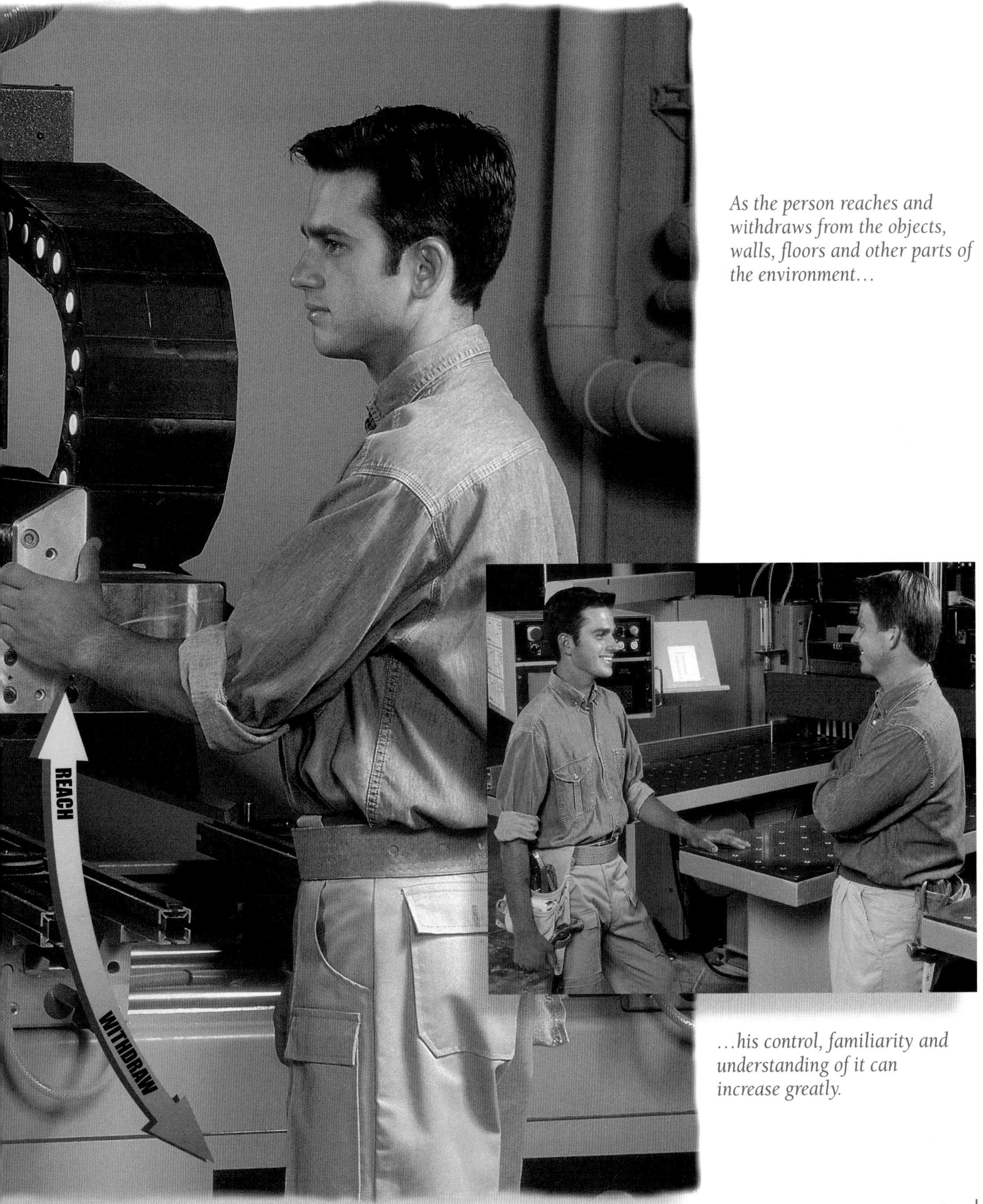

As the person reaches and withdraws from the objects, walls, floors and other parts of the environment…

…his control, familiarity and understanding of it can increase greatly.

Handling Exhaustion in the Workaday World

To work or not to work, that is the question. The answer to that question in most men's minds is exhaustion.

One begins to feel, after he has been long on a job and has been considerably abused on that job, that to work any more would be quite beyond his endurance. He is tired. The thought of doing certain things makes him tired. He thinks of raising his energy or of being able to force his way along just a little bit further, and if he does so he is thinking in the wrong channels since the answer to exhaustion has little if anything to do with energy.

Exhaustion is a very important subject, not only to an individual involved in earning his own living but to the state as well.

Scientology has rather completely established the fact that the downfall of the individual begins when he is no longer able to work. All it is necessary to do to degrade or upset an individual is to prevent him from working. Even the police have now come to recognize the basic Scientology principle that the primary thing wrong with a criminal is that he cannot work, and police have begun to look for this factor in an individual in establishing his criminality.

The subject of exhaustion is also the subject of prevented work. In the case of soldiers and sailors hospitalized during war, it is found that a few months in the hospital tends to break the morale of the soldier or sailor to such a point that he may become a questionable asset when returned to his service. This is not necessarily the result of his lowered abilities. It is the result of injury compounded by inactivity. A soldier who is wounded and cared for in a field hospital close to the front and is returned to duty the moment he can possibly support such duties will be found to retain, in a large measure, his morale. Of course the injury received has a tendency to repel him from the level of action which he once thought best but, even so, he is in better shape than a soldier who is sent to a hospital in the rear. The soldier who is sent to the hospital in the rear is being told, according to his viewpoint, that he is not particularly necessary to the war. Without actually adding up these principles, the word *exhaustion* began a general use coupled with neurosis. This was based on the fact that people with a neurosis simply looked exhausted. There was no more coordination to it than that. Actually, a person who has been denied the right to work, particularly one who has been injured and then denied the right to work, will eventually encounter exhaustion.

It has been discovered that there is no such thing as gradual diminishing by continuing contact of the energy of the individual. One does not become exhausted simply because one has worked too long or too hard. One becomes exhausted when he has worked sufficiently long to reactivate the pain and emotion of a past bad memory of some old injury.

One of the characteristics of this injury will be exhaustion. Chronic exhaustion, then, is not the product of long hours and arduous application. It is the product of the accumulation of the shocks and injuries incident to life, each of them perhaps only a few seconds or a few hours long and adding up perhaps to a totality of only fifty or seventy-five hours. But this accumulation—the accumulation of injury, repulsion and shock—eventually mounts up to a complete inability to do anything.

Exhaustion can then be trained into a person by refusing to allow him as a child to have any part in the society, or it can be beaten into a person by the various injuries or shocks he may receive incident to his particular activities. Clear up either of these two points and you have cleared up exhaustion.

Exhaustion, then, is actually the subject of a trained Scientology practitioner since only a Scientologist can adequately handle it.

There is a point, however, which is below exhaustion. This is the point of not knowing when one is tired. An individual can become a sort of hectic puppet that goes on working and working without even realizing that he is working at all, and suddenly collapses from a tiredness he was not experiencing.

Here the individual has failed to control things. Eventually he is incapable of handling anything even resembling tools of the trade or an environment of work and so is unable to inhabit such an environment or handle such tools. The individual can then have many hard words cast in his direction. He can be called lazy, he can be called a bum, he can be called criminal. But the truth of the matter is he is no more capable of righting his own condition without expert help than he is capable of diving to the center of the earth.

There are, however, some means of recovering one's energy and enthusiasm for work short of consultation with a Scientology practitioner. These are relatively simple and very easy to understand.

Extroversion and Introversion

Introversion is a simple thing. It means looking in too closely. And extroversion is also a simple thing. It means nothing more than being able to look outward.

It could be said that there are introverted personalities and extroverted personalities. An extroverted personality is one who is capable of looking around the environment. An introverted personality is only capable of looking inward at himself.

A person who is capable of looking at the world around him and seeing it quite real and quite bright is, of course, in a state of extroversion. He can look out, in other words. He can also work. He can also see situations and handle and control those things which he has to handle and control, and can stand by and watch those things which he does not have to control and be interested in them therefore.

The person who is introverted is a person who has probably passed exhaustion some way back. He has had his attention focused closer and closer to him (basically by old injuries which are still capable of exerting their influence upon him) until he is actually looking inward and not outward. He is shying away from solid objects. He does not see a reality in other people and things around him.

Now let us take the actual subject of work. Work is the application of attention and action to people or objects located in space.

When one is no longer able to face people or objects or the space in which they are located without flinching or avoiding, he begins to have a lost feeling. He begins to move in a mistiness. Things are not real to him and he is relatively incapable of controlling those things around him. He has accidents. He has bad luck. He has things turn against him simply because he is not handling them or controlling them or even observing them correctly. The future to him seems very bad, so bad sometimes that he cannot face it. This person could be said to be severely introverted.

In work his attention is riveted on objects which are usually at the most only a few feet from him. He pays his closest attention to articles which are within the reach of his hands. This puts his attention away from extroversion at least to some spot in focus in front of his face. His attention fixes there. If this is coincident with some old injury incident or operation, he is likely to fix his attention as well on some spot in former times and reactivates some past bad memory so that he gets the pains and ills and the feeling of tiredness or apathy or subapathy which he had during that moment of injury. As his attention is continuously riveted there he of course has a tendency to look only there, even when he is not working.

Let us take an accountant. An accountant's eyes are on books at fixed distances from his eyes. At length he becomes "shortsighted." Actually he doesn't become shortsighted, he becomes book-sighted. His eyes most easily fix on a certain point in distance. Now as he fixes his attention there he tends to withdraw even from that point until at length he does not quite reach even his own books. Then he is fitted with glasses so that he can see the books more clearly. His vision and his attention are much the same thing.

A person who has a machine or books or objects continually at a fixed distance from him leaves his work and tends to keep his attention fixed exactly where his work was. In other words, his attention never really leaves his work at all. Although he goes home he is still really sitting in the office. His attention is still fixed on the environment of his work. If this environment is coincident with some injury or accident (and who does not have one of these at least?), he begins to feel weariness or tiredness.

Is there a cure for this?

Of course, only a trained Scientology practitioner could clear up this difficulty entirely. But the worker does have something which he can do.

Now here is the wrong thing to do, regardless of whether one is a bookkeeper, an accountant, a clerk, an executive or a machinist. The wrong thing to do is to leave work, go home, sit down and fix attention on an object more or less at the same distance from one as one confronts continually at work. In the case of a foreman, for instance, who is continually talking to men at a certain distance away from him, the wrong thing for him to do is to go home and talk to his wife at the same distance. The next thing she knows, she will be getting orders just as though she were a member of the shop. Definitely the wrong thing to do is to go home and sit down and read a paper, eat some dinner and go to bed. If a man practiced the routine of working all day and then sitting down "to rest" with a book or a newspaper in the evening, it is certain that sooner or later he would start to feel quite exhausted and then after a while would fall even below that and would not even wonder at his unwillingness to perform tasks which were once very easy to him.

Is there a right thing to do? Yes, there is. An individual who is continually fixed upon some object of work should fix his attention otherwise after working hours.

Take a Walk

There is a Scientology procedure known as "Take a Walk." This procedure is very easy to perform. When one feels tired on finishing his work, no matter if the thought of doing so is almost all that he can tolerate without falling through the floor, he should go out and walk around the block until he feels rested. In short, he should walk around the block and look at things until he sees the things he is walking near. It does not matter how many times he walked around the block, he should walk around the block until he feels better.

In doing this it will be found that one will become a little brighter at first and then will become very much more tired. He will become sufficiently tired that he knows now that he should go to bed and have a good night's sleep. This is not the time to stop walking since he is walking through exhaustion. He is walking out his exhaustion. He is not handling the exhaustion by physical exercise. The physical exercise has always appeared to be the more important factor to people, but the exercise is relatively unimportant. The factor that is important is the unfixing of his attention from his work to the material world in which he is living.

When one is so tired that he can barely drag himself around, or is so tired that he is hectically unable to rest at all, it is actually necessary that he confront masses. It is even doubtful if there is such a thing as a "fall of physical energy." Naturally there is a limit to this procedure. One cannot work all day and walk around the block all night and go to work the next day again and still expect to feel relieved. But one should certainly spend some time extroverting after having introverted all day.

"Take a Walk" is, within reason, a near cure-all. If one feels antagonistic toward one's wife, the wrong thing to do is to beat her. The right thing to do is to go out and take a walk around the block until one feels better, and make her walk around the block in the opposite direction until an extroversion from the situation is achieved. It will be discovered that all domestic quarrels, particularly amongst working people, stem from the fact that, having been overfixed (rather than overstrained) on one's work and the situations connected with it, one has failed to control certain things in his working environment. He then comes home and seeks to find something he *can*

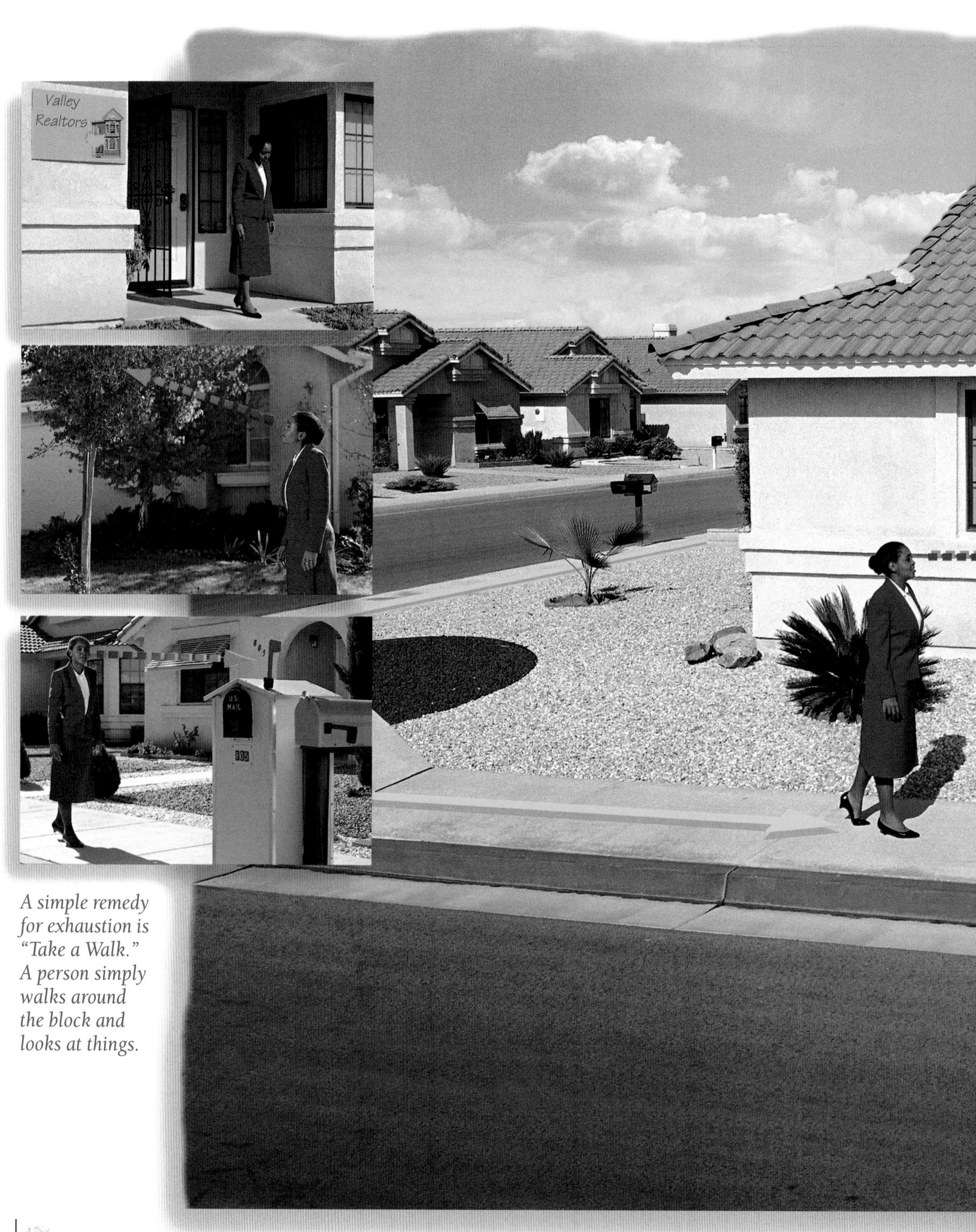

A simple remedy for exhaustion is "Take a Walk." A person simply walks around the block and looks at things.

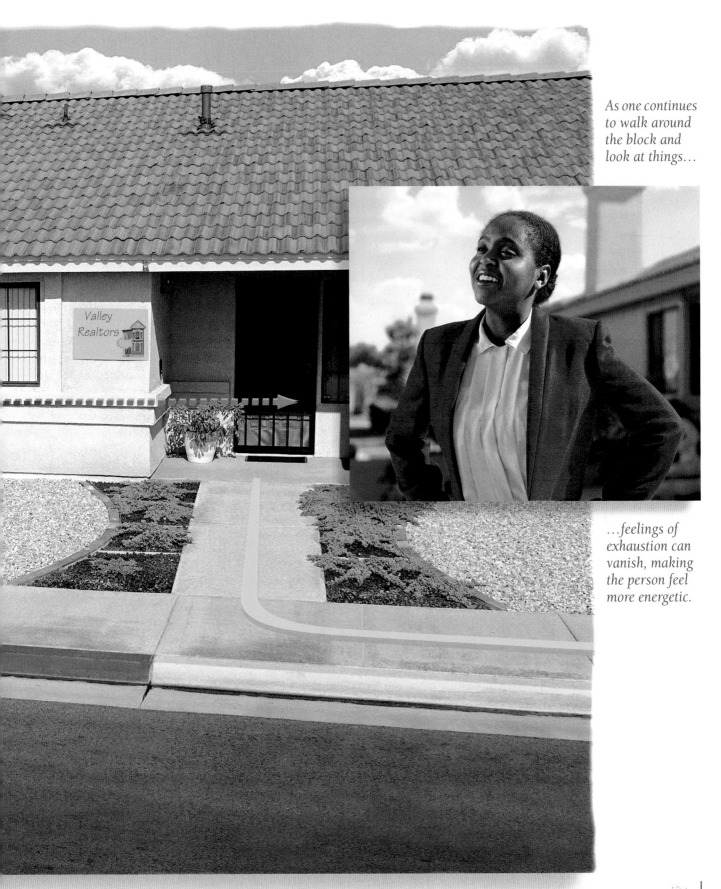

As one continues to walk around the block and look at things…

…feelings of exhaustion can vanish, making the person feel more energetic.

control. This is usually the marital partner or the children, and when one fails even there he is apt to worsen with a vengeance.

The extroversion of attention is as necessary as the work itself. There is nothing really wrong with introverting attention or with work. If one didn't have something to be interested in, he would go to pieces entirely. But if one works, it will be found that an unnatural tiredness is apt to set in. When this is found to be the case then the answer to this is not a drop into unconsciousness for a few hours as in sleep, but in actually extroverting the attention and then getting a really relaxing sleep.

These principles of extroversion and introversion have many ramifications and, although "Take a Walk" is almost laughable in its simplicity, there are many more complicated Scientology procedures in case one wished to get more complicated. However, in the main, "Take a Walk" will take care of an enormous number of difficulties attendant to work. Remember that when doing it one will get more tired at first and will then get fresher. This phenomenon has been noted by athletes. It is called the second wind. The second wind is really getting enough environment and enough mass in order to run out the exhaustion of the last race. There is no such thing as a second wind. There *is* such a thing as a return to extroversion on the physical world in which one lives.

Look Them Over

Similar to "Take a Walk" is another procedure known as "Look Them Over." If one has been talking to people all day, has been selling people all day or has been handling people who are difficult to handle all day, the wrong thing to do is to run away from all the people there are in the world. You see, the person who gets overstrained when handling people has had large difficulties with people. He has perhaps been operated upon by doctors, and the half-seen vision of them standing around the operating table identifies all people with doctors; that is to say, all people who stand still. This, by the way, is one of the reasons why doctors become so thoroughly hated in a society since they do insist on practices known as surgery and anesthesia and such incidents become interlocked with everyday incidents.

Exhaustion because of contact with people is due to one's attention having been fixated upon certain people while his attention, he felt, ought to be on other people. This straining of attention has actually cut down the number of people that he was observing.

The cure for this is a very simple one. One should go to a place that is very well populated such as a railroad station or a main street and should simply walk along the street noting people. Simply look at people—that is all. It will be found after a while that one feels people aren't so bad and one has a much kinder attitude toward them and, more importantly, the job condition of becoming overstrained with people tends to go away if one makes a practice of doing this every late afternoon for a few weeks.

This is one of the smartest things that a salesman can do, since a salesman, above and beyond others, has a vested interest in being able to handle people and get them to do exactly what he wants them to do, that is, buy what he has to sell. As he fixes his attention on just one too many customers, he gets tired of the whole idea of talking to people or selling and drops down to lower emotional levels in all of his activities and operations and begins to consider himself all kinds of a swindler and at length doesn't consider himself anything at all. He, like the others, should simply find populated places and walk along looking at people. He will find after a while that people really do exist and that they aren't so bad. One of the things that happens to people in high government is that they are being continually "protected from" the people and they at length become quite disgusted with the whole subject and are apt to do all manner of strange things. (Take, for example, the lives of Hitler and Napoleon.)

A person can become exhausted from contact with other people.

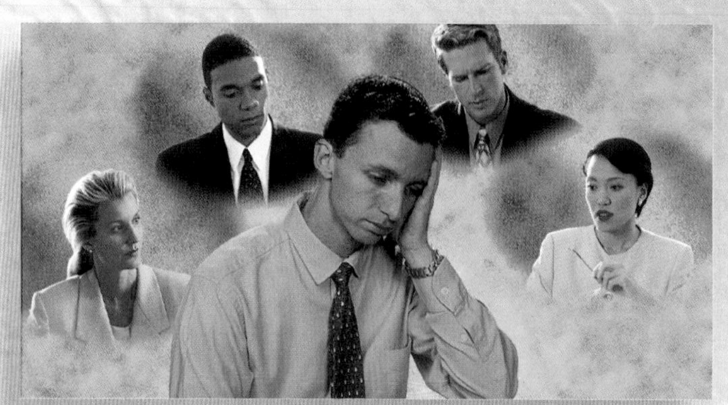

A remedy is for him to walk along a well-populated area noting people as he walks.

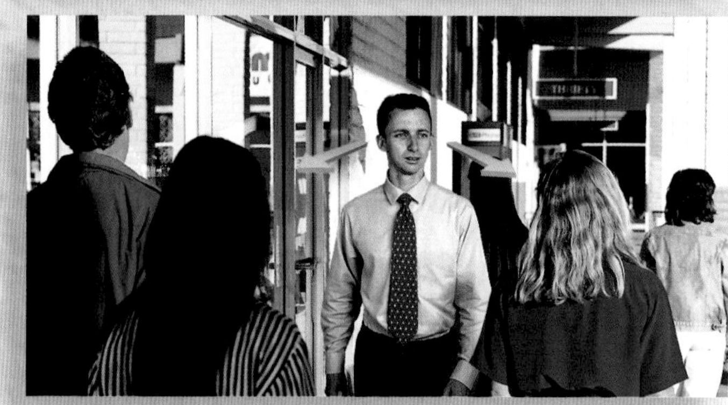

As he looks at more and more people…

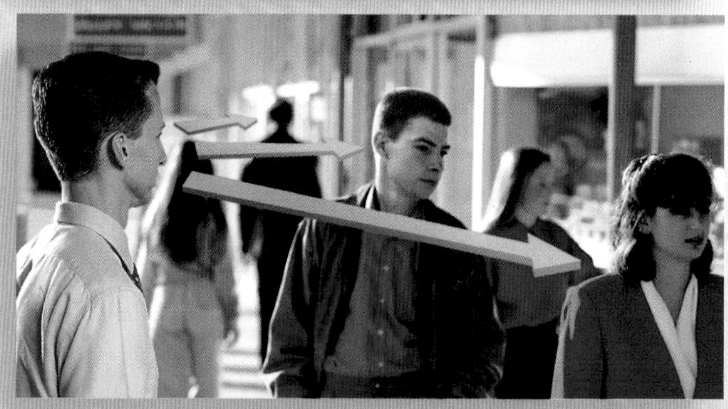

…he will find he feels kinder toward them. Any feelings of overstrain with people can go away entirely.

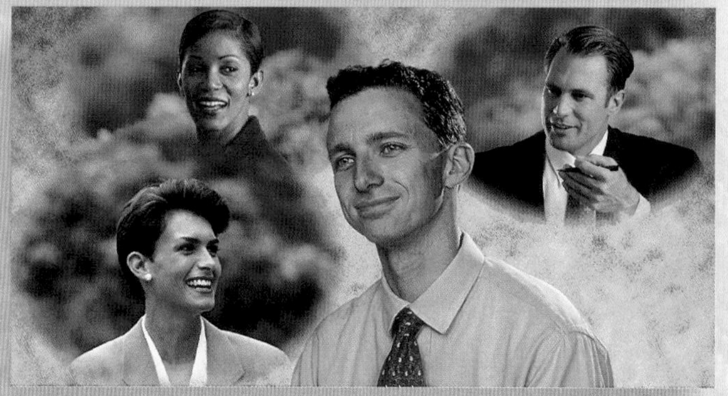

Broad Application

This principle of extroversion and introversion could go much further in a society than it does. There is something that could be done by the government and by businesses in general which would probably eradicate the idea of strikes and would increase production quite markedly. Workers who strike are usually discontented, not so much with the conditions of work, but with work itself. They feel they are being victimized, they are being pressed into working at times when they do not want to work, and a strike comes as an actual relief. They can fight something. They can do something else than stand there and fiddle with a piece of machinery or account books. Dissatisfied workers are striking workers. If people become exhausted at work, if people are not content with work, if people are upset with work, they can be counted upon to find a sufficient number of grievances to strike. And, if management is given enough trouble and lack of cooperation on the part of the people on the lower chains of command, it can be certain that management sooner or later will create situations which cause workers to strike. In other words, bad conditions of work are actually not the reason for labor troubles and disputes. Weariness of work itself or an inability to control the area and environments of work *are* the actual cause of labor difficulties.

Any management given sufficient income to do so, if that management is not terribly irrational, will pay a decent working wage. And any workman given half a chance will perform his duties cheerfully. But once the environment itself becomes overstrained, once the company itself has become introverted by harmful acts on the part of the government, once the workers have been shown that they have no control over management, there can be, after that, labor disputes. Underlying all these obvious principles, however, are the principles of introversion and extroversion. Workers become so introverted at their tasks that they no longer are capable of affinity for their leaders and are no longer capable actually of viewing the environment in which they work. Therefore someone can come along and tell them that all the executives are ogres, which is obviously not true, and on the executive level someone can come along and tell the executives that all the workers are ogres, which is obviously, on that side, not true either.

In the absence of broad treatment on individuals, which is a gargantuan (enormous) task, a full program could be worked out that would handle the principle of introversion. It is certain that if workers or managers get introverted enough they will then find ways and means of inventing irrational games such as strikes, and so disrupt production and decent relationships and living conditions within the factory, the office or the concern.

The cure would be to extrovert workers on a very broad scale. This could be done, as one solution, by making it possible for all workers to have two jobs. It would be necessary for the company, or related interests such as the government, to make available a sufficient number of public works projects to provide work for workers outside the sphere of exact application. In other words, a man who is made to work continually inside and at a very fixed task would find a considerable relief at being able to go outside and work, particularly at some disrelated task. As an example, it would be a considerable relief to an accountant to be able to dig ditches for a while. A machinist running a stationary machine would actually find it a very joyful experience to push around a bulldozer.

Such a plan then would actually take introversion and extroversion with a large hand and bring it about. Workers who are working in fixed positions with their attention very close to them would then be permitted to look more widely and to handle things which tended to extrovert them. Such a program would be very ambitious but it would be found, it is certain, to result in better labor–management relations, better production and a considerable lessening of working and public tension on the subjects of jobs and pay.

In short, there are many things that could be done with the basic principle of extroversion–introversion. The principle is very simple: When an individual is made too introverted, things become less real in his surroundings and he has less affinity for them and cannot communicate with them well. In such a condition he becomes tired easily. Introversion results in weariness, exhaustion and then an inability to work. The remedy for it is extroversion, a good look at and communication with the wider environment, and unless this is practiced, then, in view of the fact that any worker is subject to injuries or illnesses of one kind or another, a dwindling spiral will ensue which makes work less and less palatable until at length it cannot be performed at all and we have the basis of not only a nonproductive, but a criminal society.

THE IMPORTANCE OF WORK

Work is the stable datum of this society. Without something to do there is nothing for which to live. A man who cannot work is as good as dead and usually prefers death and works to achieve it.

The mysteries of life are not today, with Scientology, very mysterious. Mystery is not a needful ingredient. Only the very irrational man desires to have vast secrets held away from him. Scientology has slashed through many of the complexities which have been erected for men and has bared the core of these problems. Scientology for the first time in man's history can predictably raise intelligence, increase ability, bring about a return of the ability to play a game, and permits man to escape from the dwindling spiral of his own disabilities. Therefore work itself can become again a pleasant and happy thing.

There is one thing which has been learned in Scientology which is very important to the state of mind of the workman. One very often feels in his society that he is working for the immediate paycheck and that he does not gain for the whole society anything of any importance. He does not know several things. One of these is how few good workmen are. On the level of executives, it is interesting to note how precious any large company finds a man really is who can handle and control jobs and men. Such people are rare. All the empty space in the structure of this workaday world is at the top.

And there is another thing which is quite important, and that is the fact that the world today has been led to believe, by mental philosophies calculated to betray it, that when one is dead it is all over and done with and that one has no further responsibility for anything. It is highly doubtful that this is true. One inherits tomorrow what he died out of yesterday.

Another thing we know is that men are not dispensable. It is a mechanism of old philosophies to tell men that if they think they are indispensable they should go down to the graveyard and take a look—those men were indispensable, too. This is the sheerest foolishness. If you really looked carefully in the graveyard, you would find the machinist who set the models going in yesteryear and without whom there would be no industry today. It is doubtful if such a feat is being performed just now.

A workman is not just a workman. A laborer is not just a laborer. An office worker is not just an office worker. They are living, breathing, important pillars on which the entire structure of our civilization is erected.

They are not cogs in a mighty machine.

They are the machine itself. ■

Test Your Understanding

Answer the following questions about the information contained in this chapter. Refer back to it to check your answers. If you need to, review the chapter. Going over the material several times will increase your certainty and help you obtain better success in applying it.

- ❑ *What is a confusion?*
- ❑ *What is a stable datum?*
- ❑ *How can one use the Doctrine of the Stable Datum to handle a confusion?*
- ❑ *What is the purpose of Reach and Withdraw, and how is it done?*
- ❑ *What is the difference between good and bad control?*
- ❑ *What is introversion?*
- ❑ *What is extroversion?*
- ❑ *What causes exhaustion and how can it be remedied?*

PRACTICAL EXERCISES

The following exercises will help you understand this chapter and increase your ability to actually apply the knowledge.

1 Think of an example of a confusion you have observed or experienced. Work out for yourself how the Doctrine of the Stable Datum could have been applied to that confusion.

2 Go out and find a confusion. Using the "Doctrine of the Stable Datum," handle that confusion.

3 Practice doing Reach and Withdraw. Drill giving the commands for Reach and Withdraw to a wall, naming a part of an object in the command, pointing and acknowledging each time. Refer to the procedure as needed while drilling. Drill the procedure until you can easily do Reach and Withdraw with no uncertainty.

4 Now, do Reach and Withdraw on another person on the tools of his job or his work environment.

5 Think of an example of bad control you have observed or experienced. Note why it was bad control.

6 Think of an example of good control you have observed or experienced. Note why it was good control.

7 Think of an example you have observed or experienced where an individual was not in good communication or familiar with a machine he was operating. Note his effectiveness on the job and the quality of what he was expected to produce.

8 Think of an example you have observed or experienced where an individual was in good communication or familiar with a machine he was operating. Note his effectiveness on the job and the quality of what he was expected to produce.

9 Take a walk around the block until you feel extroverted and more alert.

10 Find a person who is feeling exhaustion from work or who is upset from a domestic quarrel, etc., and have him or her take a walk until he or she feels extroverted.

Results from Application

That Scientologists have and use technology that enables them to survive well in the workplace is reflected by the fact that more than 54 percent have positions as managers, artists, technicians, engineers, company owners or part owners, lawyers, or work in the medical profession.

But application of this data extends its effects well beyond the people who apply it—it is a positive influence on their environment and those around them, helping to create islands of sanity in the chaos of the workaday world as can be seen in the examples which follow.

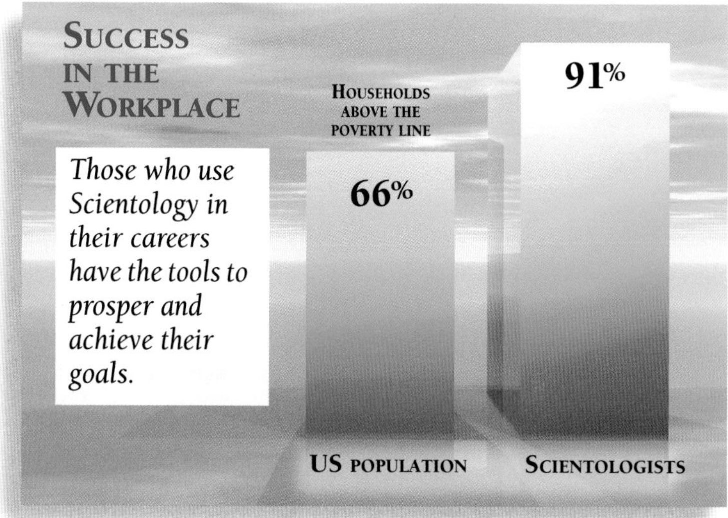
Success in the Workplace
Those who use Scientology in their careers have the tools to prosper and achieve their goals.
Households above the poverty line
66%
91%
US population
Scientologists

Frequently exhausted after his daily endeavors, a man was shown what Mr. Hubbard had written about how to handle exhaustion.

"In the past exhaustion always meant giving in and having to rest—and even rest didn't really handle the problem. The real reason for the exhaustion, and consequently the real solution, seemed to elude me. Exhaustion **can** *be handled by doing just what Mr. Hubbard says. This is most important to me. Now I can remain fresh and alert throughout the day."*

A musician receiving Reach and Withdraw on his area had considered that he was already in excellent communication with his environment. However, he was amazed at the change this simple action made in his operation.

"I had a great experience on this where I got a very clear concept of an ideal situation for creation of music and the level to which aesthetics can be raised. Only through Scientology could such an ideal be attained. What a simple and powerful piece of technology Reach and Withdraw is!"

Having learned the basic data on handling situations in the workplace, a man decided that he could do or be anything that he wanted to. So he chose to enter the catering field and promptly went out and got a position as a manager in a large catering firm that served more than 1,500 people at a new paper mill being built in South Africa.

"I had thirty-five or more staff and by applying to this job the basic Scientology I had studied, I was able to get them very productive. There were two shifts and four managers. My boss was always amazed at how smoothly my shift ran and how we were able to finish so quickly. At that time I

realized the full effectiveness of this technology and its ability to change apparently hopeless situations for the better rather rapidly."

A young woman had been working long hours for many weeks, doing the same proofreading activity day after day. One day she found that this activity, which she normally had no trouble in doing, was getting harder and harder.

"Finally, near the end of the day, my sight gave out completely and I was unable to see at all for a few seconds. My eyes were hurting and things were a bit blurry. The person I was proofreading with knew the 'Take a Walk' remedy and took me outside and we went for a walk. At first I didn't want to look around because my eyes hurt, but she made me do it. After a little while my eyes stopped hurting and I was able to look around. I became cheerful again and was able to continue proofreading with no more strain."

A businesswoman was having difficulty in getting along with her boss. A friend referred her to some basic data from Mr. Hubbard on how to get along with others in the workaday world.

"Earlier this year, I had quite a lot of trouble in my firm. My boss constantly criticized me and complained to me about every petty detail in the office. But it is completely different since I studied this data. Now when I am around he is not critical anymore and he even commends me. I know it is because of what I learned, as when I am not here, my colleagues still let him spoil their mood. But I can handle my whole environment now and for me, working conditions are very pleasant."

An executive in charge of personnel in a large Southern California company had a serious problem coping with the number of people she had to deal with.

"I had a long, long list of names of people who needed my attention and those people were constantly demanding my services. All the time I could have spent getting things done for them was being eaten up just fending off the demands. Somehow I could not get ***anything*** *done. The larger this backlog became, the more overwhelmed I was. I decided to apply the 'Doctrine of the Stable Datum.' I looked at the ideal scene and started tackling each different job from the viewpoint of taking one job and completing it and then going on to the next. Total magic! At the end of the day I was cheerful and had a feeling of freedom. I knew that I had new undone jobs, but knew how to handle, so these were no longer a problem."*

SUGGESTIONS FOR FURTHER STUDY

As part of L. Ron Hubbard's research into life and the human spirit, he developed Scientology processes and techniques specifically for use in the workplace. Applying these one can gain an increased awareness of oneself and his relation to the physical universe, and with that comes greater ability and effectiveness. The following are recommended study, no matter what one's occupation.

The Problems of Work

This is an essential reference on the use of Scientology technology in the workplace. It covers vital fundamentals including what holding a job depends on, the secret of efficiency, and the factors of freedom, barriers and purposes as they apply to the subject of work. Contains Scientology procedures that can be used directly in one's work environment, to help both oneself and others become more aware and able.

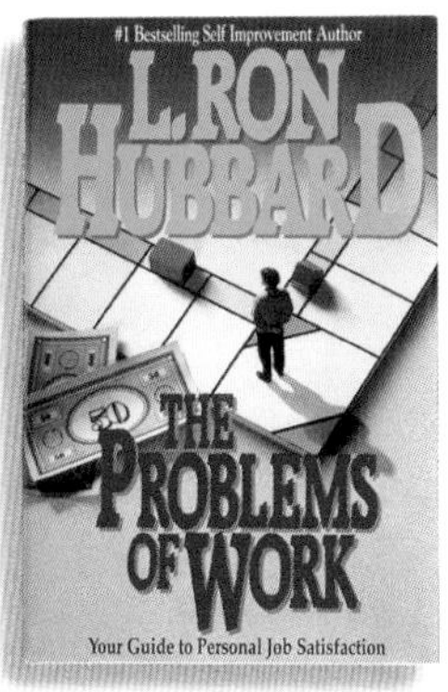

How to Make Work Easier

Based on the text of *The Problems of Work,* this Scientology Life Improvement Course provides illustrations, demonstrations and practical exercises to give the student a thorough working knowledge of the wide range of data the book contains, and certainty in its application. (Delivered in Scientology organizations.)

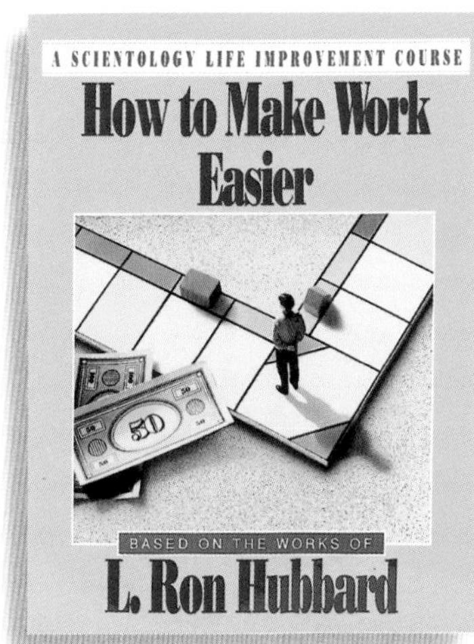

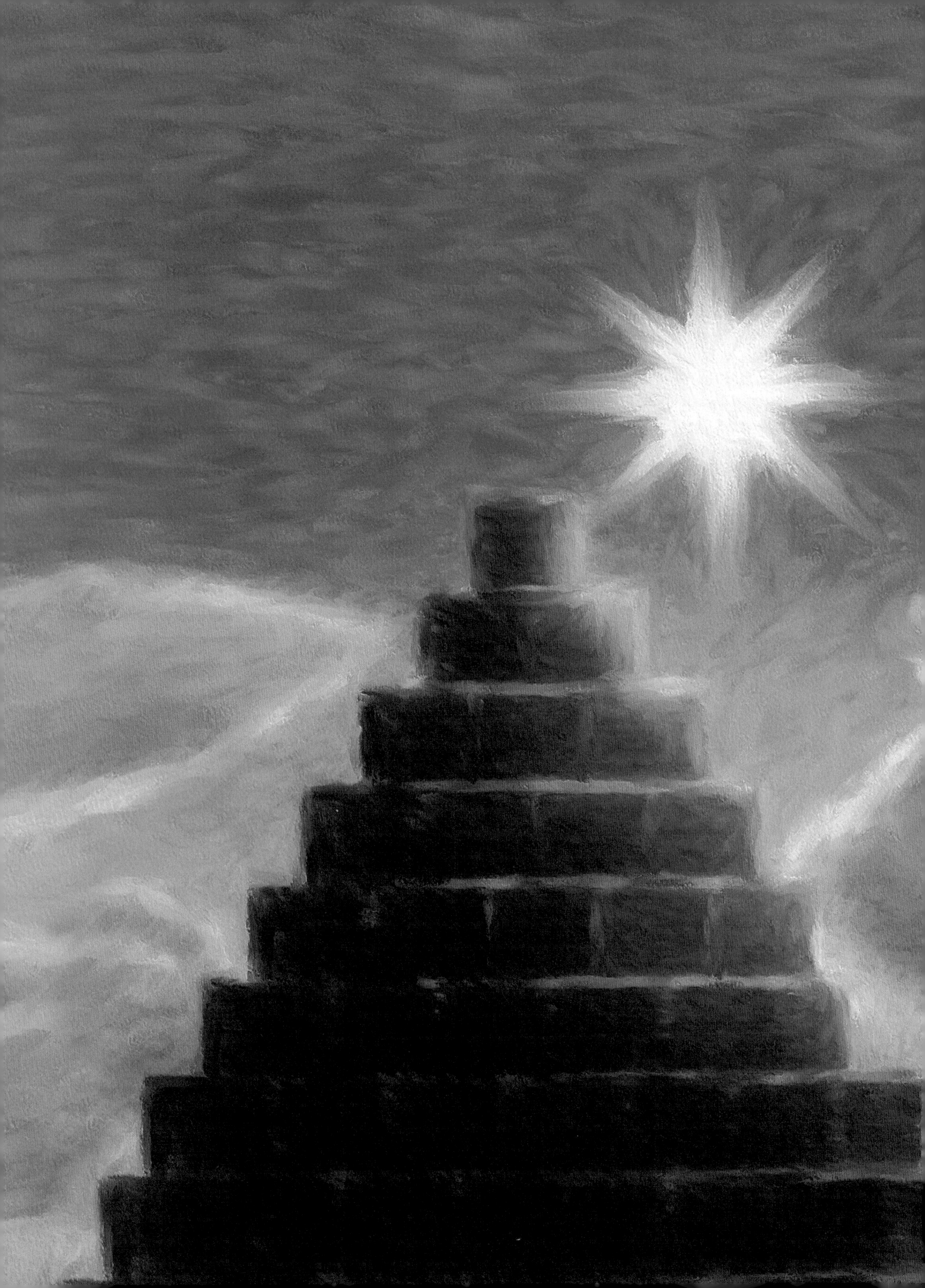

Chapter 16

BASICS OF ORGANIZING

Anybody recognizes that if things were better organized people would be better off. We have all had experiences with bureaucratic red tape, impersonal government agencies or careless commercial enterprises. The problem of poor organization is serious and costs trillions in waste, inefficiency and lowered productivity.

On a more individual level, organization is a key—and often missing—factor in personal success. It is also a necessity for a flourishing family. Attainment of one's goals, no matter how small or how large, requires a knowledge of organization. How do you most efficiently and productively manage your time, your activities and your resources? How do you minimize distractions? And how do you align your strengths in order to accomplish your purposes?

L. Ron Hubbard recognized that man was as lacking in understanding of how to organize his activities as he was about his true spiritual nature. And a sizable portion of his research was devoted to clarify the subject of organization, a task he fully accomplished.

This chapter contains only some of the most basic principles of the organizing technology he developed, but these fundamentals are, by themselves, enough to greatly enhance the activity of any endeavor, whether that of a group or an individual. Chaos and confusion are not natural conditions of life.

They only exist when natural laws are not understood and followed. Here are some of the natural laws of organization and organizing.

ORGANIZATION

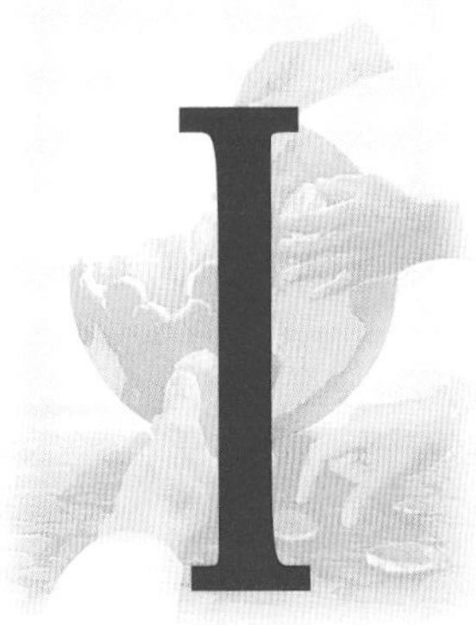

It may be that in trying to get something going, the basic of organization may be missing.

The word *organize* means to form into a whole with mutually connected and dependent parts; to give a definite and orderly structure to. From this, one gets the term *organization.*

Organization is the subdivision of actions and duties into specialized functions.

One can organize a series of actions to be done by himself or herself. This would consist of seeing what has to be done, doing what one can do first and then the remainder as a feasible series of events, all to accomplish a final completion of an action which forwards one's assigned or postulated purposes.

A group is organized so as to permit flows and accomplish specialized actions which are completed in themselves and from which small actions or completions the group purpose, assigned or specialized, is forwarded or accomplished.

There is a difference between directing and doing, which some people have trouble separating apart. A person in charge of an activity is sometimes found deficient in organizational understanding and so tries to do all the actions himself. This, if done to excess, effectively can break up a group and render it useless since all members but one have no function, having been robbed by this one-man monopoly on action.

True, an active and competent person *can* do things better. But he can really never do more than he can do. Whereas a well-organized group, each with specialized functions, coordinated by the in-charge, can accomplish many times the work only one can do.

Because it is *organized* makes a group harder to defeat than the individual.

A competent individual who has been let down too often by groups tends to take it all on himself rather than whip the group into shape and get things organized.

The correct action when faced by urgent necessity arising from incompetence of a group or other causes is to:

1. Handle it,

2. Organize the group to handle such things and do their jobs.

One can get stuck on (1) and, if he or she does, then will have trouble and overwork from there on out. Because he or she omits *also* doing (2).

The major failure of any group is to fail to organize.

Workers of the world may arise, but if they are not quickly organized before or after the fact, they will promptly be put back down!

The major cause of not organizing is just not understanding what is meant by it.

For example, an executive is told he is in charge of seeing that the X project is done. He doesn't know much about it. He has two men who do know. The incorrect action is to try to do the X project himself or issue a lot of unreal orders about it. The correct action is to call up the man who does know, give him the other as an assistant and tell them to get on with it. Then, without interfering, the executive who received the order should get more knowledgeable about the X project so *he* can be sure it is done, while still letting the designated people get on with it.

This comprehension of organization is as simple as this—put somebody on the job and let him get on with it. On a project, make a survey of all the things there are to do, group types of actions into single jobs, assign people to them, provide the routes on which communications travel between group members, materiel and liaison and let the group get on with it.

Any job, no matter how junior, has to be organized.

Anyone in charge of people has to be able to organize functions and work.

Failing that, one gets very little done and is badly overworked. And the rest of the group is wasted.

By understanding that there is a subject called organization, that the subject has been codified and that it can be learned and applied, any individual or group can succeed in its endeavors.

BASIC ORGANIZATION

What is organization?

Most people have so many associated ideas with the word "organization" that they think of one as an identity or a being, not as a dynamic activity.

Let's see what one really is.

Let us take a pile of red, white and blue beads. Let's organize them.

Now let us draw the org board. In brief, an *org board* (short for *org*anizing board) shows the functions, duties, communication routes, sequences of actions and authorities of an organization.

Let us dump the beads all on top of in-charge, all mixed up in a confusion.

Obviously in-charge must *route* them to dig himself out. So we get:

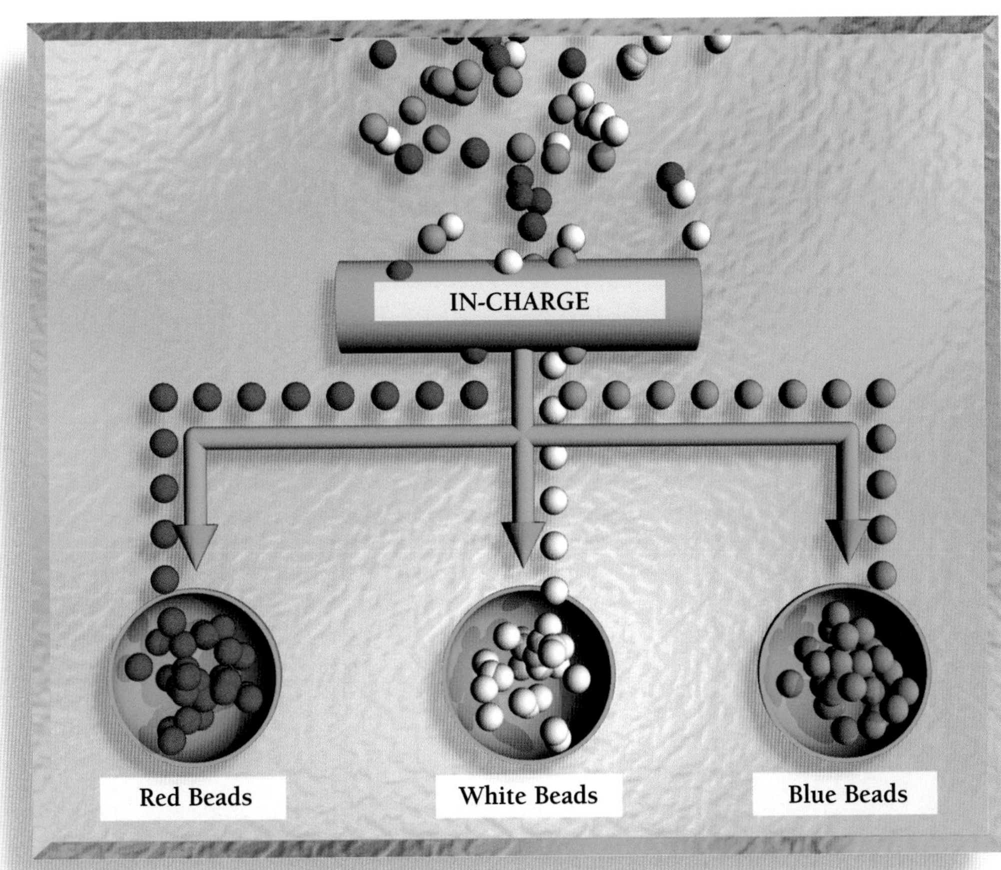

Thus we find out much of what an in-charge does. He routes. He separates into types or classes of thing or action.

This so far is a motionless organization.

We have to have products. By *product* we mean a completed thing that has exchange value within or outside the activity. This can be a service or article that has been put into the hands of someone outside the organization or another member of the organization.

Let's say the organization's products are drilled beads, strung beads, boxed beads.

We would get:

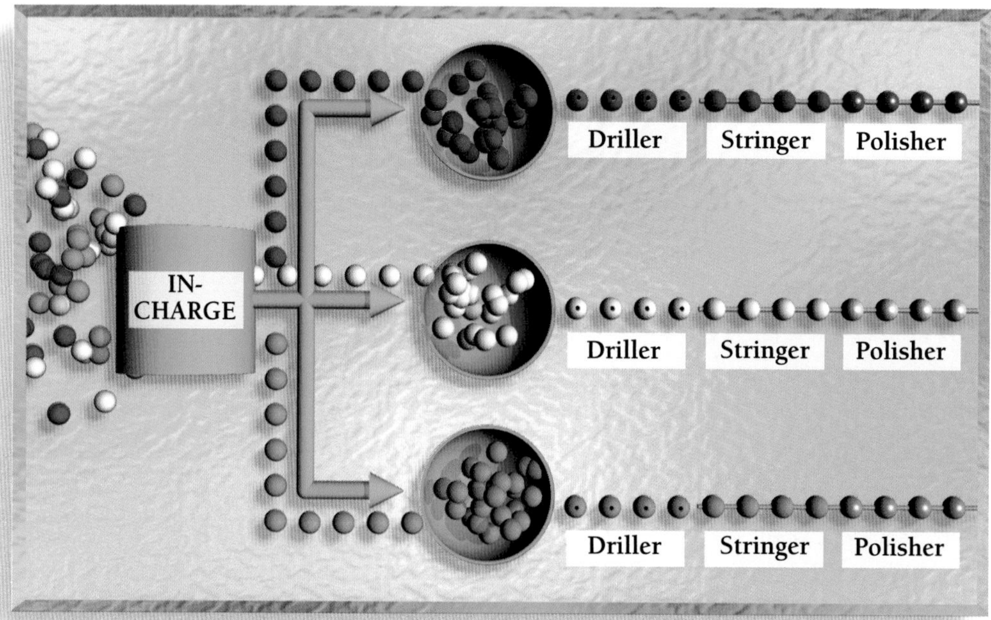

Or we would get:

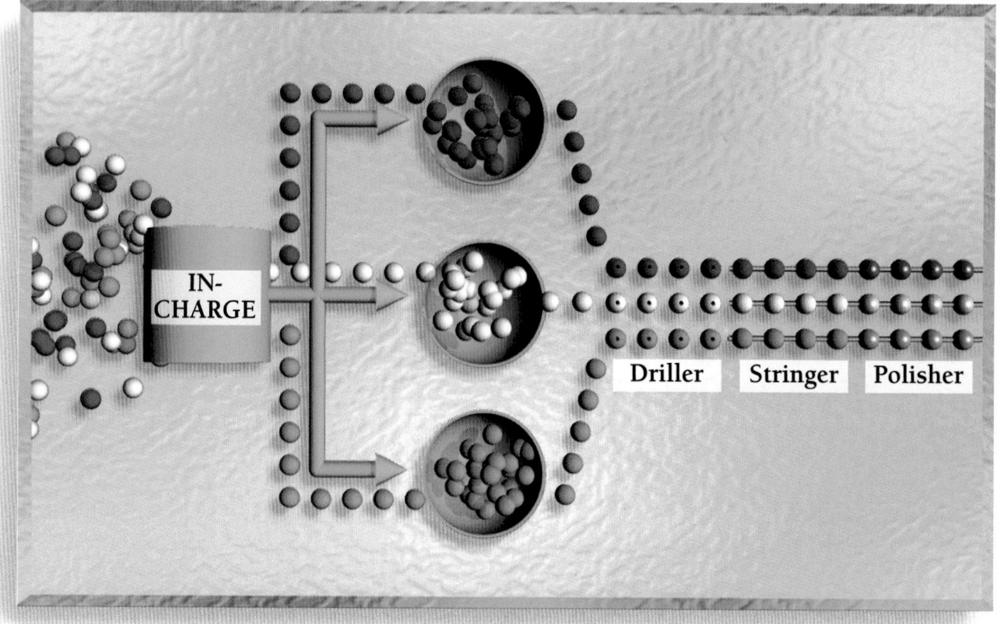

Or we would get:

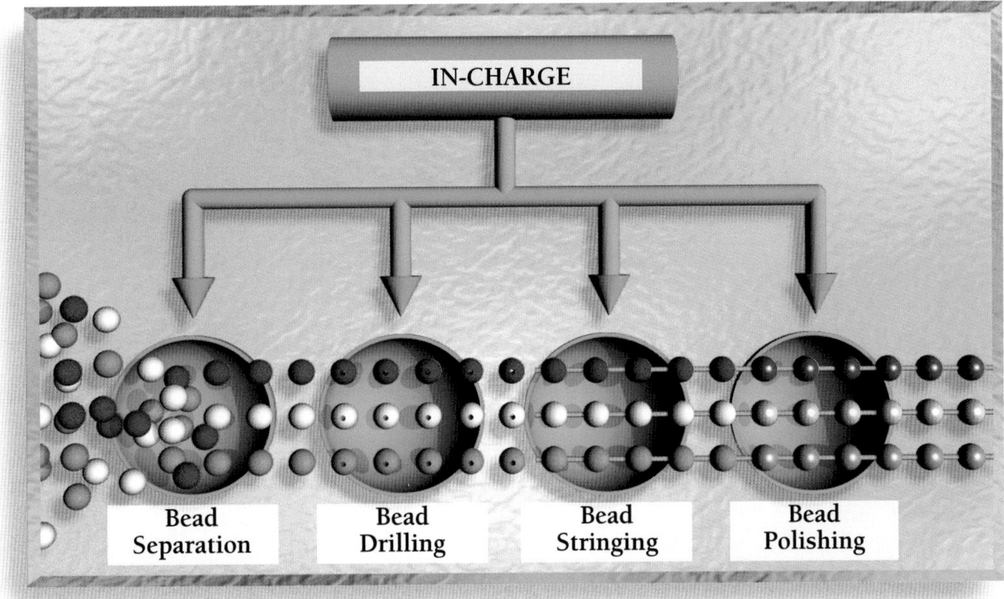

It is not particularly important which pattern of org board we use so long as it handles the volume of beads.

If we only have one person in this "organization," he would still have to have some idea of organization and a sort of org board.

If we have any volume to handle we have to add people. If we add them without an org board we will also add confusion. The organization without an org board will break down by overload and cross flows and currents. These in conflict become confusion.

All a confusion is, is unpatterned flow of particles (bodies, communications or other items). The particles collide, bounce off each other and stay IN the area. Thus there is no product, as to have a *product* something must flow OUT.

We can now note two things. We have some stable items. These are locations or posts (jobs, positions in a group or organization). And we have flow items. These are things undergoing change.

So an organization's positions change flowing particles.

Particles flow *in sequence.*

Things enter an organization, get changed, flow out of an organization.

An organization with one type of item only (red beads) is less complex than one with several types of items.

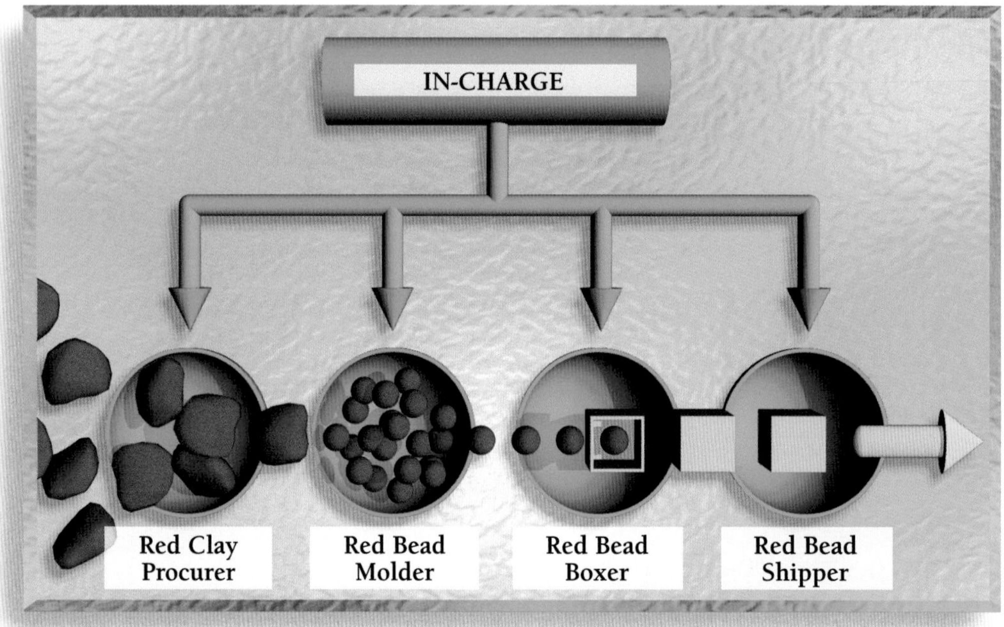

Any activity has a *sequence* of actions. It has to have stable points which do *not* flow in order to handle things which do flow.

It is not necessary to have a stable terminal do only one thing. But if so then it also has a correct sequence of actions. (By "terminal" is meant a person who sends, receives or relays communication.)

All this is true of an engine room or a lawyer's office or any organization.

In an engine room fuel flows in and is changed to motion which flows out. Somebody runs the machines. Somebody repairs the machines. It may all be done by one person but as soon as volume goes up one has to plan out the actions, classify them and put them on an org board which the people there know and abide by, or the place will not operate well.

This is done by dividing operation and repair into two actions, making two activities on the same org board.

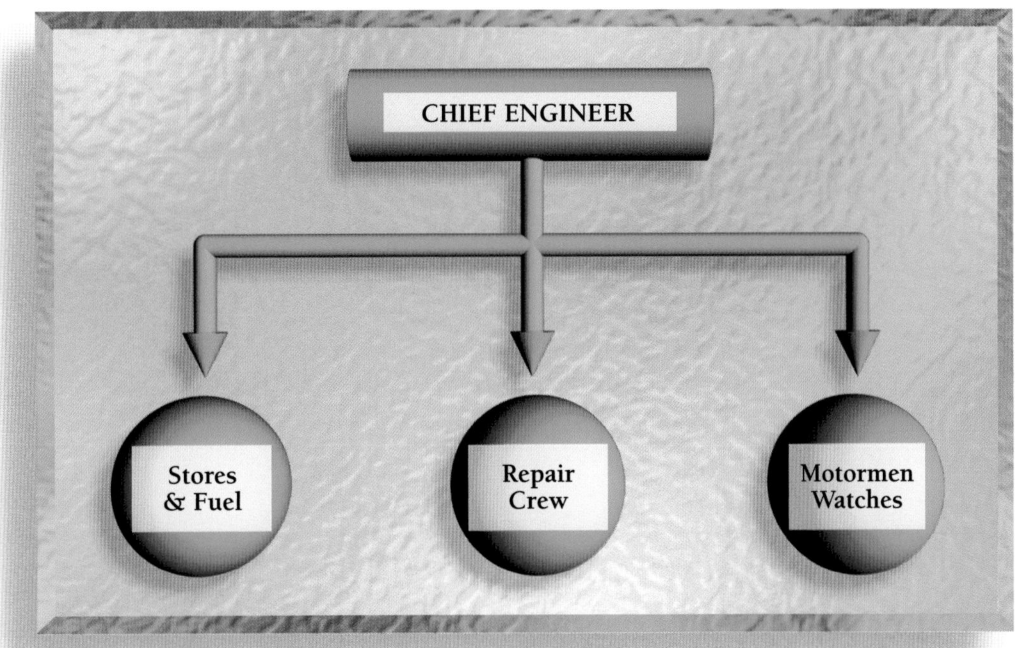

The Chief keeps the flows going and the terminals performing their actions.

In a lawyer's office we get different actions as a flow.

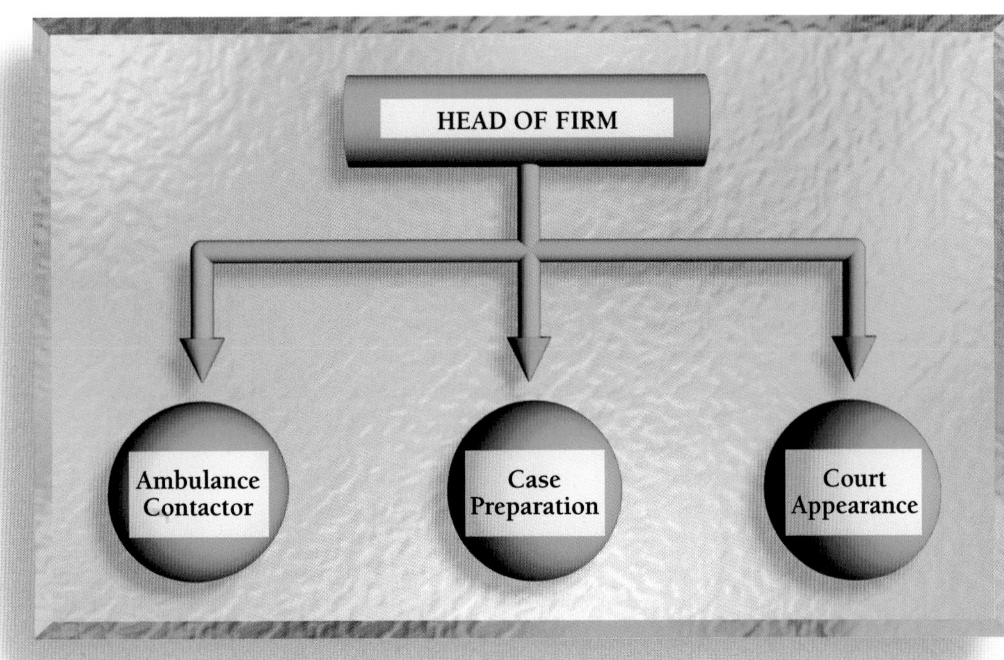

The above would be a flow pattern, possibly with a different person (with a different skill) on each point.

Or we could have a sort of motionless org board.

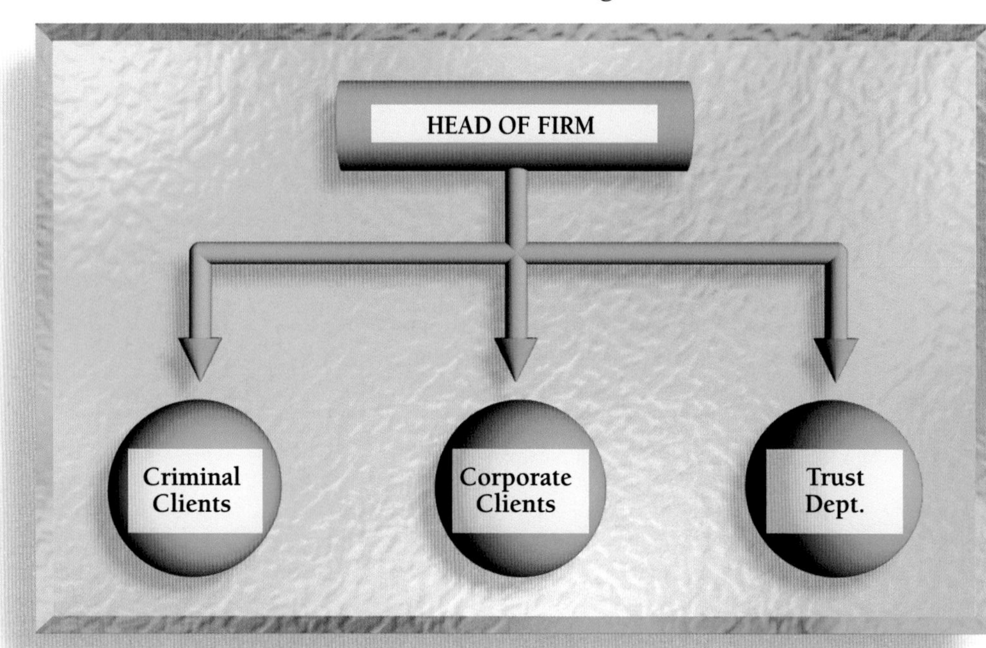

But if we did that we would have to put the motion in vertically so that flow would occur.

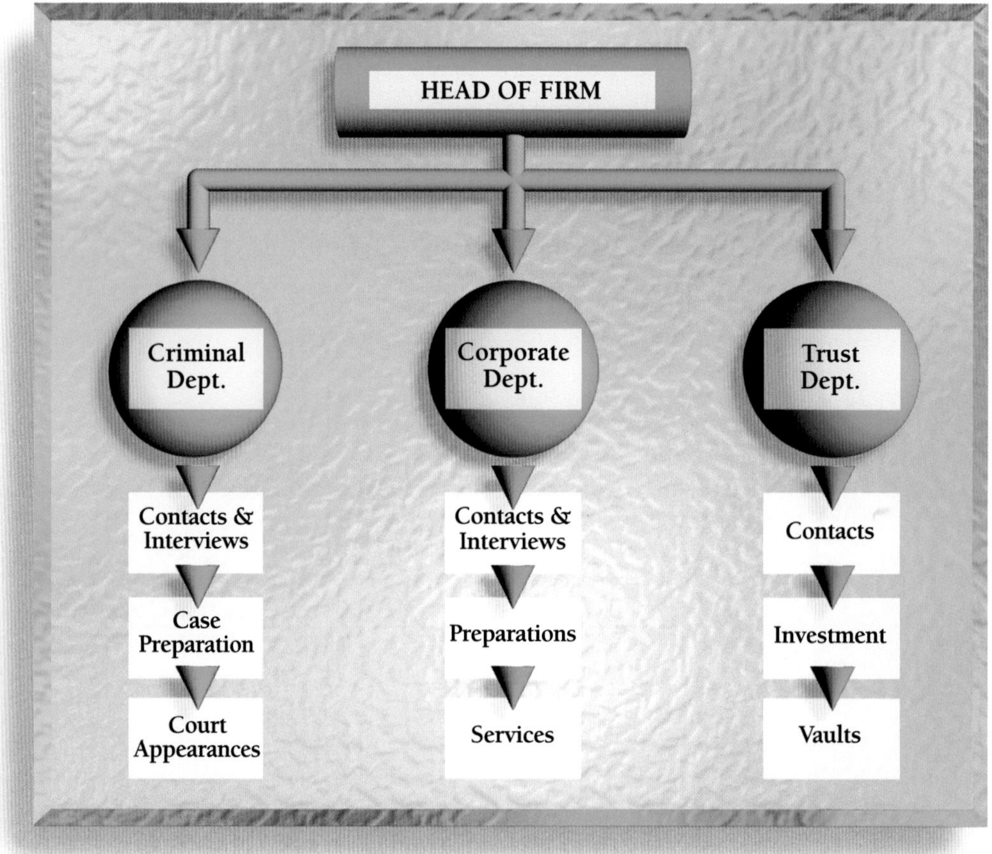

Organizing boards which only give terminals usually will not flow.

A typical army org board of yesteryear was:

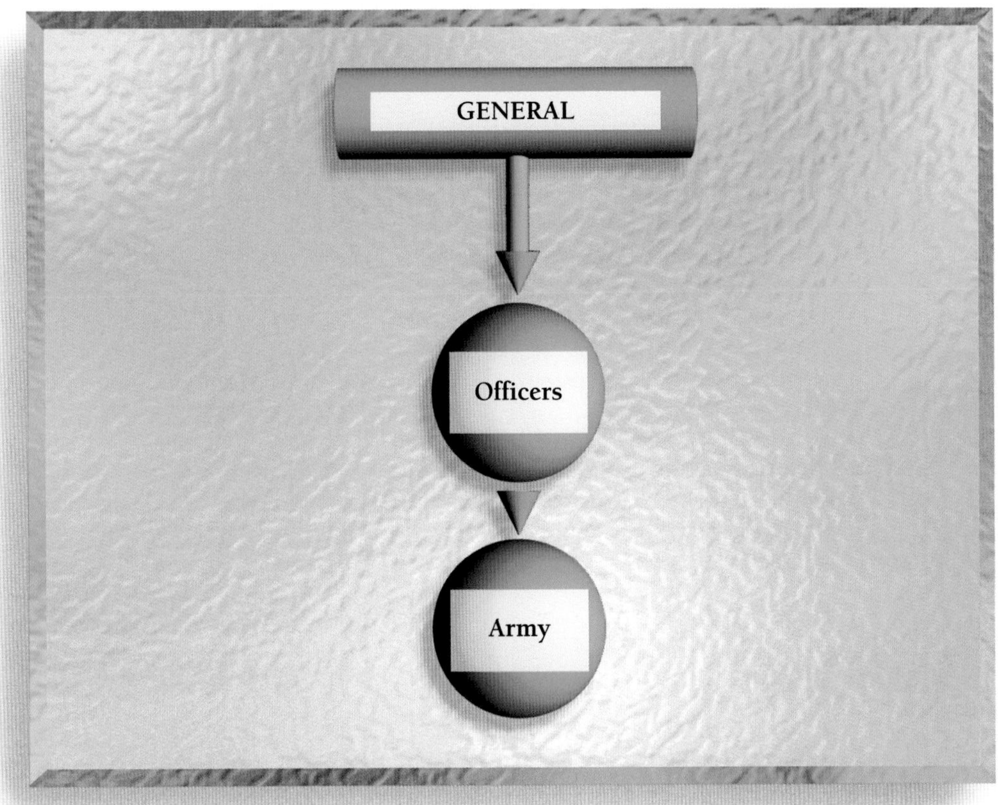

When they got into a lot more men they had to have a *flow* board.

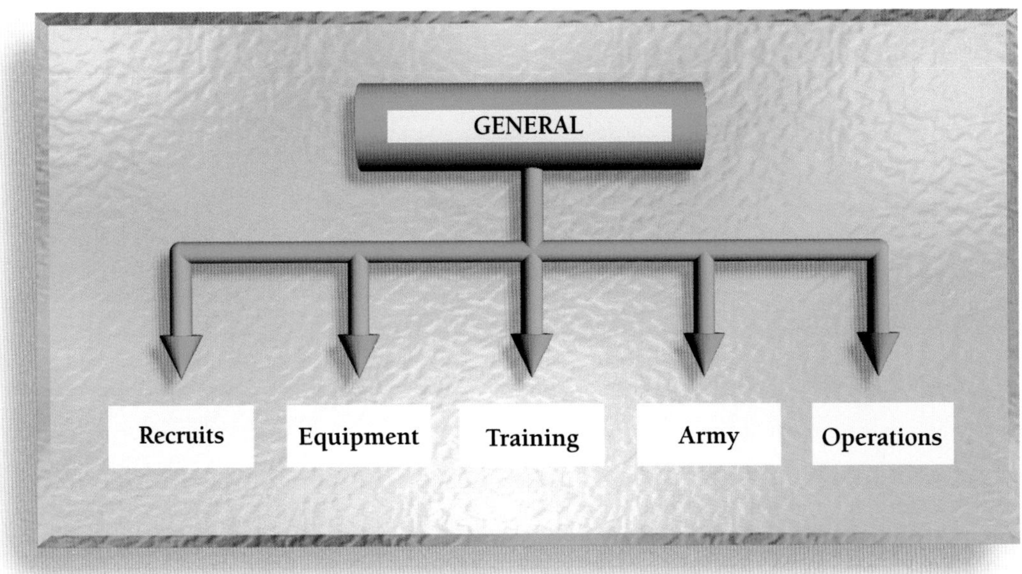

So one *organizes* by:

1. Surveying the types of particles.

2. Working out the changes desired for each to make a product.

3. Posting the terminals who will do the changing along the sequence of changes.

The board also must include a *recognition* of the types in (1) which *routes* the types to the *terminals* who *change* them and to a further *routing out* as *products*.

To be practical an org board must also provide for acquiring the materials, disposing of the product and being paid for the cycle of action (the steps done from start to finish that resulted in the product) and its supervision.

A company has various actions.

It is essentially a collection of small org boards combined to operate together as a large org board.

The basic principles you have to know to organize anything are contained in this section of the chapter.

To plan out *any* action one has to be able to visualize its sequence of flows and the changes that occur at each point. One has to be able to see where a particle (paper, body, money) comes in and where it leaves.

One has to be able to spot any point it will halt and mend that part of the flow or handle it.

A proper org board is a perpetual combination of flows which do not collide with one another and which do enter and do experience the desired change and which do leave as a product.

ORGANIZING AND HATS

The org board shows the pattern of organizing to obtain a product.

A board then is a flow chart of consecutive *products* brought about by terminals in series.

We see these terminals as "posts" or positions.

Each one of these is a hat.

The term *hat* is slang for the title and work of a post in an organization. It is taken from the fact that in many professions such as railroading the type of hat worn is the badge of the job. For example, a train crew has a conductor who wears a conductor's hat—he has charge of the passengers and collects fares.

In an organization, there is a flow along these hats.

The result of the whole board is a product.

The product of each hat on the board adds up to the total product.

Working It Out

The waste of people involved in no org board and the loss of product justify any amount of effort to work out, make known and use a proper org board.

Man instinctively uses an org board and protests the lack of one. The rawest recruit walking aboard a ship assumes the existence of an org board, if not a posted one, at least a known one. He assumes there will be somebody in charge and that different activities will be under different people. When there is no known org board he protests. He also feels insecure as he doesn't know where he fits into this organization.

Almost all revolts are manned by people who have been excluded out and are not on the country's org board. This is so true that a ridiculous circumstance occurred in the US. A president found he had "professional relief receivers." Certain people had assumed the status of "government dependent" and were giving this as their profession. It was of course a post of sorts. And because it wasn't admitted as a post by the government, there were some riots.

The effort to belong or to be part of is expressed by an org board. A person with no post is quite miserable. A person with an unreal post feels like a fraud or a mistake.

Morale then is also considerably affected by the quality of an org board or its absence.

The overall test for the group, however, is its viability, which means its ability to grow, expand, develop, etc. Viability depends on having an acceptable product. Groups which do not have an acceptable product are not likely to survive.

The volume and acceptability of a product depends in no small measure on a workable, known org board. This is true even of an individual product.

An individual or small group, to get anywhere at all, requires a very exact org board. The oddity is that the smaller the group the more vital the org board. Yet individuals and small groups are the least likely to have one. Large groups disintegrate in the absence of an org board and go nonviable in the presence of a poor one.

The quality of a product, usually blamed on individual skill only, depends to an enormous extent upon the org board. For example, one disorganized mob that was trying to make a certain product was worked to death, harassed, angry at one another and had a wholly unacceptable product at about twice the usual cost; when organized to the degree of a third, still without proper schedules, still largely untrained, they began to turn out an acceptable product at about half the effort—so even *some* organization worked.

The product volume and quality depends utterly and totally upon the org board and hats and their use. You can train individuals endlessly but unless they are operating on a workable org board they will still have a poor or small volume product.

Lack of a known and real org board can spell failure. And lack of knowledge of the *subject* of organization has to be substituted for by pure genius at every point.

Thus to make anything at all, to improve any product, sustain morale and distribute work equitably and make it count, one has to have a real and a known org board.

So how do you make one?

Hats

An org board is made up of hats.

The definition of a hat is the "beingness and doingness that attains a product." (A beingness is the assumption or choosing of a category of identity. Doingness is the act of performing some action or activity.)

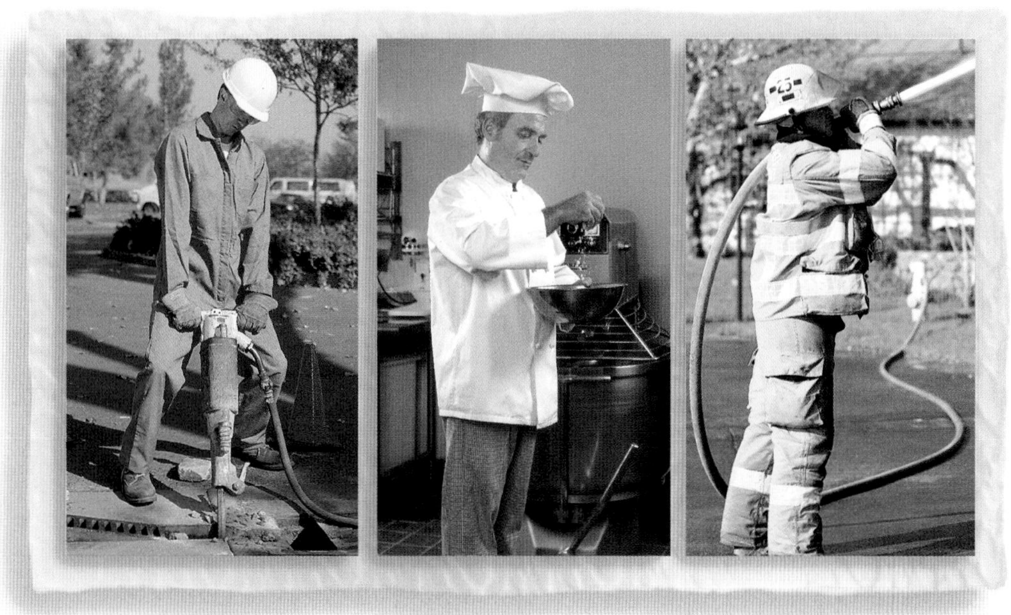

Let us take a train:

The engineer wearing his engineer hat has the title of engineer. That's the beingness.

He accepts orders, watches signals and general conditions, operates levers and valves to regulate the operation of his engine and to start, change and stop. That's the doingness.

He safely and on schedule moves the train passengers and/or freight from one location to another. A moved train and load is the product.

So how do we find out there is a hat called engineer?

As people are continually accepting or viewing already existing posts, when you ask them to dream up an org board they at first may not realize that you are asking them to *invent* the correct posts.

They don't have to invent "engineer." Everybody knows "an engineer runs a train."

So if you didn't know this? You'd have to figure it out.

One would do it this way. One would have to think along these lines:

The idea comes about because of a concept that people and goods have to be moved over distances on land. Or that a new area building up has to have transport of people and goods from and to it.

Ah. This will be viable in an economic framework because people will pay to be moved and pay for their goods to be moved.

Trains do this.

So let's use trains.

Arranging finance (or by prepayment) and obtaining a franchise for a right of way, track is laid, locomotives, train cars, stations and buildings to store and repair locomotives are built.

Now it emerges that somebody has to drive the train. So somebody had better be hired to drive the train.

So there comes into view the *post* of engineer.

How do we know this? Because we have to have a *product* of moved people and goods. That was what we were trying to do in the first place.

Therefore, the engineer hat.

So supposing now we did not have any org board at all.

The engineer hat would be the only hat. So he collects fares, runs stations, fixes his engine, buys fuel, loads the cars, sells stock....

Wait a minute. If the engineer did all that the following would happen:

1. He would be exhausted.

2. His temper would be bad.

3. He would have machinery breakdowns.

4. He might have wrecks.

5. The railroad property otherwise unhandled would disintegrate.

6. He would have a low volume of product.

7. His product would be uneven and bad as he could maintain no schedule.

8. There would shortly be no railroad.

Now let's "solve" this as it has been done in the past.

Let's appoint a person for each station and say "There we are!"

Well, it would still be a mess.

So let's hire more engineers and more station agents and more engineers and more station agents... and wind up with a confused mess, a huge payroll and a lousy product. That's how governments do it. And it is notable that current governments have no product but disaster.

No, we have to solve this in quite another way.

We do not get anywhere and we will not get a sensible org board and nothing will work or be viable unless WE COUNT THE PRODUCTS CORRECTLY AND DEVELOP HATS TO ATTAIN THEM.

When we have done this we can arrange the hats on an org board so there is a *flow* and command channels and communication channels and we've got an org board.

You cannot work out an org board until you have counted products!

As volume increases you estimate the products before the final product and hat those.

Quality of final product depends on a real org board and hats, both complete, real and trained-in and the functions DONE.

Let us see now how you break down a *final* product into the products which, put together, comprise it.

We have the final product of a railroad—viably moved loads. How many lesser products go into the big product?

There is a matter of machinery here. Any machine has two products: (a) the machine itself in good operating condition, (b) the product of the machine. A repairman and machine shop man and a repair shop keeper each has a product under (a). That is just for the machine, the engine.

Under (b) we have what the machine itself produces (hauled trains in the case of an engine).

Here we have then two major products—and these break down into lesser products, earlier in sequence to the final product.

There is even an earlier product to these—bought engines. And an earlier product to that—finance for equipment.

As for the load itself, a delivered load, accepted at the receiving end by a consignee, as you back up the sequence you will find a product—stored freight. And before that—unloaded freight. And before that—moved freight. And before that—loaded freight. And before that—freight assembled for shipment. And before that—freight contracts procured. And before that—advertising placed in public view. And before that—surveys of public freight requirement. And before that—survey for activities requiring freight service.

Each one of these products is a hat.

Surveying this again we see there's no charges or income involved so no economic viability. Thus there is an additional product, the income which is necessary for the organization's survival to pay its bills, buy the wherewithal necessary for future production and so on. This product has earlier hats of course. Some people (and a lot of executives) aren't product-minded—they think income falls into a company's lap or out of a TV set. They can't think the product sequence necessary to obtain income. So they go broke and starve. There are always a lot of prior products to the product of income. Fixated people just fixate on money itself, have no product sequence and so go broke or are poor.

Someone has to have a desirable product that is sold for more than it costs to produce and has to sell it and deliver it to have income.

Even in socialism or communism the how-does-it-support-itself question must be understood, answered, its product sequence identified, org boarded and hatted. In such a moneyless society the org boarding has to be much tighter as money adds flexibility and lack of it as a working factor makes problems that are hard to solve.

Organizing

In order to organize something one only has to:

1. Establish what is the final product.

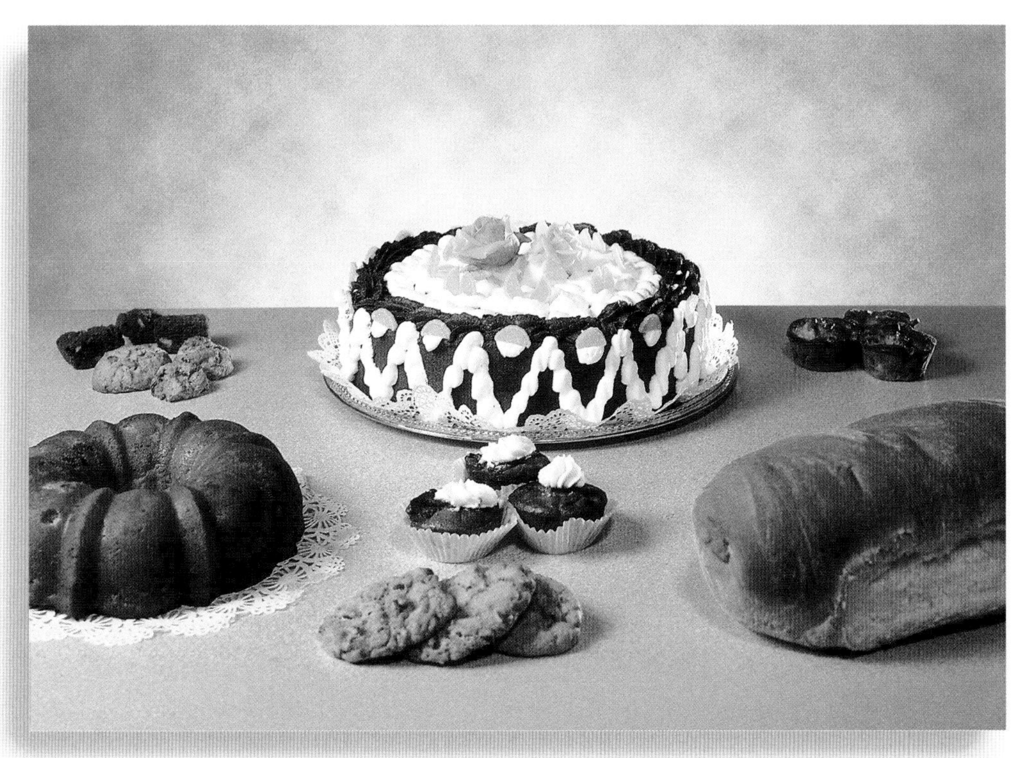

2. Work backwards in sequence to establish the earlier products necessary to make each next product and which all in a row add up to the final product.

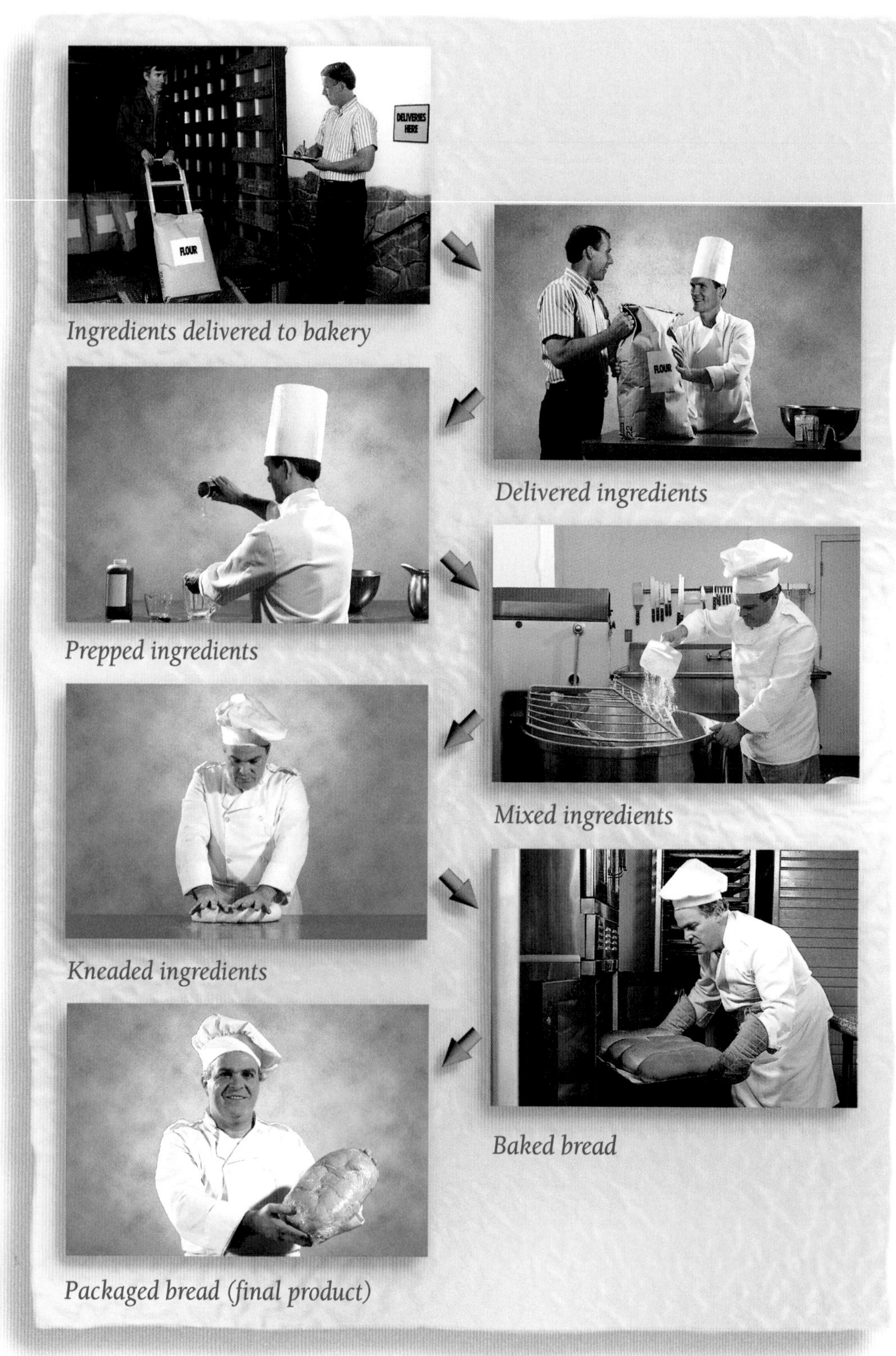

Ingredients delivered to bakery

Delivered ingredients

Prepped ingredients

Mixed ingredients

Kneaded ingredients

Baked bread

Packaged bread (final product)

3. Post it in terms of vertical greater and greater completeness of product to get command channels.

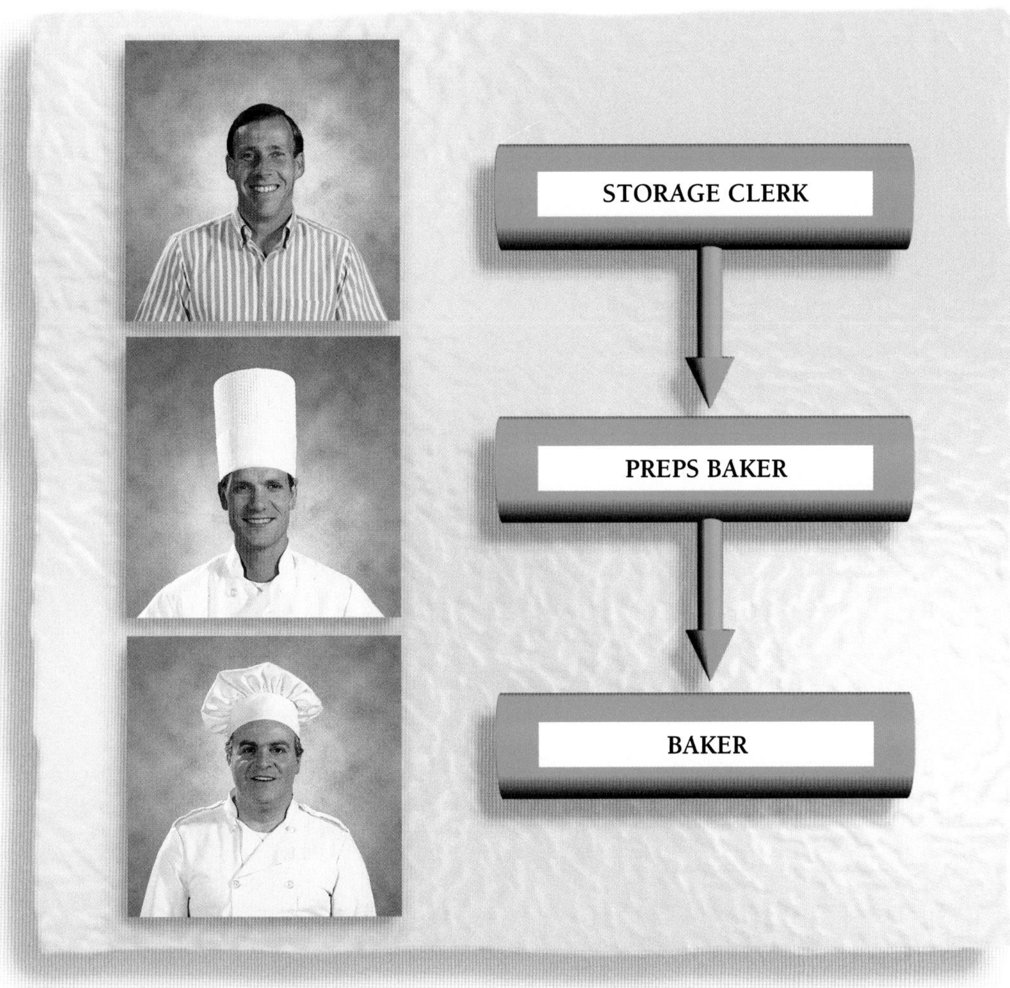

4. Adjust it for flows.

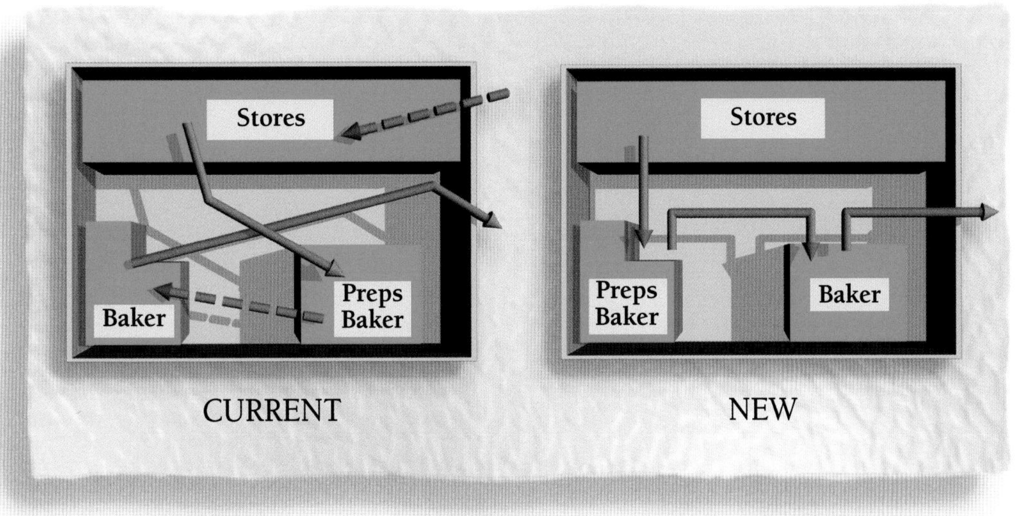

5. Assign its communication sequence.

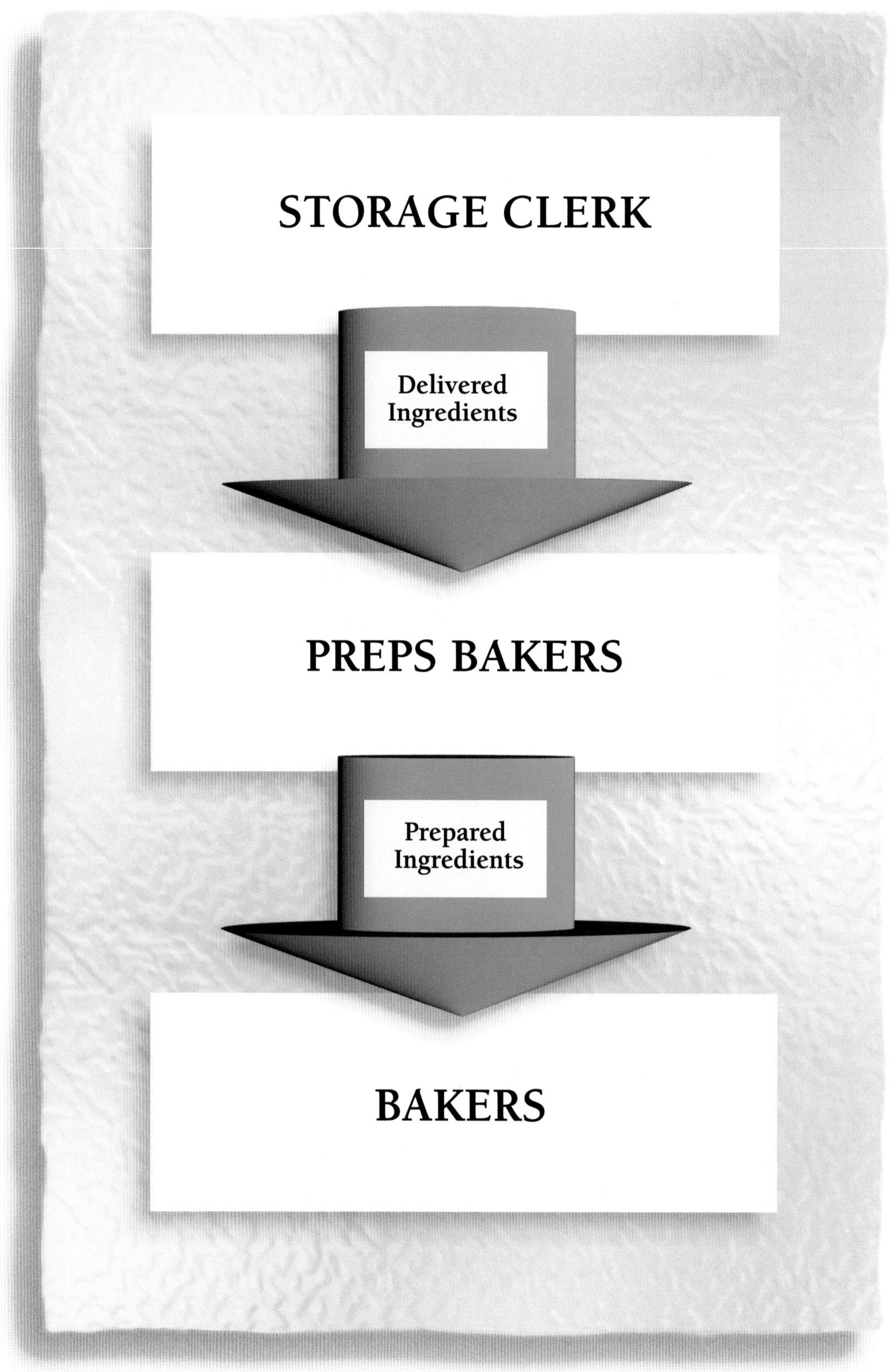

6. **Work out the doing resulting in each product. Write these as functions and actions with all skills included.**

BAKERY
FUNCTIONS AND ACTIONS

A. Stocks of ingredients ready for delivery to Preps Bakers.

Locate suppliers
Purchase ingredients
Store ingredients
Handle accounting

B. Ingredients prepared for Bakers in proper amounts.

Read recipes
Measure ingredients

C. Ingredients mixed according to recipe, baked and decorated as needed.

Read recipes
Mixing ingredients
Kneading dough
Preparing pans
Setting ovens
Decorating items

7. Name these as posts.

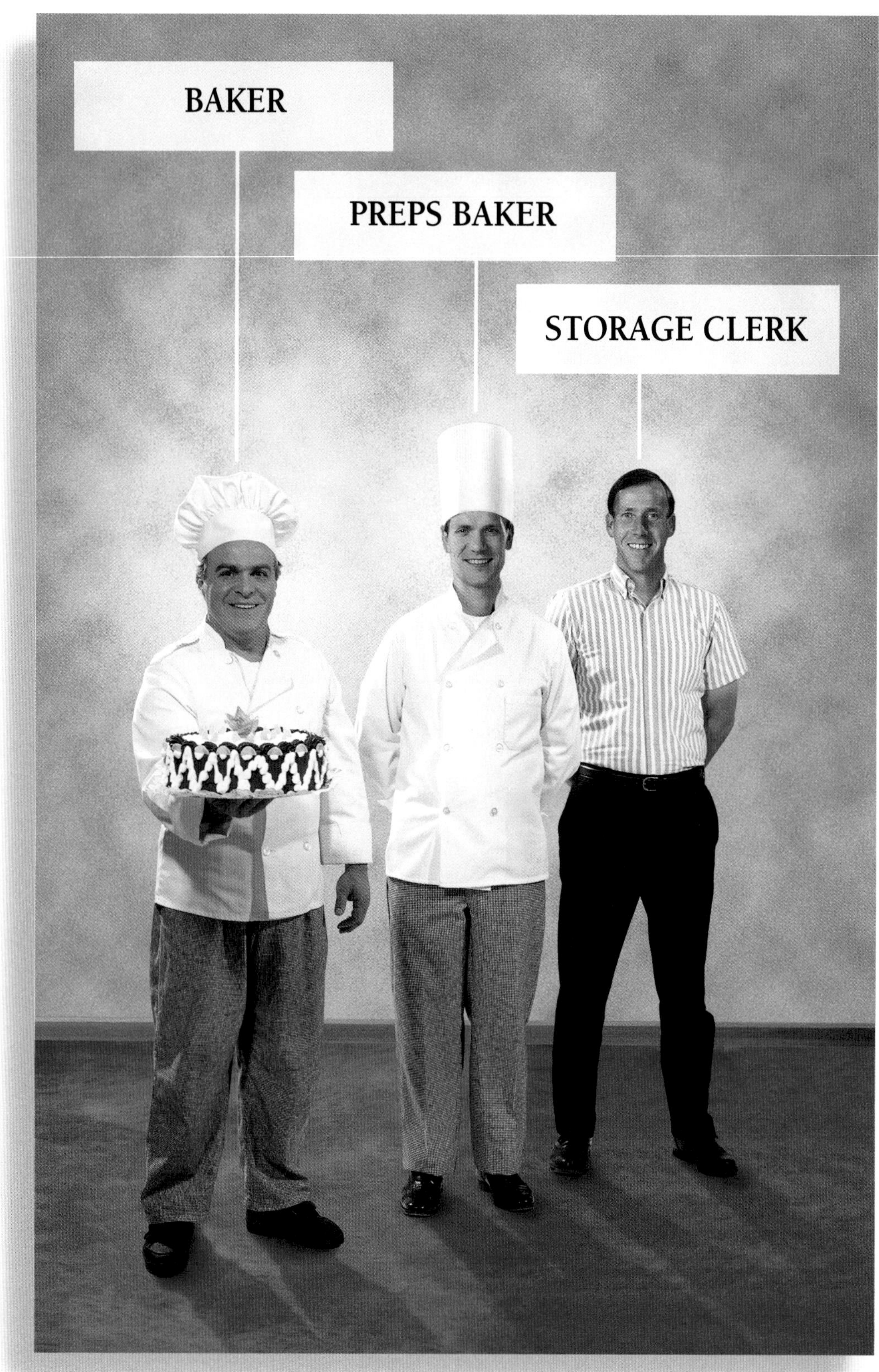

8. Post it.

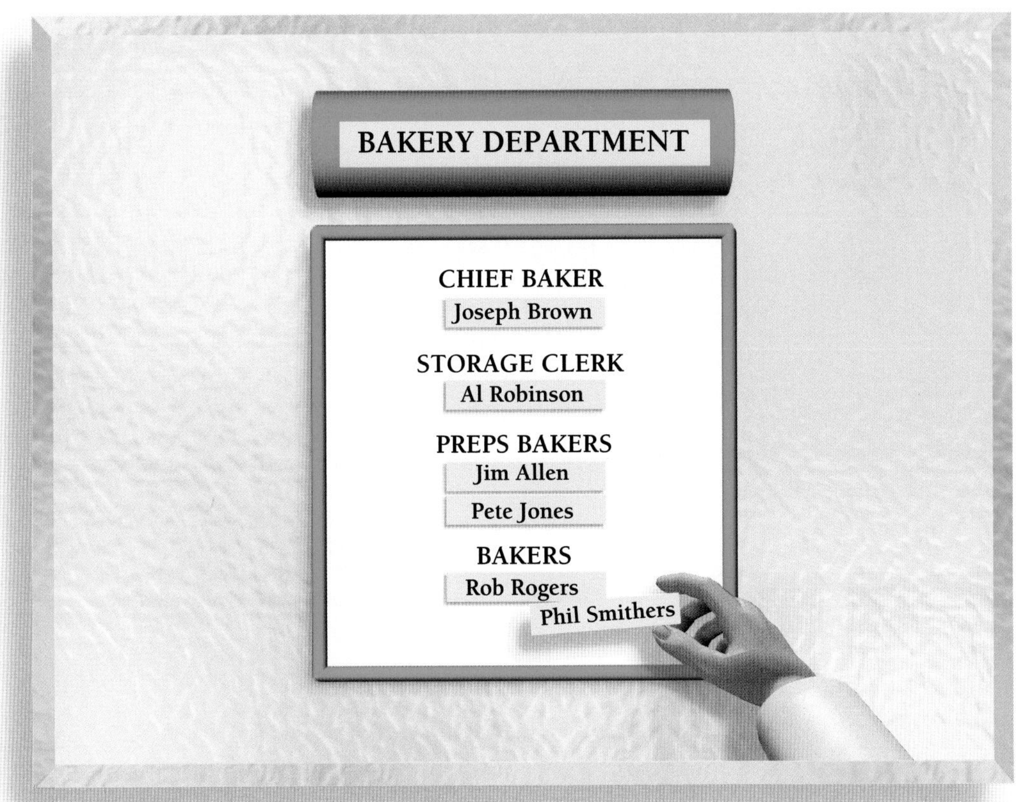

9. Drill it to get it known.

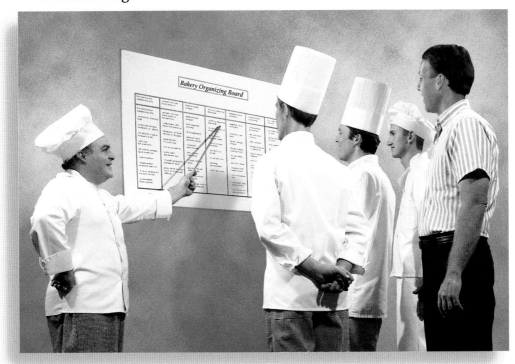

10. Assemble and issue packs of materials which describe the functions and duties of each hat.

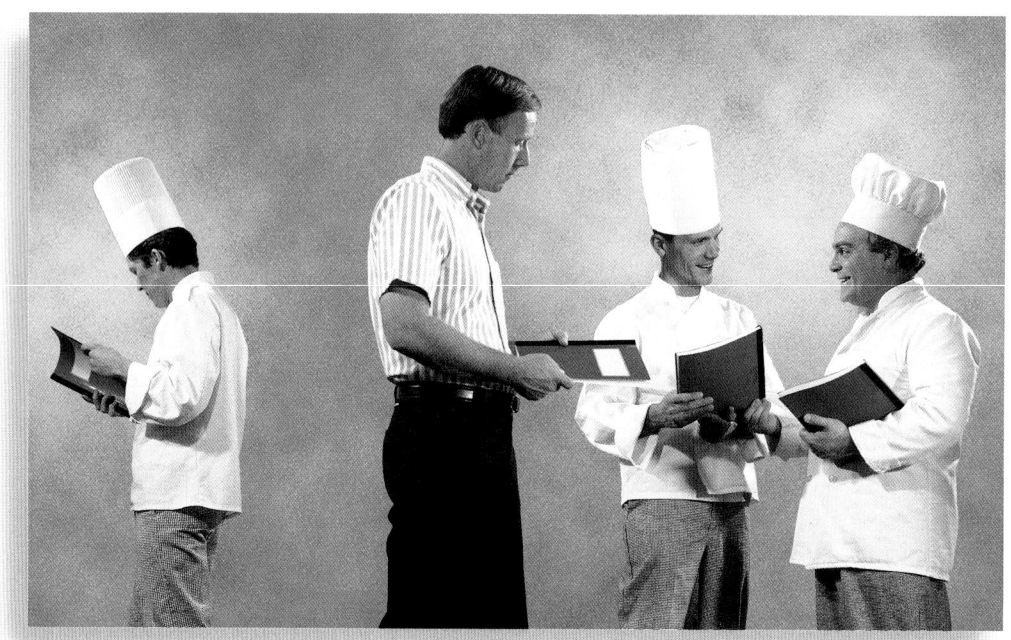

11. Get these known.

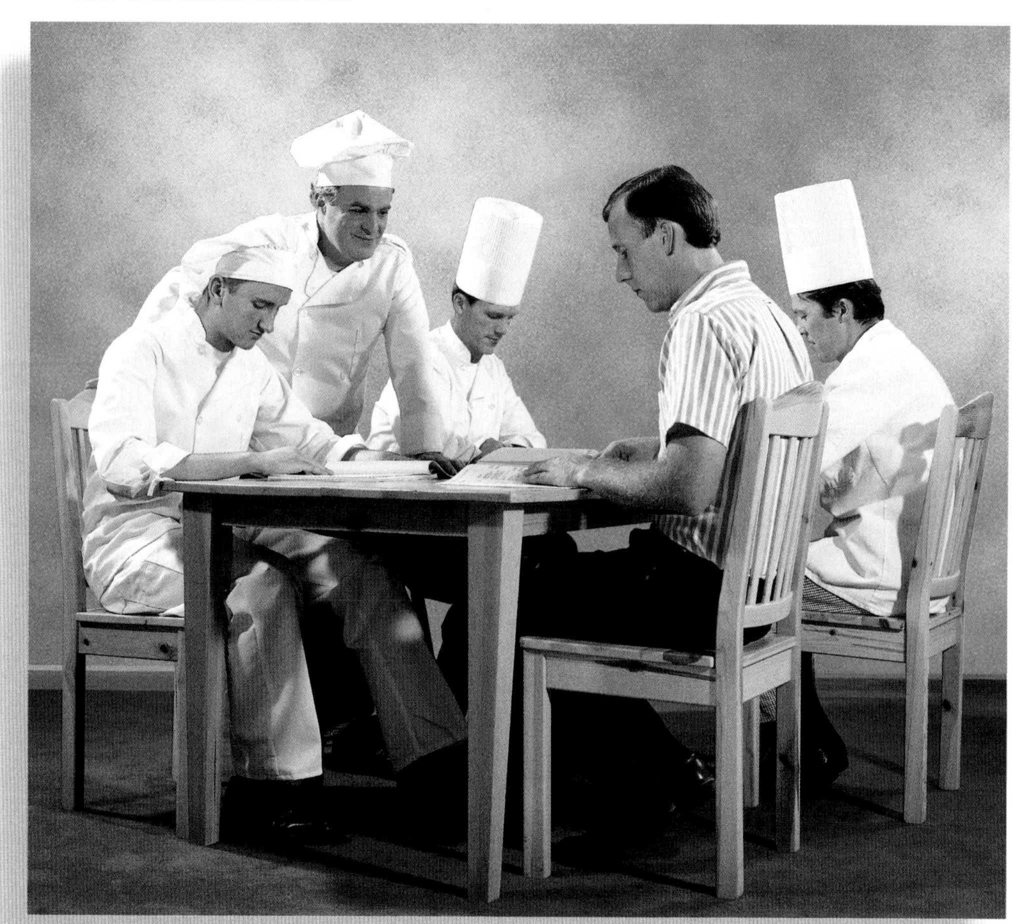

12. Get the functions done so that the products occur.

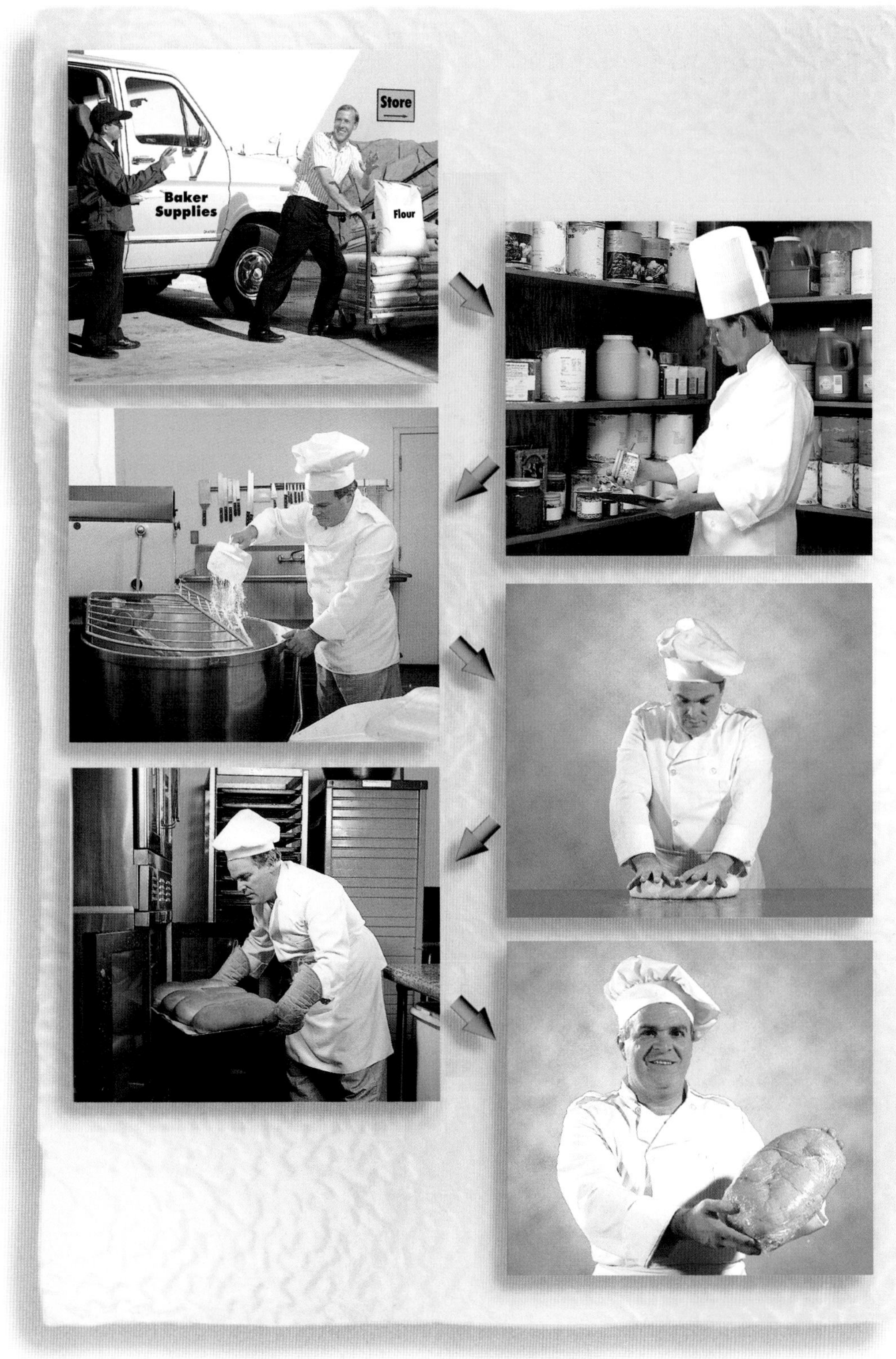

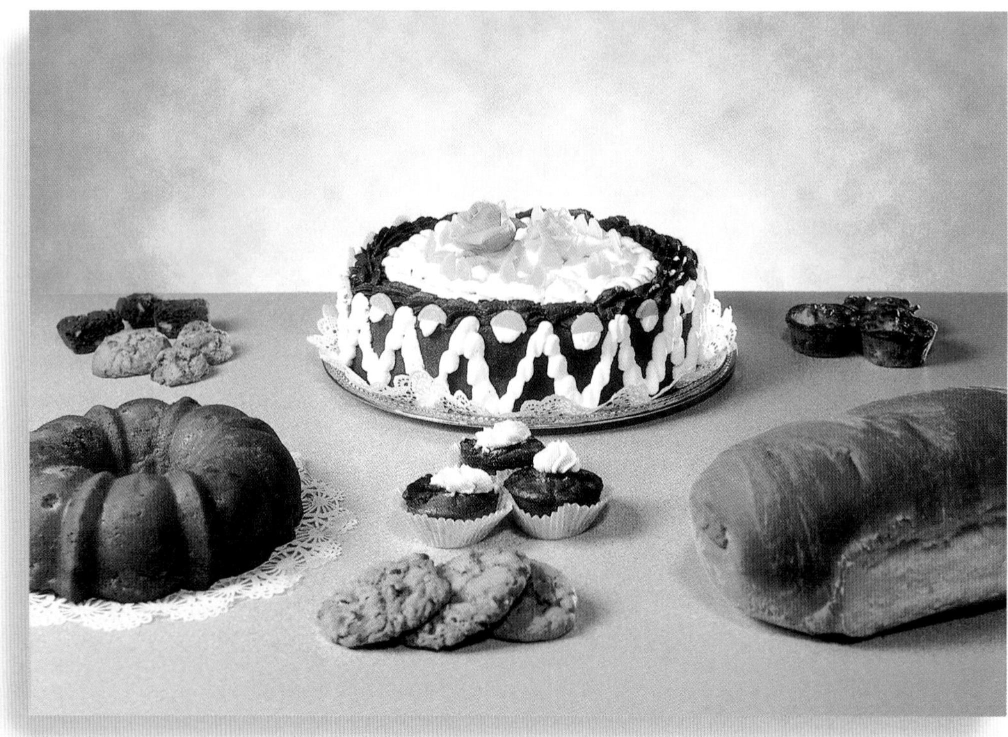

The final product results when each of the prior steps in an organized activity is done.

This is what is called "organizing."

As a comment, because railroads *didn't* fully organize, their viability decayed and they ceased to be so used.

Railroads think it's the government or airplane rivalry or many other things. It isn't. They had too many missing hats, were actually too disorganized to keep pace with the society's demands, ceased to fully deliver and declined. In fact there has never been a greater need of railroads than today. Yet, disorganized, badly org boarded and hatted, they do not furnish the service they should and so are opposed, government regulated, union hammered and caved in.

To have a quality product, organize!

To raise morale, organize!

To survive, organize!

ORGANIZING BOARD

As you have read in the previous sections of this chapter, considerable breakthroughs were made in Scientology on the subject of organizing. However, these are but a small portion of the natural laws of organization discovered and developed in Scientology during research into and discovery of the fundamental axioms of all life. With the statement of these axioms—the basics of existence itself—light was cast upon all fields.

Scientology makes the able more able. Each of its organizations has the purpose to deliver this technology to the individuals of its community so they become more able, improve their lives and the lives of those around them. As a result, the individual can accomplish his personal goals, the community as a whole grows and a new civilization free from the insanity, conflict and strife that has plagued man for millennia will be created. Ultimately, this *is* the aim of Scientology.

To make it possible to maximally service individuals and its community, it is necessary for a Scientology organization to be highly organized and efficient. Existing organizational charts were typically only command charts that showed the direction of orders from the top down, and were far from usable for the unique purposes of a Scientology organization. Needed was an organizational pattern that primarily revolved around the delivery of Scientology services and provided the other functions necessary to not only continue the organization's existence but enable it to effortlessly expand while achieving its aims. Hence, it was necessary to formulate an organizing board particularly for Scientology organizations.

Each area of a Scientology organization functions in one of two ways. Either it delivers the services the organization offers, such as its many courses, or it assists these areas by hiring and placing personnel, paying the organization's bills, caring for its staff, informing public of the services the organization offers and many, many other activities. All of the portions of a Scientology organization operate together as a unified and dedicated whole to accomplish the organization's purpose. And it is the organizing board which provides it with the vital organizational foundation to bring about success.

Though originally developed for use by Scientology organizations, the beauty of this organizing board is its flexibility in application. Based as it is on the laws of life themselves, it can be applied to any area of endeavor and by any organization, no matter its function or size; furthermore, it can even be used by an individual to organize his own life and improve his own existence.

The organizing board is divided into seven distinct areas called *divisions.* These are numbered 1 through 7. Each one performs the functions necessary to produce a product specific to that division.

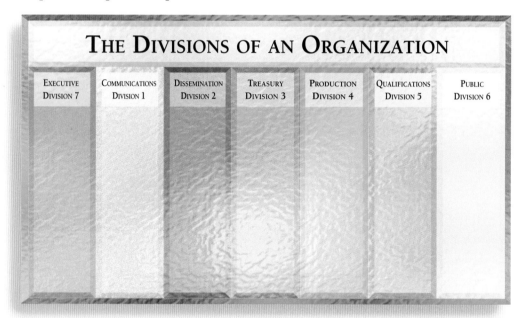

For any organization to be successful, all of the activities covered by these division names must be performed. These are: Executive, Communications, Dissemination (promoting and marketing of the organization's services and products), Treasury, Production, Qualifications (ensuring the quality of the organization's services and products), and Public (informing new public of the organization's services and products). An organization lacking one or more of these divisions will fail.

Although the seven division organizing board seems to have a number of divisions that would fit only a large group, it does, as mentioned, fit any organization of any size. The problem presented in deriving this board was how to overcome continual organizational changes because of expansion and how to apply it to organizations of different sizes. Thus this board goes from one person to thousands without change. Just fewer or more posts are occupied. That is the only change.

Unique to this organizing board is that it is entered from the left and proceeds to the right, starting with Division 1 and moving on through the divisions to Division 6, and then out. An individual or particle does not flow through Division 7—this division coordinates the activities of the rest of the organization and sees that it properly functions to accomplish its purpose. This organizing board would ideally be mounted on a large cylinder to show that it flows in a continuous circle with Division 7 meeting Division 1. To emphasize this fact, Division 7 is placed before the rest of the divisions on the board.

Divisions 1 through 7 are not arbitrarily arranged but describe a sequence known as the cycle of production. A fundamental law of this universe is that for any cycle of action to successfully complete, it must go through these exact seven main stages. In other words, for an organization or company to produce a high-quality product or service, it has to have all seven divisions properly operating. Down through the ages, innumerable civilizations, governments and groups fell prey to various ills and vanished from the face of the earth. It was a lack of one or more of these seven divisions that brought about these failures.

The direct application of this org board to an organization of any size or an individual's life is immediately evident upon inspection of it.

For instance, you would have to be in *Communication* with people about what you are doing and have your communication lines established.

Dissemination would involve telling people what you are producing, and promoting this.

You must have the physical materials to produce your product, which is *Treasury*. This includes funds to buy the materials and methods of purchasing them, as well as care for your assets.

Then there is *Production* of the product—the service being provided or item being produced.

And when the product is complete, *Qualifications* reviews it to make sure it meets the requirements of a product and if not, straightens out those involved so the product is valuable and can be exchanged. Qualifications also includes the furthering of your own education and training and that of an organization's personnel.

Once the product is qualified, the *Public* Division distributes it, creates new public who can obtain it and makes you and your products known to and desired by them.

Establishing goals and planning for the future is cared for by the *Executive* Division, which also keeps things operating and solves the various problems and bugs that may occur.

The functions performed by each division are further subdivided into *departments,* usually three in number, making twenty-one in total. Each department has a specific product or products which, when added together, result in the overall product of the division.

In a Communications Division, for example, the final product is effective, productive and ethical personnel. The first department is the Department of Routing and Personnel, which has a product of effective personnel posted and hatted. Some functions of this department are: receives individuals entering the organization and routes them to the correct terminal in the organization; hires personnel; determines the proper utilization of new staff and correctly places them to assist the organization's expansion; and sees that the organization's staff know their duties.

The Department of Communications is fully responsible for the communications into and out of the organization, as well as those which flow between organizational staff members. Its product is communications easily accepted and swiftly delivered. It answers the phones, swiftly directs calls to the correct terminal; receives incoming mail and swiftly distributes it to the staff throughout the organization; sees to it that the organization is communicating to its public in volume; establishes the organization's communications systems so its staff and executives can send and receive the communications necessary for the organization to successfully operate; and swiftly routes the internal despatches amongst the staff.

The Department of Inspections and Reports, with the product of ethical, producing personnel, is the third department. It inspects ongoing organizational projects and reports on their status to executives so, where needed, action can be taken to rectify any shortcomings; it collects and graphs the organization's statistics so these can be inspected and analyzed by its

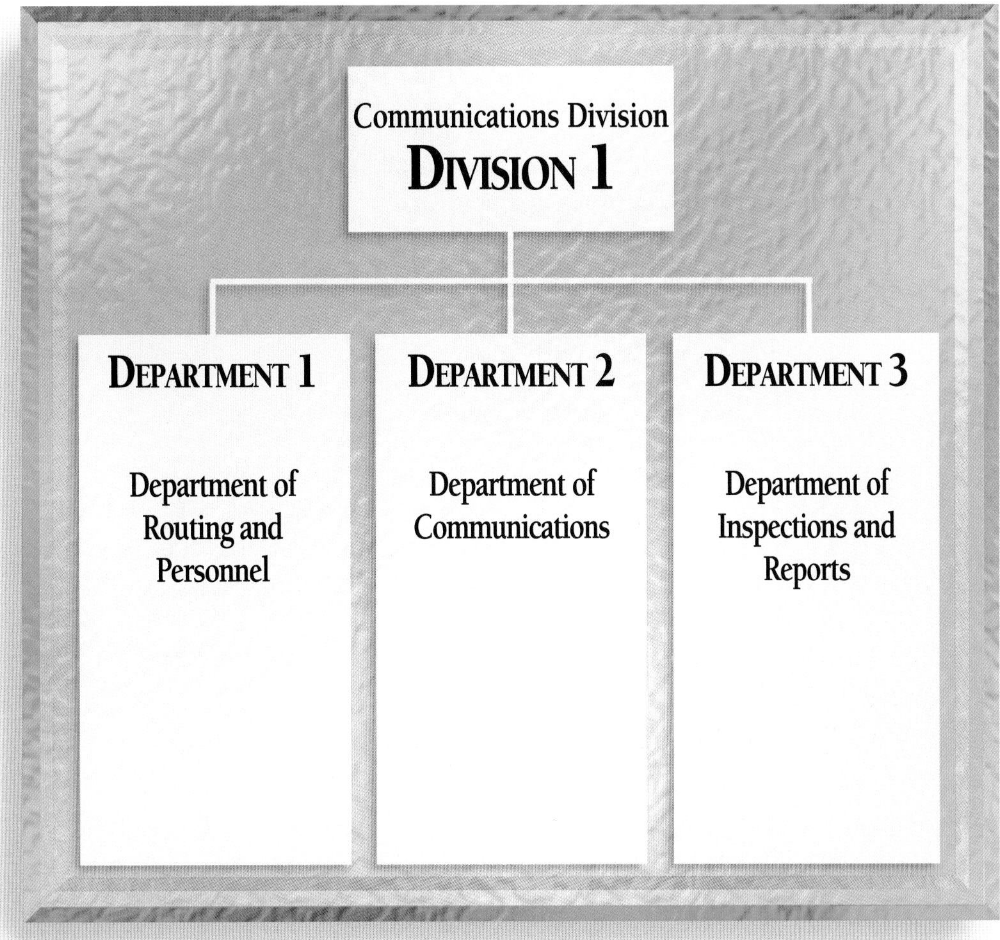

executives to improve production and effectiveness; and maintains a high level of ethical behavior in the organization.

Every individual has his twenty-one department org board. The degree to which the functions of these departments are being performed regulates his survival and success.

Applying the organizing board to one's life is quite simple. By taking up the functions done by one department and comparing these to one's own activities, he can determine if these are being done or are missing. Continuing in this fashion for the remaining departments enables one to assess what functions or even departments are missing on his own org board. He can then take action to remedy these deficiencies and improve his life.

A simplified version of the Scientology org board follows. It describes the functions of the divisions as they can be applied by any individual, organization or group.

Seven Division Organizing Board

Any organization requires an executive structure that provides supervision and coordination of the divisions' activities. On this seven division organizing board, each division is headed by a ***secretary.*** *To provide optimum guidance to the divisions, there are two* ***Executive Secretaries.*** *One supplies direction to three divisions; the other, four divisions. The entire organization is headed by an* ***Executive Director.*** *He works with and through the Executive Secretaries to see to the production and expansion of his organization.*

Communications Executive Secretary

Executive Division
Division 7
Division 7 Secretary

Office of Source | Office of External Affairs | Office of the Executive Director

This division coordinates and supervises the organization's activities so it runs smoothly, produces its products viably and delivers its products and services to individuals and the community in high quality.

Office of Source

■ Sees to it that the technology and policy of the organization is followed without deviation. In the case of a company, this office could include the office of the person who started the organization or the one who had developed the product produced by the company. Keeps the organization's premises in good repair and acquires additional space to accommodate expansion.

Office of External Affairs

■ Handles the external environment of the organization. Maintains proper governmental relations and cares for legal affairs.

Office of the Executive Director

■ Does the organization's planning. Coordinates and gets the functions of the organization done. Keeps the organization solvent, viable, producing and expanding in all its divisions and departments.

Communications Division
Division 1
Communications Secretary

Department of Routing and Personnel | Department of Communications | Department of Inspections and Reports

This division is fully responsible for the establishment of the organization.

Department of Routing and Personnel

■ Hires eligible staff and properly places them for the benefit of the individual and the organization. Gets new and existing staff hatted and apprenticed to do their jobs.

Department of Communications

■ Sets up standard communications systems and gets in established communication routes so all communications are swiftly and properly handled. Makes sure that correspondence to and from the organization's public arrives and is swiftly handled.

Department of Inspections and Reports

■ Collects and accurately graphs the organization's statistics for executive use. Maintains a high level of ethical behavior among the staff. Inspects the organization's activities so any difficulties inhibiting expansion are detected and reported upon to the proper executive for swift resolution.

Dissemination Division
Division 2
Dissemination Secretary

Department of Promotion and Marketing | Department of Publications | Department of Registration

This division makes the organization's products and services widely known and demanded, creating a high volume of public obtaining them.

Department of Promotion and Marketing

■ Does informative mailings, magazines and other promotion based on survey results, to inform the public of the organization's services and products and the published materials it offers so these are acquired in a viable quantity.

Department of Publications

■ Stocks all published materials so they are readily available for sale, and swiftly delivers these to individuals who purchase them.

Department of Registration

■ Contacts individuals who have expressed interest in the organization's products so these are obtained by them. Keeps accurate files of people who previously received service or obtained products from the organization and maintains correspondence with them so they can acquire further products and services.

Executive Director

Organization Executive Secretary

Treasury Division
Division 3
Treasury Secretary

Department of Income	Department of Disbursements	Department of Records, Assets and Materiel

This division handles the financial matters, assets and materiel of the organization so its physical body is fully cared for, enabling it to produce its products and deliver its services and remain solvent.

Department of Income

■ Handles incoming funds received in exchange for the organization's products so these are properly recorded. Accurately maintains customer accounts folders and collects all credit owed to the organization.

Department of Disbursements

■ Disburses funds for purchasing and the payment of all bills, as well as pays the staff, so its financial obligations are fulfilled and the other divisions have the wherewithal to produce their products.

Department of Records, Assets and Materiel

■ Handles the organization's supplies, keeps precise records of all financial transactions, does necessary bookkeeping and financial reports and preserves assets and reserves.

Production Division
Division 4
Production Secretary

Department of Production Services	Department of Activity	Department of Production

This division provides excellent quality products and services with no delay to its public.

Department of Production Services

■ Serves the division by prediction of what wherewithal is needed to produce and sees to its timely arrival so production can be done, and schedules production for maximum efficiency and service to the public.

Department of Activity

■ Prepares the resources needed to produce the organization's products and deliver them.

Department of Production

■ Produces the organization's product and delivers its services rapidly, in high quantity and with excellent quality so people are satisfied with results.

Qualifications Division
Division 5
Qualifications Secretary

Department of Examinations	Department of Review	Department of Certifications and Awards

This division sees that every product leaving the organization has the expected level of quality.

Department of Examinations

■ Examines the validity and correctness of products, passing these to Review or Certification so every product is certified, or corrected so it can be certified.

Department of Review

■ Reviews the organization's product to isolate the causes for any lower-than-acceptable level of quality. Also reviews staff actions and corrects them where needed so technology and policy are applied with superb results. Cares for the staff as individuals so they become fully trained in all aspects of their jobs and organizational policy and technology and become competent, contributing group members.

Department of Certifications and Awards

■ Issues and records valid attestations of skill, state and merit honestly deserved, attained and earned. Observes for any flubbed products and ensures they are corrected.

Public Division
Division 6
Public Secretary

Department of Public Information	Department of Clearing	Department of Success

This division, through all of its activities, brings knowledge of and distributes the organization's services and products to the broad public.

Department of Public Information

■ Sees to it that the appearance of the organization and its personnel is excellent. Makes the organization and its services and products well known to the community. Works with community groups and other organizations to improve the society.

Department of Clearing

■ Establishes and makes productive distribution points outside the organization which offer its services and products to new public.

Department of Success

■ Records and makes widely known to the public the successes of the organization's activities and its products.

ORGANIZING AND MORALE

The basics of organizing as found in this chapter present discoveries that can reverse the decline of any organization and bring about productivity or increase the orderly expansion of an already thriving group. They can be utilized in the home, school or the workplace—the scope of application is limitless. An individual can benefit by organizing his activities.

If you organize well and efficiently, you will have good morale. You will also have improved conditions.

Wherever morale is bad, organize!

A very careful survey of people shows that their basic protests are against lack of organization. "It doesn't run right!" is the reason they protest things.

Applying the organizing technology can smooth over these protests, bringing about increased production and thus better morale.

While they may necessitate some change in methods of operation for the individual or group, these basics of organizing are relatively simple to apply. And if success is desirable, they are well worth the effort, for they have been conclusively proven to work. By utilizing these principles any endeavor can be made to flourish. ■

TEST YOUR UNDERSTANDING

Answer the following questions about organizing technology. Refer back to the chapter to check your answers. If you need to, review the chapter. Going over the material several times will increase your certainty and help you better apply it.

- ❑ *What does "organizing" mean?*
- ❑ *What is an organizing board?*
- ❑ *What is the relationship between the posts and the particles of an organization?*
- ❑ *What is a hat?*
- ❑ *Why is it necessary for a terminal in an organization to have a hat and know it?*
- ❑ *Why does one start from the final product in organizing an activity?*
- ❑ *How does working out the lesser products of the main product enable one to organize something?*
- ❑ *What is the relationship between a division and a department?*
- ❑ *What will occur if an organization or individual has one or more divisions that are not operating?*

PRACTICAL EXERCISES

1 Write down something you want to accomplish; e.g., a clean car, a small garden planted, a room in one's house repainted, etc. This should be something that you could do in the present and in a relatively short amount of time. Then list out the series of actions that would be done to accomplish the final completion of this action. Repeat the above two more times for different things you want to accomplish.

2 Take one of the lists you wrote out in the previous exercise and actually carry the steps out to the completion of the action.

3 Write down a product of an organization or activity with which you have some familiarity. Then write down how this product is exchanged inside or outside the organization or activity.

4 Do the following steps:

a. Write down the name of a post or job with which you have some familiarity.

b. Write down the particle or particles that would be handled by this post or job.

c. Write down how the particle(s) you listed in step (b) would be changed by a person holding the job or post.

d. Repeat steps (a) to (c) for two other examples of posts or jobs.

5 Briefly describe your own hat, and write down its product(s). Repeat these two steps ten more times for other hats in organizations or activities of which you have some knowledge.

6 For one of the hats you named in the previous exercise, write a list of contents that would be included in the pack of materials that would teach an individual the actions to produce the product of the job. Do this for one other hat from the same list.

7 Do the following steps:

a. Work out and write down the final product of an organization, part of an organization or an activity with which you have some familiarity.

b. Figure out and list the lesser products earlier in sequence to the final product, working backwards in sequence.

c. Write down how you would post it to get command channels.

d. Repeat steps (a)–(c) for two other organizations or activities that you have familiarity or knowledge of.

8 Write down the name of an activity, organization or part of an organization you have observed or been part of which had flows in need of adjustment. Draw out as best you can what the existing flows are. Then draw out how the flows should be adjusted to improve its organization and production.

9 Pick one of the lesser products you listed in #7 above. Write down three examples of the functions and actions that would be done to bring about that lesser product. Repeat this for two other lesser products.

10 Using the data you wrote up in Exercise #7, write down for yourself three examples of posts that would do the functions to bring about the lesser products and final products.

11 With the data in the previous two practicals and in Exercise #7, work out the organization's or activity's Production Division. Refer to the materials in this chapter to carry out the steps necessary to do this. Sketch out the Production Division, showing the different posts by name.

12 Write down a realistic example of an action you could do that would be part of the Communications Division in an organization or activity. Repeat this for each of the remaining six divisions: Dissemination, Treasury, Production, Qualifications, Public and Executive.

13 Get a large piece of paper, or tape several sheets together to make a large sheet of paper. Using the seven division organizing board given in this book, sketch out an outline of a twenty-one department organizing board. Do this as follows: (a) Lay the paper on a flat surface, turned in such a way that the long length is lying from left to right in front of you. (b) Draw vertical dividing lines for the seven divisions. Use up the whole width of your paper except for small margins on each side. Each division is to be approximately the same width, equally spaced across the paper. Draw horizontal lines across the top and bottom of the vertical lines you drew. Leave about five inches of space at the top of the page. (c) Draw in the three departments for each division, each department approximately the same width. (d) Write in the names of the divisions and departments along the top of each in the sketch. Go on to the next exercise.

14 As the final exercise, work out a twenty-one department org board for your own life. To do this, use the twenty-one department org board outline you drew in the previous exercise and the seven division organizing board on pages 602–603. Compare your life to the functions of the divisions and departments to locate those which are missing. Take up the functions given for Department 1 and determine which are being performed in your life and which are not. Where you find one is missing (not being performed in your life), write it down in the Department 1 column on your org board outline. Then go on to the next department. Continue in this fashion until you have analyzed your life against the entire organizing board. Utilize what you found in this analysis to get in the missing functions and departments in your life.

RESULTS FROM APPLICATION

Dramatic and lasting changes have been made by individuals, family members and executives through using the basic tools of organizing as formulated by Mr. Hubbard. Organizing technology left the dark ages forever with the discoveries he made. The ease and effectiveness of application create daily miracles in the companies and corporations of those who use them. Its application in the home has made for much more fulfilling and productive familial activities. Business stress and its accompanying array of illnesses become a thing of the past replaced by well-being and a true enjoyment of production. This technology even combats the unpredictability of future survival for oneself and one's group endeavors. The resultant raised productivity and satisfaction gained from being able to causatively direct the course of organizational affairs is reflected in the accounts of application below.

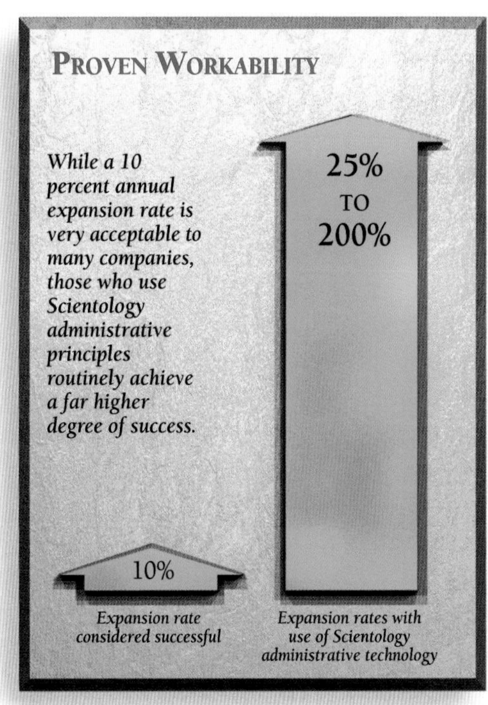

PROVEN WORKABILITY
While a 10 percent annual expansion rate is very acceptable to many companies, those who use Scientology administrative principles routinely achieve a far higher degree of success.
25% TO 200%
10%
Expansion rate considered successful
Expansion rates with use of Scientology administrative technology

As the president of an environmental company in Burbank, California, a man has used L. Ron Hubbard's administrative technology for the entire twelve years the company has been operating.

"We have grown from one small office with an individual founder to a 26,000-square-foot corporate headquarters with two hundred staff and ten offices throughout California. Our company has been listed for three years in a row in the top five hundred fastest growing private corporations in the United States. This is a direct result of L. Ron Hubbard's administrative technology on organizing boards and other subjects, all designed to get results. After majoring in business at Illinois University, I knew very little about the actual operation of a company. I can attribute the success of this company to the use of Mr. Hubbard's technology and to that alone."

A young sailor had the goal to work in the music industry. He worked on this but didn't really get anywhere until he became familiar with Mr. Hubbard's technology on organizing boards:

"I had been dealing with professional music all my life before I became a sailor and wanted to go back to work with music. I really tried to make it happen, but this had

been going on for the better part of five years with no result. Then I learned about Mr. Hubbard's technology concerning org boards and started applying specifically the data on Divisions 4 and 6. I suddenly found my skills in demand. Less than a month after beginning to apply this data, I was approached by a personnel director from a music company who wanted me to start working in a very advanced music studio. While waiting to get started, I got into production as a music composer and continued my personal promotion. I was hired and am now where I want to be. The turning point for all this was without doubt the application of the technology about org boards. Doing this made everything fall into place."

An executive in Washington, DC was put in charge of a major operation and luckily knew Mr. Hubbard's technology about organizing. She applied it and got the following result:

"By using L. Ron Hubbard's technology on organizing I was able to get a unit of twenty-five people organized up with lines and terminals and getting out products on a twenty-four-hour basis. (This was an unusual situation where the night crew had to prepare materials throughout the night and have them ready to go for the day crew each morning by 7 A.M.) I used the exact data on organizing, followed it to the letter and drilled the crew on everything. It took me a day or two to prepare the drilling but once it was applied, the whole thing worked like magic. The drilled crew was there, knew exactly what to do, what their other team members were doing, and it went off like clockwork."

A young woman's experience with organizing an activity demonstrated to her the value of Mr. Hubbard's organizational principles:

"Some time ago I went with fifteen other people to do a major convention in Florida, in which we had over two hundred people receiving services. We were not organized properly ***at all****, had not given specific hats to each person and so were stumbling over each other, had complaints about slow service, and were running ourselves into the ground trying to keep track of everything. We didn't want to repeat our errors at the next convention we did in England, and so we decided to learn something from our earlier mistakes. We worked out a simple org board for the upcoming convention detailing who was going to take care of what functions and assigned specific hats to the people who were there. The result? We serviced several hundred people with less personnel and had far less confusion than the first convention. This couldn't have been accomplished had we not used Mr. Hubbard's technology on organizing boards."*

SUGGESTIONS FOR FURTHER STUDY

L. Ron Hubbard found that the fundamental truths which apply to the spiritual advancement of the *individual* could be applied to the survival of a *group*. From these basics of the Scientology philosophy he developed group technology. The laws and axioms of Scientology give an insight into working within a group that no one ever had before. The following are key materials on this subject.

How to Live Though an Executive

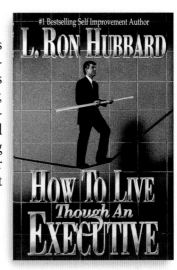

Using his discoveries about communication and its importance in life, Mr. Hubbard developed communication systems for use by groups. In this book he covers such subjects as the importance of applying affinity, reality and communication within a group, the relationship of communication to matter, energy, space and time, and group goals and their attainment. By knowing and applying this material, any individual can better lead a group, improving his own survival as well as that of his group.

Increasing Efficiency

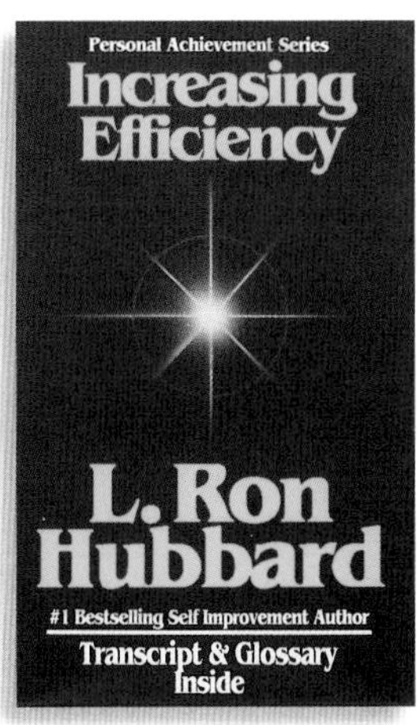

Inefficiency is a major barrier to success. Scores of systems, programs, calendars, memory aids, card files and other gimmicks have been put forward to overcome it. In this lecture from the Personal Achievement Series, Mr. Hubbard emphasizes the most important element for improvement of your efficiency: *you*. Here are the factors proven to boost efficiency, effectiveness and productivity.

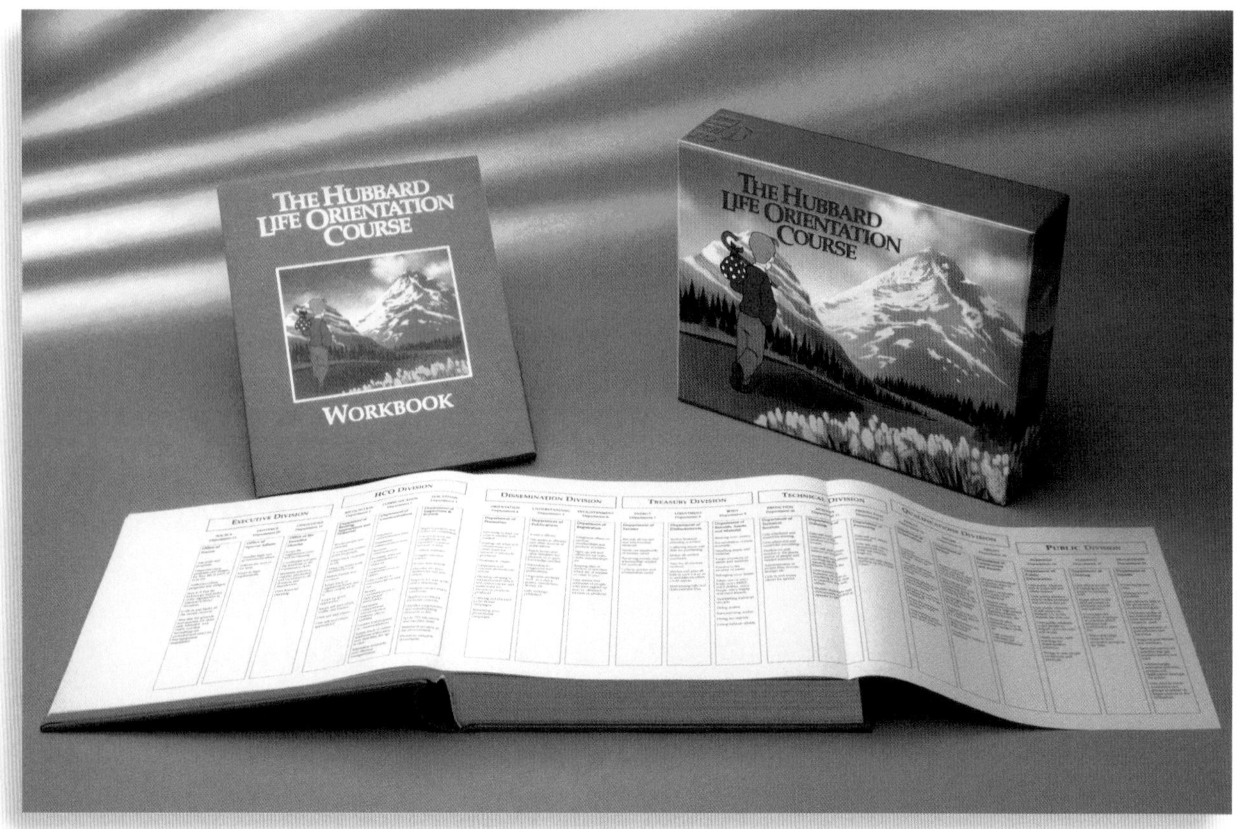

Hubbard Life Orientation Course

One can be truly productive—and therefore happy—in life if he understands and is following his true purpose. This four-week course helps one analyze and sort out every single area of his life and bring all its factors into alignment. Any person's life contains all the functions given on the organizing board. The Life Orientation Course brings these into view and clarifies them. One is also provided with tools and technology he can apply in everyday life to obtain his products successfully. The result is a person who has his life organized, knows where he is headed in life and has the understanding and tools to get where he wants to go. The Life Orientation Course is a route *into* the activity of living. (Delivered in Scientology organizations.)

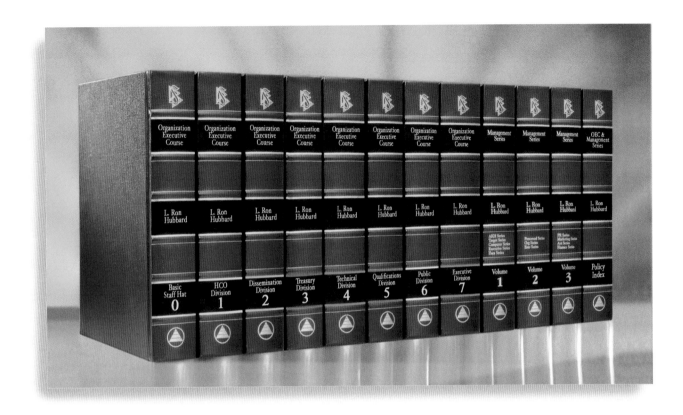

The Organization Executive Course Volumes and Management Series Volumes

Throughout several decades of research, applying his discoveries about the mind and spirit to the subject of groups, L. Ron Hubbard formulated the laws of group survival. Twelve large volumes contain thousands of individual writings which detail these principles. The *Organization Executive Course* (OEC) *Volumes* cover the theory and application of subjects such as communication and communication lines, levels of awareness and how these apply to a group, ethics and ethical codes, and many others. An individual cannot survive well if he has no knowledge or understanding of group technology. The laws of life must be known and applied, if one is going to have a group in this universe that survives and wins through its obstacles.

As part of his development of Scientology group technology, Mr. Hubbard applied the axioms of life and the human spirit to the subject of management. The three *Management Series Volumes* contain numerous writings on such topics as how to organize different types of projects and activities, how to help group members learn their jobs better, and ways to attain targets and goals.

Courses using the OEC and *Management Series Volumes* are available in Scientology organizations.

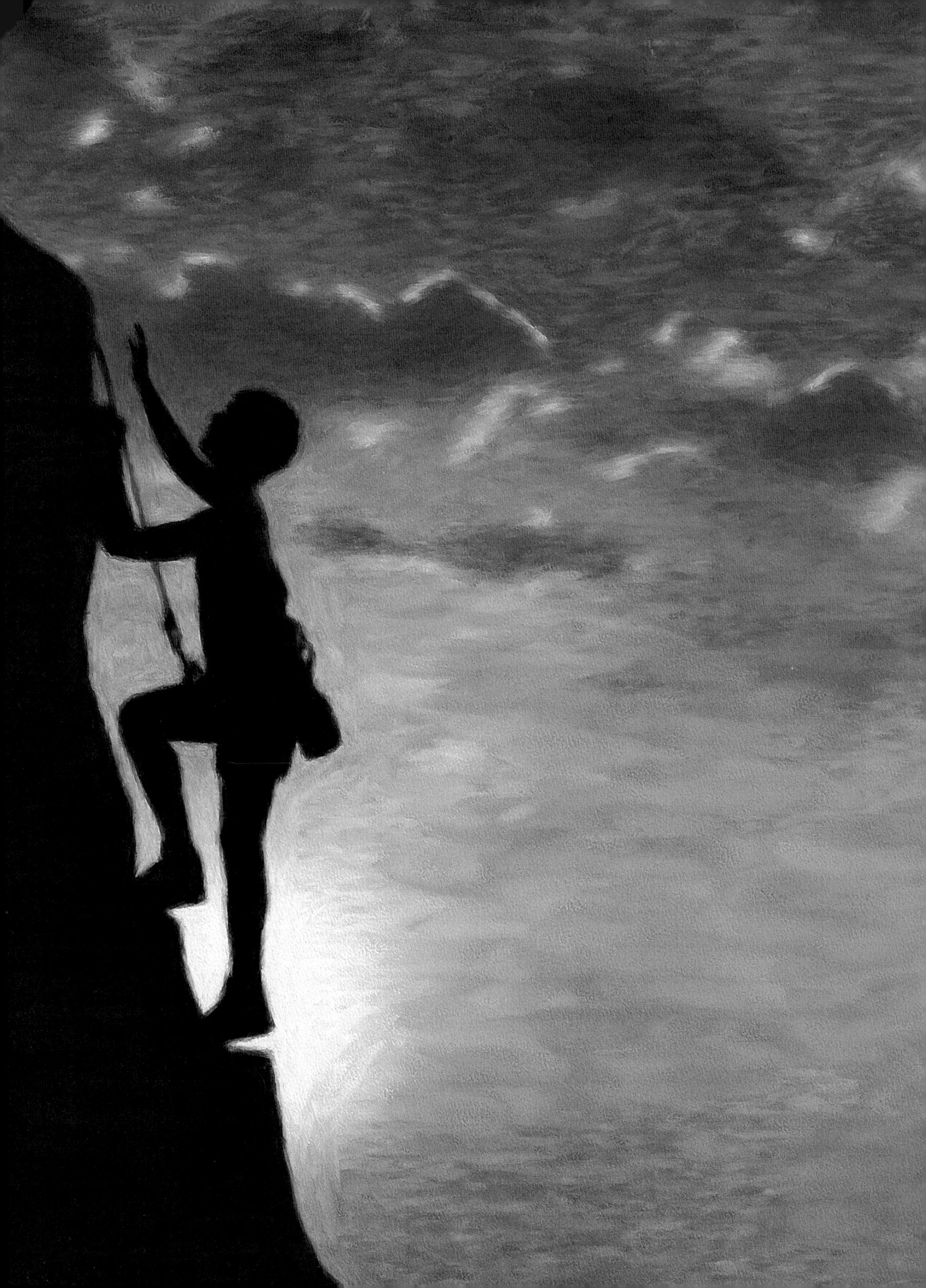

Chapter 17

Targets and Goals

How does one get things done? How does one make a dream a reality or carry a plan through to completion? Many of us seem to have unrealized goals or incomplete plans and many of us face tasks that appear overwhelming, even impossible to achieve. This is true not only of individuals, but of companies and even countries. History is filled with failed projects.

In examining the subject of organization, L. Ron Hubbard developed an enormous body of technology to ensure the success of any group. In doing so, he also provided a solution to the most common of failings: the lack of ability to execute plans.

In this chapter, you will discover how to attain literally any goal, large or small. Plans **can** *be carried through to fruition, but a number of vital steps must be taken, one after the other. You'll learn what these steps are and how to apply them to anything—a personal ambition, a family, a group, a business and more. You'll learn that your dreams can become real.*

ADMINISTRATIVE SCALE

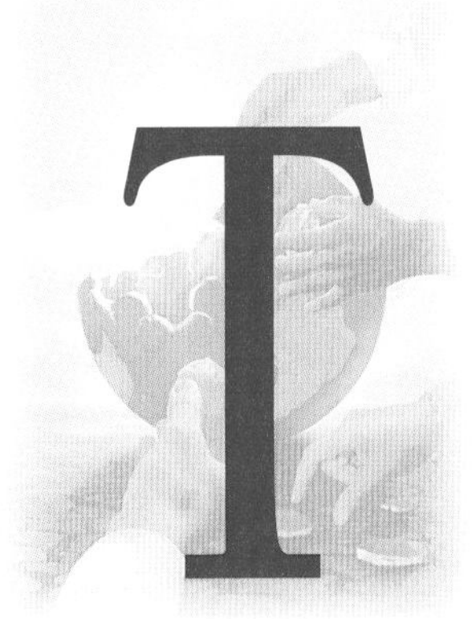

The achievement of one's goals, no matter how large or small the endeavor, relies on goals, purposes and activities being aligned and organized.

A goal is not something that one decides upon which then miraculously comes to fruition, just because one decided it would. The attainment of a goal necessitates that certain actions be carried out in the real world which effect some change for the better and a step closer toward its accomplishment.

One can be working toward a goal, but discover that his actions do not yield any forward progress. This occurs not only for an individual in his life, but also for an organization, state or country of any size. This can be a result of the plans, actions and other factors not being aligned to attain the goal.

There are actually a number of subjects that make up an activity. Each of these must operate in a coordinated manner to achieve success in the intended accomplishment of the envisioned goal.

A scale has been developed in Scientology which gives a sequence (and relative seniority) of subjects relating to organization.

GOALS	A *goal* is a known objective toward which actions are directed with the purpose of achieving that end.
PURPOSES	A *purpose* is a lesser goal applying to specific activities or subjects. It often expresses future intentions.
POLICY	*Policy* consists of the operational rules or guides for the organization which are not subject to change.
PLANS	A *plan* is a short-range broad intention thought up for the handling of a broad area to remedy it or expand it, or to obstruct or impede an opposition to expansion.
PROGRAMS	A *program* is a series of steps in sequence to carry out a plan.
PROJECTS	A *project* is a sequence of steps written to carry out *one* step of a program.
ORDERS	An *order* is a verbal or written direction to carry out a program step or apply general policy.
IDEAL SCENES	An *ideal scene* expresses what a scene or area ought to be. If one has not envisioned an ideal scene with which to compare the existing scene, he will not be able to recognize departures from it.
STATISTICS	A *statistic* is a number or amount compared to an earlier number or amount of the same thing. Statistics refer to the quantity of work done or the value of it.
VALUABLE FINAL PRODUCTS	A *valuable final product* is a product that can be exchanged for the services or goods of the society.

This scale is worked up and worked down UNTIL IT IS (EACH ITEM) IN FULL AGREEMENT WITH THE REMAINING ITEMS.

In short, for success, all these items in the scale must agree with all other items in the scale on the same subject.

Let us take "golf balls" as a subject for the scale. Then all these scale items must be in agreement with one another on the subject of golf balls. It is an interesting exercise.

The scale also applies in a destructive subject. Like "cockroaches."

When an item in the scale is *not* aligned with the other items, the project will be hindered, if not fail.

The skill with which all these items in any activity are aligned and gotten into action is called MANAGEMENT.

Group members only become upset when one or more of these points are not aligned to the rest and at least some group agreement.

Groups appear slow, inefficient, unhappy, inactive or quarrelsome only when these items are not aligned, made known and coordinated.

Any activity can be improved by debugging or aligning this scale in relation to the group activity.

As lack of agreement breeds lessened communication and lessened affinity, it follows that unreal items on the scale (not aligned) produce upsets and disaffection.

It then follows that when these scale items are well aligned with each other and the group, there will be high agreement, high communication and high affinity in the group.

Group mores aligned so and followed by the group gives one an ethical group and also establishes what will then be considered as harmful, contrasurvival acts in the group by group members.

This scale and its parts and ability to line them up are one of the most valuable tools of organization.

MAKING PLANNING AN ACTUALITY

For an individual, group or organization to achieve an intended goal requires knowledge of certain principles on the subject of organization.

When we look at organization in its most simple form, when we seek certain key actions or circumstances that make organization work, when we need a very simple, very vital rundown to teach people that will produce results, we find only a few points we need to stress.

The purpose of organization is TO MAKE PLANNING BECOME ACTUALITY.

An actuality is a state or thing that exists in reality.

Organization is not just a fancy, complex system, done for its own sake. That is bureaucracy at its worst. Graphs for the sake of graphs, rules for the sake of rules, only add up to failures.

The only virtue (not always a bad one) of a complex, unwieldy, meaningless bureaucratic structure is that it provides jobs for the friends of those in control. If it does not also bring about burdensome taxation and threatened bankruptcy by reason of the expense of maintaining it, and if it does not saddle a people or production employees with militant (aggressive) inspections and needless control, organization for the sake of providing employment is not evil but beyond providing employment is useless, and only when given too much authority is it destructive.

The kings of France and other lands used to invent titles and duties to give activity to the hordes of noble hangers-on to keep them at court, under surveillance, and out of mischief out in the provinces where they might stir up their own people. "Keeper of the Footstools," "Holder of the Royal Nightgown" and other such titles were fought for, bought, sold and held with ferocity.

Status-seeking, the effort to become more important and have a personal reason for being and for being respected, gets in the road of honest efforts to effectively organize in order to get something done, in order to make something economically sound.

Organization for its own sake, in actual practice, usually erects a monster that becomes so hard to live with that it becomes overthrown. Production losses, high taxes, irritating or fearsome interference with the people or actual producers invites and accomplishes bankruptcy or revolt, usually both, even in commercial companies.

Therefore to be meaningful, useful and lasting, an organization (corporation, company, business, group, etc.) has to fit into the definition above:

TO MAKE PLANNING BECOME ACTUALITY.

In companies and countries there is no real lack of dreaming. All but the most depraved (morally bad or corrupt) heads of companies or states wish to see specific or general improvement. This is also true of their executives and, as it forms the basis of nearly all revolts, it is certainly true of workers. From top to bottom, then, there is, in the large majority, a desire for improvement.

More food, more profit, more pay, more facilities and, in general, more and better of whatever they believe is good or beneficial. This also includes less of what they generally consider to be bad.

Programs which obtain general support consist of more of what is beneficial and less of what is detrimental. "More food, less disease," "more beautiful buildings, less hovels," "more leisure, less work," "more activity, less unemployment," are typical of valuable and acceptable programs.

But only to have a program is to have only a dream. In companies, in political parties, useful programs are very numerous. They suffer only from a lack of execution.

All sorts of variations of program failure occur. The program is too big. It is not generally considered desirable. It is not needed at all. It would benefit only a few. Such are surface reasons. The basic reason is lack of organization know-how.

Any program, too ambitious, partially acceptable, needed or not needed, could be put into effect if properly organized.

The five-year plans of some nations which were in vogue were almost all very valuable and almost all fell short of their objectives. The reason was not that they were unreal, too ambitious or generally unacceptable. The reason for any such failure was and is lack of organization.

It is not man's dreams that fail him. It is the lack of know-how required to bring those dreams into actuality.

Good administration has two distinct targets:

1. To perpetuate (prolong the existence of) an existing company, culture or society,

2. To make planning become actuality.

Given a base on which to operate—which is to say land, people, equipment and a culture—one needs a good administrative pattern of some sort just to maintain it.

Thus (1) and (2) above become (2) only. The plan is "to continue the existing entity." No company or country continues unless one continues to put it there. Thus an administrative system of some sort, no matter how crude, is necessary to perpetuate any group or any subdivision of a group. Even a king or headman or manager who has no other supporting system to whom one can bring disputes about land or water or pay is an administrative system. The foreman of a labor gang that only loads trucks has an astonishingly complex administrative system at work.

Companies and countries do not work just because they are there or because they are traditional. They are continuously put there by one or another form of administration.

When a whole system of administration moves out or gets lost or forgotten, collapse occurs unless a new or substitute system is at once moved into place.

Changing the head of a department, much less a general manager and much, much less a ruler, can destroy a portion or the whole since the old system, unknown, disregarded or forgotten, may cease and no new system which is understood is put in its place. Frequent transfers within a company or country can keep the entire group small, disordered and confused, since such transfers destroy what little administration there might have been.

Thus, if administrative shifts or errors or lack can collapse any type of group, it is vital to know the basic subject of organization.

Even if the group is at effect—which is to say originates nothing but only defends in the face of threatened disaster—it still must plan. And if it plans, somehow it must get the plan executed or done. Even a simple situation of an attacked fortress has to be defended by planning and doing the plan, no matter how crude. The order "Repel the invader who is storming the south wall" is the result of observation and planning no matter how brief or unthorough. Getting the south wall defended occurs by some system of administration even if it only consists of sergeants hearing the order and pushing their men to the south wall.

A company with heavy debts has to plan even if it is just to stall off creditors. And some administrative system has to exist even to do only that.

The terrible dismay of a young leader who plans a great and powerful new era only to find himself dealing with old and weak faults is attributable not to his "foolish ambition" or "lack of reality" but to his lack of organizational know-how.

Even elected presidents or prime ministers of democracies are victims of such terrible dismay. They do not, as is routinely asserted, "go back on their campaign promises" or "betray the people." They, as well as their members of parliament, simply lack the rudiments (fundamentals) of organizational know-how. They cannot put their campaign promises into effect, not because they are too high-flown (sounding grand or important) but because they are politicians, not administrators.

To some men it seems enough to dream a wonderful dream. Just because they dreamed it they feel it should now take place. They become very provoked when it does not occur.

Whole nations, to say nothing of commercial firms or societies or groups, have spent decades in floundering turmoil because the basic dreams and plans were never brought to fruition (successful completion).

Whether one is planning for the affluence of the Appalachian Mountains or a new loading shed closer to the highway, the gap between the plan and the actuality will be found to be lack of administrative know-how.

Technical ignorance, finance, even lack of authority and unreal planning itself are none of them true barriers between planning and actuality.

PLANS AND PROGRAMS

There is, however, much to know of the techniques employed to draw up planning which will bring one's dreams to realization. An initial step would be to comprehend the basic terms relating to the subject.

A *plan* is a description of the short-range broad intentions as to what one sees is required to handle a specific area. A plan would be expected to remedy nonoptimum circumstances in an area or expand it or to obstruct or impede an opposition to expansion.

For a plan to be carried out requires it be broken down into the specific actions necessary to accomplish what the plan intends to do. This is done by use of a *program.*

A *program* is a series of steps in sequence to carry out a plan. To write a program requires that a plan exist beforehand, even if only in the mind of the person writing the program. A step of a program is called a *target.*

A program is composed of targets. A *target* is an action which should be undertaken in order to achieve a desired objective.

There are several *values* of targets. Not all targets are the same value or importance. Each of these is described below.

Major Target

A *major target* is the desirable overall ambition being undertaken. This is highly generalized, such as "to become a trained Scientology practitioner."

Other examples in different fields would be:

"To get all machinery and equipment in the company operational."

"To acquire, set up, make ready and use a suitable property and facilities at reasonable low cost."

"To get books being distributed to mail order customers and any stores or distributors."

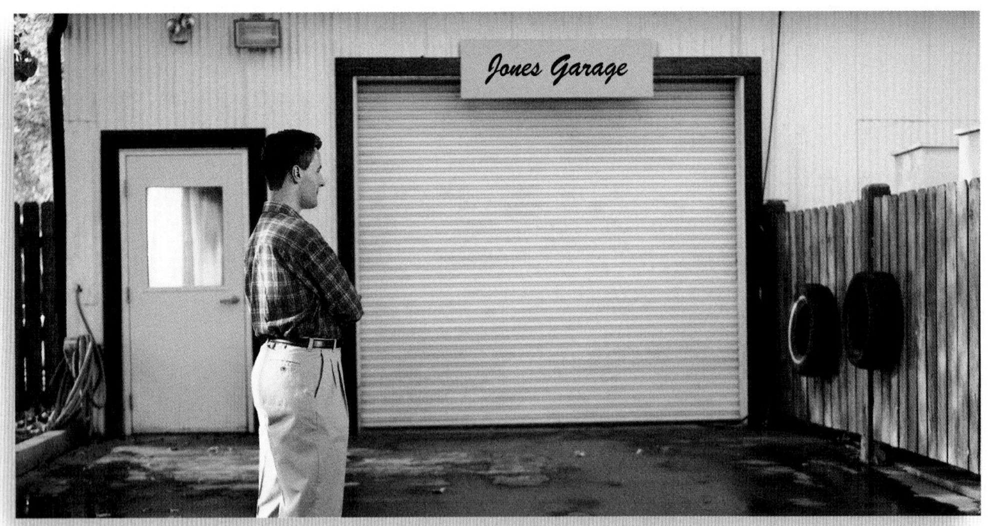

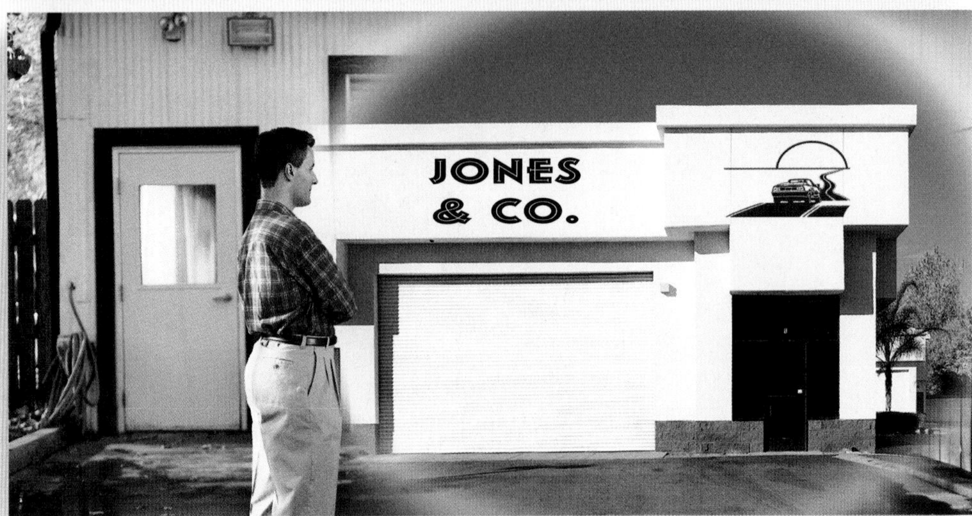

A ***major target*** *is the overall objective.*

Primary Targets

A *primary target* is one which deals with the organizational, personnel and communication-type steps that have to be kept in. These are a group of "understood" targets which, if overlooked, bring about inaction.

The first of these is: SOMEBODY THERE

Then: WORTHWHILE PURPOSE

Then: SOMEBODY TAKING RESPONSIBILITY FOR THE AREA OR ACTION

Then: FORM OF ORGANIZATION PLANNED WELL

Then: FORM OF ORGANIZATION HELD OR REESTABLISHED

Then: ORGANIZATION OPERATING

If we have the above "understood" targets, we can go on; *but if these drop out or are not substituted for,* then no matter what targets are set thereafter they will go rickety or fail entirely.

In the above there may be a continual necessity to reassert one or more of the "understood" targets WHILE trying to get further *targets* going.

Some examples of primary targets would be:

"Accept the job to which one is being assigned."

"Read and understand the program which you will be doing."

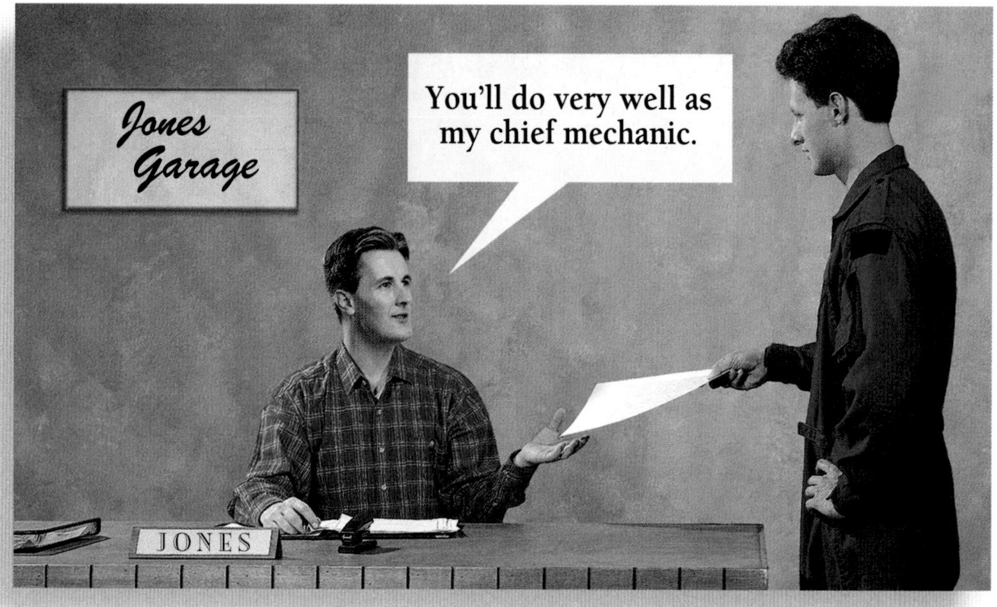
Jones Garage
You'll do very well as my chief mechanic.
JONES

Somebody there is an example of a primary target.

Vital Targets

A *vital target* is something that must be done to operate at all.

This requires an inspection of both the area one is operating into and the factors or materiel or organization with which we are operating.

One then finds those points (sometimes *while* operating) which stop or threaten future successes. And sets the overcoming of the vital ones as targets.

Some examples of these would be:

"Look into the circumstances one is inspecting with your own eyes; don't accept another's report."

"Accept no orders from anyone other than your direct senior."

"Do not let the supply of books falter in the country while the campaign is ongoing."

"Maintain a high level of ethical behavior and set an excellent example in doing so."

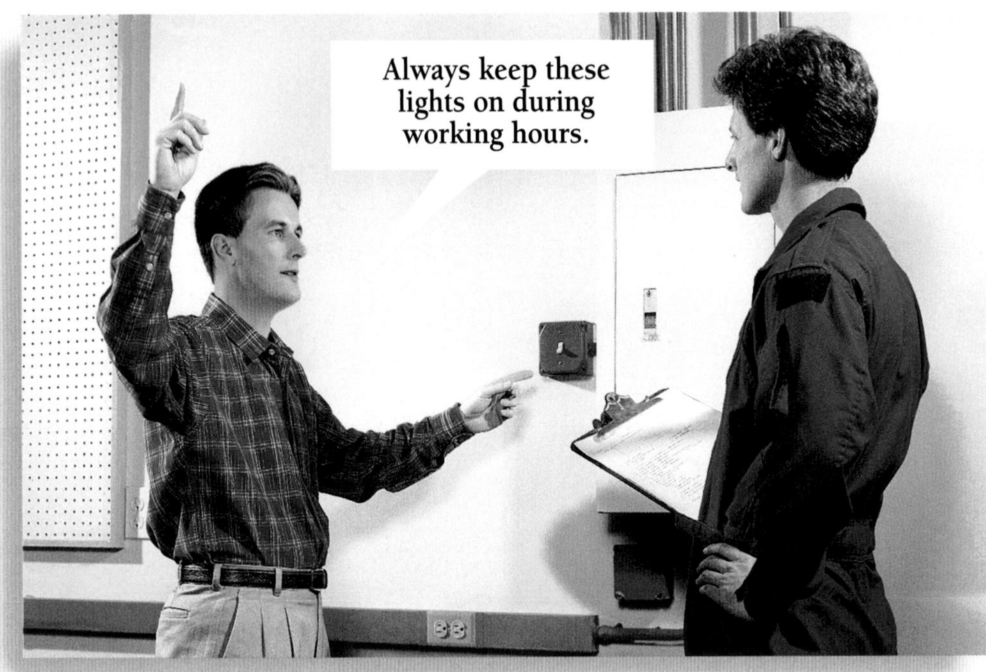
Always keep these
lights on during
working hours.

A vital target must be in to operate successfully.

Conditional Targets

A *conditional target* is one which is done to find out data, or if a project can be done, where it can be done, etc.

You've seen chaps work all their lives to "get rich" or some such thing in order to "tour the world" and never make it. Some other fellow sets "tour the world" and goes directly at it and *does* it. So there is a type of target known as a *conditional* target: If I could just _______ then we could _______ and so accomplish _______. This is all right of course until it gets unreal.

There is a whole class of conditional targets that have no IF in them. These are legitimate targets. They have lots of WILL in them, "We *will* _______ and then _______."

Sometimes sudden "breaks" show up and one must quickly take advantage of them. This is only "good luck." One uses it and replans quickly when it *happens*. One is on shaky ground to count on "good luck" as a solution.

A valid conditional target would be:

"We will go there and see if the area is useful."

Another example of a conditional target is:

"If there is a backlog of filing, then organize a short time period each day where the company's employees assist in filing the particles in the correct files."

All conditional targets are basically actions of gathering data first, and if it is okay, then go into action.

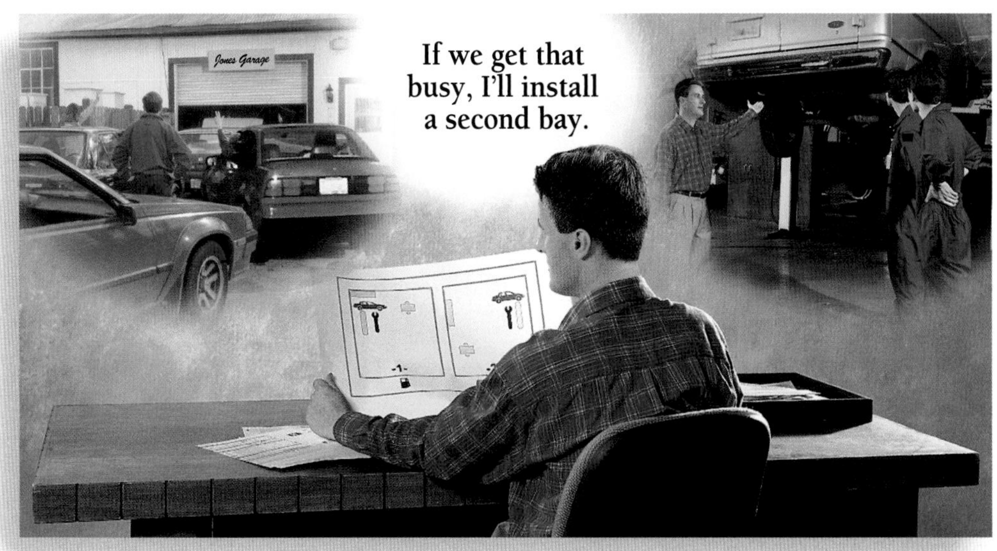
Jones Garage
If we get that busy, I'll install a second bay.

*All **conditional targets** are basically actions of gathering data first, and if it is okay, then go into action.*

Operating Targets

An *operating target* is one which would set the *direction* of advance and qualify it. It normally includes a scheduled *time* by which it has to be complete so as to fit into other targets.

Sometimes the time is set as "BEFORE." And there may be no time for the event that it must be done "before." Thus it goes into a rush basis "just in case."

Examples of operating targets would be:

"Advertise books in local magazines which are subscribed to by the type of audience who would be interested in these books."

"Hire local labor to make adobe bricks for the walls."

"Establish how the company newsletter can be most inexpensively mailed to the branch offices."

"Clean up the President's suite."

"Send a courier with the return mail direct to the home office."

*An **operating target** would set the direction of advance and qualify it.*

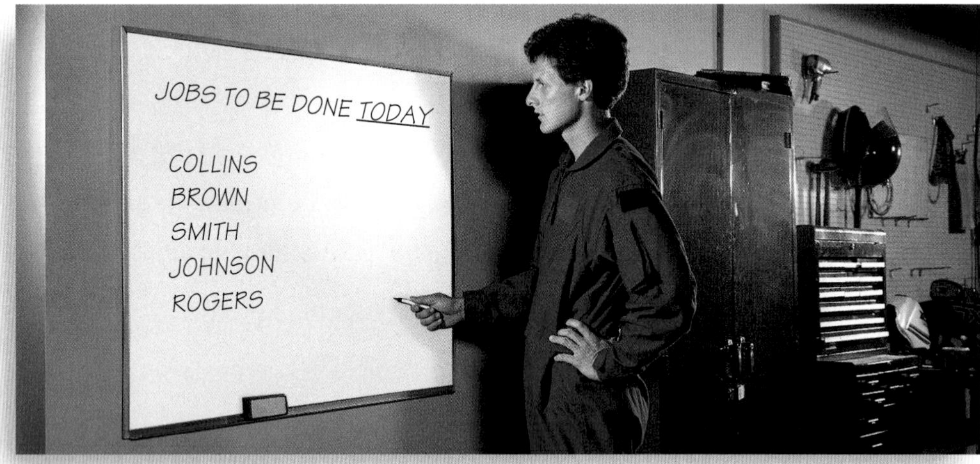

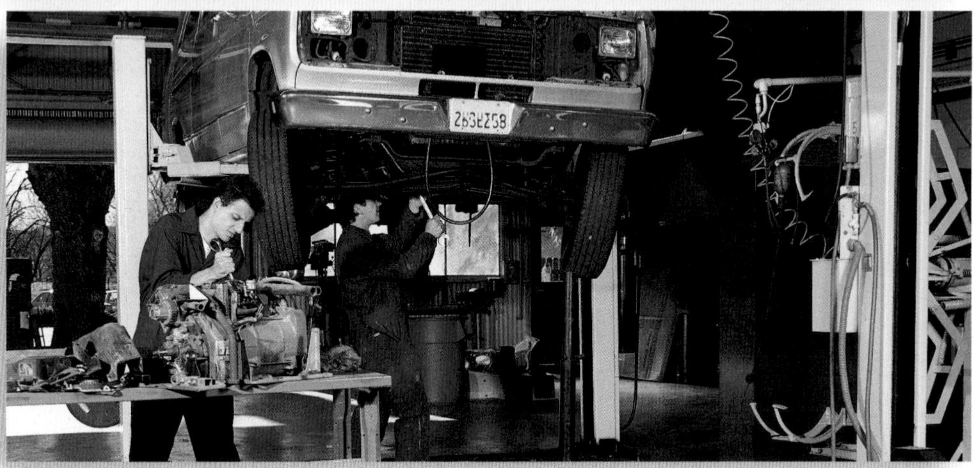

Production Targets

Setting quotas, usually against time, are *production* targets.

Examples of production targets would be:

"Next year's tuition set aside by June."

"Fifty thousand books bound by next month."

As *statistics* most easily reflect production, an organization or activity can be so PRODUCTION TARGET conscious that it fails to set conditional, operating or primary targets. When this happens, then production is liable to collapse for lack of planning stated in other types of targets.

Production as the only target type can become so engulfing that conditional targets even when set are utterly neglected. Then operating and primary targets get very unreal and statistics go DOWN.

YOU HAVE TO INSPECT AND SURVEY AND GATHER DATA AND SET OPERATING AND PRIMARY TARGETS BEFORE YOU CAN SET PRODUCTION TARGETS.

A normal reason for down statistics on production is the vanishment of primary targets. These go out and nobody notices that this affects production badly. Production depends on other prior targets being kept *in*.

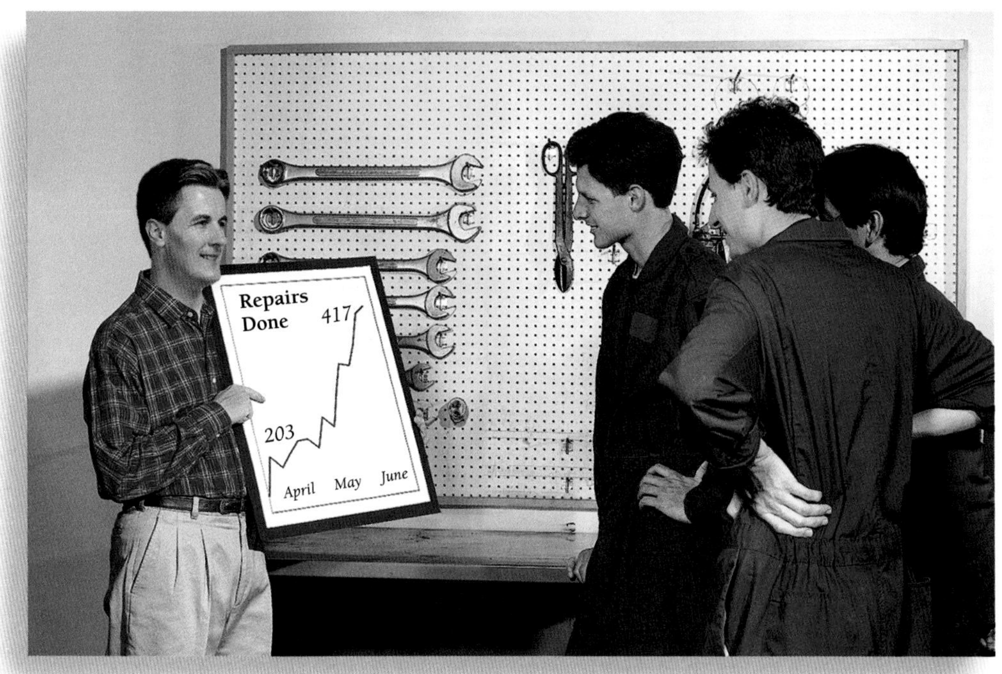

*Setting quotas, usually against time, are **production targets**.*

The following is a concise summary of the different types of targets which make up a program.

Types of Targets

MAJOR TARGETS	The broad general ambition, possibly covering a long, only approximated period of time. Such as "To attain greater security" or "To get the organization up to fifty employees."
PRIMARY TARGETS	The organizational, personnel, communication-type targets. These have to be kept *in*. These are the type of targets which deal with the terminals, communication routes, materiel and organizing boards. Example: "To put someone in charge of organizing it and have him set remaining primary targets." Or "To reestablish the original communication system which has dropped out."
VITAL TARGETS	Those which must be done to operate at all, based on an inspection of the area in which one is operating.
CONDITIONAL TARGETS	Those which set up EITHER/OR, to find out data or if a project can be done or where or to whom.
OPERATING TARGETS	Those which lay out directions and actions or a schedule of events or timetable.
PRODUCTION TARGETS	Those which set quantities like statistics.

WRITING PROGRAM TARGETS

A few data must be kept in mind when writing targets for a program. Applying these will assist one to get his programs done and bring his plans to actuality.

When writing operating targets, the first one must require the person, area or organization increase its level of production.

However, in actual fact, you can't write an operating target that is pure production. It would be impossible to write such a target because somebody would have to do it, and the moment that you have somebody there to do it, you have organization. So there is a certain amount of organization that comes into it.

For example, in handling a department responsible for collecting the organization's income, one would have to include in it, as its second target, beefing up the department. The first target would be for the department to do anything it could to handle its collections. And the second target would be to beef up that department forthwith. Otherwise, the production would not continue.

So there has to be immediate organization for production.

Terminable Targets

Now, how do you like a target like this: "Maintain friendly relations with the environment." How do you like that target? It is utterly, completely not a target that gets the person to carry out an action. It isn't a target at all!

Now, if it said, "Call on so and so, and so and so, and make them aware of your presence..." and so forth, it could have a DONE on it.

Targets should be terminable—doable, finishable, completable. This will contribute to the success of one's programs.

Sample Programs

Having learned the types of targets and how to write them, one can then formulate programs.

On the following pages you will find two sample programs. They clearly show the interrelationship and sequence of the different target types which make up a standard program. Each sample has a specific purpose: with the first, one learns how to do a project; with the second, one learns about production. One can do these two programs, target by target, and understand the orderliness and workability of programs and above all, what the types of targets are and how they work together.

By doing these programs, you will then be able to write and carry out your own programs and that will set you firmly on the road to accomplishing your goals and purposes.

Sample Program #1

Purpose: To learn to do a program.

Major Target: To get it done.

Primary Target:

1. Read this program.

Vital Targets:

1. Be honest about doing this.
2. Do all of it.
3. Check off each one when done.

Operating Targets:

1. Take off your right shoe. Look at the sole. Note what's on it. Put it back on.
2. Go get a drink of water.
3. Take a sheet of paper. Draw three concentric circles on it. Turn it over face down. Write your name on the back. Tear it up and put the scraps in a book.
4. Take off your left shoe. Look at the sole. Note what is on it. Put it back on.
5. Go find someone and say hello. Return and write a message to yourself as to how they received it.
6. Take off both shoes and bang the heels together three times and put them back on.
7. Write a list of projects in your life you have left incomplete or not done.
8. Write why this was.
9. Check this program carefully to make sure you have honestly done it all.
10. List your realizations, if any, while doing this program.
11. Decide whether you have honestly done this program.

Sample Program #2

Purpose: To learn about production.

Major Target: To actually produce something.

Primary Targets:

1. Get a pencil and five sheets of paper.
2. Situate yourself so you can do this program.

Vital Targets:

1. Read an operating target and be sure to do it all before going on.
2. Actually produce what's called for.

Operating Targets:

1. Look very busy without actually doing anything.
2. Do it again but this time be very convincing.
3. Work out the product of your job or activity. Get help from another person as needed.
4. Straighten up the papers on your desk.
5. Take sheet 1 as per primary targets above. Write whether or not No. 4 was production.
6. Find a paper or message that doesn't contribute in any way to your getting out your own product.
7. Answer it.
8. Take the second sheet called for in the primary target. Write on it why the action in 7 is perfectly reasonable.
9. Take the third sheet of paper and draw out how you receive communication on your job.
10. Get out one correct product for your job, complete, of high quality.
11. Deliver it.
12. Review the operating targets and see which one made you feel best.
13. Take the fourth sheet of paper and write down whether or not production is the basis of morale.
14. Take the fifth sheet of paper, use it for a cover sheet and write a summary of the program.
15. Realize you have completed a program.

PLANNING AND TARGETS

All manner of plans can be drawn up to accomplish desirable ends. However, they are just plans. Until the when and how they will be done and by whom has been established, scheduled, authorized or agreed upon, they will not be completed.

This is why planning sometimes gets a bad name.

You could *plan* to make a million dollars but if when, how and who were not set in program form as targets of different types, it just wouldn't happen. A brilliant plan is drawn as to *how* to convert Boston Harbor into a fuel tanker area. It could be on drawings with everything perfectly placed. One could even have models of it. Ten years go by and it has not been started much less completed. You have seen such plans. World's fairs are full of them.

One could also have a plan which was targeted in program form—who, when, how—and if the targets were poor or unreal, it would never be completed.

One can also have a plan which had no CONDITIONAL TARGET ahead of it and so no one really wanted it and it served no purpose really. It is unlikely it would ever be finished. Such a thing existed in Corfu (an island off Greece). It was a half-completed Greek theater which had just been left that way. No one had asked the inhabitants if they wanted it or if it was needed. So even though very well planned and even partially targeted and half-completed, there it is—half-finished. And has remained that way.

A plan, by which is meant the drawing or scale modeling of some area, project or thing, is of course a vital necessity in any construction and construction fails without it. It can even be okayed *as a plan*.

But if it was not the result of findings of a conditional target (a survey of what's needed or feasible), it will be useless or won't fit in. And if no funds are allocated to it and no one is ordered to do it and if no scheduling of doing it exists, then on each separate count it won't ever be done.

Where one has worked out a plan and is devising a program requiring approval, to get them okayed, one would have to show it as:

a. A result of a conditional target (survey of what's wanted and needed),

b. The details of the thing itself, meaning a picture of it or its scope plus the ease or difficulty in doing it and with what persons or materials,

c. Classification of it as vital or simply useful,

d. The primary targets of it showing the organization needed to do it,

e. The operating targets showing its scheduling (even if scheduled not with dates but days or weeks) and dovetailing with other actions,

f. Its cost and whether or not it will pay for itself or can be afforded or how much money it will make.

The program would have to include the targets.

A *plan* would be the *design* of the thing itself.

Thus we see why some things don't come off at all and why they often don't get completed even when planned. The plan is not put forward in its *target* framework and so is unreal or doesn't get done.

Sometimes a conditional target fails to ask what obstacles or opposition would be encountered or what skills are available and so can go off the rails in that fashion.

But if these points are grasped, then one sees the scope of the subject and can become quite brilliant and achieve things hitherto out of reach or never thought of before.

STRATEGIC PLANNING

No study of planning and targets is complete without examining the subject of strategic planning. It is of such vital importance that it merits an in-depth study as to its definition and use as well as its relationship to other aspects of management.

The term "STRATEGY" is derived from the Greek words:

strategos, which means "general,"

stratos, which means "army,"

agein, meaning "to lead."

STRATEGY, therefore, by dictionary definition, refers to a plan for the overall conduct of a war or sector of it.

By extrapolation (inferring from known facts), it has also come to mean a plan for the skillful overall conduct of a large field of operations, or a sector of such operations, toward the achievement of a specific goal or result.

This is planning that is done at upper-echelon level, as, if it is to be effective, it must be done from an overview of the broad existing situation.

It is a statement of the intended plans for accomplishing a broad objective and inherent in its definition is the idea of clever use of resources or maneuvers for outwitting the enemy or overcoming existing obstacles to win the objective.

It is the central strategy worked out at the top which, like an umbrella, covers the activities of the echelons below it.

That tells us what strategic planning is.

What It Does

What strategic planning does is provide direction for the activities of all the lower echelons. All the tactical plans and programs and projects to be carried out at lower echelons in order to accomplish the objective stream down from the strategic plan at the top. It is the overall plan against which all of these are coordinated.

This gives a clear look at why strategic planning is so vitally important and why it must be done by the upper-level planning body if management is to be effective and succeed.

What happens if strategic planning is missing? Well, what happens in the conduct of a war if no strategic planning is done?

Key troops can be left unflanked and unsupported in key areas while other troops fight aimless battles at some minor outpost. Supplies and ammunition could be deployed (positioned for use) to the wrong area or not forwarded at all. Conflict of orders, jammed lines and maneuvers, wasted resources and lost battles all result. With the lack of a plan, coordination is missing and it's a scene of confusion and dispersal. In short, disaster.

What a difference between this and a strong, coordinated, positive thrust toward attaining the objective!

Transposing all of this over into our own activity gives an even clearer look at why strategic planning must be done at the upper levels of management. The key word here is "done." It cannot be neglected or dropped out. It cannot be *assumed* to be done. Strategic planning must be done and stated and made known at least to the next lower levels of management so coordination and correct targeting can take place.

Purpose and Strategic Planning

A strategic plan begins with the observation of a situation to be handled or a goal to be met.

It always carries with it a statement of the definite purpose or purposes to be achieved.

Once the purpose has been established, it is possible to derive from it various strategic plannings.

In fact, STRATEGY CAN BE SAID TO BE HOW ONE IS GOING TO ACTUALLY EFFECTIVELY AND SWIFTLY GET A PURPOSE MANIFESTED AND ROLLING IN THE REAL PHYSICAL UNIVERSE AT SPEED AND WITH NO FLUBS.

Any strategic plan can encompass a number of major actions required from one or more different sectors in order to achieve the purpose. These are expressed in highly general terms as they are a statement of the initial overall planning that has been done. From them one can then derive tactical plannings. But all of these things have to fit together.

Example:

Situation: The ABC Paper Company, though continuing to produce its formerly successful line of paper products, is also continuing to concentrate solely on its regular, already-established clientele while neglecting a number of its potential publics. The company is rapidly going broke and losing its execs to companies where there is "more opportunity for expansion."

Purpose: Put a full-blown paper company there which reaches all of its potential public for volume sales of existing and new products, while it also continues to sell and service its regular clientele in volume, and thus restore the company's solvency and build its repute as a lucrative, progressive concern with opportunities for expansion.

Strategic Plan: The strategic planning, based on the situation and established purpose, might go something like this:

1. The most immediate and vital action needed to arrest the losses is to (without interrupting any ongoing business or taking down or destroying any other unit) set up and get functioning a new sales unit (alongside the existing one) which will have as its first priority the development of immediate new clients for the current line of products from among (a) retail paper outlets, (b) wholesale paper outlets, and (c) direct mail order. Clean, experienced salesmen will need to be procured to head up each of these sections, and other professional salesmen will need to be located in volume. These can be hired at very low retainer and make the bulk of their money on commissions. This operation can then be expanded over broader areas using district managers, salesmen who start other salesmen and even door-to-door salesmen. As a part of this plan, commission systems, package sales kits and promotion and

advertising will need to be worked out. Getting this going on an immediate basis will boost sales and offset losses and very shortly expand the company into the field of stellar profits.

2. While the immediate holding action is going in, current sales and servicing of clients must be maintained. At the same time, sales and production records of existing staff will need to be reviewed as well as a thorough accounting done of company books to find where the losses are coming from. Any unproductive personnel will need to be dismissed and those who do produce retained. Should any embezzlement or financial irregularity be found this will need to be handled with appropriate legal action. In other words, the current operation is to be fully reviewed, cleaned up and its production not only maintained but stepped up all possible, with production targets set and met.

3. A program is to be worked out whereby surveys are done of all publics to find out what new paper products the publics want or will buy. Based on these survey results, a whole new line of paper products (additional to the old established line) can then be developed, produced, promoted and sold broadly. The program for establishing the new line of goods will need to cover financing, the organizing of the new production unit (including clean executives, competent designers, any needed additional workmen) as well as any additional machinery or equipment required. It will also need to cover broad PR, promotion and sales campaigns that push the new products as well as the old for volume sales of both. Inherent in this planning would be a campaign to enhance the company's image as pioneers in the field of new paper products with opportunities for expansion-minded executives.

Such a strategic plan not only corrects a bad situation but turns it around into a highly profitable and expanding scene for the future of the whole company.

What one is trying to accomplish is digging the scene out of the soup and expanding it into a terrific level of viability.

From this strategic plan, tactical planning would be done, taking the broad strategic targets and breaking them down into precise and exactly targeted actions which get the strategic planning executed.

One would have many people working on this and it would be essential that they all had the purpose straight and that there be no conflicting internal spots in the overall campaign. Somebody reading over such plans might not see the importance of it unless they understood the situation and had a general overall riding purpose from which they could refine their tactical planning.

It is quite common in tactical execution of a strategic planning to find it necessary to modify some tactical targets or add new ones or even drop out some as found to be unnecessary.

The tactical management of a strategic planning is a bit of an art in itself so this is allowed for.

Given a good purpose, then, against which things can be coordinated, the strategic action necessary to accomplish it can then be worked out and the tactical plans to bring the strategic plans into existence can follow.

This way a group can flourish and prosper. When all strengths and forces are aligned to a single thrust a tremendous amount of power can be developed.

So one gets the purpose stated and from that works out what strategy will be used to accomplish the purpose and this then bridges the purpose into a tactical feasibility.

When the strategic plan, with its purpose, has been put forward, it is picked up by the next lower level of command and turned into tactical planning.

Strategic Versus Tactical Planning

Strategy differs from tactics.

This is a point which must be clearly understood by the various echelons of management.

There is a very, very great difference between a strategic plan and a tactical plan.

While tactical planning is used to win an engagement, strategic planning is used to win the full campaign.

While the strategic plan is the large-scale, long-range plan to ensure victory, a tactical plan tells exactly who to move what to where and exactly what to do at that point.

The tactical plan must integrate into the strategic plan and accomplish the strategic plan. And it must do this with precise, doable targets.

And that, in essence, is management.

Bridging Between Purpose and Tactical

One error that is commonly made by untrained personnel is to jump from purpose to tactical planning, omitting the strategic plan. And this won't work. The reason it won't work is that unless one's targeted tactical plan is aligned to a strategic plan it will go off the rails.

The point to be understood here is that strategic planning *creates* tactical planning. One won't get one's purpose achieved unless there is a strategy worked out and used by which to achieve it. And, based on that strategy, one works out the tactical moves to be made to implement the strategy. But jumping from purpose to tactical, ignoring the strategy, one will miss.

So, between purpose and tactical there is *always* the step of strategic planning. We could say that by a strategic plan is meant some means to get the purpose itself to function.

It is actually a plan that has to do with cleverness.

One might be well aware of the purpose and might come up with a number of tactical targets having to do with it. And possibly the targets will work, in themselves. But the purpose is to get a situation handled and, lacking a strategic means to do this, one might still find himself facing the same problem.

Putting the actual bridge there between purpose and tactical, which bridge is the strategic side of it, the purpose will have some chance of succeeding.

Battle Plans

One accomplishes his goals by formulating plans and programs, which are then done target by target. An individual or group has daily and weekly actions he must do that will result in completed targets and programs. A tool one can employ to get his programs done, plans completed and goals accomplished is *battle plans.*

A "battle plan" is defined as:

A list of targets for the coming day or week which forward the strategic planning and handle the immediate actions and outnesses which impede it. (An outness is a condition or instance of something being wrong, incorrect or missing.)

Some people write "battle plans" as just a series of actions which they hope to get done in the coming day or week. This is fine and better than nothing and does give some orientation to one's actions. In fact, someone who does not do this is quite likely to get far less done and be considerably more harassed and "busy" than one who does. An orderly planning of what one intends to do in the coming day or week and then getting it done is an excellent way to achieve production. But this is using "battle planning" in an irreducible-minimum form as a tool.

Let us take up definitions. Why is this called a "battle plan" in the first place? It seems a very harsh military term to apply to the workaday world of administration. But it is a very apt term.

A war is something that happens over a long period of time. The fate of everything depends on it. A battle is something which occurs in a short unit of time. One can lose several battles and still win a war. Thus one in essence is talking about short periods of time when one is talking about a battle plan.

This goes further. When one is talking about a war, one is talking about a series of events which will take place over a long period of time. No general, or captain for that matter, ever won a war unless he did some strategic planning. This would concern an overall conduct of a war or a sector of it.

This is the big, upper-level idea sector. It is posed in high generalities, has definite purposes and applies at the top of the Admin Scale.

Below strategic planning one has tactical. In order to carry out a strategic plan one must have the plan of movement and actions necessary to carry it out. Tactical planning normally occurs down the org board in an army and is normally used to implement strategic planning. (An *org board,* short for *organizing board,* is a board which displays the functions, duties, sequences of action and authorities of an organization.) Tactical planning can go down to a point as low as "Private Joe is to keep his machine gun pointed on clump of trees 10 and fire if anything moves in it."

"Middle management"—the heads of regiments right on down to the corporals are covered by this term—is concerned with the implementation of strategic planning.

The upper planning body turns out a strategic plan. Middle management turns this strategic plan into tactical orders. They do this on a long-term basis and a short-term basis. When you get on down to the short-term basis you have battle plans.

A battle plan therefore means turning strategic planning into exact doable targets which are then executed in terms of motion and action for the immediate period being worked on. Thus one gets a situation whereby a good strategic plan, turned into good tactical targets and then executed, results in forward progress. Enough of these sequences carried out successfully gives one the war.

This should give you a grip on what a battle plan really is. It is the list of targets to be executed in the immediate short-term future that will implement and bring into reality some portion of the strategic plan.

One can see then that management is at its best when there is a strategic plan and when it is known at least down to the level of tactical planners. And tactical planners are simply those people putting strategic plans into targets which are then known to and executed from middle management on down. This is very successful management when it is done.

Of course the worthwhileness of any evolution depends on the soundness of the strategic plan.

But the strategic plan is dependent upon programs being written in target form and which are doable within the resources available.

What we speak of as "compliance" is really a done target. The person doing the target might not be aware of the overall strategic plan or how it fits into it; however, it is very poor management indeed whose targets do not *all* implement to one degree or another the overall strategic plan.

When we speak of coordination, we are really talking about conceiving or overseeing a strategic plan into the tactical version and at the lower echelon (level of responsibility in an organization) coordinating the actions of those who will do the actual things necessary to carry it out so that they all align in one direction.

All this comes under the heading of *alignment*. As an example, if you put a number of people in a large hall facing in various directions and then suddenly yelled at them to start running, they would, of course, collide with one another and you would have a complete confusion. This is the picture one gets when strategic planning is not turned into smooth tactical planning and is not executed within that framework. These people running in this hall could get very busy, even frantic, and one could say that they were on the job and producing but that would certainly be a very large lie. Their actions are not coordinated. Now if we were to take these same people in the same hall and have them do something useful such as clean up the hall, we are dealing with specific actions of specific individuals having to do with brooms and mops—who gets them, who empties the trash and so forth. The strategic plan of "Get the hall ready for the convention" is turned into a tactical plan which says exactly who does what and where. That would be the tactical plan. The result would be a clean hall ready for the convention.

But "Clean up the hall for the convention" by simple inspection can be seen to be what would be only a small portion of an overall strategic plan. In other words the strategic plan itself has to be broken down into smaller sectors.

One can see then that a battle plan could exist for the head of an organization which would have a number of elements in it which in their turn were turned over to subexecutives who would write battle plans for their own sectors which would be far more specific. Thus we have a gradient scale of the grand overall plan broken down into segments and these segments broken down even further.

The test of all of this is whether or not it results in worthwhile accomplishments which forward the general overall strategic plan.

If you understand all the above, you will have mastered the elements of coordination.

Feasibility enters into such planning. This depends upon the resources available. Thus a certain number of targets and battle plans, to an organization which is expanding or attempting big projects, must include organizational planning and targets and battle plans so that the organization stays together as it expands. One writes a battle plan, not on the basis of, "What am I going to do tomorrow?" or, "What am I going to do next week?" (which is fine in its own way and better than nothing), but on the overall question, "What exact actions do I have to do to carry out this strategic plan to achieve the exact results necessary for this stage of the strategic plan within the limits of available resources?" Then one would have the battle plan for the next day or the next week.

There is one thing to beware of in doing battle plans. One can write a great many targets which have little or nothing to do with the strategic plan and which keep people terribly busy and which accomplish no part of the overall strategic plan. Thus a battle plan can become a liability since it is not pushing any overall strategic plan and is not accomplishing any tactical objective.

So what is a "battle plan"? It is the doable targets in written form which accomplish a desirable part of an overall strategic plan.

The understanding and competent use of targeting in battle plans is vital to the overall accomplishment that raises production, income, delivery or anything else that is a desirable end.

It is a test of an executive whether or not he can competently battle plan and then get his battle plan executed. This tool can also be applied by persons in all walks of life and in any activity.

One accomplishes goals by formulating plans. To implement the plans one does programs and projects, which get completed through the use of battle plans. This aligns to the Admin Scale.

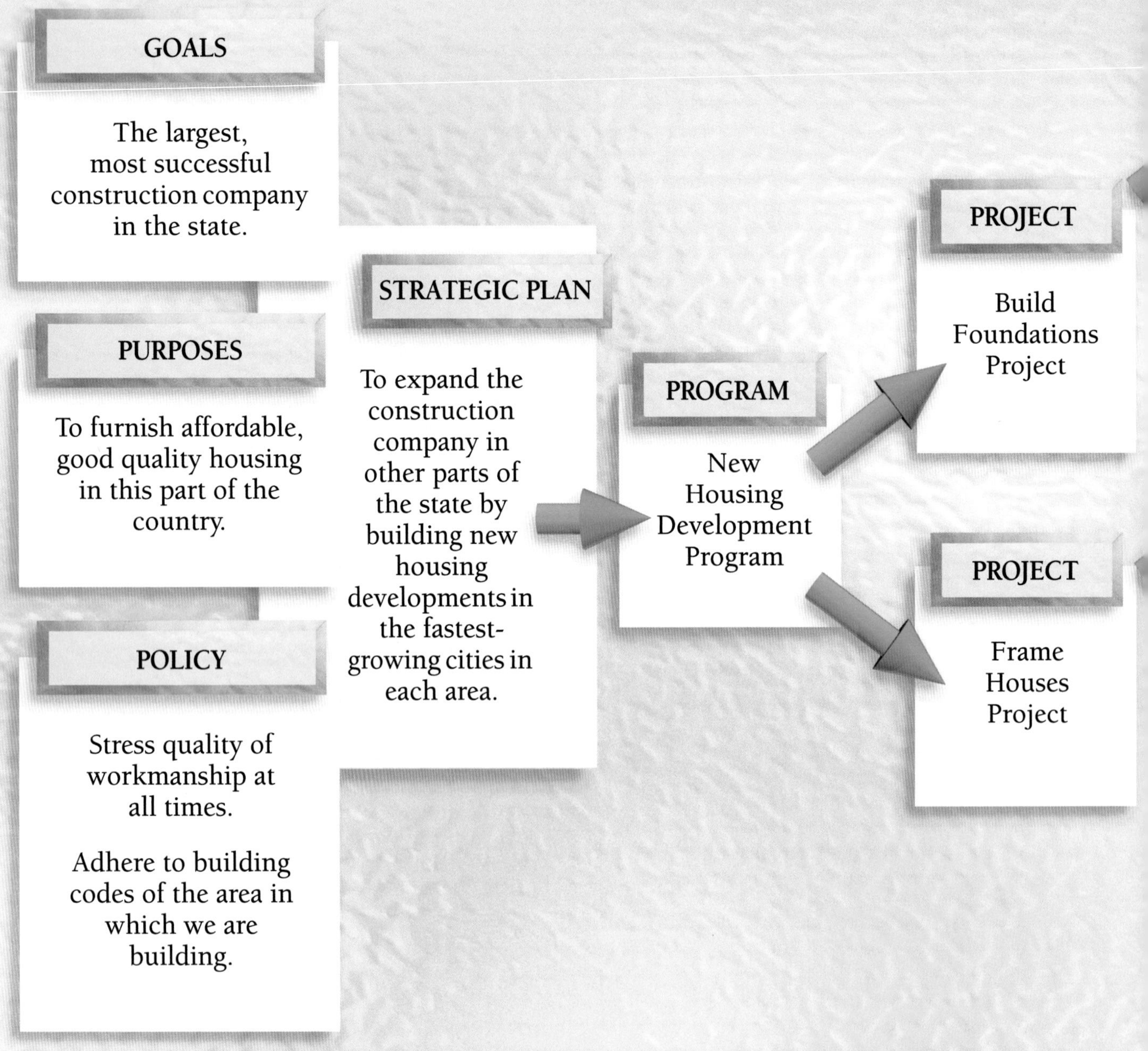

GOALS

The largest, most successful construction company in the state.

PURPOSES

To furnish affordable, good quality housing in this part of the country.

POLICY

Stress quality of workmanship at all times.

Adhere to building codes of the area in which we are building.

STRATEGIC PLAN

To expand the construction company in other parts of the state by building new housing developments in the fastest-growing cities in each area.

PROGRAM

New Housing Development Program

PROJECT

Build Foundations Project

PROJECT

Frame Houses Project

IDEAL SCENE

Houses being constructed on time and within budget.

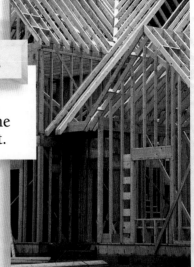

ORDERS

Dig the trench for the south wall of the foundation for lot #27.

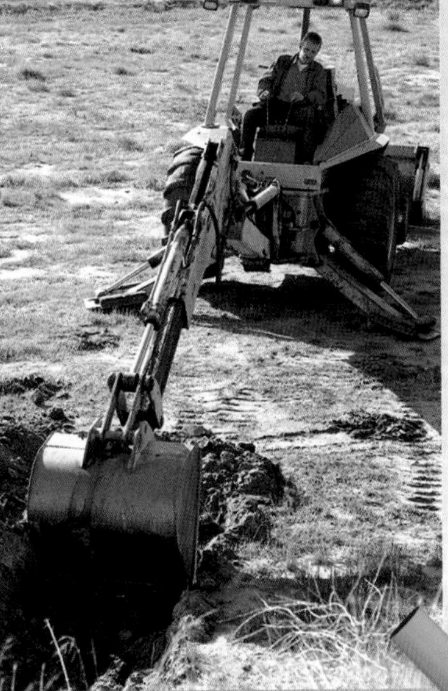

MONDAY BATTLE PLAN

1. Lay out foundations for lots 27–31.
2. Excavate foundations for lots 27–31.
3. Schedule the concrete pour for lots 27–31 for Tuesday.
4. Report target #5 of project complete.

STATISTICS

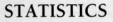

# of Houses Built

ORDERS

Nail the wood supports with 3½" nails.

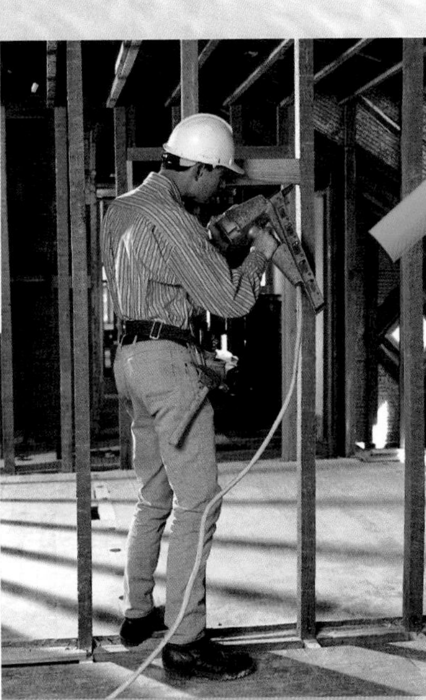

MONDAY BATTLE PLAN

1. Cut all lumber to length for units 18–22.
2. Lay out the walls for units 18–22.
3. Assemble the four main walls for units 18–22.
4. Erect and brace the four main walls for units 18–22.
5. Report target #11 of project as done.

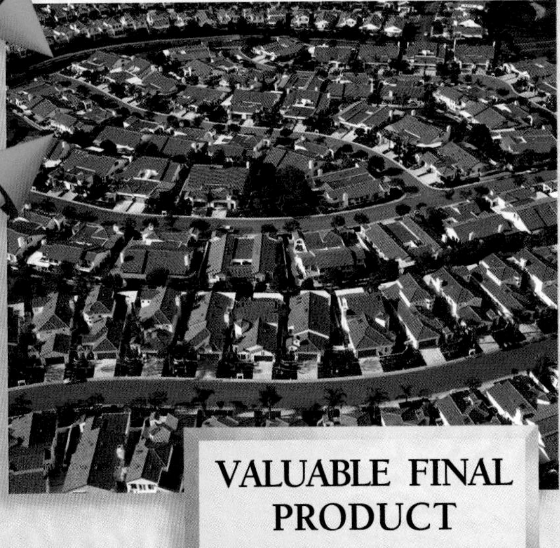

VALUABLE FINAL PRODUCT

MAXIMS OF PROGRAMING

Programing is important enough to pay a lot of attention to. And there is a lot of information about it. And the facts all add up to no matter how many programs you have, each one consists of certain parts. And if you don't assemble those parts and run the program in an orderly fashion, then it just won't spark off. These are some of the principles about programs.

If you don't know these facts of life, here they are:

Maxim One: Any idea, no matter if badly executed, is better than no idea at all.

Maxim Two: A program, to be effective, must be executed.

Maxim Three: A program put into action requires guidance.

Maxim Four: A program running without guidance will fail and is better left undone. If you haven't got the time to guide it, don't do it; put more steam behind existing programs because it will flop.

Maxim Five: Any program requires some finance. Get the finance into sight before you start to fire, or have a very solid guarantee that the program will produce finance before you execute it.

Maxim Six: A program requires attention from somebody. An untended program that is everybody's child will become a juvenile delinquent.

Maxim Seven: The best program is the one that will reach the greatest number of dynamics and will do the greatest good on the greatest number of dynamics. (A dynamic is an urge to survive along a certain course. There are eight dynamics: first, self; second, sex and the family unit; third, groups; fourth, mankind; fifth, life forms; sixth, physical universe; seventh, spirits; and eighth, Supreme Being. These dynamics embrace all the goals of survival an individual has and all the things for which he survives.)

Maxim Eight: Programs must support themselves financially.

Maxim Nine: Programs must *accumulate* interest and bring in other assistance by the virtue of the program interest alone or they will never grow.

Maxim Ten: A program is a bad program if it detracts from programs which are already proving successful or distracts staff people or associates from work they are already doing that is adding up to successful execution of other programs.

Maxim Eleven: Never spend more on a program than the income from one person can repay.

Maxim Twelve: Never permit a new program to inhibit the success of a routine one or injure its income.

Programing requires execution. It requires carry-through. It requires judgment enough to know a good program and carry it on and on and to recognize a bad one and drop it like hot bricks.

Programs extend in time and go overdue to the extent the various types of targets are not set or not pushed home or drop out. They fail only because the various types of targets are not executed or are not kept in.

You can get done almost anything you want to do if types of targets are understood, set with reality, held in or completed.

One can readily accomplish the intended goals either for himself or for his group by adherence to good, steady programing that wins.

This is the way to make planning an actuality, to achieve goals. It is as true for an individual as it is for a large group. All people can benefit from this technology. ■

TEST YOUR UNDERSTANDING

Answer the following questions about targets and goals. Refer back to the chapter to check your answers. If you need to, review the chapter. Going over the materials several times will increase your certainty and help you better apply it.

- ❑ *What is a target?*
- ❑ *What is the difference between a plan and a program?*
- ❑ *When would a conditional target be used?*
- ❑ *What is strategic planning?*
- ❑ *How does purpose relate to strategic planning?*
- ❑ *What is a battle plan?*
- ❑ *How does one use a battle plan to get something done?*
- ❑ *When is a program considered a bad program?*

PRACTICAL EXERCISES

Here are some practical exercises to increase your knowledge and skill in applying the basic data on programs and targets to achieve your goals.

1 Work out and write down a realistic goal you want to achieve in some area of your life, job, etc.

2 Write up an example of strategic planning you would do to accomplish the goal you set in the previous practical exercise.

3 Write down two examples of each of the following target types. Each example is to be one that could be on a program you would write and do.

a. major target

b. primary target

c. vital target

d. operating target

e. conditional target

f. production target

4 Do the program given as Sample Program #1 in this chapter. Actually carry out its steps as directed in the program.

5 Do the program given as Sample Program #2 in this chapter. Actually carry out its steps as directed in the program.

6 Write a program to take a walk. Use the target types you learned in this chapter to do so.

7 Write a program to get ready for the day. Lay out the steps you take to prepare for your day of work, study or whatever. Use the target types you learned in this chapter to do so.

8 Write a program that would be done to accomplish the strategic planning you set down in doing Practical Exercise #2 above. Utilize the materials you read in this chapter and the skills you gained in doing the above practical exercises.

9 Write up a battle plan for the day which will forward the strategic planning and program you have written in exercises 2 and 8 above.

RESULTS FROM APPLICATION

Failure to accomplish one's goals—personal, familial or organizational—has been a heavy burden many people have had to bear. L. Ron Hubbard's discoveries on the subject of target attainment, however, can provide any individual with methods to lift this weight and thus create a more fulfilling life. In fact, those who have studied and applied these tenets have attained success, where such seemed difficult or impossible to reach before. Below you will find just a few tributes to the workability of Mr. Hubbard's developments in this field.

A young woman from Italy got a job that consisted of carrying out long-term projects. She said about it:

"I used to not be able to confront doing big jobs that would take many weeks to get done and required a lot of steps to get the overall job done. Then I found out about target types and how to use them. Now, when I have a big project in front of me, I sit down and I break it down into targets and as I get each of them done I know I am getting closer and closer to achieving the complete product. Every target done is a win."

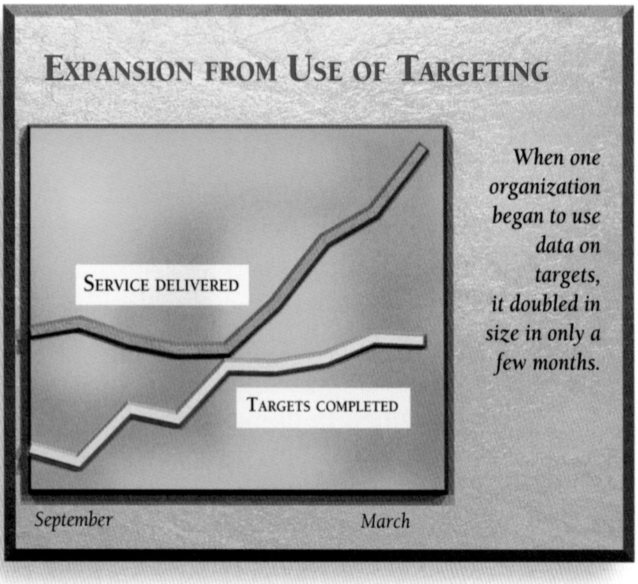

EXPANSION FROM USE OF TARGETING

SERVICE DELIVERED

TARGETS COMPLETED

September

March

When one organization began to use data on targets, it doubled in size in only a few months.

Employed as Communications Officer in a large US corporation, a man was made responsible for the international communication lines. When first starting the job, he found a situation where many units in his charge had antiquated communication systems or even none at all. This is how he went about handling it:

"My knowledge of this area was almost nonexistent and the financial budget was limited. This involved, altogether, fifty units that had to be handled.

"From this I worked out the exact plan for the fifty units and how to get all these units equipped with proper, fast-running communications systems. I then wrote programs using Mr. Hubbard's technology on targets and with this series of programs, I was able to procure, install and make these systems functional. In addition I wrote a program for the nine main areas to give them directions for better operation in their respective areas.

"Pushing the targets through to completion, with dogged persistence, I accomplished what had not been done before and every unit ended up with a computerized fast-running communications system. The best ever. It would have been almost impossible to get this done in the time it was done without the use of targeting technology."

One lady, whose family and many of her friends were in another state, was still able to continue her relationships and help them by use of targets and goals:

"I set goals last year to accomplish certain things with my family. I decided what I wanted to do to help my parents and my friends. I set the major targets that we wanted to accomplish, then we set the other different types of targets and I went over this with them. We agreed we would do these things, small things or large, to help us get closer together.

"Now my son can read and is very proud of this. My husband has completed things in his life he has long planned to do and is doing much better as a result. My family is moving closer to where I live and we have had time together and helped each other despite the distance in the meanwhile. My friends are each doing better and I have helped them through support and other small things to really push those targets through that they had set for themselves. These small things add to and make my life full and keep me in balance.

"Sure, I target for production on the job and for business projects. But being able to help someone else to complete targets in their lives gives me a great feeling of knowing I helped. Knowing this technology, I can get things done on a long-distance line and accomplish targets that bring my family closer together."

An executive for personnel in the Los Angeles area had a major task to perform in order to build up a second unit for a film studio. Here is how she handled this:

"I was given a specific deadline to hire a large number of staff and professionals in a very short time period.

"At first, I didn't really know how to go about getting this done within the time frame I had, or if I could get it done at all. I knew it was important to complete it within the amount of time I had. In fact, four people prior to me had attempted to achieve the same deadline that I had just been given.

"I worked with other employees; I tried to get them to achieve this over and over but I wasn't getting anywhere. Finally, I realized that there must be some technology that I wasn't applying.

"I looked to L. Ron Hubbard's targeting technology.

"I then really figured out what exactly I had to do to get the product. I named who I wanted to hire and I wrote a program with the exact targets that I had to do in order to get all of these people actually arrived to work. I then met with every person, giving each one an exact project to execute so all of them would arrive within the required time.

"This worked. The whole team knew exactly what part of the product they were responsible for, how much time they had to get their part of the product produced and I got each step to hire each person done one by one and this made it possible for us to attain our goal!

"We achieved our major target! We got the whole program done within the needed amount of time. I couldn't have

done this without knowing and applying this technology."

An executive in a Southern California construction project found Mr. Hubbard's technology on programs and targets of immense value in accomplishing his intended goals:

"We had to get new buildings constructed as they were badly needed to dramatically improve the facilities of our organization. Our construction plans required approval by a specific time to ensure our success. L. Ron Hubbard's discoveries on target types and programs were used to isolate the exact actions that had to be accomplished and in what sequence. What I personally found of tremendous help was that Mr. Hubbard discovered and differentiated the different types of targets. This technology allows one to go from wherever he is to where he wants to go by properly using each type of target.

"We had to obtain agreement for the construction plan from the local community. Our program had targets to find out what the community leaders wanted so we could provide this and obtain the authorizations we needed. Had we not done this, we would not have been able to build what we wanted. But because we were applying Mr. Hubbard's technology on programs and targets, we easily handled what was required and obtained full approval. As a result, everyone won.

"Anyone trying to get anything done in this world is going to run aground unless he knows and uses Mr. Hubbard's technology on target types and programs. It is based on natural laws. It is *how one gets something accomplished. It will help spot and handle the potential pitfalls before one is stopped by them. It points out the things that, if not maintained throughout executing the construction plan, would snarl up the whole plan.*

"Anything can be done using this tech. Literally anything!"

SUGGESTIONS FOR FURTHER STUDY

The axioms and laws of life and the universe as contained in Scientology apply not only to the survival of the individual, but also to the survival of groups and the attainment of group purposes and goals. The following materials are recommended for further study by anyone who is interested in getting things done and achieving one's objectives.

The Problems of Work

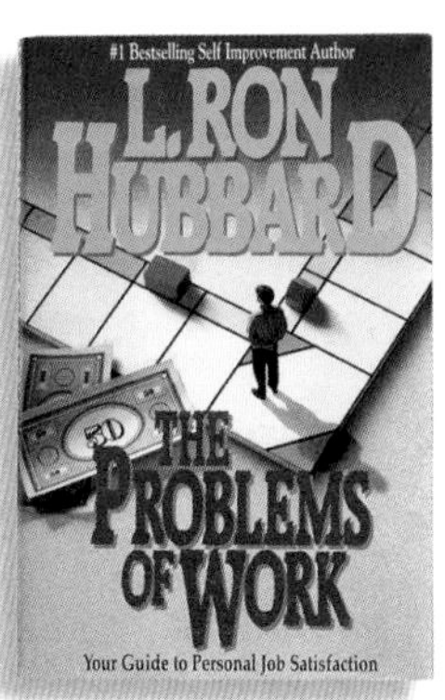

Mr. Hubbard analyzes the subject of work itself and provides practical data to help one succeed at his job and make his working hours calmer, less confusing and more enjoyable. The book presents the application of Scientology principles to the world of work and gives solutions to exhaustion from work, how to speed recovery from injuries sustained on the job, how to handle confusions and many other key data.

How to Make Work Easier

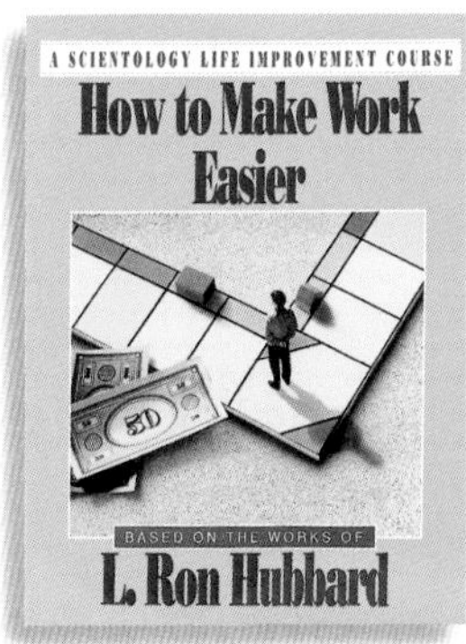

Based on the text of *The Problems of Work,* this Scientology Life Improvement Course provides illustrations, demonstrations and practical exercises to give the student a thorough working knowledge of the wide range of data the book contains, and certainty in its application. (Delivered in Scientology organizations.)

Management Series Volumes

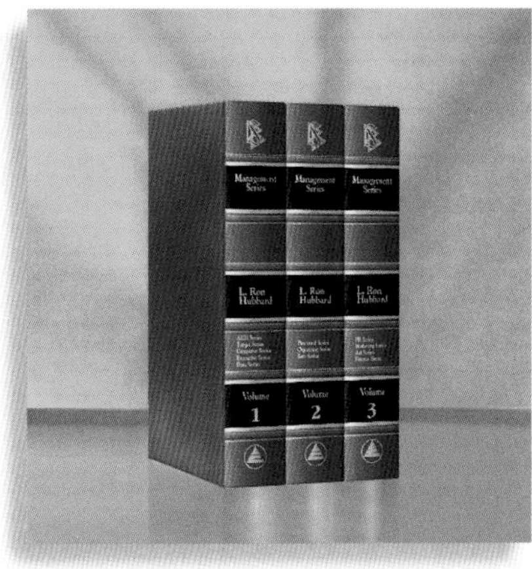

Mr. Hubbard developed group technology from the fundamental principles of the Scientology philosophy on the mind, life and the human spirit. The forces inherent in life forms can succeed only when channeled and aligned with one another. Using the basics of Scientology this can be accomplished, with the result of increased awareness and greater survival for both the individual and the group. A three-volume set, the *Management Series Volumes* contain vital data on such topics as how to help group members learn their jobs better, how to set objectives for a group, ways to attain targets and goals, how to best organize different types of projects and activities, and many more.

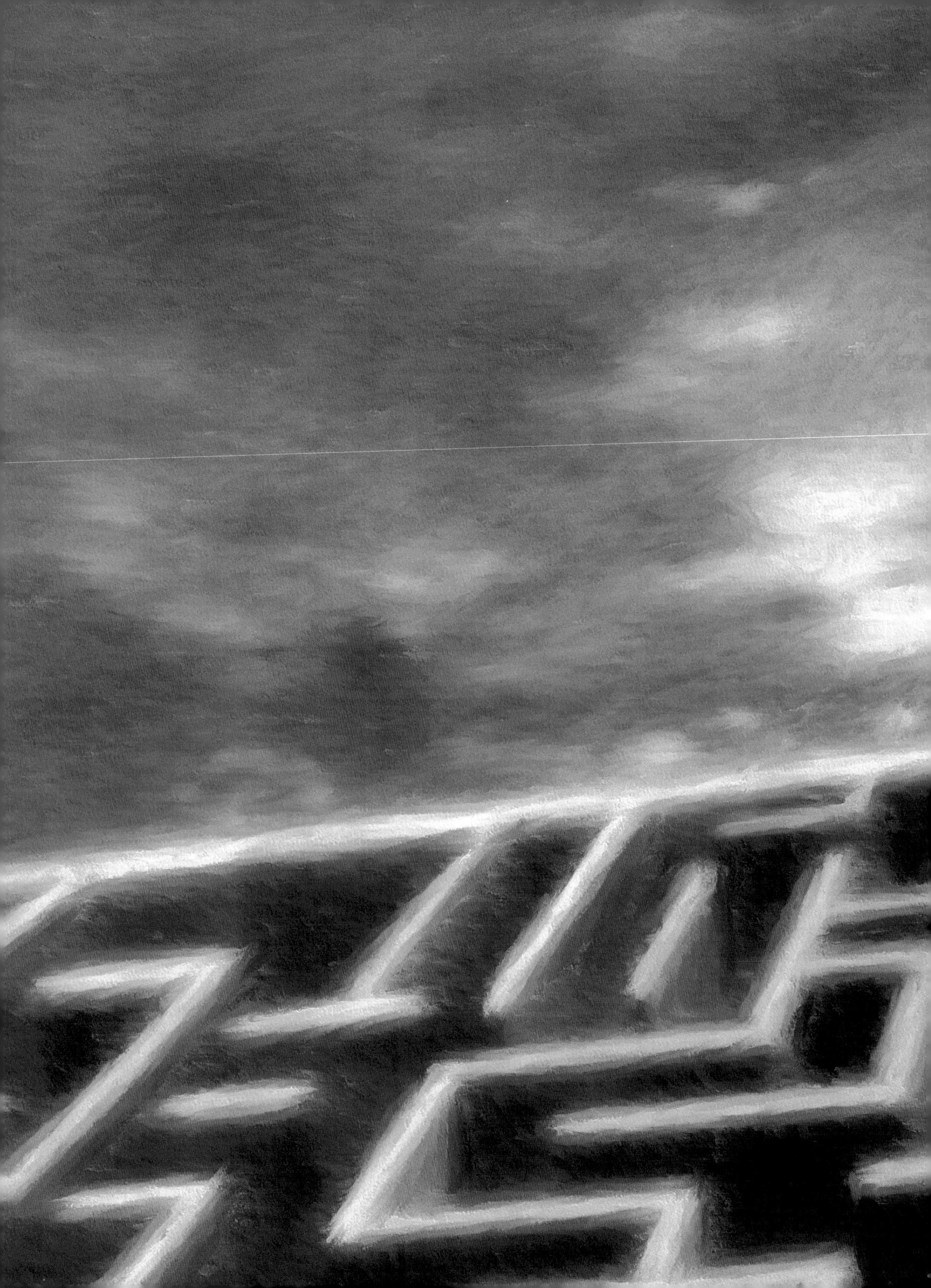

Chapter 18

INVESTIGATIONS

Many people go through life in a rather hit-or-miss fashion, casting about for ideas to explain why their projects improve or decline, why they are successful or why they are not. Guessing and "hunches," however, are not very reliable. And without the knowledge of how to actually investigate situations, good or bad, and get the true facts, a person is set adrift in a sea of unevaluated data.

Accurate investigation is, in fact, a rare commodity. Man's tendency in matters he doesn't understand is to accept the first proffered explanation, no matter how faulty. Thus investigatory technology had not actually been practiced or refined. However, L. Ron Hubbard made a breakthrough in the subject of logic and reasoning which led to his development of the first truly effective way to search for and consistently find the actual causes for things.

Knowing how to investigate gives one the power to navigate through the random facts and opinions and emerge with the **real** *reasons behind success or failure in any aspect of life. By really finding out why things are the way they are, one is therefore able to remedy and improve a situation—any situation. This is an invaluable technology for people in all walks of life.*

INVESTIGATION AND ITS USE

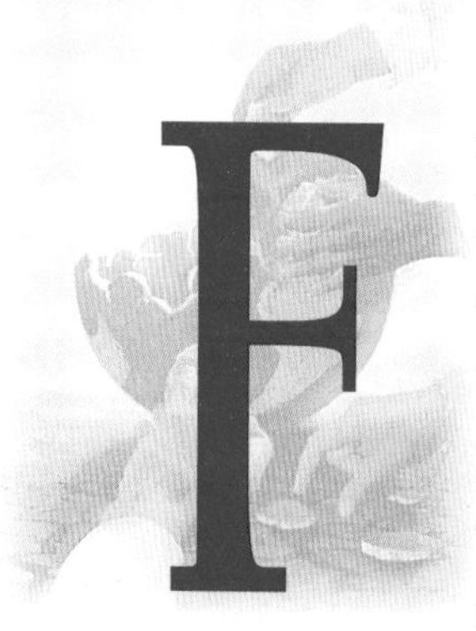

From day to day and week to week, one can face many less-than-desirable circumstances in his life. Somehow one manages to slog through these situations, convinced there is not much he can do to improve his lot. Perhaps a project planned for months at work doesn't come off with the expected success; productivity in the office has declined sharply during the past quarter; or the addition to one's house takes longer than first envisioned. Such situations are common enough occurrences for many of us.

But these need not be the usual state of affairs. People can live a happy existence and accomplish their goals in any area of life—individually, with the family, the job and so on. The aims an individual once visualized for himself can be accomplished.

If such goals are not being attained or if one is in a situation that has deteriorated or worsened, there is a valid, locatable cause for this. This concept is one people often do not realize—things are actually *caused.* They don't just happen. There are reasons behind every situation—reasons that people themselves can control.

Without knowing this, man often relies upon "fate," superstition, fortunetelling or astrology to determine his destiny or future. Many just hope vainly that nothing else will go wrong or they deceive themselves with the belief that life is ordinarily a struggle.

For example, a farmer with a very poor crop one year has no credible explanation for it. He has no concept that he himself caused this condition. However, looking into it, one would find that he had earlier failed to keep seed grain secure for the spring planting, and thus it fell prey to insects. Not knowing this, he might come up with all sorts of odd "reasons" or just blame it on bad luck.

In a factory with low production, management could be shifting personnel, hiring new workers, etc., in an attempt to raise productivity before the organization goes under. But executives might not have the skills needed to really examine the company's own operations to find the cause of the situation. Upon inspection, one could discover that the suppliers of its raw materials refused to deliver because the company's accounting office wasn't paying the bills.

To look into, handle and improve any such situation in any area of life requires skill in *investigation*—the ability to think logically and get to the bottom of things.

Investigation is the careful discovery and sorting of facts. In investigating, one is searching out and examining the particulars of something in an attempt to learn the facts, especially in an attempt to find a cause.

A proper investigation gets to the bottom of the state of affairs facing one. For instance, in any organization, one could observe that its production was down. This is a nonoptimum situation which should be investigated and the cause located. Investigations can also be utilized in an individual's personal life to improve conditions.

In doing an investigation, you are asking the question, "What don't I understand?" with regard to the existing conditions. You'll find that two facts don't agree—they contradict themselves and can't be understood. So you try to rationalize these two facts: you question these two facts and you will get another point you don't understand. And when you try to get *this* point understood, you will now find another fact that you don't understand. And someplace along the way, you will find the reason for the circumstances you are investigating.

Any investigation should proceed along these lines. Sometimes many questions have to be asked, sometimes it only takes a "What's that noise?" to lead one to the source of a difficulty. Here is an example of an investigation done on a rapid, emergency basis: An engineer is on duty in a ship's engine room. He has normal but experienced perception: is observing his area. Hears a hiss that shouldn't be—something contradictory to the expected conditions in an engine room. Scans the area and sees nothing out of order but a small white cloud. Combines sight and hearing. Moves forward to get a better look. Sees valve has broken. Shuts off steam line.

In a nutshell, (a) one finds an imperfect functioning of some portion of an organization or whatever he is investigating and then (b) finds something that one doesn't understand about it and then (c) questions the individuals in that portion connected with the imperfect functioning or looks into the area to get more data.

Following this sequence isolates the cause of the trouble which can then be handled so the area properly operates again. In an organization, one can apply just these three steps over and over again, and it will usually be quite enough to keep it running quite smoothly.

Statistics play a role in investigations. A statistic shows the production of an activity, area or organization, as compared to an earlier moment in time. It reflects whether or not the area is achieving its purpose—if statistics are up, it is more closely accomplishing what is intended for the area. In doing an investigation, one looks for *down* statistics. These aren't understandable, of course, so one questions the people concerned. In their answers there will be something that doesn't make sense at all to the person doing the investigation—for example, "We can't pay the bills because Josie has been doing a course." The investigator is only looking for something he himself can't reconcile. So he questions the person who gave this data *and* Josie. Sooner or later the real reason shows up.

As one is going down the trail of things he can't understand, one of two things will happen. Either it is a dead end and it doesn't go any further, at which time he returns to the main line of the investigation, or it produces further material. And if it produces further material, one will find more things he can't understand.

The trick of this procedure is to find a piece of string sticking out—something one can't understand and, by questioning, pull on it. A small cat

In encountering two facts that contradict, one questions on these two facts and gets another point he doesn't understand. He continues on this path of things he doesn't get until the real reason is located.

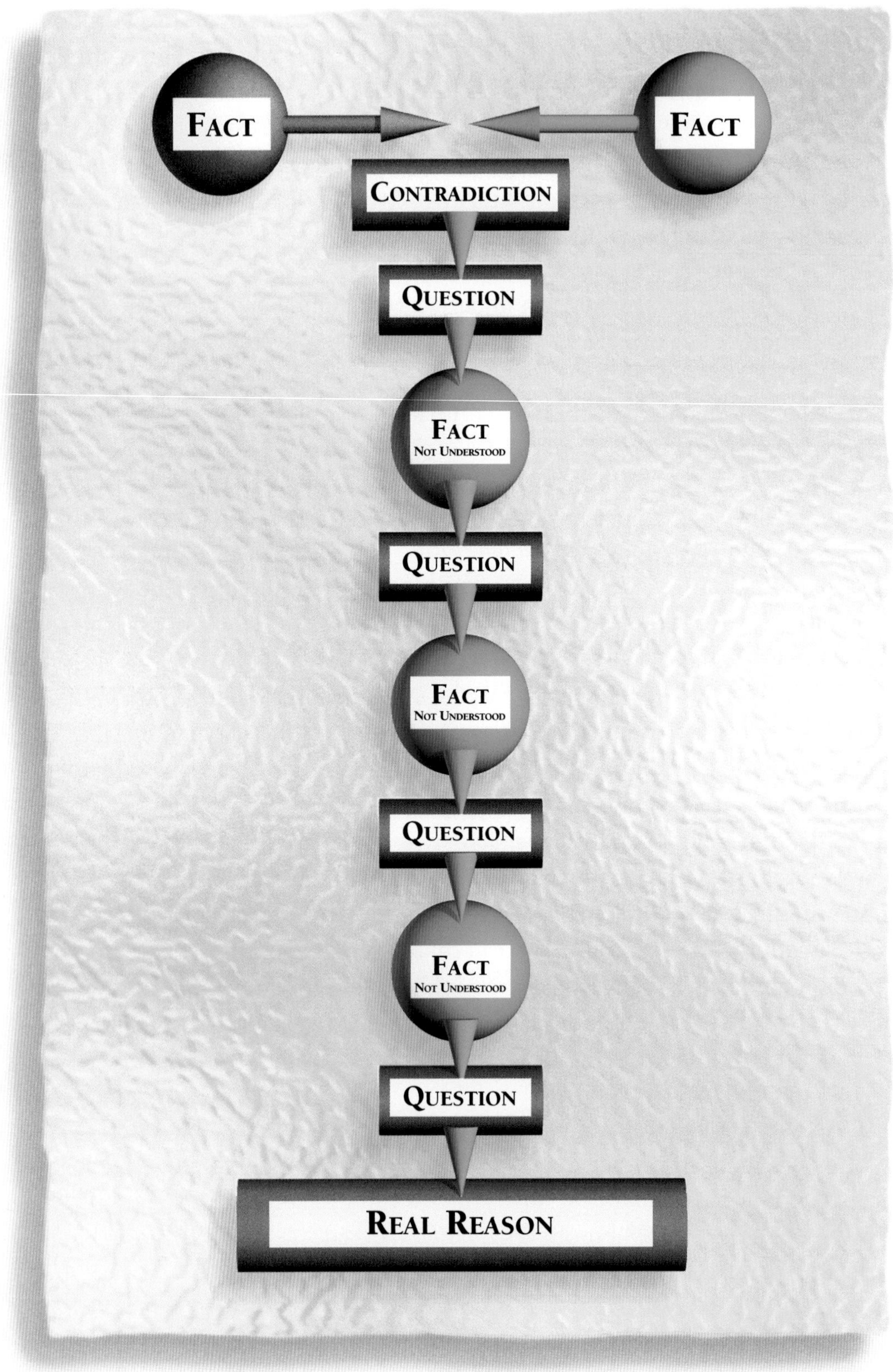

shows up. Pull on the string by asking more questions. A baby gorilla shows up. Pull some more. A tiger appears. Pull again and wow! You've got a General Sherman tank!

It *isn't* reasonable for people to be lazy or stupid. At the bottom you find the *real* cause of no action in a portion of an organization or continuous upset.

When you have your "General Sherman tank," you can take action.

There's always a *reason* behind a bad statistic. Question those involved until you *have the real reason* in view. It will never be "Agnes isn't bright." It is more likely, Agnes was hired as a typist but never knew how to type. Or the executive over the area simply never comes to work.

The real explanation of a down statistic is always a very easily understood thing. If you question enough, you'll get the real explanation and then you can act.

This technique of investigation, while elementary, is highly effective. It can be applied when faced with simple or complex situations to get to the bottom of them, and therefore enables one to resolve them and improve conditions in life.

Investigatory skills improve with practice. They can be sharpened and made more effective so that one is able to instantly spot something he doesn't understand. This ability is not innate in people but can be easily acquired. To make investigations even more rapid and effective, one should be able to understand and apply the principles of logic—a subject that until now has not only been misunderstood but has been made unnecessarily complex.

Logic

The subject of logic has been under discussion for at least three thousand years without any clean breakthrough of real use to those who work with data.

"Logic" means the subject of reasoning. Some in ages past have sought to label it a science. But that can be discarded as pretense and pompousness.

If there were such a "science," men would be able to think. And they can't.

The term itself is utterly forbidding. If you were to read a text on logic, you would go quite mad trying to figure it out, much less learn how to think.

Yet logic or the ability to reason is vital to an organizer or administrator. If he cannot think clearly, he will not be able to reach the conclusions vital to make correct decisions.

Many agencies, governments, societies, groups capitalize upon this lack of logic and have for a very long time. A population that is unable to think or reason can be manipulated easily by falsehoods and wretched causes.

Thus logic has not been a supported subject, rather the opposite.

Even Western schools have sought to convince students they should study geometry as "that is the way they think." And of course it isn't.

The administrator, the manager, the artisan and the clerk each have a considerable use for logic. If they cannot reason, they make costly and time-consuming errors and can send the entire organization into chaos and oblivion.

Their stuff in trade are data and situations. Unless they can observe and think their way through, they can reach wrong conclusions and take incorrect actions.

Modern man thinks mathematics can serve him for logic and most of his situations go utterly adrift because of this touching and misplaced confidence. The complexity of human problems and the vast number of factors involved make mathematics utterly inadequate.

Computers are at best only crutches to the mind. Yet the chromium-plated civilization today has a childish faith in them. It depends on who asks the questions and who reads the computer's answers whether they are of any use or not. And even then their answers are often madhouse silly.

Computers can't *think* because the rules of live logic aren't fully known to man and computer builders. One false datum fed into a computer gives one a completely wrong answer.

If people on management and work lines do not know logic, an organization can go adrift and require a fabulous amount of genius to hold it together and keep it running.

Whole civilizations vanish because of lack of logic in its rulers, leaders and people.

So this is a very important subject.

Unlocking Logic

Scientology contains a way to unlock logic. This is a breakthrough which is no small win. If by it a formidable and almost impossible subject can be reduced to simplicity, then correct answers to situations can be far more frequent and an organization or a civilization far more effective.

The breakthrough is a simple one:

BY ESTABLISHING THE WAYS IN WHICH THINGS BECOME ILLOGICAL, ONE CAN THEN ESTABLISH WHAT IS LOGIC.

In other words, if one has a grasp of what makes things illogical or irrational (or crazy, if you please) it is then possible to conceive of what makes things logical.

Illogics

There are specific ways for a relay of information or a situation to become illogical. These are the things which cause one to have an incorrect idea of a situation. Each different way is called an *outpoint,* which is any one datum that is offered as true that is in fact found to be illogical. Each one of these is described below.

Omitted Data

An omitted anything is an outpoint.

This can be an omitted person, terminal (person who sends, receives and relays communication), object, energy, space, time, form, sequence or even an omitted scene. Anything that *can* be omitted that *should* be there is an outpoint.

This is easily the most overlooked outpoint as it isn't there to directly attract attention.

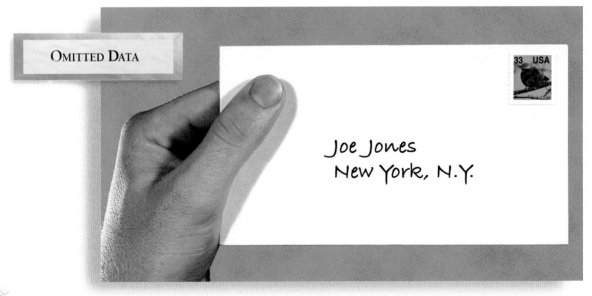

Altered Sequence

Any things, events, objects, sizes, in a wrong sequence is an outpoint.

The number series 3, 7, 1, 2, 4, 6, 5 is an altered sequence, or an incorrect sequence.

Doing step two of a sequence of actions before doing step one can be counted on to tangle any sequence of actions.

The basic outness is no sequence at all. (An *outness* is a condition or state of something being incorrect, wrong or missing.) This leads into FIXED IDEAS. It also shows up in what is called disassociation, an insanity. Things connected to or similar to each other are not seen as consecutive. Such people also jump about subjectwise without relation to an obvious sequence. Disassociation is the extreme case where things that are related are not seen to be and things that have no relation are conceived to have.

"Sequence" means linear (in a line) travel either through space or time or both.

A sequence that should be one and isn't is an outpoint.

A "sequence" that isn't but is thought to be one is an outpoint.

A cart-before-the-horse out of sequence is an outpoint.

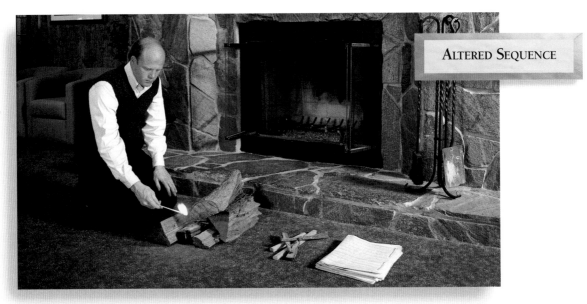
ALTERED SEQUENCE

One's hardest task sometimes is indicating an inevitable sequence into the future that is invisible to another. This is a consequence. "If you saw off the limb you are sitting on you will of course fall." Police try to bring this home often to people who have no concept of sequence; so the threat of punishment works well on well-behaved citizens and not at all on criminals since they often are criminals because they can't think in sequence—they are simply fixated. "If you kill a man you will be hanged," is an indicated sequence. A murderer fixated on revenge cannot think in sequence. One has to think in sequences to have correct sequences.

Therefore, it is far more common than one would at first imagine to see altered sequences since persons who do not think in sequence do not see altered sequences in their own actions or areas.

Visualizing sequences and drills in shifting attention can clean this up and restore it as a faculty.

Motion pictures and TV were spotted by a writer as fixating attention and not permitting it to travel. Where one had TV-raised children, it would follow, one possibly would have people with a tendency to altered sequences or no sequences at all.

Dropped Time

Time that should be noted and isn't would be an outpoint of "dropped time." It is a special case of an omitted datum.

Dropped time has a peculiarly ferocious effect that adds up to utter lunacy.

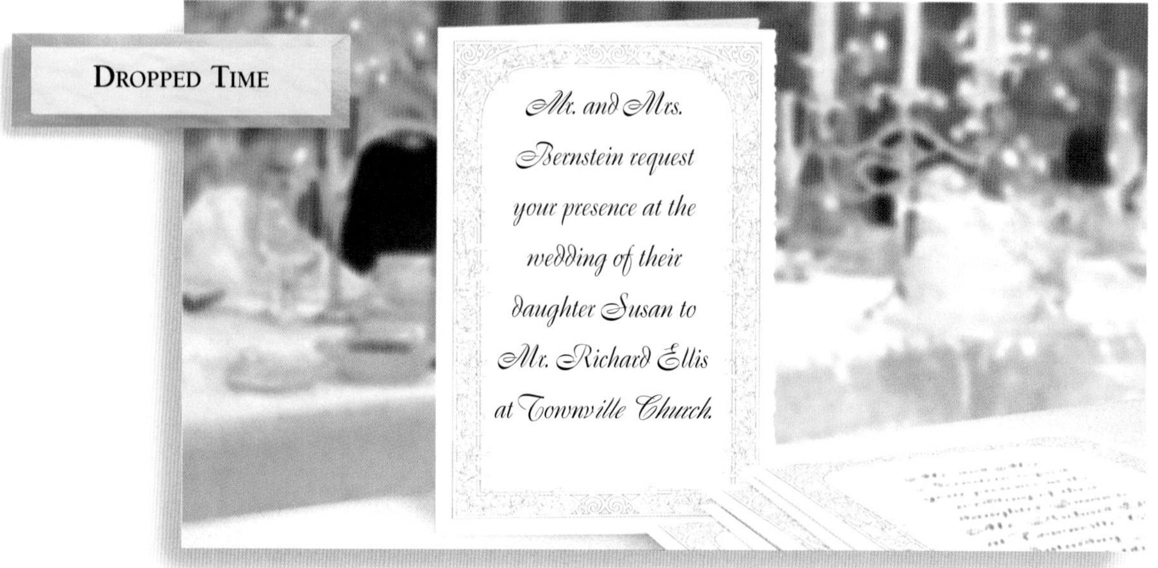
Dropped Time
Mr. and Mrs.
Bernstein request
your presence at the
wedding of their
daughter Susan to
Mr. Richard Ellis
at Townville Church.

A news bulletin from 1814 and one from 1922 read consecutively without time assigned produces otherwise undetectable madness.

A summary report of a situation containing events strung over half a year without saying so can provoke a reaction not in keeping with the current scene.

In madmen the present is the dropped time, leaving them in the haunted past. Just telling a group of madmen to "come up to present time" will produce a few miraculous "cures." And getting the date of an ache or pain will often cause it to vanish.

Time aberrations (illogicalities) are so strong that dropped time well qualifies as an outpoint.

Falsehood

When you hear two facts that are contrary, one is a falsehood or both are.

Propaganda and other activities specialize in falsehoods and provoke great disturbance.

Willful or unintentional, a falsehood is an outpoint. It may be a mistake or a calculated or defensive falsehood and it is still an outpoint.

A false anything qualifies for this outpoint. A false being, terminal, act, intention, anything that seeks to be what it isn't is a falsehood and an outpoint.

Fiction that does not pretend to be anything else is of course not a falsehood.

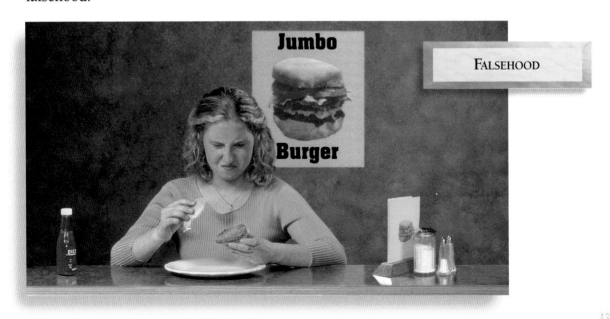

FALSEHOOD

So the falsehood means "other than it appears" or "other than represented."

One does not have to concern oneself to define philosophic truth or reality to see that something stated or modeled to be one thing is in actual fact something else and therefore an outpoint.

Altered Importance

An importance shifted from its actual relative importance, up or down, is an outpoint.

Something can be assigned an importance greater than it has.

Something can be assigned an importance less than it has.

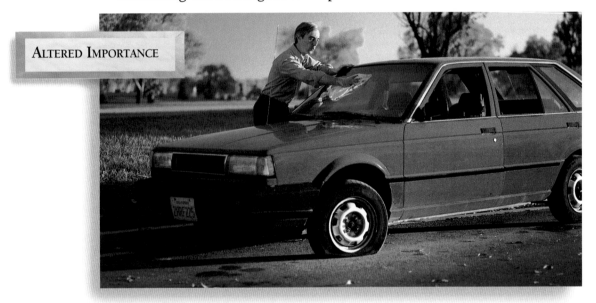
ALTERED IMPORTANCE

A number of things of different importances can be assigned a monotone of importance.

These are all outpoints, three versions of the same thing.

All importances are relative to their actuality.

Wrong Target

A mistaken objective wherein one believes he is or should be reaching toward A and finds he is or should be reaching toward B is an outpoint.

This is commonly mistaken identity. It is also mistaken purposes or goals.

"If we tear down X we will be okay" often results in disclosure that it should have been Y.

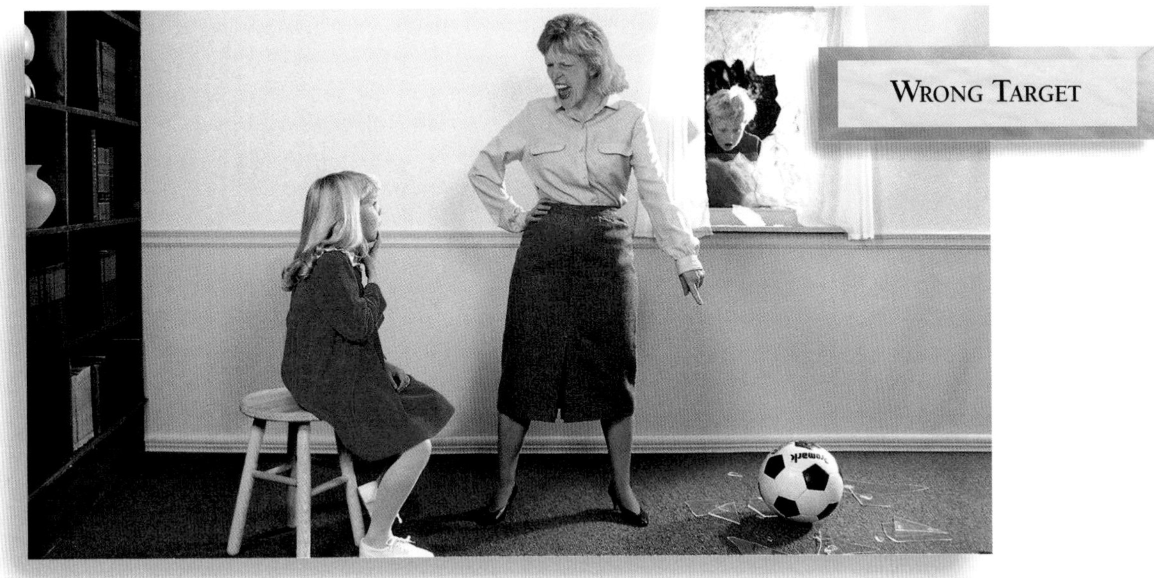

Killing the king to be free from taxation leaves the tax collector alive for the next regime.

Injustice is usually a wrong target outpoint.

Arrest the drug consumer, award the drug company would be an example.

Military tactics and strategy are almost always an effort to coax the selection of a wrong target by the enemy.

And most dislikes and spontaneous hates in human relations are based on mistaken associations of Bill for Pete.

A large sum of aberration is based on wrong targets, wrong sources, wrong causes.

Incorrectly tell a patient he has ulcers when he hasn't and he's hung with an outpoint which impedes recovery.

The industry spent on wrong objectives would light the world for a millennium.

Wrong Source

"Wrong source" is the other side of the coin of wrong target.

Information taken from wrong source, orders taken from the wrong source, gifts or materiel (supplies) taken from wrong source all add up to eventual confusion and possible trouble.

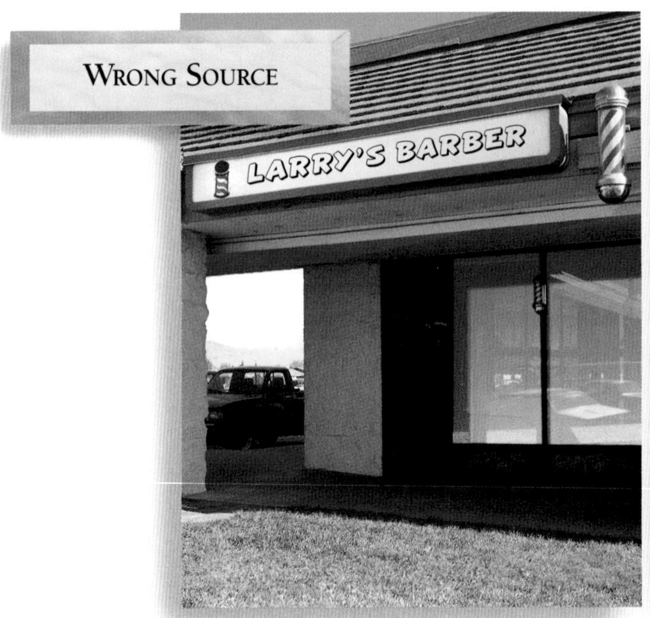
WRONG SOURCE
LARRY'S BARBER

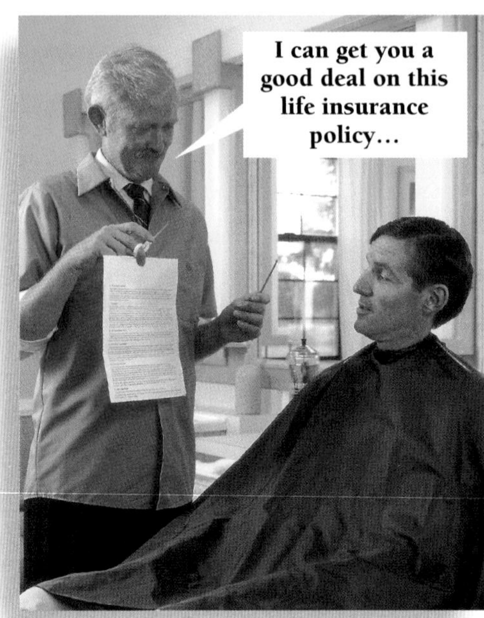
I can get you a good deal on this life insurance policy...

Unwittingly receiving from a wrong source can be very embarrassing or confusing, so much so that it is a favorite intelligence trick. Department D in East Germany, the Department of Disinformation, had very intricate methods of planting false information and disguising its source.

Technology can come from wrong source. For instance, Leipzig University's school of psychology and psychiatry opened the door to death camps in Hitler's Germany. Using drugs, these men apparently gave Hitler to the world as their puppet. At the end of World War II these extremists formed the "World Federation of Mental Health," which enlisted the American Psychiatric Association and the American Medical Association and established "National Associations for Mental Health" over the world. These became the sole advisors to the US government on "mental health, education and welfare" and the appointers of all health ministers through the civilized world. This source is so wrong that it is destroying man, having already destroyed scores of millions.

Not only taking data from wrong source but officialdom from it can therefore be sufficiently aberrated as to result in planetary insanity.

In a lesser level, taking a report from a known bad hat (corrupt or worthless person) and acting upon it is the *usual* reason for errors made in management.

Contrary Facts

When two statements are made on one subject which are contrary to each other, we have "contrary facts."

This illogic could be classified as a falsehood, since one of them must be false.

But in investigatory procedure one cannot offhand distinguish which is the false fact. Thus it becomes a special outpoint.

"The company made an above average income that week" and "They couldn't pay the employees" occurring in the same time period gives us one or both as false. We may not know which is true but we do know they are contrary and can so label it.

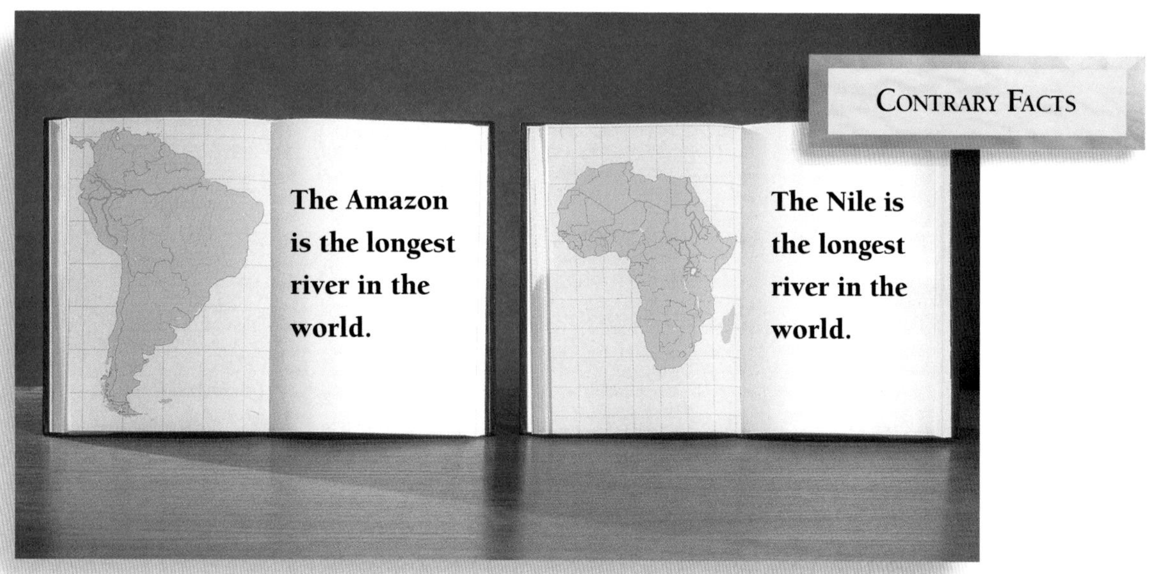

CONTRARY FACTS
The Amazon is the longest river in the world.
The Nile is the longest river in the world.

In interrogation this point is so important that anyone giving two contrary facts becomes a prime suspect for further investigation. "I am a Swiss citizen" as a statement from someone who has had a German passport found in his baggage would be an example.

When two "facts" are contrary or contradictory, we may not know which is true but we do know they can't both be true.

Issued by the same organization, even from two different people in that organization, two contradictory "facts" qualifies as an outpoint.

Added Time

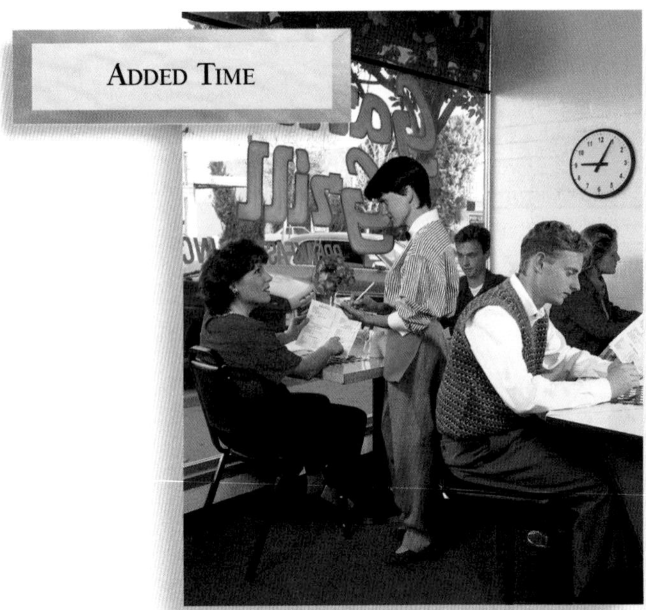

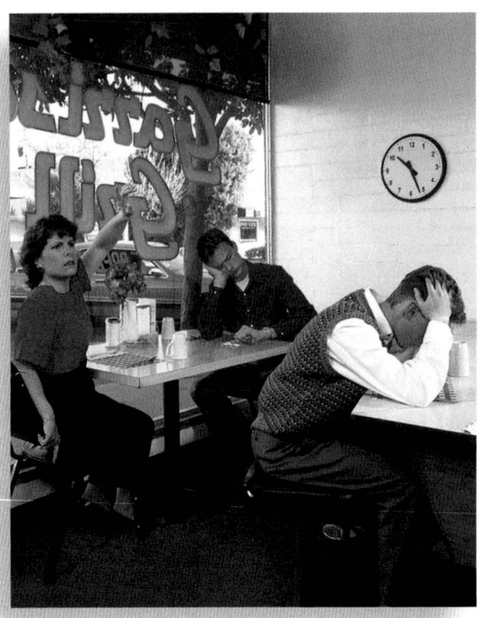

Added Time

In this outpoint we have the reverse of dropped time. In added time we have, as the most common example, something taking longer than it possibly could. To this degree it is a version of conflicting data—for example, something takes three weeks to do but it is reported as taking six months. But added time must be called to attention as an outpoint in its own right for there is a tendency to be "reasonable" about it and not see that it *is* an outpoint in itself.

In its most severe sense, added time becomes a very serious outpoint when, for example, two or more events occur at the same moment involving, let us say, the same person who could not have experienced both. Time had to be *added* to the physical universe for the data to be true. Like this: "I left for Saigon at midnight on April 21, 1962, by ship from San Francisco." "I took over my duties at Saigon on April 30, 1962." Here we have to add time to the physical universe for both events to occur as a ship would take two or three weeks to get from San Francisco to "Saigon."

Another instance, a true occurrence and better example of added time, happened when a checklist of actions it would take a month to complete was sent to a junior executive and compliance was received in full in the next return mail. The checklist was in her hands only one day! She would have had to add twenty-nine days to the physical universe for the compliance report to be true. This was also dropped time on her part.

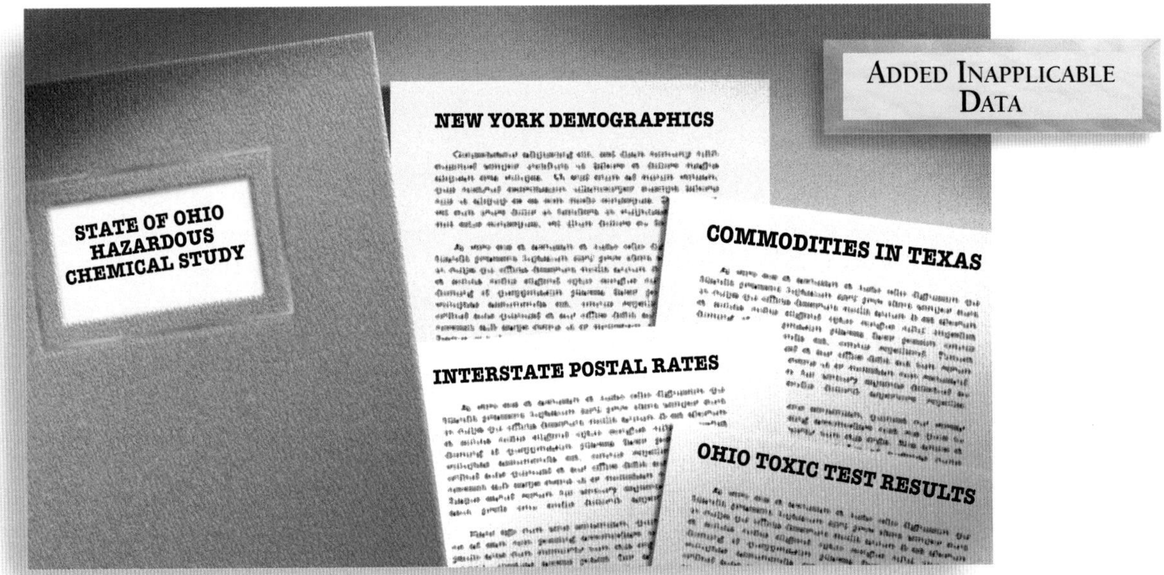

Added Inapplicable Data

Just plain added data does not necessarily constitute an outpoint. It may be someone being thorough. But when the data is in no way applicable to the scene or situation and is added, it is a definite outpoint.

Often added data is put there to cover up neglect of duty or mask a real situation. It certainly means the person is obscuring something.

Usually added data also contains other types of outpoints like wrong target or added time.

In using this outpoint be very sure you also understand the word *inapplicable* and see that it is only an outpoint if the data itself does not apply to the subject at hand.

Incorrectly Included Datum

There is an outpoint called *incorrectly included datum,* which is a companion to the omitted datum as an outpoint.

This most commonly occurs when, in the mind, the scene itself is missing and the first thing needed to classify data (scene) is not there.

An example is camera storage by someone who has no idea of *types* of cameras. Instead of classifying all the needful bits of a certain camera in one box, one inevitably gets the lens hoods of *all* cameras jumbled into one box marked

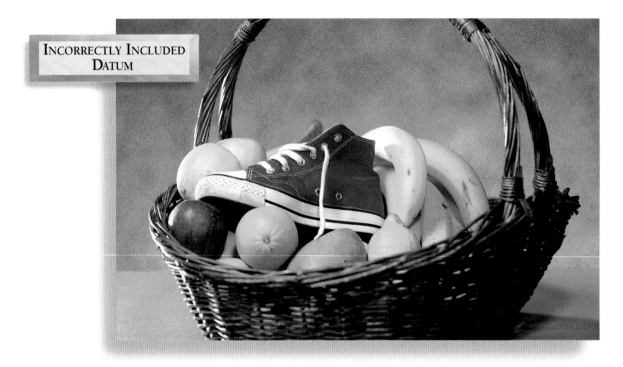
Incorrectly Included Datum

"lens hoods." To assemble or use the camera one spends hours trying to find its parts in boxes neatly labeled "camera backs," "lenses," "tripods," etc.

Here, when the scene of what a set-up camera looks like and operates like, is missing, one gets a closer identification of data than exists. Lens hoods are lens hoods. Tripods are tripods. Thus a wrong system of classification occurs out of scene ignorance.

A traveler unable to distinguish one uniform from another "solves" it by classifying all uniforms as "porters." Hands his bag to an arrogant police captain and that's how he spent his vacation, in jail.

Lack of the scene brings about too tight an identification of one thing with another.

A newly called-up army lieutenant passes right on by an enemy spy dressed as one of his own soldiers. An experienced sergeant right behind him claps the spy in jail accurately because "he wasn't wearing 'is 'at the way we do in our regiment!"

Times change data classification. In 1920 anyone with a camera near a seaport was a spy. In 1960 anyone not carrying a camera couldn't be a tourist so was watched!

So the scene for one cultural period is not the scene for another.

There are three other types of outpoints which should be known for use in an investigation. These are as follows:

ASSUMED "IDENTITIES"
ARE NOT IDENTICAL

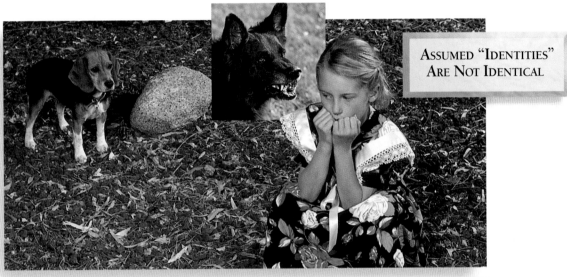

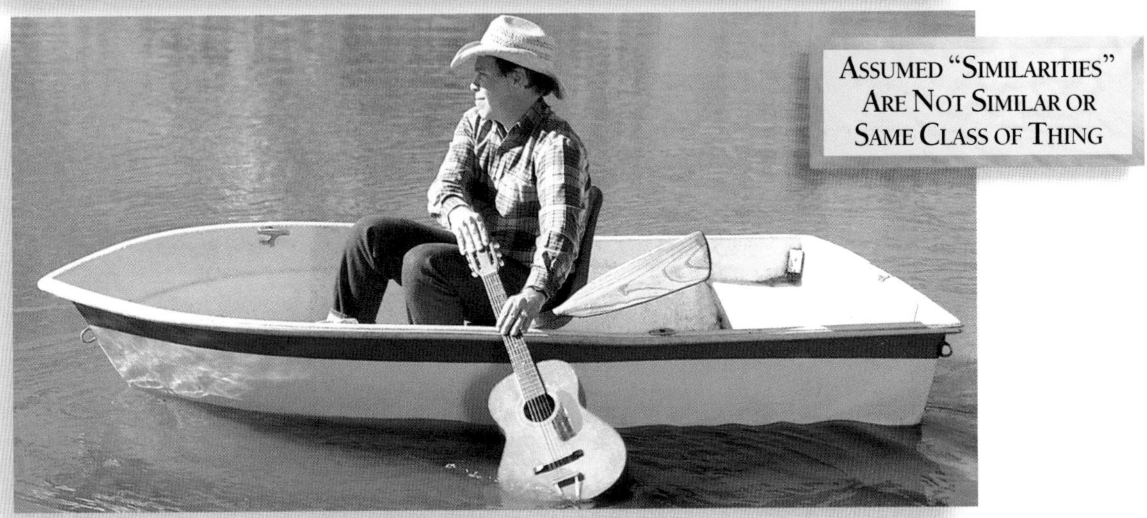
ASSUMED "SIMILARITIES"
ARE NOT SIMILAR OR
SAME CLASS OF THING

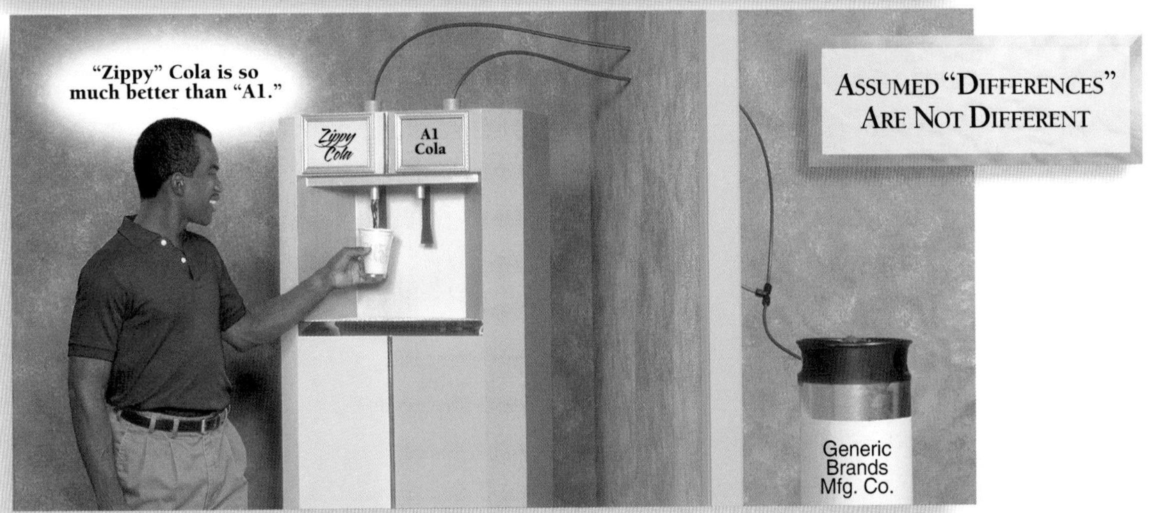

Handling Data

There are hundreds of ways these mishandlings of data can then give one a completely false picture.

When basing actions or orders on data which contains one of the above, one then makes a mistake.

REASON DEPENDS ON DATA.

WHEN DATA IS FAULTY (as above) THE ANSWER WILL BE WRONG AND LOOKED UPON AS UNREASONABLE.

There are a vast number of combinations of these data. More than one (or all) may be present in the same report.

Observation and its communication may contain one of these illogics.

If so, then any effort to handle the situation will be ineffective in correcting or handling it.

Use

If any body of data is given the above tests, it is often exposed as an invitation to acting illogically.

To achieve a logical answer one must have logical data.

Any body of data which contains one or more of the above faults can lead one into illogical conclusions.

The basis of an unreasonable or unworkable order is a conclusion which is made illogical by possessing one or more of the above faults.

Pluspoints

There are one or more conditions which exist when a situation or circumstance is logical. These are called pluspoints. A *pluspoint* is a datum of truth found to be true when compared to the following list of logical conditions.

Pluspoints show where *logic* exists and where things are going right or likely to.

Where things get better or there is a sudden improvement in an area or organization, the cause for this should be found to reinforce what was successful. Such an investigation is done by use of pluspoints.

The pluspoints are as follows:

RELATED FACTS KNOWN. (All relevant facts known.)

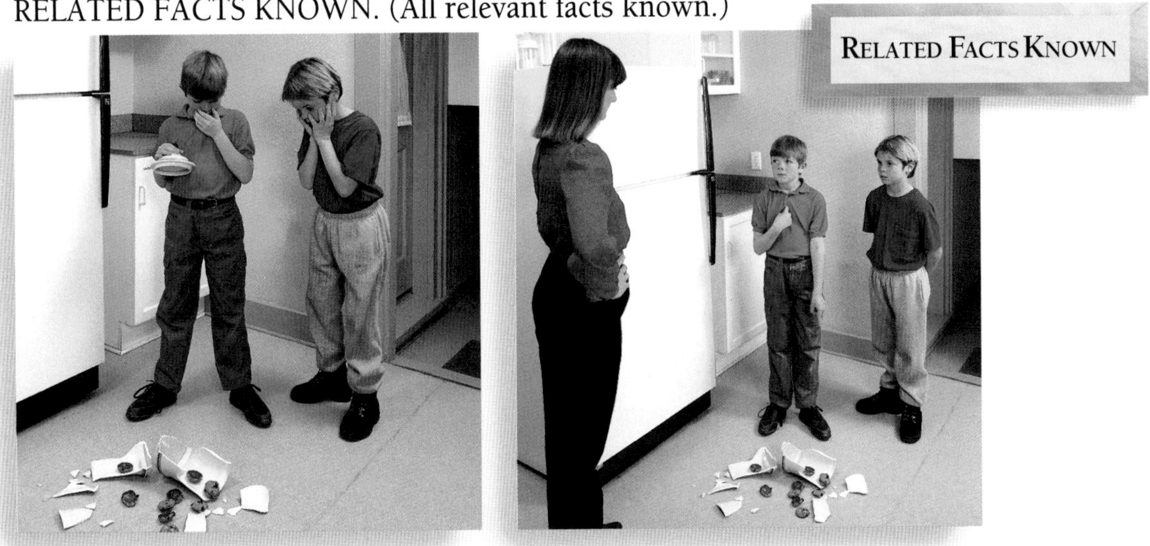

EVENTS IN CORRECT SEQUENCE. (Events in actual sequence.)

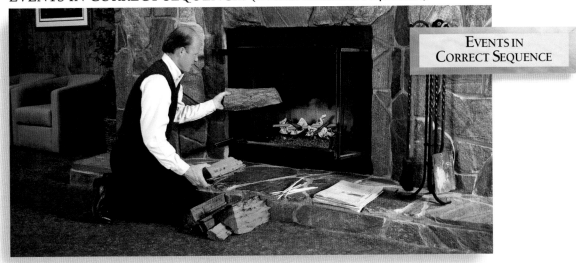

TIME NOTED.
(Time is properly noted.)

DATA PROVEN FACTUAL.
(Data must be factual, which is to say, true and valid.)

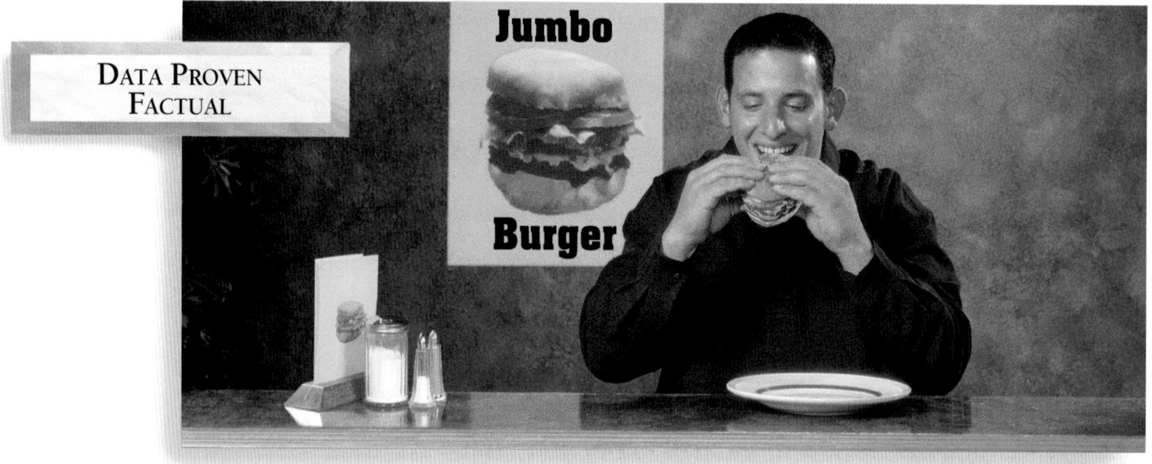

CORRECT RELATIVE IMPORTANCE.
(The important and unimportant are correctly sorted out.)

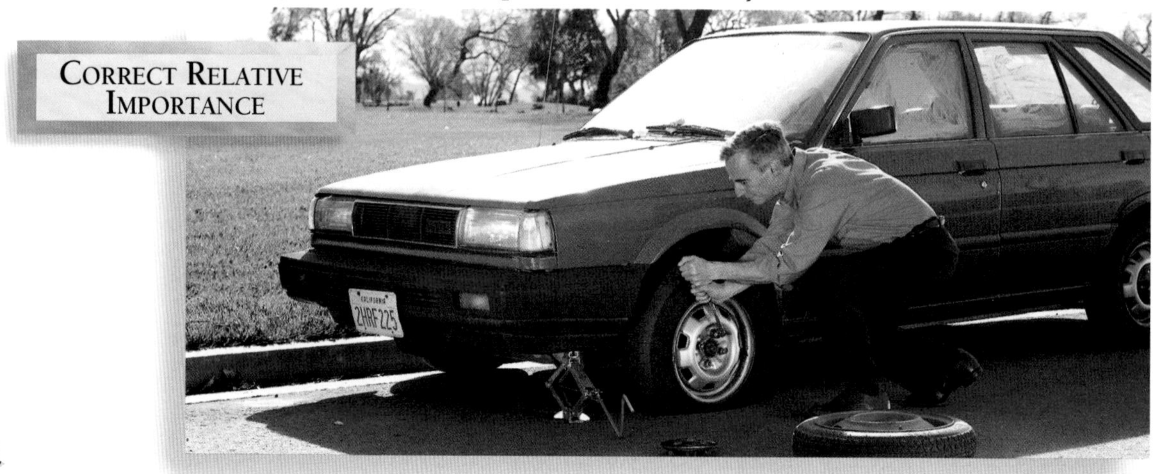

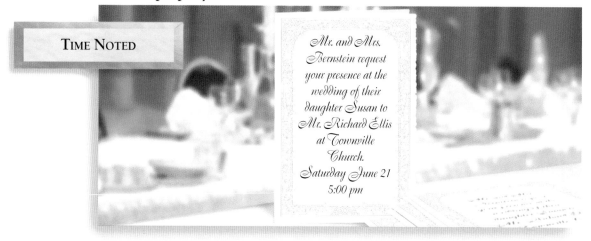

EXPECTED TIME PERIOD. (Events occurring or done in the time one would reasonably expect them to be.)

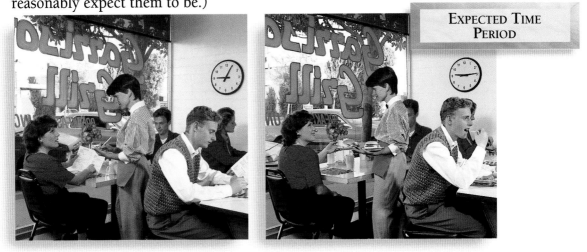

ADEQUATE DATA. (No sectors of omitted data that would influence the situation.)

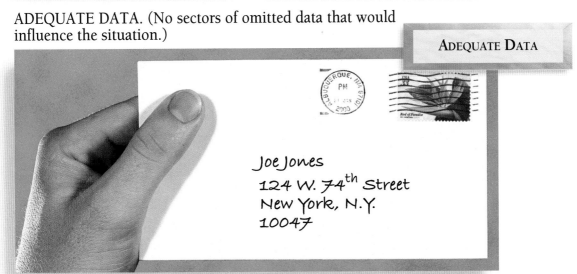

APPLICABLE DATA. (The data presented or available applies to the matter in hand and not something else.)

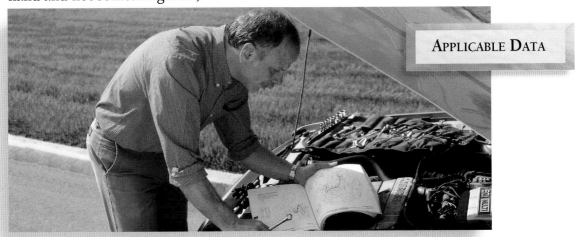

CORRECT SOURCE.
(Not wrong source.)

CORRECT TARGET.
(Not going in some direction that would be wrong for the situation.)

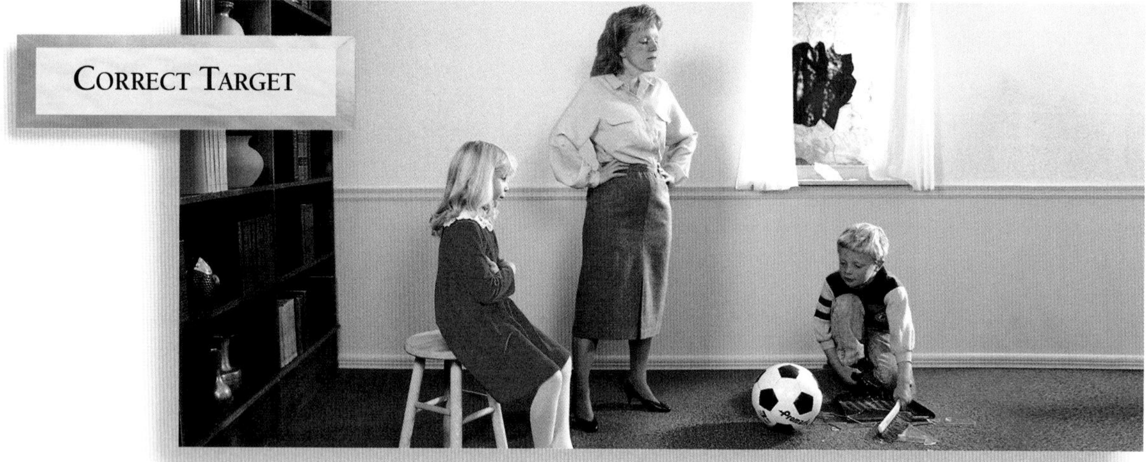

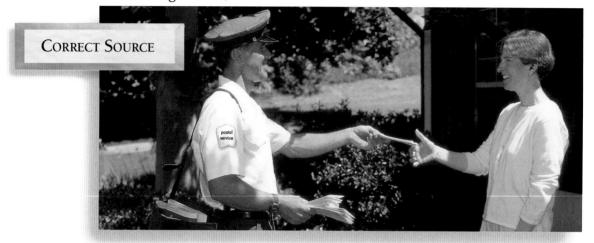

DATA IN SAME CLASSIFICATION. (Data from two or more different classes of material not introduced as the same class.)

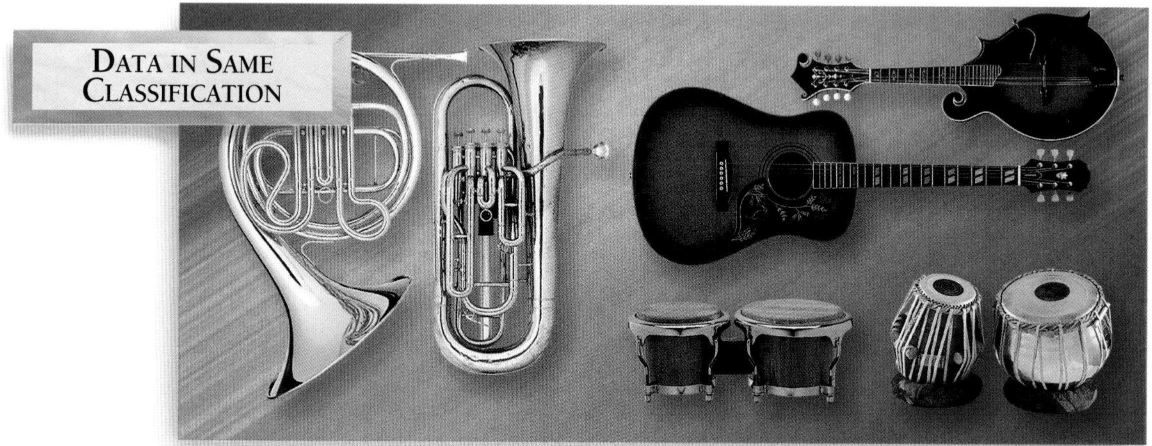

IDENTITIES ARE IDENTICAL.
(Not similar or different.)

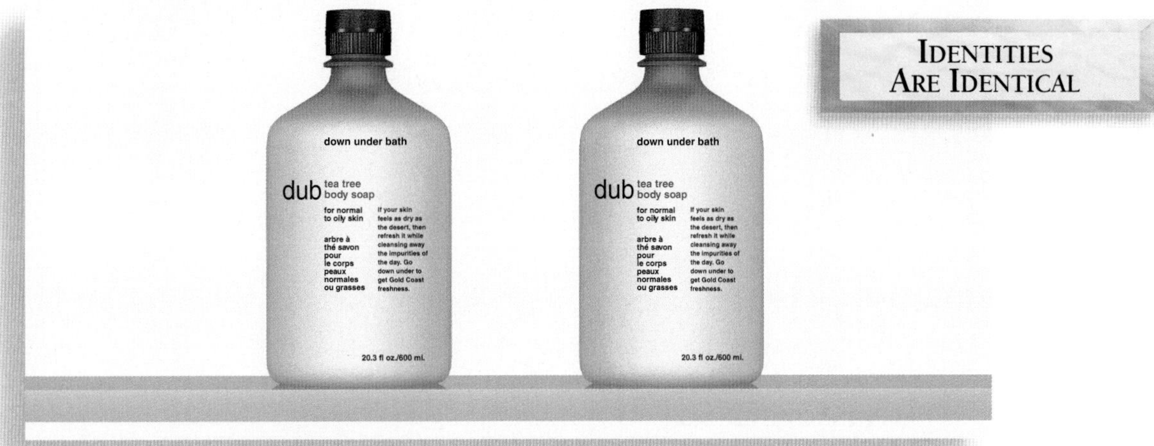

SIMILARITIES ARE SIMILAR.
(Not identical or different.)

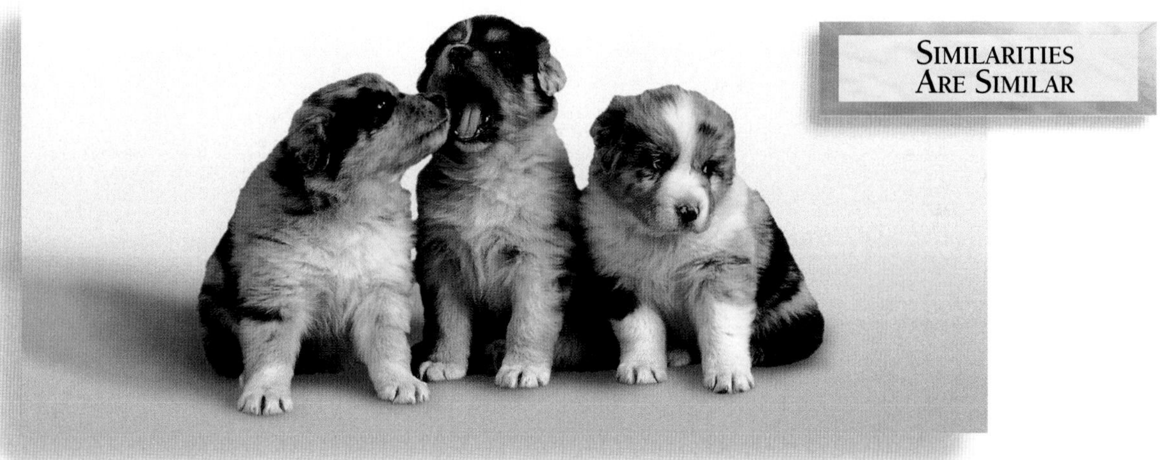

DIFFERENCES ARE DIFFERENT.
(Not made to be identical or similar.)

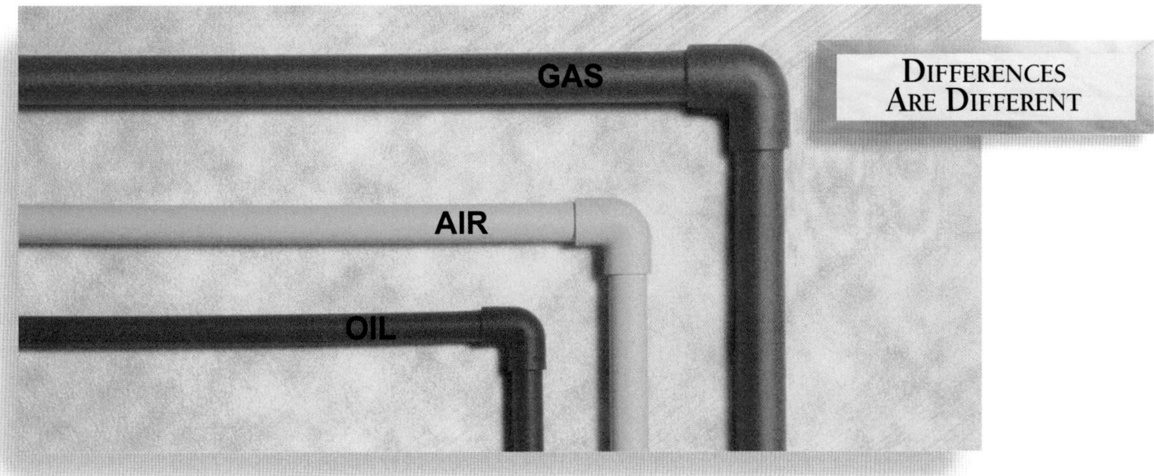

In finding out why things got better so they can be repeated, it is vital to use the actual pluspoints by name as above.

Pluspoints are, after all, what make things go right.

Not Know

One can always know something about anything.

It is a wise man who, confronted with conflicting data, realizes that he knows at least one thing—that he doesn't know.

Grasping that, he can then take action to find out.

If he evaluates the data he does find out against the things above, he can clarify the situation. Then he can reach a logical conclusion.

Drills

It is necessary to work out your own examples of the violations of logic described herein.

By doing so, you will have gained skill in sorting out the data of a situation.

When you can sort out data and become skilled in it, you will become very difficult to fool and you will have taken the first vital step in grasping a correct estimate of any situation.

DATA AND SITUATION ANALYZING

That one gains an excellent understanding of logic and a good grasp of the types of outpoints and pluspoints is vital to investigation. With this as a foundation, the two general steps one has to take to "find out what is really going on" are:

1. Analyze the data,

2. Using the data thus analyzed to analyze the situation.

The term *data* is defined as facts, graphs, statements, decisions, actions, descriptions, which are supposedly true. *Situation* is defined as the broad general scene on which a body of current data exists.

The way to analyze *data* is to compare it to the outpoints and see if any of those appear in the data.

The way to analyze the *situation* is to put in its smaller areas each of the data analyzed as above.

Doing this gives you the locations of greatest error or disorganization and also gives you areas of greatest effectiveness.

Example: There is trouble in the Refreshment Unit. There are three people in the unit. Doing a data analysis on the whole area gives us a number of outpoints. Then we assign these to employees A, B and C who work in the unit and find B had the most outpoints. This indicates that the trouble in the Refreshment Unit is with B. B can be handled in various ways such as training him on the duties of his job, his attendance, etc. Note we analyzed the *data* of the main area and assigned it to the bits in the area, then we had an analyzed situation and we could handle.

Example: We analyze all the data we have about the Bingo Car Plant. We assign the data thus analyzed as out (outpoints) to each function of the Bingo Car Plant. We thus pinpoint what function is the worst off. We then handle that function in various ways, principally by organizing it and training its executives and personnel.

There are several variations.

WE OBTAIN AN ANALYSIS OF THE SITUATION BY ANALYZING ALL THE DATA WE HAVE AND ASSIGNING THE OUTPOINT DATA TO THE AREAS OR PARTS. THE AREA HAVING THE MOST OUTPOINTS IS THE TARGET FOR CORRECTION.

In confronting a broad situation to be handled, we have of course the problem of finding out what's wrong before we can correct it. This is done by data analysis followed by situation analysis.

We do this by grading all the data for outpoints (illogics). We now have a long list of outpoints. This is data analysis.

We sort the outpoints we now have into the principal areas of the scene. The majority will appear in *one* area. This is situation analysis.

We now know what area to handle.

Example: Seventy data exist on the general scene. We find twenty-one of these data are irrational (outpoints). We slot the twenty-one outpoints into the areas they came from or apply to. Sixteen came from area G. We handle area G.

Experience

The remarkable part of such an exercise is that the data analysis of the data of a period of one day compares to three months operating *experience.*

Thus data and situation analysis is an instant result where experience takes a lot of time.

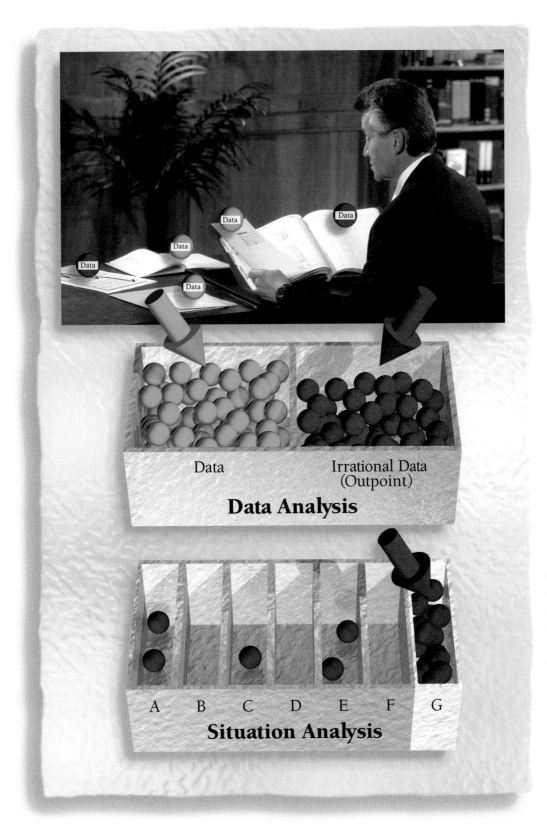

One obtains an analysis of a situation by analyzing all the data one has and assigning the outpoint data to the areas or posts. The area having the most outpoints is the target for correction.

The quality of the data analysis depends on one knowing the ideal organization and purpose on which the activity is based. This means one has to know what its activities are *supposed* to be from a rational or logical viewpoint.

A clock is supposed to keep running and indicate time and be of practical and pleasant design. A clock factory is supposed to make clocks. It is supposed to produce enough clocks cheaply enough that are good enough to be in demand and to sell for enough to keep the place solvent. It consumes raw materials, repairs and replaces its tools and equipment. It hires workmen and executives. It has service firms and distributors. That is the sort of thing one means by *ideal* or theoretical structure of the clock company and its organization.

Those are the *rational* points.

From the body of actual current today data on the clock company one spots the outpoints for a *data analysis.*

One assigns the outpoints to the whole as a *situation analysis.*

One uses his admin know-how and expertise to repair the most aberrated subsection.

One gets a functioning clock factory that runs closer to the ideal.

Military, political and PR situations, etc., are handled all in the same way.

We call these two actions:

DATA ANALYSIS

SITUATION ANALYSIS

FAMILIARITY

If one has no familiarity with how a scene (area) ought to be, one cannot easily spot outpoints (illogical data) in it.

This is what also could be called an *ideal* scene or situation. If one doesn't know the *ideal* scene or situation then one is not likely to observe nonideal points in it.

Let us send a farmer to sea. In a mild blow, with the sails and their gear creaking and water hitting the hull, he is sure the ship is about to sink. He has no familiarity with how it should sound or look so he misses any real outpoints and may consider all pluspoints as outpoints.

Yet on a calm and pretty day he sees a freighter come within five hundred feet of the side and go full astern and thinks everything is great.

An experienced officer may attempt madly to avoid collision and all the farmer would think was that the officer was being impolite! The farmer, lacking any familiarity with the sea and having no *ideal* as to what smooth running would be, would rarely see real outpoints unless he drowned. Yet an experienced sailor, familiar with the scene in all its changing faces sees an outpoint in all small illogicals.

On the other hand, the sailor on the farm would completely miss disease in the wheat and an open gate and see no outpoints in a farm that the farmer knew was about to go bust.

The rule is:

A PERSON MUST HAVE AN IDEAL SCENE WITH WHICH TO COMPARE THE EXISTING SCENE.

If a staff hasn't got an idea of how a real organization should run, then it misses obvious outpoints.

One sees examples of this when an experienced organization executive visiting an organization tries to point out to a green staff (which has no ideal or familiarity) what is out. The green staff grudgingly fixes up what he says to do but lets go of it the moment he departs. Lacking familiarity and an ideal of a perfect organization, the green staff just doesn't see anything wrong or anything right either!

The consequences of this are themselves illogical. One sees an untrained executive firing all the producers and letting the bad hats (corrupt or worthless people) alone. His erroneous ideal would be a quiet organization, let us say. So he dismisses anyone who is noisy or demanding. He ignores statistics. He ignores the things he should watch merely because he has a faulty ideal and no familiarity of a proper scene.

Observation Errors

When the scene is not familiar one has to look hard to become aware of things. You've noticed tourists doing this. Yet the old resident "sees" far more than they do while walking straight ahead down the road.

It is easy to confuse the novel with the "important fact." "It was a warm day for winter" is a useful fact only when it turns out that actually everything froze up on that day or it indicated some other outpoint.

Most errors in observation are made because one has no ideal for the scene or no familiarity with it.

However there are other error sources.

"Being reasonable" is the chief offender. People dub in (presume or have a false, delusory perception of) a missing piece of a sequence, for instance, instead of seeing that it *is* missing. A false datum is imagined to exist because a sequence is wrong or has a missing step.

It is horrifying to behold how easily people buy dub-in. This is because an illogical sequence is uncomfortable. To relieve the discomfort they distort their own observation by ignoring the outpoint and concluding something else.

Accurate Observation

There are certain conditions necessary for accurate observation.

First is a means of *perception* whether by remote communication by various communication lines or by direct looking, feeling, experiencing.

Second is an *ideal* of how the scene or area should be.

Third is *familiarity* with how such scenes are when things are going well or poorly.

Fourth is understanding *pluspoints* or rightnesses when present.

Fifth is knowing *outpoints* (all types) when they appear.

Sixth is rapid ability to *analyze data.*

Seventh is the ability to *analyze* the *situation.*

Eighth is the willingness to *inspect* more closely the area of outness.

Then one has to have the knowledge and imagination necessary to *handle.*

One could call the above the *cycle of observation.* If one calls *handle* number nine it would be the Cycle of Control.

If one is trained to conceive all variations of outpoints (illogics) and studies up to conceive an ideal and gains familiarity with the scene or type of area, his ability to observe and handle things would be considered almost supernatural.

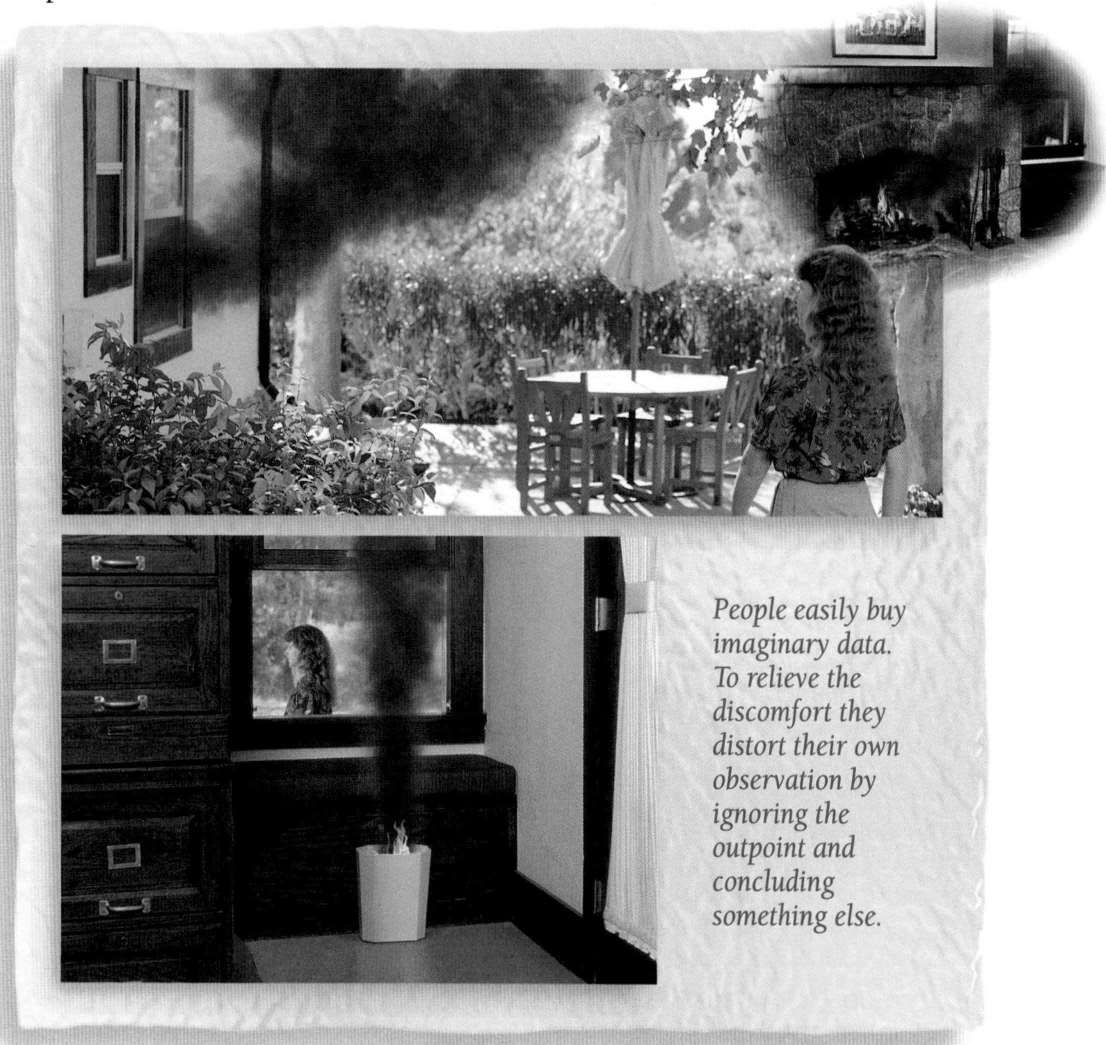

People easily buy imaginary data. To relieve the discomfort they distort their own observation by ignoring the outpoint and concluding something else.

INVESTIGATORY ACTIONS

Correction of things which are not wrong and neglecting things which are not right puts the tombstone on any organization or civilization.

This boils down to *correct investigation.* It is not a slight skill. It is *the* basic skill behind any intelligent action.

Suppressive Justice

When justice goes astray (as it usually does) the things that have occurred are:

1. Use of justice for some other purpose than public safety (such as maintaining a privileged group or indulging a fixed idea) or

2. Omitted use of investigatory procedure.

All suppressive use of the forces of justice can be traced back to one or the other of these.

Aberrations and hate very often find outlet by calling them "justice" or "law and order." This is why it can be said that man cannot be trusted with justice.

This or just plain stupidity bring about a neglect of intelligent investigatory procedures. Yet all group sanity depends upon correct and unaberrated (rational) investigatory procedures. Only in that way can one establish causes of things. And only by establishing causes can one cease to be the effect of unwanted situations.

It is one thing to be able to observe. It is quite another to utilize observations so that one can get to the basis of things.

Sequences

Investigations become necessary in the face of outpoints or pluspoints.

Investigations can occur out of idle curiosity or particular interest. They can also occur to locate the cause of pluspoints.

Whatever the motive for investigation, the action itself is conducted by sequences.

If one is incapable mentally of tracing a series of events or actions, one cannot investigate.

Altered sequence is a primary block to investigation.

At first glance, omitted data would seem to be the block. On the contrary, it is the end product of an investigation and is what pulls an investigation along—one is looking for omitted data.

An altered sequence of actions defeats any investigation. Examples: We will hang him and then conduct a trial. We will assume who did it and then find evidence to prove it. A crime should be provoked to find who commits them.

Any time an investigation gets back-to-front, it will not succeed.

Thus, if an investigator himself has any trouble with seeing or visualizing sequences of actions, he will inevitably come up with the wrong answer.

Reversely, when one sees that someone has come up with a wrong or incomplete answer, one can assume that the investigator has trouble with sequences of events or, of course, did not really investigate.

One can't really credit that Sherlock Holmes would say, "I have here the fingerprint of Mr. Murgatroyd on the murder weapon. Have the police arrest him. Now, Watson, hand me a magnifying glass and ask Sgt. Doherty to let us look over his fingerprint files."

If one cannot visualize a series of actions, like a ball bouncing down a flight of stairs, or if one cannot relate in proper order several different actions with one object into a proper sequence, he will not be able to investigate.

If one can, that's fine.

Investigations

All betterment of life depends on finding out pluspoints and why and reinforcing them, locating outpoints and why and eradicating them.

This is the successful survival pattern of living. A primitive who is going to survive does just that and a scientist who is worth anything does just that.

The fisherman sees sea gulls clustering over a point on the sea. That's the beginning of a short sequence, point number one. He predicts a school of fish, point number two. He sails over as sequence point number three. He looks down as sequence point number four. He sees fish as point number five. He gets out a net as point number six. He circles the school with the net, number seven. He draws in the net, number eight. He brings the fish on board, number nine. He goes to port, number ten. He sells the fish, number eleven. That's following a pluspoint—cluster of sea gulls.

A sequence from an outpoint might be: Housewife serves dinner. Nobody eats the cake, number one; she tastes it, number two; she recognizes soap in it, number three. She goes to kitchen, number four. She looks into cupboard, number five. She finds the soapbox upset, number six. She sees the flour below it, number seven. She sees cookie jar empty, number eight. She grabs young son, number nine. She shows him the setup, number ten. She gets a confession, number eleven. And number twelve is too painful to describe.

Discoveries

All discoveries are the end product of a sequence of investigatory actions that begin with either a pluspoint or an outpoint.

Thus all knowledge proceeds from pluspoints or outpoints observed.

And all knowledge depends on an ability to investigate.

And all investigation is done in correct sequence.

And all successes depend upon the ability to do these things.

WHYS

One uses the above knowledge and skill to track down the real reason for the positive or nonoptimum situation. This is called a "Why."

Why = that basic outness found which will lead to a recovery of statistics.

Wrong Why = the incorrectly identified outness which when applied does not lead to recovery.

A *mere explanation* = a *"Why"* given as *the* Why that does not open the door to any recovery.

Example: A mere explanation: "The statistics went down because of rainy weather that week." So? So do we now turn off rain? Another mere explanation: "The staff became overwhelmed that week." An order saying "Don't overwhelm staff" would be the possible "solution" of some manager. BUT THE STATISTICS WOULDN'T RECOVER.

The *real* Why when found and corrected leads straight back to improved stats (statistics).

A wrong Why, corrected, will further depress stats.

A mere explanation does nothing at all and decay continues.

Here is a situation as it is followed up:

The stats of an area were down. Investigation disclosed there had been sickness two weeks before. The report came in: "The statistics were down because people were sick." This was a mere explanation. Very reasonable. But it solved nothing. What do we do now? Maybe we accept this as the correct Why. And give an order, "All people in the area must get a medical exam and unhealthy workers will not be accepted and unhealthy ones will be fired." As it's a correction to a wrong Why, the stats *really* crash. So that's not it. Looking further we find the real Why. In the area, a boss gives orders to the wrong people which, when executed, then hurt their individual stats. We organize the place, train the boss and we get a stat recovery and even an improvement.

The correct Why led to a stat recovery. Here is another one. Statistics are down in a school. An investigation comes up with a mere explanation: "The students were all busy with sports." So management says "No sports!" Statistics go down again. A new investigation comes up with a wrong Why: "The students are being taught wrongly." Management sacks the dean. Statistics really crash now. A further, more competent investigation occurs. It turns out that there were 140 students and only the dean and one instructor! And the dean had other duties! We return the dean to his job and hire two more instructors making three. Statistics soar. Because we got the right Why.

Management and organizational catastrophes and successes are *all* explained by these three types of Why. An arbitrary, a false order or datum entered into a situation, is probably just a wrong Why held in by law. And if so held in, it will crash the place.

One really has to understand logic to get to the correct Why and must really be on his toes not to use and correct a wrong Why.

In world banking, where inflation occurs, finance regulations or laws are probably just one long parade of wrong Whys. The value of the money and its usefulness to the citizen deteriorate to such an extent that a whole ideology can be built up (as in Sparta by Lycurgus [a Greek lawgiver] who invented iron money nobody could lift in order to rid Sparta of money evils) that knocks money out entirely and puts nothing but nonsense in its place.

Organizational troubles are greatly worsened by using mere explanations (which lead to no remedies) or wrong Whys (which further depress stats). Organizational recoveries come from finding the real Why and correcting it.

The test of the real Why is "When it is corrected, do stats recover?" If they do that was it. And any other remedial order given but based on a wrong Why would have to be cancelled quickly.

DOING AN INVESTIGATION

When one begins to apply data analysis, he is often still trying to grasp the data about data analysis rather than the outpoints in the data. The remedy is just become more familiar with the materials of this chapter.

Further, one may not realize the ease with which one can acquire the knowledge of an ideal scene. An outpoint is simply an illogical departure from the ideal scene. By comparing the existing scene with the ideal scene, one easily sees the outpoints.

To know the ideal scene, one has only to work out the correct products for it. If these aren't getting out, then there is a departure. One can then find the outpoints of the various types and then locate a Why and in that way open the door to handling. And by handling, one is simply trying to get the scene to get out its products.

Unless one proceeds in this fashion (from product back to establishment), one can't analyze much of anything. One merely comes up with errors.

An existing scene is as good as it gets out its products, not as good as it is painted or carpeted or given public relations boosts.

So for *any* scene, manufacturing or fighting a war or being a hostess at a party, there are *products*.

People who lead pointless lives are very unhappy people. Even the idler or dilettante is happy only when he has a product!

There is always a product for any scene.

Standard Action

A beginner can juggle around and go badly adrift if he doesn't follow the pattern:

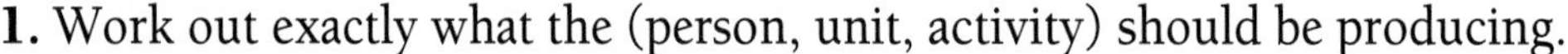
1. Work out exactly what the (person, unit, activity) should be producing.

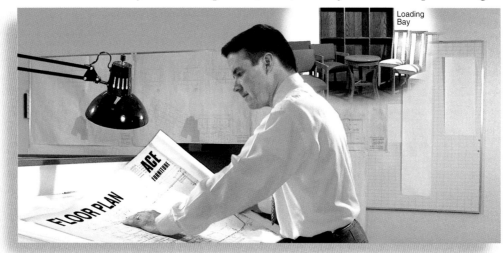

2. Work out the ideal scene.

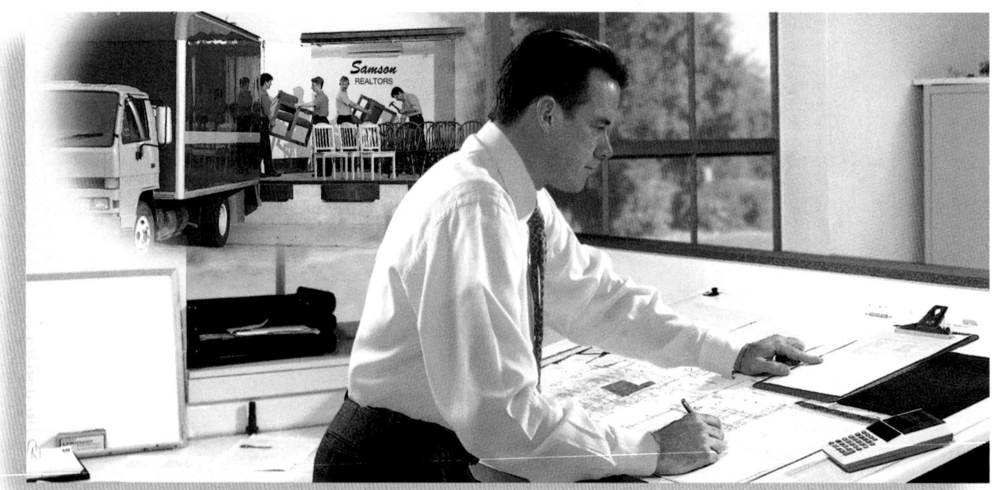

3. Investigate the existing scene.

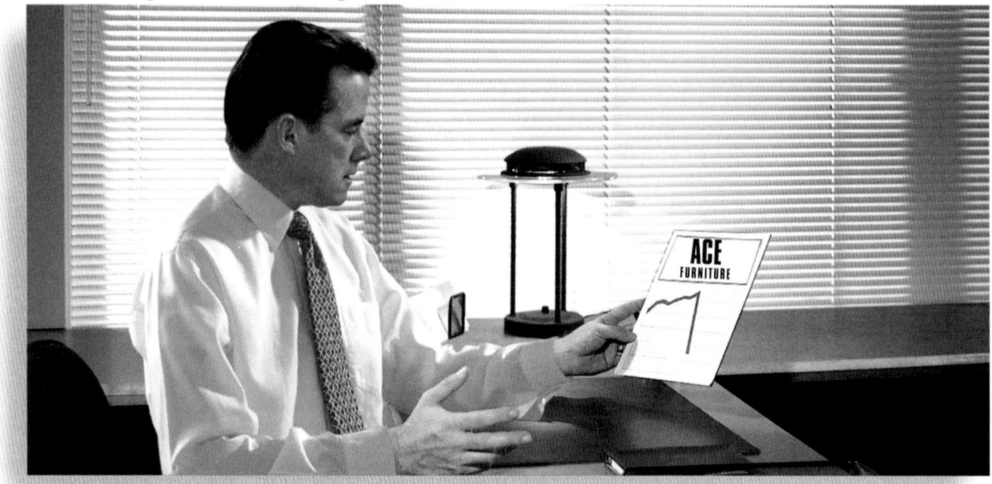

4. Follow outpoints back from ideal to existing.

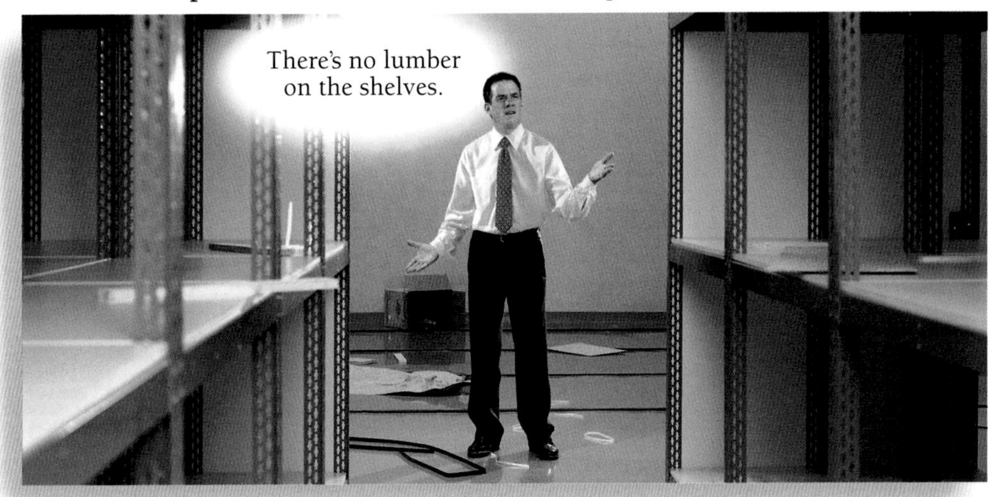
There's no lumber
on the shelves.

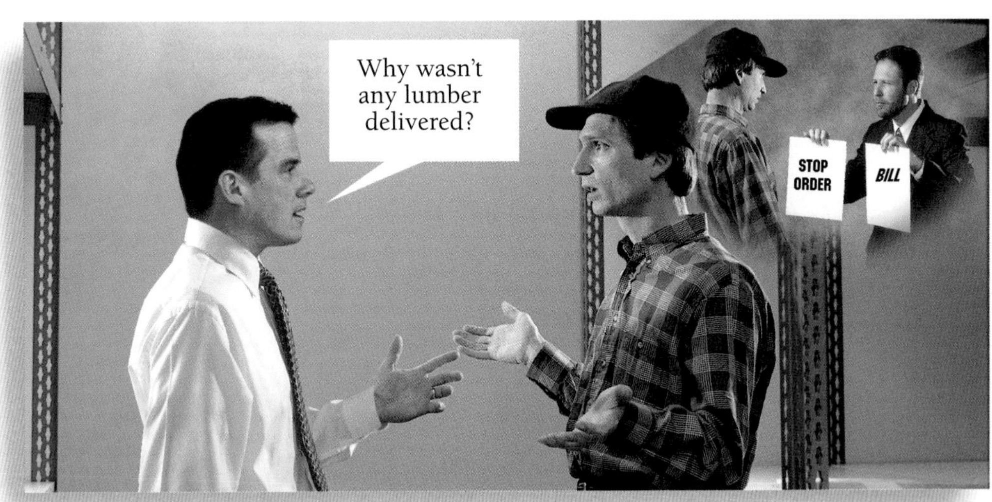
Why wasn't
any lumber
delivered?
STOP
ORDER
BILL

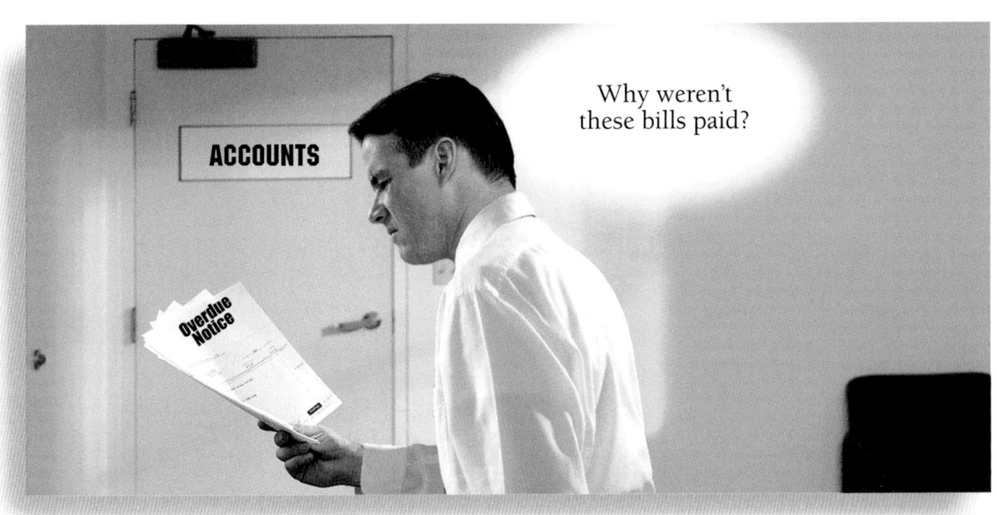
Why weren't
these bills paid?
ACCOUNTS
Overdue
Notice

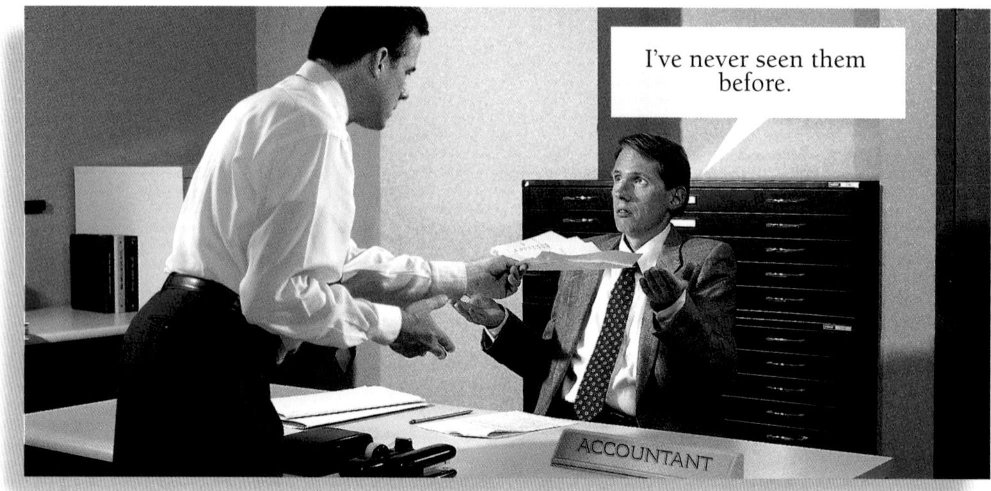
I've never seen them before.
ACCOUNTANT

5. Locate the real Why that will move the existing toward ideal.

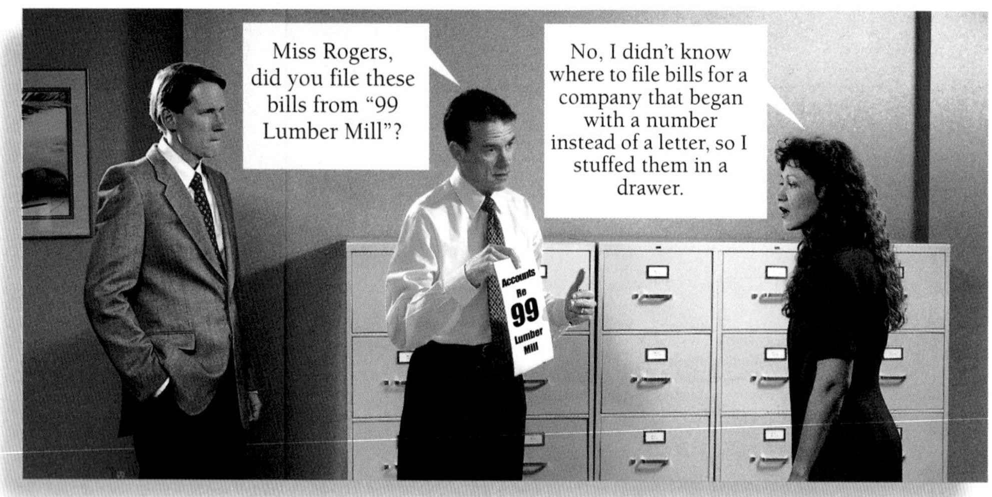
Miss Rogers, did you file these bills from "99 Lumber Mill"?
No, I didn't know where to file bills for a company that began with a number instead of a letter, so I stuffed them in a drawer.
Accounts Re 99 Lumber Mill

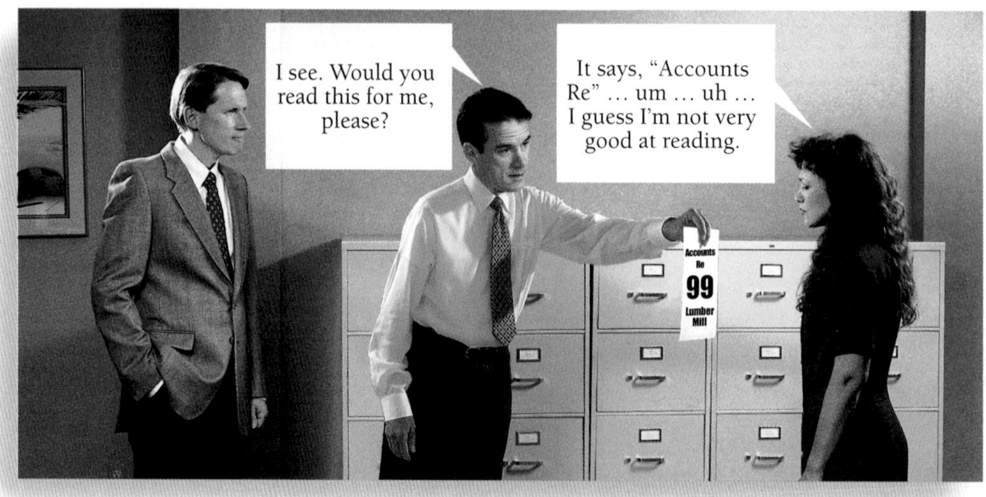
I see. Would you read this for me, please?
It says, "Accounts Re" ... um ... uh ... I guess I'm not very good at reading.
Accounts Re 99 Lumber Mill

6. Look over existing resources.

7. Get a bright idea of how to handle.

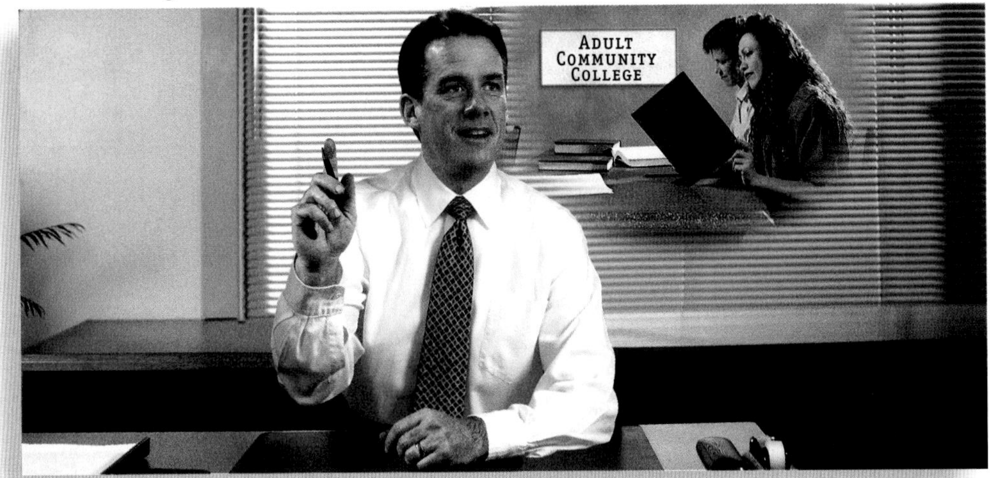

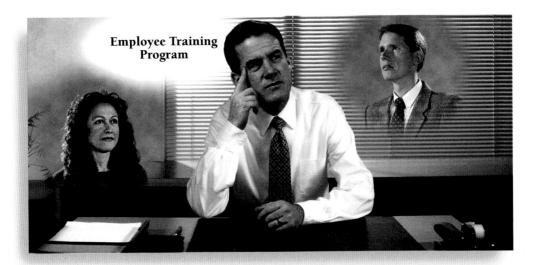

8. Handle or recommend handling so that it stays handled.

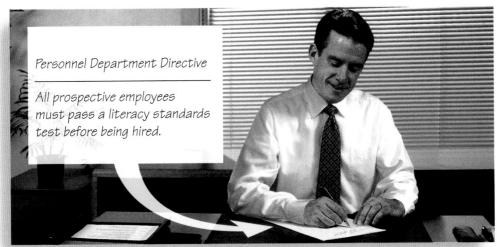

This is a very surefire approach.

If one just notes errors in a scene, with no product or ideal with which to compare the existing scene, he will not be doing data analysis and situations will deteriorate badly because he is finding wrong Whys.

Thinking

One has to be able to think with outpoints. A crude way of saying this is "learn to think like an idiot." One could also add "without abandoning any ability to think like a genius."

If one can't tolerate outpoints at all or confront them, one can't *see* them.

A madman can't tolerate pluspoints and he doesn't see them either.

But there can be a lot of pluspoints around and no production. Thus, one can be told how great it all is while the place edges over to the point of collapse.

One who listens to people on the scene and takes *their* Whys runs a grave risk. If these *were* the Whys, then things would be better.

A far safer way is to talk only insofar as finding what the product is concerned and investigating.

One should observe the existing scene through data or through observers or through direct observation.

One often has to guess what the Why might be. It is doing that which brings up the phrase "Learn to think like an idiot." The Why will be found at the end of a trail of outpoints. Each one is an aberration when compared to the ideal scene. The biggest idiocy which then explains all the rest and which opens the door to improvement toward the ideal scene is the Why.

One also has to learn to think like a genius with pluspoints.

Get the big peak period of production (now or in the past). Compare it to the existing scene just before.

Now find the pluspoints that were entered in. Trace these and you arrive at the Why as the biggest pluspoint that opened the door to improvement.

But once more one considers resources available and has to get a bright idea.

So it is the same series of steps as above but with pluspoints.

SUCCESSFUL INVESTIGATIONS

Correct investigations depend on correct Whys. You can understand a real *Why* if you realize this:

A REAL WHY OPENS THE DOOR TO HANDLING.

If you write down a Why, ask this question of it: "Does this open the door to handling?"

If it does not, then it is a wrong Why.

When you have a right Why, handling becomes simple. The more one has to beat his brains for a bright idea to handle, the more likely it is that he has a wrong Why.

So if the handling doesn't leap out at you then THE WHY HAS NOT OPENED THE DOOR and is probably wrong.

A right Why opens the door to improvement, enabling one to work out a handling which, if correctly done, will attain the envisioned ideal scene. Investigatory Technology can be applied to situations good or bad, large or small, dispelling many of life's puzzles and making real solutions possible. ■

TEST YOUR UNDERSTANDING

Answer the following questions about investigations. Refer back to the chapter to check your answers. If you need to, review the chapter. Going over the materials several times will increase your certainty and help you better apply it.

- ❑ *How does one "pull a string"?*
- ❑ *What is logic?*
- ❑ *What is a pluspoint?*
- ❑ *What is an outpoint?*
- ❑ *How is a data analysis done?*
- ❑ *What is a situation?*
- ❑ *How does one use situation analysis to determine the area to investigate?*
- ❑ *What is the difference between an ideal scene and an existing scene?*
- ❑ *How does one formulate an ideal scene?*
- ❑ *How does "being reasonable" affect one's ability to investigate?*
- ❑ *What is a Why?*
- ❑ *How does one know when he has a right Why when doing an investigation?*
- ❑ *What does one do when he follows outpoints back from an ideal scene to an existing scene?*

PRACTICAL EXERCISES

Here are some practical exercises to increase your knowledge and skill in applying the basic data on investigations.

1 Using a newspaper or newsmagazine, find two data which you don't understand. Then write down the question you would ask to clear up the contradiction. Repeat this five other times.

2 For each of the following outpoints, write down three examples that you could observe or that could occur in your life:

Omitted Data	Altered Sequence
Dropped Time	Falsehood
Altered Importance	Wrong Target
Wrong Source	Contrary Facts
Added Time	Added Inapplicable Data
Incorrectly Included Datum	Assumed "Identities" Are Not Identical
Assumed "Similarities" Are Not Similar	Assumed "Differences" Are Not Different

3 For each of the following pluspoints, write down three examples that you could observe or that could occur in your life:

Related Facts Known	Events in Correct Sequence
Time Noted	Data Proven Factual
Correct Relative Importance	Expected Time Period
Adequate Data	Applicable Data
Correct Source	Correct Target
Data in Same Classification	Identities Are Identical
Similarities Are Similar	Differences Are Different

4 By observation of your environment or by looking at newspapers, magazines, etc., find twenty outpoints. For each, write down the type of outpoint.

5 By observation of your environment or by looking at newspapers, magazines, etc., find twenty pluspoints. For each, write down the type of pluspoint.

6 In your environment, newspapers, magazines and so on, locate two conflicting data. Then write down how you would find what you didn't know so as to resolve the conflict between the data. Repeat this three more times.

7 Using the data in a newspaper or magazine, do a data analysis. Then, using this, do a situation analysis. Repeat these steps two more times.

8 Do the following:

a. Write down an activity with which you have good familiarity.

b. Write down an ideal scene one could have for that activity.

c. Repeat steps (a) and (b) four more times for different activities.

9 Describe an example you observed or experienced where someone was "being reasonable." Include the data or circumstances the person was faced with, and the outpoint(s) being ignored. Repeat this for two other examples.

10 Write down a sequence which describes in proper order several different actions with one object. Repeat this for four other sequences.

11 Using a newspaper or newsmagazine, find three examples of a wrong Why. For each one, write down the reason it is a wrong Why.

12 Using a newspaper or magazine, find three examples of a mere explanation. For each one, write down the reason it is a mere explanation.

13 Using an area or activity with which you are very familiar, apply steps 1–8 of the subsection, "Standard Action" (pages 699–703) and do the following:

a. Write down what the person, area or activity should be producing.

b. Using what you wrote up in step (a), write down its ideal scene.

c. Write down the existing scene for this area or activity.

d. Using the materials you studied in this chapter, investigate the existing scene. Write down what you find.

e. Follow outpoints you find in this area or activity back from the ideal scene to the existing scene.

f. Locate the real Why of the area or activity being investigated. Apply the materials in the chapter to confirm this is a right Why by asking the following question of it: "Does this open the door to handling?"

g. Based on what you found in steps (a)–(f) above, look over the existing resources and get a bright idea of how to handle. Write down these resources and your bright idea. Then list out the steps you would do to handle the area or activity to move it toward the ideal scene.

RESULTS FROM APPLICATION

The technology of investigation has been successfully used in many different areas of human endeavor. One does not have to be a professional investigator to benefit from this data. Many use it on their jobs to find out why there has been a slump, or what caused a recent increase in statistics in order to ensure the expansion of an organization. Use in the home makes for increased accord amongst family members and a happier family. The ability to think clearly and act sanely as a result of accurate investigation is key to survival. Some examples of the use of this technology follow:

Investigatory Technology can be used with amazing success to improve the quality of life in any area. Here is an example:

"I moved into a new neighborhood where people seemed to be always getting sick—routinely coming down with colds and other illnesses. Using L. Ron Hubbard's Investigatory Technology, I narrowed down the probable cause area to a pond that was heavily infested with insects. Bugs, especially flies, easily carry disease. Further investigation disclosed the unbelievable: the pond was being covertly used as a dump site and thousands of gallons of waste were being pumped into it weekly! I forced officials to handle the situation. The insect population immediately died down, illness in our community dramatically reduced, and the pond reverted to its original natural beauty."

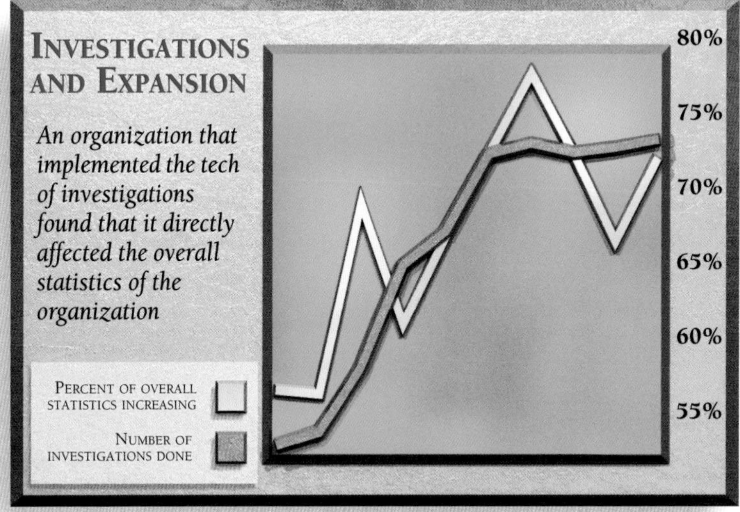

INVESTIGATIONS AND EXPANSION
An organization that implemented the tech of investigations found that it directly affected the overall statistics of the organization
PERCENT OF OVERALL STATISTICS INCREASING
NUMBER OF INVESTIGATIONS DONE
80%
75%
70%
65%
60%
55%

Having the technology of outpoints and the ability to find a right Why is essential according to an executive in a Los Angeles management company.

"It makes it possible to perceive what's in front of you as well as what went before that—it brings everything into alignment. Then you can see the outpoints and pluspoints immediately as you have a complete understanding of the situation."

An attorney in California found that the administrative technology of investigations made his job considerably easier.

"With this data, I find that situations I see in my job are easier to understand. When I look at a situation I can see the outpoints, but I also look for the ideal scene and this is invaluable in sorting out legal situations. For example, I had a client who thought he had an incredible

problem with his partner. We looked at the outpoints and determined that it wasn't the partner at all—the problem was coming from another part of the company entirely! He was then able to apply the proper handling to the situation, which was of course, quite different than the one he had anticipated."

Trained in investigatory procedure as developed by Mr. Hubbard, an individual said the following about its use:

"I can't say enough about L. Ron Hubbard's Investigatory Technology. Not only have I used it successfully on my job, but I use it in everyday situations I encounter to make life go more smoothly for myself and my friends. Using this Investigatory Technology I have found lost children, located misplaced money, figured out and corrected the reason my computer would not work and have even discovered the Why behind a terrible tasting dessert! Hardly a day goes by without being able to use this technology to make life better."

A business consultant had a client who ran an auto repair business. The business was struggling and the client himself was not doing well in life. The consultant used Investigatory Technology to handle this:

"Initially it didn't make sense that this business was not doing well. My client was a smart man and had done well in the past. I started looking into this to find out what the Why was. Coincident with the beginning of the business slump, I found that he had employed a 'silent partner' to do his books. So I looked into this fellow carefully and discovered that he was not being wholly honest in his bookkeeping and, in fact, was ripping my client off! Because this man had posed as a professional and as someone who knew what he was doing, my client had not looked into this area at all as a possible reason for his failing. Simply by applying Mr. Hubbard's technology on investigations, the answer fell into my lap. My client was more than relieved. He took back over the business in full and his statistics took off. He himself is back to battery, and once again I marvel at the simplicity of Investigatory Technology."

SUGGESTIONS FOR FURTHER STUDY

The fundamentals of logic and reason are covered in this chapter, but the data included here only scratches the surface of the full body of technology that L. Ron Hubbard developed on this subject. His breakthroughs in this area encompass a whole new way to think. Study of the following materials will increase your understanding of and ability to apply this technology.

Management Series Volumes

Mr. Hubbard applied his discoveries about life and the basic truths of Scientology to the subject of management. Contained within these three volumes is the complete body of technology on logic and how to apply it with precision to find the Why of any situation. Studying these books also provides one with knowledge in organizing, handling personnel, operating as an executive, public relations, attaining targets and many other subjects vital to the optimum survival of any group.

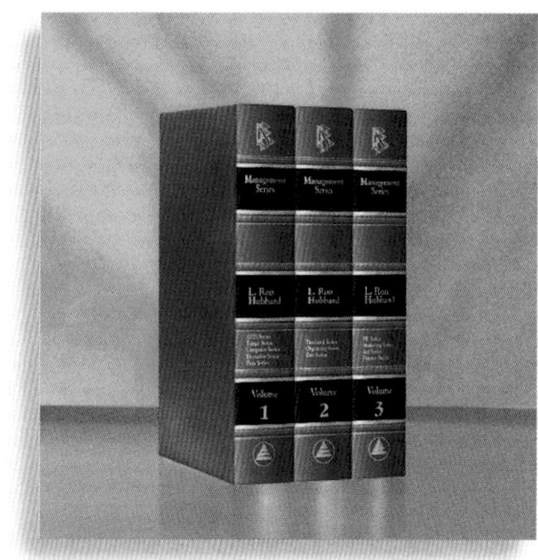

Hubbard Elementary Data Series Evaluator's Course

The Data Series is Mr. Hubbard's complete writings on finding what is logical and illogical about any situation, determining its ideal scene and revealing the greatest departure from this ideal which, when handled, will dramatically improve the circumstances. An *evaluator* is one trained in these materials. An individual's survival and success relies on his operating on correct Whys and then handling what was found. This course provides one with these skills and puts him in a causative position with regard to any state of affairs he could encounter in life. (Delivered in Scientology organizations.)

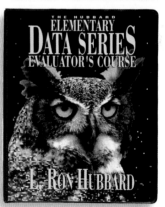

The Professional Product Debug Course

As part of the body of group technology, Mr. Hubbard developed the means to unsnarl or *debug* stops or slows in getting an activity carried through to completion. *Debug technology* utilizes fundamental maxims of life and its relationship to the physical universe. With it one can unsnarl or *debug* those factors preventing or blocking the handling of a Why. The Professional Product Debug Course covers the complete array of debug technology, including how to locate and clear up misunderstood concepts and terminology, how to find and handle false data from earlier studies, and much more. (Delivered in Scientology organizations.)

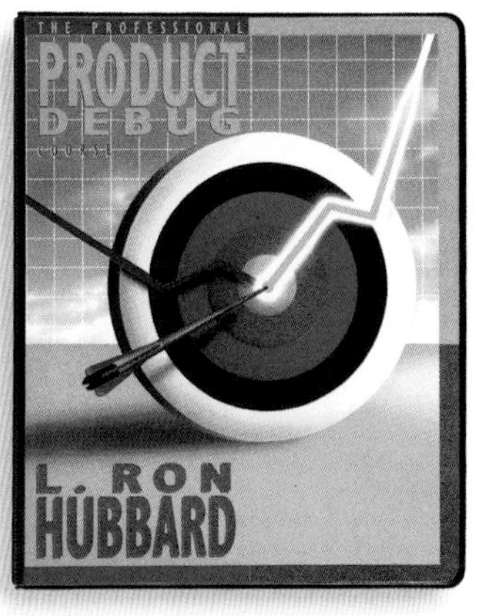

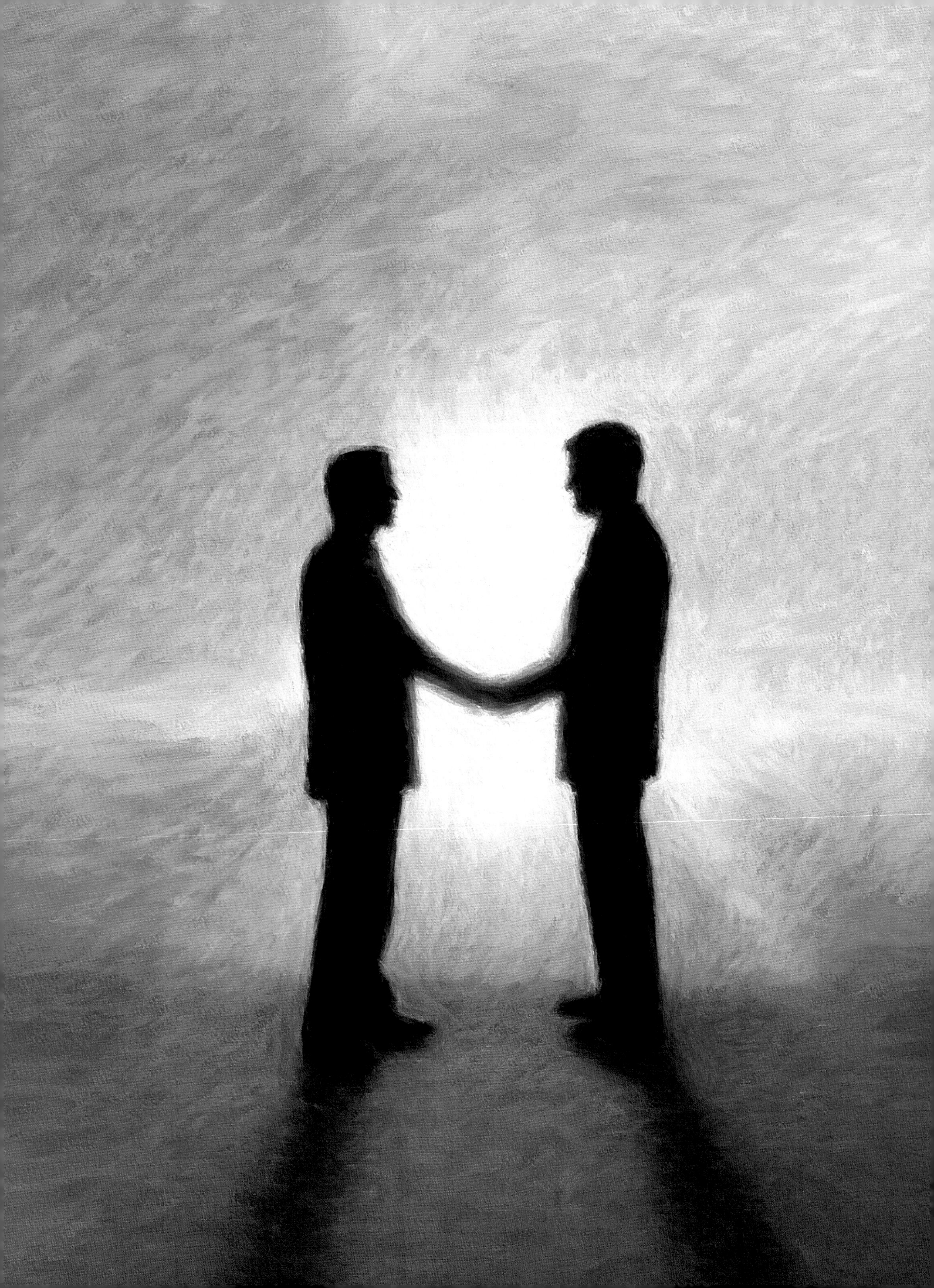

Chapter 19

Fundamentals of Public Relations

Public relations provides the means to communicate your ideas and get them accepted—a skill vitally necessary when dealing with new ideas. It is a way to gain support for your projects and endeavors.

Generally considered a method to gain publicity, public relations has previously been subjected to severe limitations. This was a practice that lacked certain key elements. Now, because of some important discoveries in Scientology, advances have made the entire activity significantly more useful and effective.

L. Ron Hubbard's refinement of public relations not only makes it essential for any group and any individual, but removes the previously inherent limitations. Although the full technology is extensive, the basic principles covered here will be of immense value to anyone with a worthwhile purpose.

PUBLIC RELATIONS

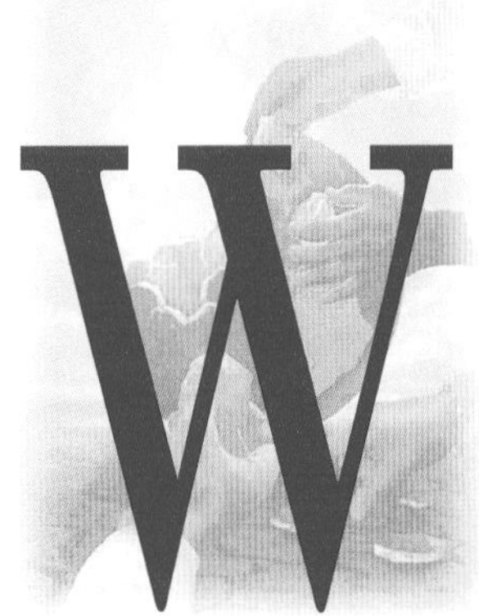

When one is dealing with others to gain their agreement or cooperation or support for something, he has entered the field of public relations, or PR for short.

The definition of PR is: GOOD WORKS WELL PUBLICIZED.

Doing good works is not enough, one has to actually publicize it to gain cooperation or agreement.

In public relations one is essentially reaching people with an idea of some kind and gaining their agreement. One's success in dealing with others, then, is effective to the degree that he can reach them with the idea he intends them to have.

Public relations is an indispensable tool to help one get his ideas across, and any person who is making the world a better place would benefit greatly from its use.

No matter what you do—from taking actions to improve education in an area, to helping people get off drugs—by using the tools of public relations you can reach others with the correct message and gain their agreement on it. Thus it opens the door to acceptance of the activity you want to do.

Public relations is not new. It existed as a formal subject in Roman times, when it was employed for the purpose of electing senators. Even then, political campaign slogans were written on the walls of the Colosseum for people to see.

Through the centuries PR has remained only partially developed as a subject, suppressed in its development by the ill-intentioned who were only interested in using it to serve their ulterior motives.

It wasn't until Scientology, with its discoveries about communication and the true nature of man, that public relations actually became a complete subject of benefit to the society and to the individual.

Public relations is a technology. It has its own laws.

To begin to learn the techniques of public relations, you must start with an understanding of the basic factors or ingredients which make up the subject.

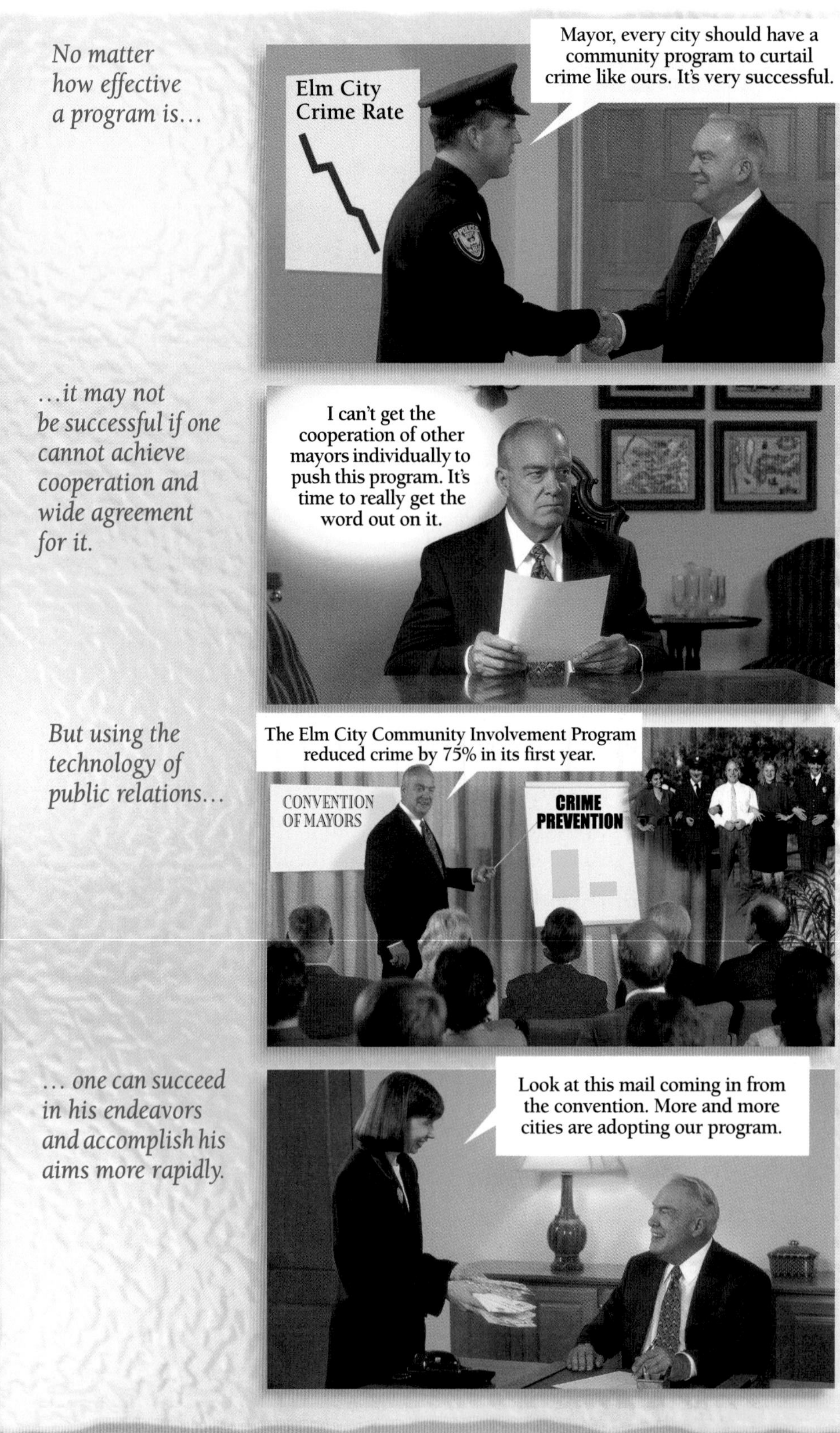
No matter how effective a program is...
Elm City Crime Rate
Mayor, every city should have a community program to curtail crime like ours. It's very successful.
...it may not be successful if one cannot achieve cooperation and wide agreement for it.
I can't get the cooperation of other mayors individually to push this program. It's time to really get the word out on it.
But using the technology of public relations...
The Elm City Community Involvement Program reduced crime by 75% in its first year.
CONVENTION OF MAYORS
CRIME PREVENTION
... one can succeed in his endeavors and accomplish his aims more rapidly.
Look at this mail coming in from the convention. More and more cities are adopting our program.

THE MISSING INGREDIENT

There has been a missing ingredient in the technology of public relations for as long as this subject has existed. This omission has been one of the key factors that has rendered public relations incomplete as a subject and, consequently, something of potential liability to its user.

This ingredient is *reality*.

The things which we perceive with our senses are real. Reality is essentially *agreement* upon perceptions and data in the physical universe. It is the degree of agreement reached between people. You are either in agreement with your fellows or in disagreement with your fellows, and as you agree or disagree, thus is your reality.

Those things upon which you and your fellows agree are real. Those things upon which you disagree are not real.

It was discovered in Scientology that reality is interconnected with two other components: affinity and communication.

The term *affinity* is fairly close in meaning to the word *like*. However, affinity is a two-way proposition. Not only do you *like* something but you feel that it likes you. Affinity is also very much like the word *love* when *love* is used in the universal sense. It includes both *love* and *like* and is broader than both.

Communication is the interchange of ideas across space. A man's impact on the world has been directly proportionate to his development of a means of communication. Communication in its broadest sense, of course, includes all the ways in which a person or thing becomes aware of, or becomes aware to, another person or thing.

These three components—affinity, reality and communication—form the ARC (pronounced A-R-C) triangle of Scientology and together these form the component parts of understanding.

If one corner of this triangle (say A) is raised, the other two will rise. If one corner is lowered, the other two are as well.

Thus with high affinity, one also has a high reality and a high communication. With a low affinity one has also a low reality and a low communication.

With a high or low R one has a high or low A and C.

And so it goes. The whole triangle rises and lowers as one piece. One cannot have a low R and a high A and C.

Public relations is supposed to be a *communication* technique. It communicates ideas. Suppose one were to try to communicate an out-the-bottom R. In such a case the communication would possibly at first reach, but then it would recoil due to its R.

This whole interrelationship of affinity, reality and communication is of course an advance in the technology of Scientology. It was not available to early pioneers of PR. So they talked (and still talk) mainly lies.

Older PR practitioners *preferred* lies. They used circus exaggeration or covert attacks using slander and falsehoods on persons' reputations. They sought to startle or intrigue and the easiest way to do it was with exclamation point "facts" which were in fact lies.

"Mental health" public relations men dreamed up out of whole cloth the "statistics" of the insane. "Nine out of every fifteen Englishmen will go insane at some period of their lives" is a complete lie. Streams of such false statistics gush from PR lobbyists to get a quick pound from Parliament.

The stock in trade of public relations people, whether hired by Stalin, Hitler, the US president or the International Bank, has been black, baldfaced lies.

A US president once gave two different figures of the percentage of increased government cost per year in two months. His public relations man was trying to influence Congress.

The "Backfire 8" as the "Car of the Century" and the parachute exhibition "record delayed drop" and the ambassador's press conference on "Middle East Aims" are all public relations functions—and salted throughout with lies.

You pick up a newspaper or listen in the street and you see PR—PR—PR—all lies.

A battle cruiser makes a "goodwill visit" to a town it is only equipped to crush and you have more lies.

The tremendous power of newspapers, magazines, radio, TV and modern "mass media" communication is guided by the PR men of special interests and they guide with lies.

Thus public relations is corrupted to "a technique of lying convincingly."

It makes a cynical world. It has smashed idealism, patriotism and morality.

Why?

When an enforced communication channel carries only lies, then the affinity caves in and you get hate. For the *R* is corrupted.

Public relations, dedicated to a false reality of lies, then becomes low A, low C and recoils on the user.

So the first lesson we can learn that enables us to use PR safely is to KEEP A HIGH R.

The more lies you use in public relations the more likely it is that the PR will recoil.

Thus the law:

NEVER USE LIES IN PR.

The trouble with public relations then was its lack of *reality*. A lie of course is a false reality.

The trouble with PR was R!

In getting out a press release on a new can opener that opens cans easily, and you want to say "A child could use it," find out if it's a fact. Give one to a child and have him open a can. So it's true. So use the line and say what child. Don't call it the "Can Opener of the Century." It won't communicate.

Just because radios, TVs and press pour out does not mean they communicate. Communication implies that somebody is reached.

Any lie will either blunt the C (communication) or end the C off one day with revulsion.

So there *is* a technique known as public relations. And it has the high liability of abuse through lies and the degrade of its practitioner.

But if one strictly attends to the values of truth and affinity, he will be able to communicate and can stand up to the strain.

Knowing this, public relations becomes a far more useful and mature subject.

The next thing to know about this is "who" or what "public" one is trying to communicate with. Lack of this knowledge can lead to fruitless public relations efforts.

PUBLICS

What is a "public"?

One hears "*the* public," a star says "*my* public." You look in the dictionary and you find "public" means an organized or general body of people.

There is a specialized definition of the word *"public"* which is not in the dictionary but which is used in the field of public relations. *"Public"* is a professional term to public relations people. It doesn't mean the mob or the masses. It means "a *type of audience.*"

The broad population to PR professionals is divided up into separate *publics.* Possibly the early pioneers in public relations should have begun to use "audiences" back in 1911 when some of the first texts on PR were written. But they didn't. They used the word "publics" to mean different types of audiences for their communications.

So you won't find this in the dictionaries as a public relations professional term. But you sure better wrap your wits and tongue around this term for *use.* Otherwise, you'll make more PR errors than can easily be computered.

Wrong public sums up about 99 percent of the errors in public relations activities and adds up to the majority reason for PR failures.

So what's a "public"?

In PRese (public relations slang) use "public" along with another word always. There is no single word form for "public" in public relations. A public relations professional never says THE public.

There is the "community public," meaning people in the town not personally grouped into any other special public. There is the "employee public," meaning the people who work for the firm. There's the "shareholder public," meaning the people who own shares in the company. There's the "teenage public," meaning the under-twenty people. There's the "doctor public," meaning the MD audience one is trying to reach.

There are hundreds of different types of publics.

An interest in common or a professional or social class characteristic in common—some similarity amongst a special group—determines the type of public or audience.

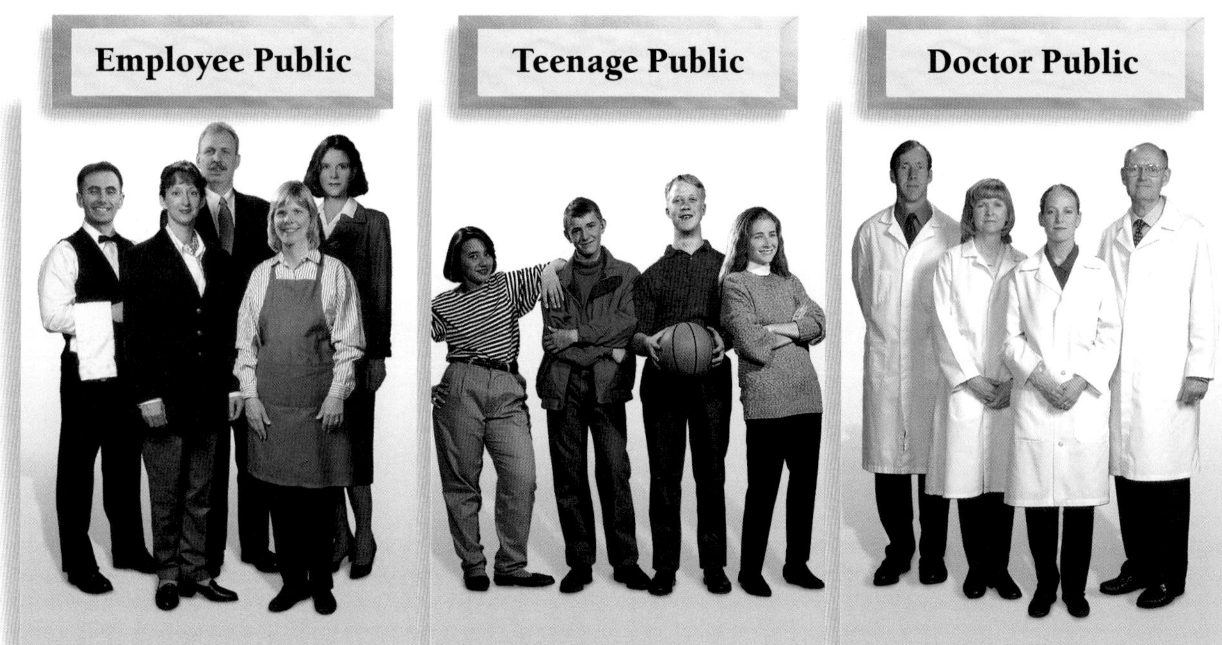

A person applying public relations needs this grouping as he can expect each different type of public to have different interests. Therefore his promotion to them must be designed especially for each type of public.

"Public" is a professional term to PR people. It doesn't mean the mob or the masses. It means "a type of audience."

In the public relations world there aren't kids—there is a "child public." There aren't teenagers—there's a "teenage public." There aren't elderly people—there's an "elderly public."

Someone using public relations does not think in huge masses. He thinks in group types within the masses.

Public relations is an activity concerned with *presentation* and *audience.* Even when he writes a news release, he "slants" it for a publication that reaches a type of audience and he writes it *for* that audience.

In order to do this, he first has to have an idea of the opinions or reality of that public or audience. He finds that out by conducting a survey.

A *survey* is a sampling, or partial collection, of facts, figures or opinions taken and used to approximate or indicate what a complete collection and analysis might reveal.

For instance, there is a group of three thousand teachers in one area and you want to find out what they want from the school board. By asking two hundred of those teachers, selected at random, you can get a good idea of where the whole group of teachers stands on that particular question.

A user of PR techniques *surveys* in terms of special publics. Then he presents his material so as to influence *that* particular public.

He doesn't offer stories about wheelchairs to the teenage public or Mickey Mouse prizes to the elderly public.

All things being offered to the public should be designed to reach a special public.

When you mix it up, you fail.

When you get it straight and survey it, you succeed.

Someone who did not understand this concept of publics could miss completely. If some PR man tried to promote the "praises of John Dillinger" to the "police public," he would certainly not get a response. Likewise, the "criminal public" isn't going to go into raptures over the "heroes in blue"!

All expert public relations is aimed at a specific, carefully surveyed, special audience called a "__________ public."

When you know that, you can grasp the subject of public relations.

When you can use it expertly, you are a professional in the field of public relations.

Anyone using PR has to figure out his precise publics. There may be several distinct types.

Then he has to survey and look over the reactions of each different type.

He then plans and designs his communication and offerings for each one.

He sends the right message to the right public in each case. There may be a dozen different messages if there are a dozen different publics. Each one is right for that public.

Someone using public relations is after a result, a call-in, a reply, a response.

The right message in the right form to the right public gets the result.

A wrong message to the wrong public simply costs lots of money and gets no result.

Knowing the right public, one can then survey them and communicate to them with reality.

If you want to obtain results, know who your publics are.

SURVEYS

As you read earlier in this chapter, it is important to use reality in PR and to know the reality level of the public you are addressing.

Surveys accomplish this.

In public relations terminology, "survey" means to carefully examine public opinion with regard to an idea, a product, an aspect of life or any other subject. By examining in detail (person to person surveying) one can arrive at a whole view of public opinion on a subject by tabulating highest percentage of popular response.

But what does this mean to an individual on his own? Certainly he cannot rush out and hire polling experts or a research company to tell him all about the neighbors in the new neighborhood he just moved into or what students think in class or what fellow employees at work think about his project.

The fact is, a person can do his own surveys very easily.

A survey is done in order to find what *buttons* a group has. In surveying, the word *button* means the subject or phrase or concept that communicates the reality of a specific public. It is something that is real to the majority of persons in that group and which can be used to get a response and gain agreement. The term came from the early 1900s expression "press the button" which means, in a figurative sense, "to perform an action that automatically brings about the required state of affairs." In public relations the state of affairs one wants is agreement and cooperation with one's actions.

In a survey, you question people to get their opinion on something. A *button* is the primary datum you get from this action. It is the answer given the most number of times to your survey question. It is what will elicit agreement and response.

Surveys can also be designed to tell you what people detest.

With a knowledge of a public's reality as gained through surveys, one has opened the door to informing them of the ideas one wants them to accept—in other words he can get his *message* across.

The *message* is the communication, the thought, the significance you want to get across to an audience or public.

A *button* is used to get the public's agreement to hear the message.

A message and a button are *not* the same thing.

By doing a survey and finding the right button, you can then use that button to elicit agreement and thereby get response.

To do a proper survey and to then use its results effectively requires an understanding of the purpose of surveys, and of ARC and the ARC triangle. It requires an understanding of what reality is.

One uses the ARC triangle in conducting a survey initially and, following that, one applies the ARC triangle in putting the survey results to use.

It goes like this: One *communicates* to an audience or public (via a survey) with *affinity* to find out what the *reality* of that audience is. Reality is agreement as to what is. The reason you do a survey is to find out what that audience or public will agree with.

One then approaches the public with that *reality* in a promotional piece or some other communication to get the public's agreement to hear the message. And thus one raises the public's *affinity* for the item one is promoting.

That is the simplicity of it. But it will only be simple to the person who understands the ARC triangle. Without reality or some agreement, communication will not reach and affinity will be absent.

Thus, surveys are done to get agreement. Surveys are not done for any other purpose. They're done to establish agreement with an audience.

You ask ten or ten hundred people what they would most want or expect of an automobile tire and seven or seven hundred of them tell you

SURVEY EXAMPLE

Here is an example of an actual survey. A group of Scientologists in South Africa was interested in finding out how best to reach children in rural townships with an educational program using Scientology Study Technology. They saw that in order to do this they first needed to determine what children considered to be the major barriers facing them.

The questions asked and the top answers with their percentages were:

1. Who do you take advice from?

73% Parents

13% Brother or sister

5% Teacher

2. What do you feel is the biggest problem in the world today?

50% Violence, war

15% Nothing, no problem

10% Education

3. What could be done to change that?

23% Stop it

15% Nothing, no problem

10% Education

4. What in your life would you like to change the most?

25% Violence, hatred

18% The situation, everything

15% Education

5. What in your life is going the best?

33% Education

30% Nothing

15% Everything

6. What thing in your life do you look forward to the most?

58% School, education

10% Don't know

10% Everything, anything

"durability." That's the button. That's the reality, the point of agreement on automobile tires among that public. So you use that button with that public and you've established reality; you've got agreement and they will then listen to what you have to say about automobile tires.

Buttons have their use but we are not so much interested in them as we are in *message.* The message is the real essence of any promotional piece or PR communication. Buttons are just the grease to use to get your message through.

A survey like the one in the example just given would be of great use in reaching children with tools by which they can learn and receive a meaningful education.

Buttons found from the survey include:

Parents—these children listen to their parents.

Violence, war—this came up as their biggest problem and something they would most like to change.

Education and school was the part of their lives which they most look forward to.

Having conducted such a survey, the results could then be used by this group to get their program better known and accepted. Their basic message is that workable methods of education exist and will help them. Using these survey results they could state their message so it would be better accepted. They could say, for example, "Education is the solution to violence and a better life for you, and our program will help you get a valuable education."

How to Conduct a Survey

The actions involved in doing a survey are simple and few. The first thing is to establish the questions you are going to ask the public to find out what is wanted and needed, popular or unpopular or whatever.

After the questions are established, they are written or typed on a piece of plain paper for the surveyor to refer to. If one were doing a survey in a city where large numbers of people were interviewed, survey forms might be most practical. However, all that is needed for most surveys is a clipboard with plenty of plain paper and several ballpoint pens (so running out of ink in the middle of the survey doesn't cause interruption). The survey question page is then placed on top of the pad of paper and flipped back while taking notes of the interview.

To begin a survey, you simply walk up to a person and in a friendly manner introduce yourself (if a stranger) and ask to survey them. If the person asks for more information about the survey or why it is being done, his questions are answered and the survey is begun.

Ask the person the first question, flip back the question page and take down the answer. Be sure to number the answers corresponding to the question number being asked. You needn't write down every word as the person speaks to you, but get the most important points. You will find, after practice surveying, you can write almost everything down.

After the person has answered the first question, thank him or her and go to the next question.

At the end of the survey, thank the person. The person will most likely be thanking you at this point as people love to be asked their opinion of things. And having another person listen attentively is a rare and valuable experience to many.

Then go to the next person and repeat the same procedure. This is all there is to the mechanical action of surveying.

Tabulation of Surveys

Once a survey is done, the responses have to be tabulated in order to be usable.

The word "tabulate" is defined by *Webster's New World Dictionary* as, "to put (facts, statistics, etc.) in a table or columns; arrange systematically."

In tabulating survey responses, you are arranging the data gathered systematically in order to permit analysis of those results. The definition of "analysis" could be stated as "examination in detail so as to determine the nature or tendencies of."

The most commonly used format for survey tabulations is to list each question, with the categories of responses and their percentages laid out from highest percentage to lowest under each question.

In order to accomplish public relations that are effective and which communicate one's message and make one's good works well known, it is essential that one know what his publics want or will accept, what they will agree with and what they will believe.

Surveys, then, give one the reality of one's public. Without them, one is going at it blindly in a hit-or-miss fashion that will not get him very far.

TABULATION PROCEDURE

1. Count all the surveys.

2. Establish various categories of answers for each question by listing answers briefly but accurately as you go through the survey responses.

3. When categories have been established, you will be able to simply mark a slant next to the appropriate category, meaning one more answer of a similar nature.

4. Once all the responses have been tabulated, count up the number of responses in each category for each question.

5. Work out the percentage for each category under each question. This is done by dividing the number of surveys and multiplying by 100. Let's say you had 1,500 answers of a similar nature to one question and your total number of surveys is 2,500.

$$1{,}500 \div 2{,}500 = 0.6 \times 100 = 60$$

This means 60 percent gave that similar type of answer.

6. The only mistake you can make is not to realize the similarity of answers and so have a great diversity of categories.

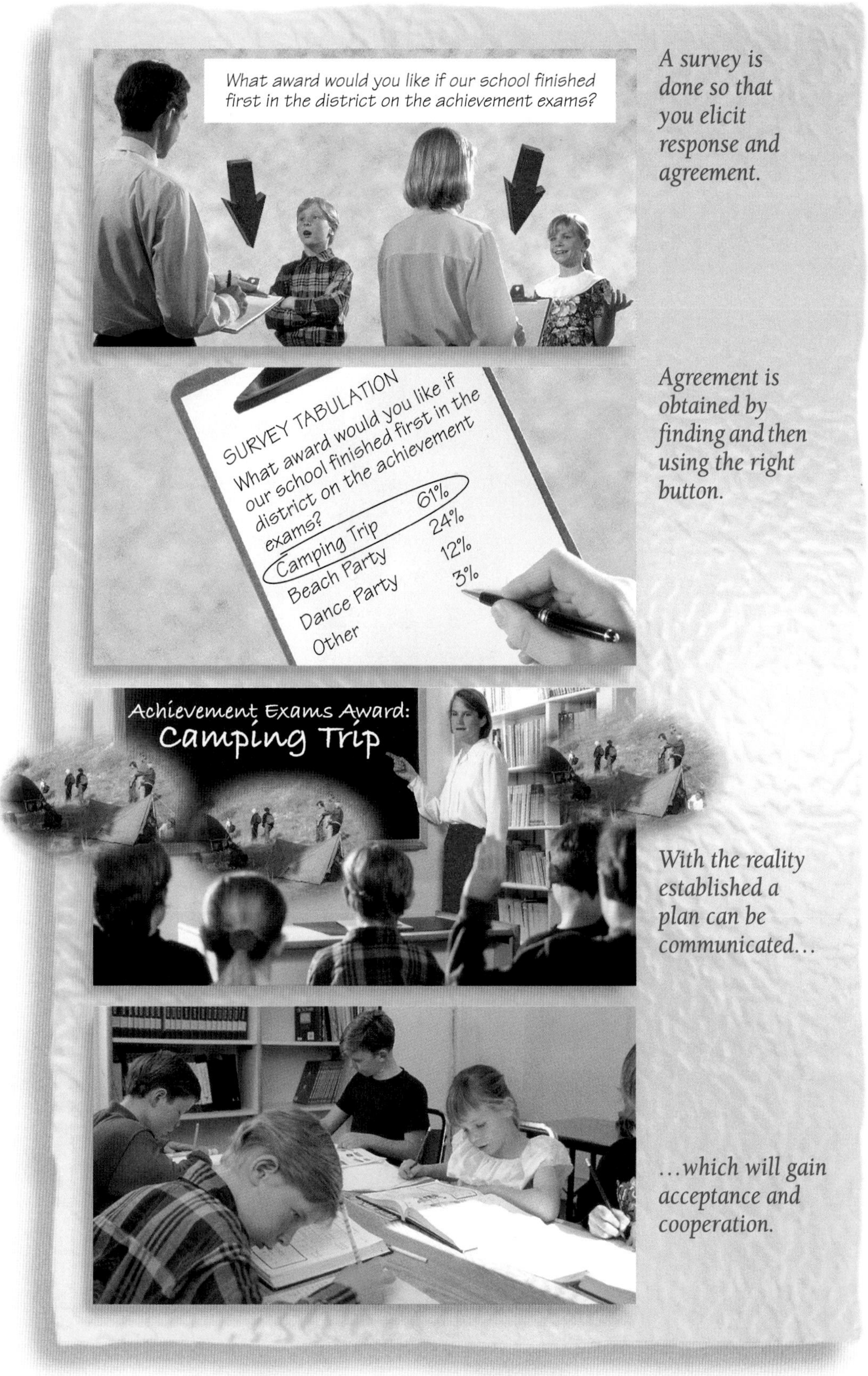

A survey is done so that you elicit response and agreement.

Agreement is obtained by finding and then using the right button.

With the reality established a plan can be communicated…

…which will gain acceptance and cooperation.

HOW TO HANDLE RUMORS AND WHISPERING CAMPAIGNS

There may be times when one's reputation comes under attack by rumor or gossip, giving one a false reality and making him unreal and out of agreement with the people he is in contact with. This situation is the opposite of what good public relations is supposed to accomplish. It amounts to "bad works falsely publicized."

Often a person just shrugs and accepts this as part of life; this is the way it is and there is no trusting human nature. Others bitterly fight to defend their reputations and, lacking the technology of public relations that can show one how to deal with such circumstances, go about it in such a way that their denials only make matters worse.

Slander does not just happen to celebrities or political figures. Rumors and lies can make life unpleasant in any social circle.

What does one do when threatened with such attacks upon one's good name?

There are standard public relations solutions to this problem that one should know and apply if this type of situation ever arises.

"Black propaganda" (black = bad or derogatory; propaganda = pushing out statements or ideas) is the term used to describe the technique employed to destroy reputation or public belief in persons, companies or nations.

The technique of black propaganda seeks to bring a reputation so low that the person, company or nation is denied any rights whatever by "general agreement." It is then possible to destroy the person, company or nation with a minor attack if the black propaganda itself has not already accomplished this.

Vicious and lying gossip by old women was the earlier form of this tactic and was so bad that some areas put them in public stocks (neck yokes) or drove them out of town.

In modern times there is no such check on black propaganda. Difficulties and costs of libel and slander suits, abuse of press privilege, and so forth, lay anyone open to such a campaign.

All one needs is an enemy. And there are few men in history who have been without enemies.

There are random individuals in the society who do not understand very much.

This is expressed as a sort of malicious glee about things. Such pass on slanderous rumors very easily. In an illiterate society such people abound. Since they cannot read, the bulk of knowledge is denied to them. Since they do not know very many words, much of what is said to them is not understood.

This is not isolated to the illiterate only.

What they do not understand they substitute for with imaginary things.

Thus such persons not only listen to slander but also corrupt and twist even it.

Thus a rumor can go through a society that has no basis in truth.

When numbers of such rumors exist and are persistent, one suspects a "whispering campaign." This is not because people whisper these things but because like an evil wind it *seems* to have no source.

Black propaganda makes use of such a willingness to pass on and amplify falsehoods.

Much black propaganda is of course more bold and appears blatantly in irresponsible (or covertly controlled) newspapers and radio and television.

But even after a bad press story has appeared or a bad radio or TV broadcast has been given, the "whispering campaign" is counted upon by black propagandists to carry the slander through the society.

Thus any person, any being, is at risk.

A person comes to fear bad things being said about him. In the face of a whispering campaign, real or imagined, one tends to withdraw, tends to become less active and reach less.

This is equally true of companies and even nations.

Thus, unless one knows how to handle such an attack, one can in fact be made quite miserable and ill.

The Law of the Omitted Data

There is a natural law at work that unfortunately favors black propaganda.

WHERE THERE IS NO DATA AVAILABLE PEOPLE WILL INVENT IT.

This is the Law of the Omitted Data.

A vacuum tends to fill itself. Old philosophers said that "nature abhors a vacuum." Actually the surrounding pressure flows into an area of no pressure.

It is this way with a person, company or nation.

Hit by lies the person tends to withdraw. This already tends to pull things in.

The person does not then wish to put out data. He becomes to some degree a mystery.

To fill that mystery people will invent data.

This is true of persons, companies or nations.

This is where *public relations is a necessity*.

Essentially public relations is the art of making good works well known.

It is a fatal error to think good works speak for themselves. They do not. They must be publicized.

Essentially this is what public relations is. And this is *why* it is—to fill that vacuum of omitted data. In the midst of a black propaganda campaign one is denied normal communication channels. The press media along which the campaign is being conducted will *not* run favorable comment. One is mad if he thinks it will as it is serving other masters that mean to destroy the repute of the target.

"Authoritative" utterances push plain truth out of sight.

Thus public relations people have to be very expert in their technology when they confront black propaganda.

The Handling

When one is not fighting a battle against black propaganda, public relations is easy.

One hires a reporter who gets to work thinking up ideas and turning out releases. That's why reporters are often thought of as public relations people, which they are not.

In the face of a black propaganda campaign, such releases are twisted, refused and that is the end of it.

There is far more to the art than this.

These are some of the rules that apply:

Fill the Vacuum

First of all, cease to withdraw. It is proven conclusively that in public relations handling of black propaganda, only the outflow of information pays off. Saying nothing may be noble in a character but it is fatal in public relations.

Blunt denial is crude and can be used against one as a sort of confirmation.

You don't have to announce or spread a flap and never should. Public relations men often *make* the flap.

But don't interpret this as "silence is necessary." Get in a safe place and speak up.

Use any channel to speak up. But don't seek channels that will corrupt what you say in repeating it.

Don't stay on the same subject that you are being attacked on.

An example of speaking up without denying and thus confirming might be:

STATEMENT: "I read your company went broke last month."

REBUTTAL: "My God. You're telling me! If we hadn't got out of that contract we really would have gone broke. There was a hell of a row in the boardroom. But McLinty won. Scotch to the core. He said, 'I won't sign it!' Like to have tore the president's head off. Hell of a row. Seems like we got 80 million buried somewhere and McLinty is in charge of it and he won't *move an inch* on it."

The interrogator's conclusion is you're not broke. He's got data. The vacuum is filled with a story of board rows and 80 million mysterious reserves.

Disprove False Data

This consists of disproving utterly the false statement with documents or demonstration or display. One has to have a kit (a collection of documents) or the ability to demonstrate or something to display.

STATEMENT: "I've been told you are in trouble with the County Board of Health."

REBUTTAL: "Here's our recently issued health certificate and a letter of commendation from the Board of Health." Displays same.

Result? Whoever told him that is now discredited with him as an accurate informer.

When the person makes some disprovable statement, find *who* to fix his mind on it and then produce the rebuttal.

STATEMENT: "I hear you aren't married to the man you're living with."

REBUTTAL: "*Who* told you that?"

STATER: "I forget."

REBUTTER: "Well, you remember and I'll show you some proof."

STATER: "Well, it was a man...."

REBUTTER: "*Who?*"

STATER: "Joe Schmo."

REBUTTER: "Okay. Here's my marriage certificate. Who's the Joe Schmo nut anyway?"

Now it's Joe Schmo who's the mystery. How come he lies? What's in it for him?

When one hasn't got the document but can get it, one can say, "You tell me the name of whoever said that and next time I see you I'll show you something *very* interesting about it."

And be sure to get the document and see him again.

There are a billion variations. "It won't fly." Fly it. "Place is empty." Show him it's full.

The subject matter of this is *proof* in whatever form.

You only challenge statements you *can* prove are false and in any conversation let the rest slide.

Disprove Every Rumor

Proving negatives is almost impossible. "How do I know you aren't a CIA man?" Well, how can one prove that? One can't whip out a KGB badge as that would be just as bad. No one ever wrote a document, "Bill Till is not a member of the CIA." Useless. It is a denial. Who'd believe it?

Sometimes "You don't" works.

But the right answer to a negative (no proof) is to "fill the vacuum."

And once in a while you *can* prove a negative. Accused of drug smuggling one can show he's a member of the antidrug league. The counter in a negative proof must be *creditable.*

A million million variations exist.

Where there is no data available people will invent it. This law unfortunately favors black propaganda.

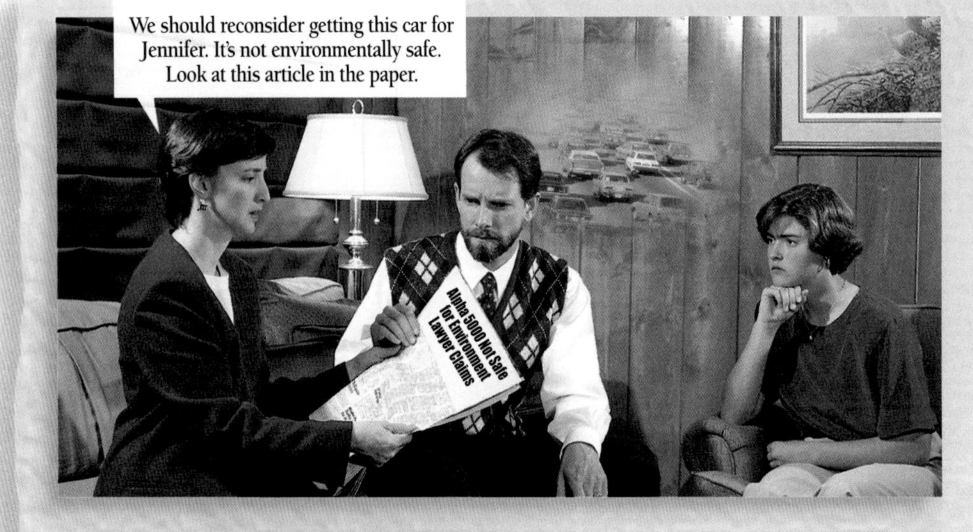
We should reconsider getting this car for Jennifer. It's not environmentally safe. Look at this article in the paper.
Alpha 5000 Not Safe for Environment Lawyer Claims

If the vacuum is filled by true data…

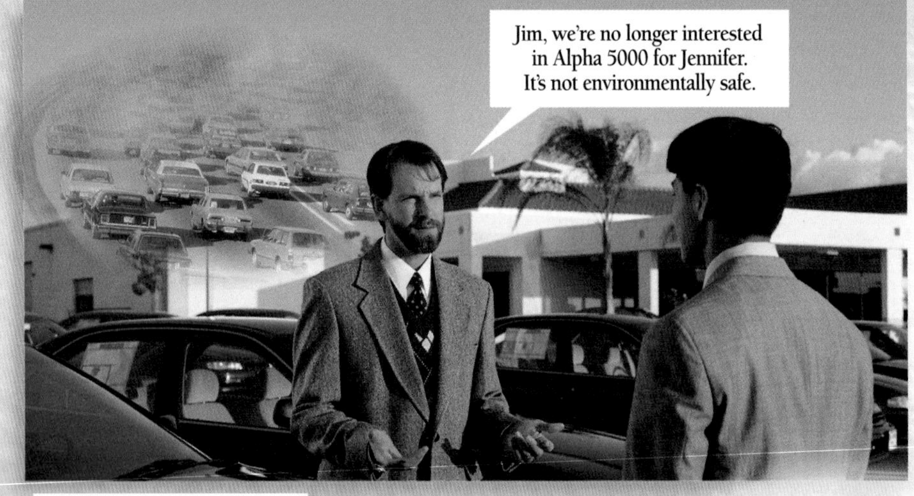
Jim, we're no longer interested in Alpha 5000 for Jennifer. It's not environmentally safe.

…the black propaganda is seen to be a lie and vanishes.

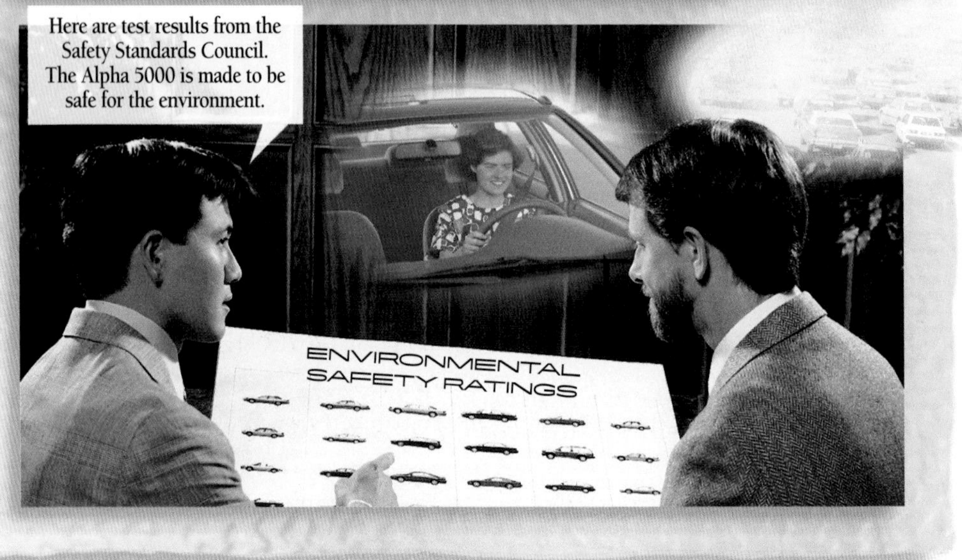
Here are test results from the Safety Standards Council. The Alpha 5000 is made to be safe for the environment.
ENVIRONMENTAL SAFETY RATINGS

The basis of it is *not* to be the thing rumored and to be able to prove it fast.

Continue to Fill the Vacuum

Continuous good works and effective release of material about one's good works is vital.

Pamphlets, brochures, press releases, one's own newspaper and magazine, these and many more, must be supplied with *a comprehensible identity of self.*

Distributing or using these, one publicizes one's own good works.

And one must also *do* good works. One must, through his good works and actions at least, be visible.

So a continual, truthful and artful torrent of public relations pieces must occur.

Then one day there is no enemy.

And one's repute is high.

There may be other attacks but now one can handle them as small fires and not as a whole burning forest.

You can see that black propaganda is a covert attack on the reputation of a person, company or nation, using slander and lies in order to weaken or destroy.

Defense presupposes that the target is not that bad.

One does not have to be perfect to withstand such an attack, but it helps.

But even if one *were* perfect it would be no defense. Almost all the saints in history have been subjected to such attacks. And most of them died of it.

The answer is public relations *technology skillfully applied.*

To be skillful in anything, one has to know it and be experienced in it and *do* it.

EASING HUMAN RELATIONS

There is another basic element of public relations that is often overlooked and given far too little importance, but when applied correctly can give one a foundation for success in dealing with others.

The original procedure developed by man to oil the machinery of human relationships was "good manners."

Various other terms that describe this procedure are politeness, decorum, formality, etiquette, form, courtesy, refinement, polish, culture, civility, courtliness and respect.

Even the most primitive cultures had highly developed rituals of human relationship. A study of twenty-one different primitive races shows the formalities which attended their interpersonal and intertribal and interracial relationships to be quite impressive.

Throughout all races, "bad manners" are condemned.

Those with "bad manners" are *rejected.*

Thus the primary technology of public relations was "manners."

Therefore, a person or team of people applying the techniques of public relations who have not drilled and mastered the manners accepted as "good manners" by those being contacted will fail. Such a person or team may know all the senior PR technology and yet fail miserably on the sole basis of "exhibiting bad manners."

"Good manners" sum up to:

(a) granting importance to the other person and

(b) using the two-way communication cycle.

In dealing with people, it is impossible to get one's ideas across and gain any acceptance without a two-way communication cycle.

By "cycle" is meant a span of time with a beginning and an end. In a cycle of communication we have one person originating a communication to a second person who receives the communication, understands it and acknowledges it, thus ending the cycle. In a *two-way* communication cycle, the second person now originates a communication to the first person who receives it, understands it and acknowledges it. In other words, the two-way communication cycle is a normal cycle of a communication between two people. It is not a two-way communication cycle if either person fails, in his turn, to originate a communication when he should.

Whatever motions or rituals there are, these two factors—granting importance to the other person, and using the two-way communication cycle—are involved. Thus a person violating them will find himself and his program rejected.

Arrogance and force may win dominion and control but will never win acceptance and respect.

For all his "mental technology" the psychiatrist or psychologist could never win applause or general goodwill because they are personally (a) arrogant beyond belief (b) hold others in scathing contempt ("man is an animal," "people are all insane," etc.).

They just don't have "good manners"; i.e., they do not (a) consider or give others a feeling of importance and (b) they are total strangers to a communication cycle.

Successful PR

All successful public relations, then, is built upon the bedrock of good manners, as these are the first technology developed to ease human relations.

Good manners are much more widely known and respected than public relations technology. Therefore *no* public relations technology will be successful if this element is omitted.

Brushing off "mere guards" as beneath one's notice while one goes after a contact with their boss can be fatal. Who talks to their boss? These "mere guards."

Making an appointment and not keeping it, issuing an invitation too late for it to be accepted, not offering food or a drink, not standing up when a lady or important man enters, treating one's subordinates like lackeys in public, raising one's voice harshly in public, interrupting what someone else is saying to "do something important," not saying thank you or good night—these are all "bad manners." People who do these or a thousand other discourtesies are mentally rejected by those with whom they come into contact.

As public relations is basically acceptance then bad manners defeat it utterly.

To apply the techniques of PR successfully, a person has to have good manners.

This is not hard. One has to assess his attitude toward others and iron it out. Are they individually important? And then he has to have his two-way communication cycle so perfect and natural, it is never noticed.

Given those two things, a person can now learn the bits of ritual that go to make up the procedure that is considered "good manners" in the group with which he is associating.

Then given public relations technology correctly used, one has successful PR.

Importance

You have no idea how important people are. There is a reversed ratio—those at the bottom have a self-importance *far* greater than those at the top who *are* important. A charlady's (cleaning woman's) concept of her own importance is far greater than that of a successful general manager!

Ignore people at your peril.

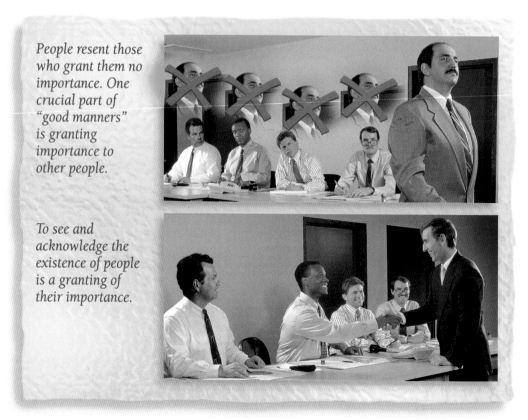

People resent those who grant them no importance. One crucial part of "good manners" is granting importance to other people.

To see and acknowledge the existence of people is a granting of their importance.

Flattery is not very useful, is often suspect, as it does not come from a sincere belief and the falsity in it is detectable to all but a fool.

A person's importance is made evident to him by showing him respect, or just by assuring him he is visible and acceptable.

To see and acknowledge the existence of someone is a granting of their importance.

To know their name and their connections also establishes importance.

Asserting one's *own* importance is about as acceptable as a dead cat at a wedding.

People have value and are important. Big or small they are important.

If you know that, you are halfway home with good manners.

Thus public relations can occur.

Communication

The two-way communication cycle is more important than the content.

The content of the communication, the meaning to be put across to another or others, is secondary to the fact of a two-way communication cycle.

Communication exists to be replied to or used.

Communication, with the communication cycle present first, must exist before it carries any message.

Messages do not travel on no communication line. The line or route along which a communication travels from one person to another must be there.

Advertising is always violating this. "Buy Beanos!" into the empty air. Other things must establish the line. And the line must be such as to obtain an answer, either by use or purchase or reply.

A funny example was a salesman who without preamble or reason wrote to people and told them to buy a multithousand-dollar product without even an explanation of its use or value. Response zero. No communication line. He was writing to a name but not really to anyone.

In social intercourse a communication cycle must be established before any acceptance of the speaker can occur. Then one might get across a message.

A communication which travels in one direction only never establishes a two-way communication cycle. In social situations, acceptance of the person won't occur without it.

Good manners require a two-way communication cycle between oneself and the other person.

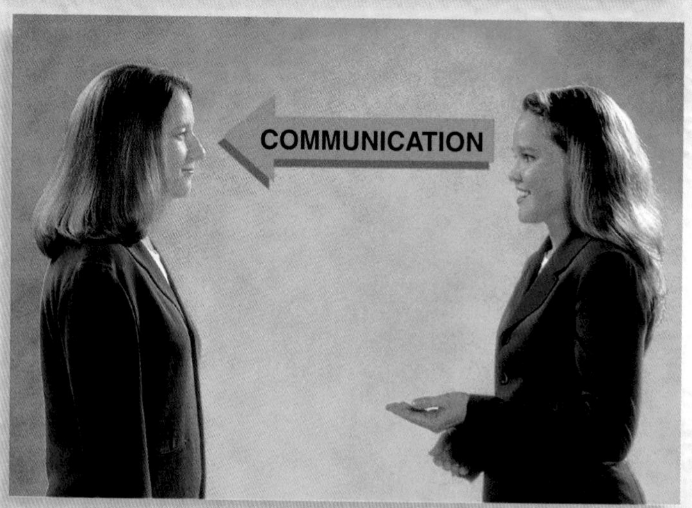

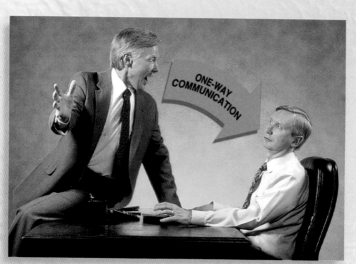

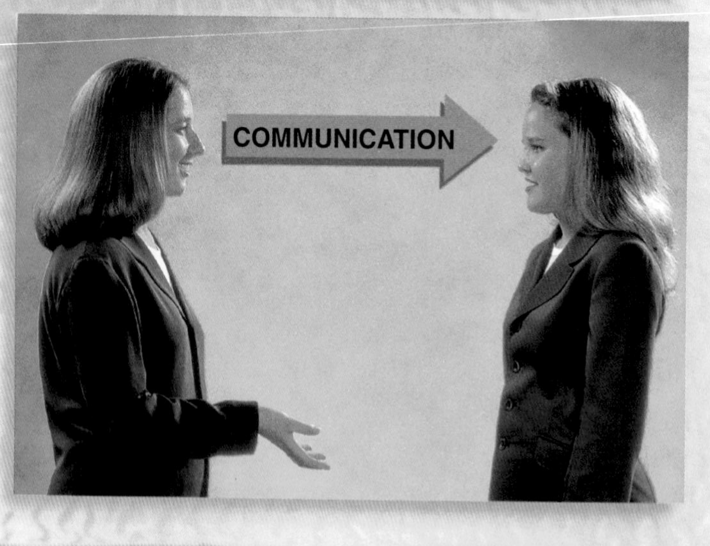

Good manners require a two-way communication cycle. This is even true of social letters and phone calls.

Out of this one gets "telling the hostess good night as one leaves."

One really has to understand the two-way communication cycle to have really good manners.

Without a two-way communication cycle, public relations is pretty poor stuff.

Rituals

If an American Indian's ritual of conference was so exact and complex, if a thousand other primitive races had precise social conduct and forms of address, then it is not too much to ask modern man to have good manners as well.

But "good manners" are less apparent in our times than they once were. This comes about because the intermingling of so many races and customs have tended to destroy the ritual patterns once well established in the smaller units.

So one appears to behold a sloppy age of manners.

This is no excuse to have bad manners.

One can have excellent manners by just observing:

a. Importance of people

b. Two-way communication cycle

c. Local rituals observed as proper conduct

These are the first musts of someone applying PR technology.

On that foundation can be built an acceptable public relations presence that makes PR succeed.

PR TECHNOLOGY

One can influence the community as a whole with public relations technology.

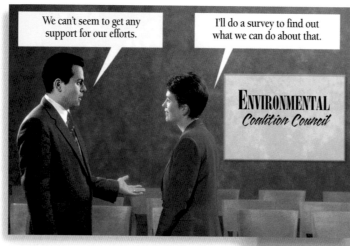

We can't seem to get any support for our efforts.

I'll do a survey to find out what we can do about that.

ENVIRONMENTAL Coalition Council

A survey done on sufficient numbers of the public…

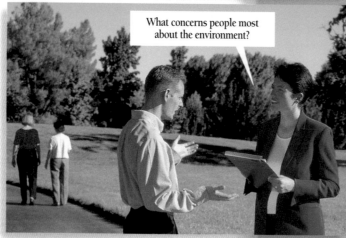

…discloses the concern that is most real to them.

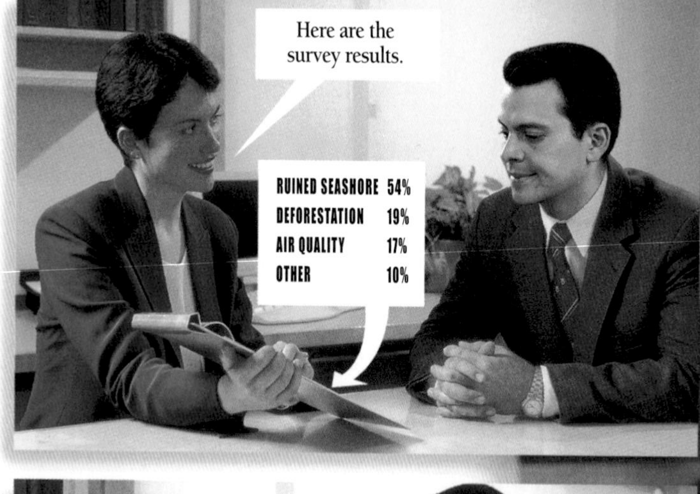

A program can then be drawn up for the group that forwards their goals and which now gains community support.

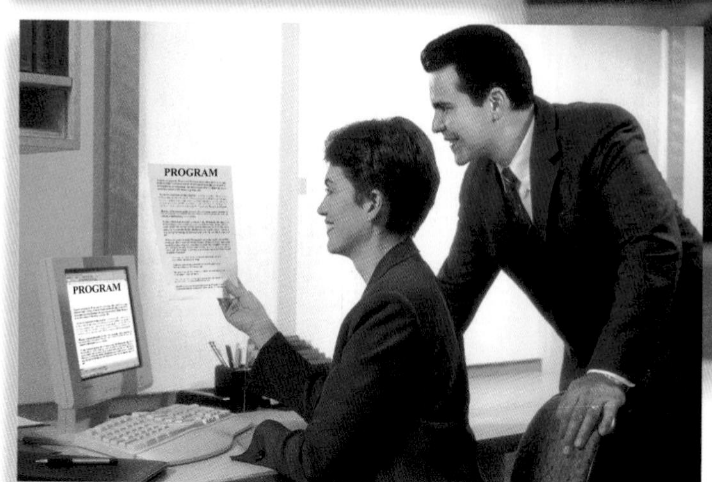

HELPS YOU MAKE A BETTER WORLD

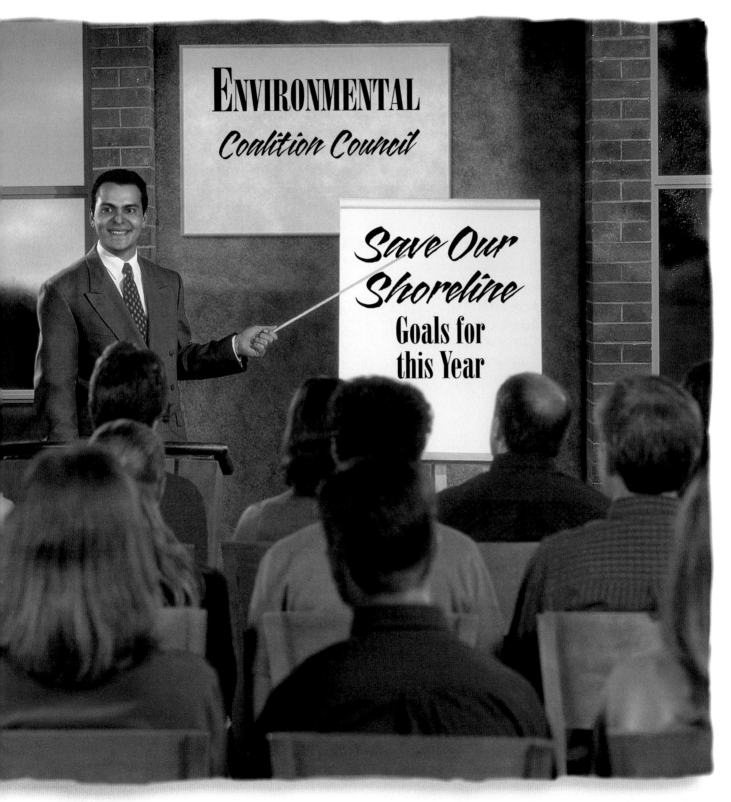

The result is increased cooperation with actions that improve conditions in society and the world.

PUBLIC RELATIONS APPLICATION

No matter how worthwhile your purpose or activity, you can't just depend on the agreement and cooperation of others. Unless your purposes are made known and real, there is little reason for others to support your efforts.

Public relations is the method one can use to get that support.

There are many PR tools available. For instance, one has surveys to discover his publics and the reality and acceptance level of each. One has the ARC triangle with the two-way cycle of communication to raise affinity and reality. There is the knowledge of manners, granting importance to others and observing their rituals, which will help one successfully interact with them.

The tools are numerous, but they must be well known and skillfully applied in order to gain the agreement of others.

There are many worthy purposes that will help this world become a better place. But no man stands alone in society, and if one wants his purposes accomplished, the cooperation of others is always necessary.

If you have a purpose to help others and improve society, you can utilize public relations to make your task easier.

Many other people have similar goals to yours, and with this technology, you can reach them. Anything that is truly worthwhile is worth getting done—and you are not likely to accomplish it by yourself. PR is how you get others to work with you. ■

TEST YOUR UNDERSTANDING

Answer the following questions about public relations. Refer back to the chapter to check your answers. If you need to, review the chapter. Going over the material several times will increase your certainty and help you better apply it.

- ❑ *What is public relations?*
- ❑ *What was the missing ingredient in earlier studies of public relations?*
- ❑ *What is a "public"?*
- ❑ *How can one use surveys in PR?*
- ❑ *How does one tabulate a survey?*
- ❑ *What is "black propaganda"?*
- ❑ *How does one handle "black propaganda"?*
- ❑ *What do "good manners" sum up to?*

PRACTICAL EXERCISES

Here are exercises relating to public relations. Doing these will increase your understanding of the data.

1 Look around your environment and name as many different "publics" as possible. Do this until you are certain you can correctly determine various publics who would be addressed with a separate PR message.

2 Choose a specific group or public in an area or activity which you have some familiarity with. Conduct a survey on that group or public to establish their reality on some subject.

3 Tabulate the responses to the survey you did in the previous exercise, using the data in this chapter on tabulating survey responses.

4 Write down an example from your own observation or experience of the Law of the Omitted Data: "WHERE THERE IS NO DATA AVAILABLE PEOPLE WILL INVENT IT." Then give specific ways in which the person or persons involved could handle the situation using the data on PR covered in this chapter. Repeat this as many times as needed until you are certain you can correctly observe examples of the Law of the Omitted Data and know how to handle them using PR technology.

5 Find several local rituals observed as proper conduct in your area which should be observed if one is to have "good manners."

6 Go out and practice "good manners" by just observing:

a. Importance of people

b. Two-way communication cycle

c. Local rituals observed as proper conduct

Do this until you can practice good manners with certainty.

RESULTS FROM APPLICATION

The technology of public relations and surveys, as developed by L. Ron Hubbard, can open any door. People who have studied this data have been amazed at its simplicity and applicability. With it, causes can be fought for and won. Ideas can be accepted where they wouldn't have been before and real production can occur unhindered. As the successes below illustrate, PR is an indispensable tool.

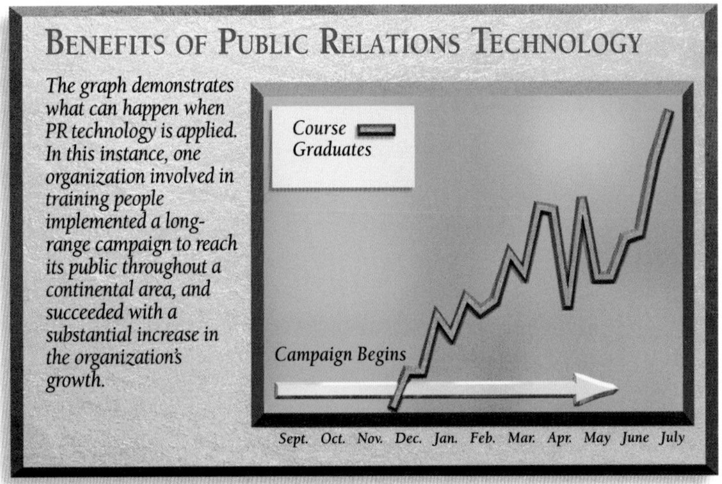

BENEFITS OF PUBLIC RELATIONS TECHNOLOGY
The graph demonstrates what can happen when PR technology is applied. In this instance, one organization involved in training people implemented a long-range campaign to reach its public throughout a continental area, and succeeded with a substantial increase in the organization's growth.
Course Graduates
Campaign Begins
Sept. Oct. Nov. Dec. Jan. Feb. Mar. Apr. May June July

A woman in South America found that the female police in the city were having difficulty in getting along with the people in their district. After speaking to several of these police officers, she isolated their problem to a lack of technology on communication. She then gave a series of lectures on this subject to the female police in the city, including the basic data on "manners" and the ARC triangle. As a result she received the following acknowledgment from the Second Superintendent Commander of the Female Police who presented a plaque saying:

"In the name of the General Secretariat of Protection and Public Traffic of the Federal District Department, we acknowledge you for the valuable and altruistic promotion of the technology of L. Ron Hubbard. For giving the female police a better relationship with the citizens by the use of affinity, reality and communication, thus improving our image in the society."

A newly appointed public relations director used Scientology technology to establish goodwill for a company which had just moved to a new location. Here are his results:

"As the newly appointed public relations director for a company which had just moved to a new location, my first assignment was to establish goodwill for the company in the local community. New to the area myself, my first action was to apply L. Ron Hubbard's technology on public relations. I had surveys done in the local neighborhood to find out what the residents thought was important or needed and wanted in the area. It soon became evident that crime was of major concern and the community wanted something effective done. With this data to hand I then met with the local police. In coordination with them, I used Mr. Hubbard's data on targets and programs and worked out a neighborhood crime watch program. Volunteers from the company, who were also concerned about crime, spent a few hours each day to help

implement the targets of the program by canvassing the local area getting each resident to participate in the program. Thanks to the effectiveness of this program, the crime rate in the area plummeted considerably within a matter of weeks. Not only was something actually done to handle the crime problem in that area (which was very much appreciated), but good relations with the community were established for the company as well."

Being newly employed in the complaints department of a large company became a challenge for a California woman as she found that its repair service department had broken promises to customers about the return of repaired appliances. She had studied Mr. Hubbard's technology of PR and used it to totally change the area and handle the past bad standing the company had with its customers.

"Initially I regularly got complaints. The public did not know when they would get their repairs done. That their electrical appliances were being handled in forty-eight hours was a pleasant surprise to all.

"I did have a customer on the phone at one point who had called because her appliance had been in repair for more than forty-eight hours. When I checked, I found that a special part was being gotten to improve the appearance of the appliance. I told her what was being done, where exactly the appliance was on the repair line and when she could expect it. She thanked me and was really thrilled that she was basically getting back a brand-new electrical appliance.

"I have created excellent public relations for my company—our customers now know they can trust me and my company to deliver what is promised. The managing director knows that he never has to bother about the repairs, delivery and unhandled complaints, whereas earlier these matters were always on his plate. The importance of honesty and PR is now completely real to me—this technology makes my job a pleasure."

The country of Colombia has been torn by civil violence and unrest for several years. Resolving to draw wide attention to efforts to reduce violence in their country, a group of concerned citizens utilized L. Ron Hubbard's Public Relations Technology to determine how best to make the point that violence has no part in their society. They then began a campaign to raise the level of honesty in the community, using Scientology principles of integrity and right and wrong. As a result, they got hundreds of Colombian youth gathered at an amusement park and demonstrated their desire for a country without war and violence by tossing toy guns into a fire. Their demonstration was broadcast to the entire country and had a major impact. A few weeks later, a letter was received from the president's office, endorsing the group's actions which was made known to the nation through radio and television. It said, in part:

"A few weeks later, a Colombian guerrilla group followed suit by publicly laying down their weapons (real ones), burning them and saying no to violence, murder and destruction and saying yes to peace, happiness and survival."

SUGGESTIONS FOR FURTHER STUDY

The data in this chapter represents only a fraction of L. Ron Hubbard's materials that are applicable to the subject of public relations. All basic books on the Scientology philosophy are applicable to the subject of relations between people, but the following books in particular are recommended as further study.

Dianetics 55!

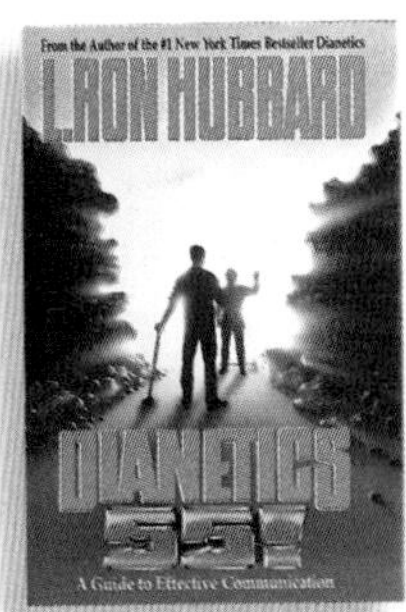

Contains Mr. Hubbard's most complete description of communication, its components and use in life, with thorough explanations of all its aspects. It is the complete manual on communication and essential for those who wish to fully understand the subject.

Science of Survival

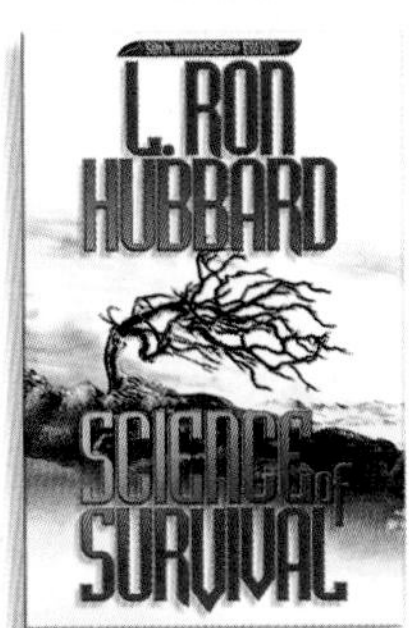

Provides the most complete description of human behavior ever written, making it an indispensable text for anyone who deals with people. One can use the book to accurately predict what another will do in any situation in life. This vital Scientology technology has been used for more than forty years by people in all walks of life, to help them better understand others and attain greater affinity, reality and communication.

Scientology 8-8008

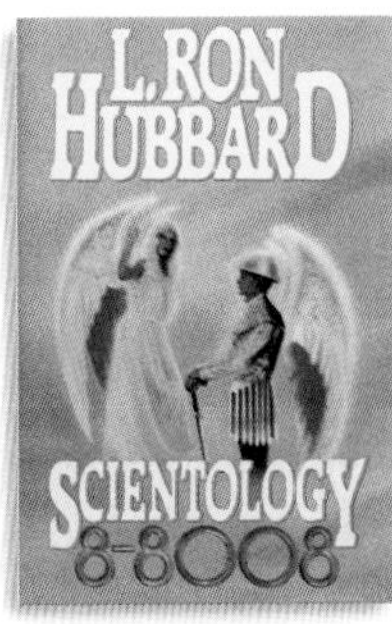

This book contains a wealth of information about human behavior. It fully covers affinity, reality and communication and other fundamental concepts that lead to a more profound understanding of life and the universe. This advanced book on Scientology principles is invaluable to anyone dealing with people in any capacity.

Management Series Volumes

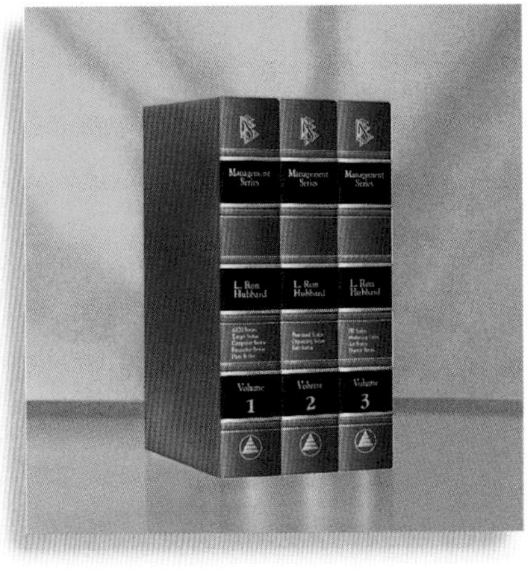

Mr. Hubbard applied his discoveries about the spirit and life to the survival of groups, and developed a whole body of technology to help both individuals and groups attain their goals. A three-volume set, the *Management Series Volumes* contain vital data on such topics as how to apply the ARC triangle and the cycle of communication in handling personnel, how to help group members learn their jobs better, how to set objectives for a group, ways to attain targets and goals, and how to best organize different types of projects and activities, and many more.

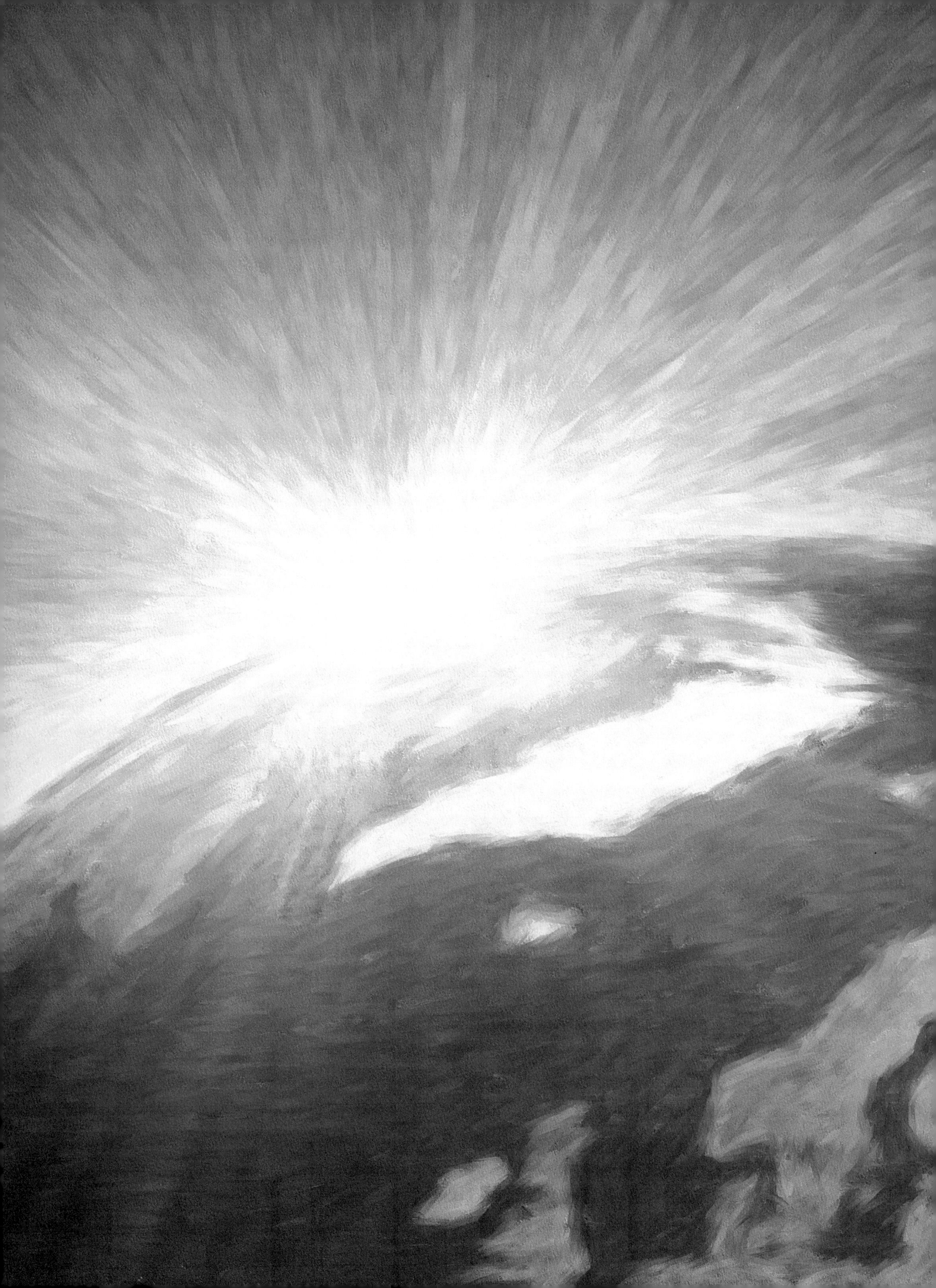

You, Scientology and the World

Building a Better World

Imagine a world where people have the technology to change conditions and create happier, more productive lives.

Where pain and suffering are rapidly alleviated.

Where people have the tools necessary to organize their activities and achieve their goals.

Where the source of conflicts is rapidly detected and those quarrels are easily resolved.

Where destructive antisocial personalities are recognized for who they are.

Where, in fact, there is no insanity, no criminals or war, where the able prosper and honest beings have rights, and where man is free to rise to greater heights.

Such a world not only can exist, but it is within our reach, for the technology is available.

And for such a world to actually become a reality, all it would take is for people to apply this technology.

All good is done by individuals, as are all evils. In fact, as has been pointed out in this book, the social ills of man are chiefly a composite of his personal difficulties. And it is the combined dishonesties of individuals that add to the formidable total of mankind's problems.

Yet, formidable as they may appear, the resolution of these ills lies in their very composition. For if individuals can create them, then individuals can resolve them. In fact, the truth is that *only* the actions of individuals will change conditions. And the tools an individual needs to do just that can be found in the pages of this handbook.

You have probably read much of this book by now. And, possibly, you have even applied some of the knowledge to yourself or people around you. Perhaps you have given an assist to a neighbor or a child. Or utilized the principles of affinity, reality and communication to bring about a better understanding with someone. If so, you have clearly seen that what has been presented here is not simply theory dreamed up in some ivory tower, but *practical wisdom that works.*

In the event you have not yet applied this knowledge, do so. You have nothing to lose and much to gain. It is true that man has been fooled so often with promises of help that he tends to doubt them all. Nor can he be blamed for doing so. But the simplicity of Scientology is that it promises nothing, it asks only that you apply its principles exactly as presented and see if they work for you.

And after you have done this, you will find yourself facing a rather startling realization:

Within your hands you have a technology you can use to actually help yourself and others, methods you can apply to improve the conditions you see around you.

You, an individual, have the tools to bring about change.

Turning the Tide

You have read about the dynamics of life, eight in all, beginning with the first dynamic, self, and expanding to the eighth, the infinity dynamic. You read also that a man is as well off as he enhances the survival of all these dynamics.

Which brings up an interesting question: What responsibility does an individual have for knowledge? If you have discovered the workability of the knowledge contained in Scientology and have developed a certainty that it could help your fellow man, what responsibility do you have for that?

If no dynamic other than the first existed, you would have no responsibility other than to help yourself. But there are seven more dynamics and, as you have read, if you reduce them to nothing, sooner or later the first dynamic reduces to nothing. Therefore, one cannot sit back and watch his family, his work environment, his community, even his society or culture go downhill. The most wrong thing one can do is to do nothing.

Unfortunately, many people choose to live under the delusion that others are already taking care of the problems that face society. The police are taking care of crime. Doctors are taking care of disease. Educators are taking care of education. And someone is taking care of the environment.

Why then, with all these problems being taken care of by others, are they not disappearing? Why are they instead snowballing into explosive crises that threaten the survival of not only our society but the world we live in? Obviously, they are not being resolved.

It is important to understand that bad conditions don't just happen. The cultural decay we see around us isn't haphazard. It was caused. Unless one understands this he won't be able to defend himself or reach out into society with effectiveness.

The real solution, of course, is to let a man know he is himself a spiritual being, that he is capable of the power of choice and has the right to aspire to greater wisdom. With this, you have started him up a higher road.

Yet the time to bring chaos under control is before it is well begun. And we are slightly late as it is. The world is facing several crises of magnitude.

Only wisdom can reverse this situation. Wisdom held by many, not one man or some priestly elite. Wisdom held and used by individuals like you. As you have seen, however, this is not theoretical wisdom merely to be studied between pages of a book. It is practical knowledge for application.

You are encouraged to utilize *The Scientology Handbook* to learn and then use these basics to relieve your fellows of their sufferings and problems.

The fundamental ingredients needed to do this are simple: the decision to do something and a strong purpose to help others.

Can the formidable tide of cultural decay and societal insanity be changed?

Of course. Not only by highly trained Scientologists, but also by those who take it upon themselves to apply this data, those who read this book.

What You Can Do

Your first step should be to help the best friend you have. As Mr. Hubbard said, "Probably the most neglected friend you have is you. And yet every man, before he can be a true friend to the world, must first become a friend to himself."

Become a friend to yourself by using this handbook to put order into your own life. Apply the data to areas you feel could be improved.

Whether you use the technology of communication in your dealings with others or use an assist to recover from an injury or the data on organization to structure your activities, you will soon notice a difference. Things will begin to change—perhaps gradually or perhaps suddenly—but they *will* improve.

There truly is no better way to find out how well Scientology works than to try it on yourself. Once you gain familiarity with the tools and the fact of their workability becomes more real to you, you will feel much more confident applying them to others.

You should know that the key to the handling of any area, to improve it, is to *bring order.* But there is a datum about this: Every time you put some order into an individual's life or a group or society, a little confusion blows off. It appears, then dissipates.

Ignore the confusion. It is transitory. Order is not. It *stays.* The wrong thing to do is give up. Persist with what you are doing to put in order and it will begin to resolve the situation. Start with one thing. Resolve it. Then move to the next and resolve that. Step by step, you will master the situation.

It is important to know this data about disorder, as it will help you through any rough spots you encounter. If you follow this basic rule and persist, you will succeed.

The technology of Scientology works when honestly and correctly applied. It is a workable system. Study it well and then apply it *exactly* as it is presented in this book. You *will* get the results.

To begin applying this technology, you need meet no more people than you already know. You'll soon discover that many have need of help in different areas of their lives.

The best way to gain confidence and certainty with any of these tools is to use them and use them again. By all means, review the text of this book between uses. But remember, no action, where action is needed, leaves a situation in place—and it will only worsen. Situations do not "go away" by themselves. They are either handled or they worsen.

Perhaps you have friends with marital problems. By having them study the data in the marriage chapter, helping them clean up their overts and withholds and providing them with the basic data about communication, there is much you could do to help them.

It is not unlikely that you know someone with a drug or alcohol problem. By utilizing the information you now have on drug rehabilitation, you could salvage a life.

Whatever the need, start with the individuals you care for and, step by step, you will expand your ability to improve your environment.

It is important that as many people as possible who now have this technology increase their spheres of action by getting it applied more broadly on the communication lines of the world. The neighborhoods, the factories, the marts of trade, the schools, the hospitals, the halls of government will all benefit from your presence with this technology.

When you make a company win, the whole world wins. When you make a neighborhood win, we all win.

There are many activities you can become involved in. These could include:

Joining local clubs and community groups.

Delivering seminars or lectures based on chapters of this handbook to various groups of people such as company employees, community associations and so forth.

Helping your local schools, organizing the parents and upgrading standards of education by implementing Study Technology.

Organizing a community group to make your neighborhood safer.

Applying Ethics Technology to help troubled teenagers sort out their lives.

These and many similar activities will do much to bring about change and improvement in any areas you choose to address.

One person can do much, but a group can do more.

The individuals you help should not be allowed to just drift away. There is so much more that could be done to help them better deal with life. And once they have started to improve their own lives, many will be anxious to help others. For this reason, you should invite those you have helped to form the core of a group. Together, you can accomplish a great deal for your community. Using surveys, you can find what people in the community want improved and form a group to handle this with the technology in this book. Or you can help an existing group with worthwhile purposes achieve its goals.

People will not participate if there is an absence of purpose *they* can understand. Therefore it is important to have a clear and stated purpose. For example, you can announce a program to raise personal efficiency. This would be the agreed-upon purpose. Or you can initiate a program to tutor local children who are having difficulty with their studies, or another to rid your neighborhood of crime. There are many such purposes people will be willing to contribute to.

As your group grows, and as your members get more and more training from this book and the many courses available in Scientology churches and missions, its impact upon the environment will increase. You will find there is no more rewarding activity than helping others.

THE VOLUNTEER MINISTER

Through the application of Scientology we are taking effective steps to arrest and reverse the deterioration of the world.

The activities described here are the traditional domain of religion, as Mr. Hubbard says, to "help civilize society, bring it conscience and kindness and love and freedom from travail by instilling into it trust, decency, honesty and tolerance."

More specifically, this is the function of the minister: to administer help to alleviate the tortured troubles of man. Thus, in Scientology we have the Volunteer Minister.

Thousands of Volunteer Ministers use Scientology to help their fellows in communities throughout the world.

Anyone of any denomination can train to become a Volunteer Minister. You can go to your nearest Scientology church or mission and do a course based on this book. If that is not practical, you can do an extension course by mail to help you become more skilled in these procedures.

A Volunteer Minister understands that something needs to be done about the world and though he may not be a professionally trained Scientology auditor, he nevertheless wants to do what he can for those around him. By training as a Volunteer Minister he learns basic tools he can then use to help people he knows or meets in life. And by joining with like-minded individuals he can participate in a wide variety of community projects and bring about even greater change.

To become able to handle more complex situations and, in fact, to fully handle *any* situation in life, you need to train further and become an auditor. This training is done in Scientology churches.

However, simply by using this handbook now, you will get results. More than were ever available to you before. But further training will expand your effectiveness.

In your own life, among families, in neighborhoods and towns, among community groups and governments, whether working together with others or alone, it is individuals like you who are using the practical wisdom of Scientology to improve a troubled world.

Becoming a Volunteer Minister

Volunteer Ministers willingly supply help in areas wherever it is needed. They do this on a part-time volunteer basis, fully realizing the necessity to contribute toward bettering conditions in the world around them.

A full study of the **Scientology Handbook** *is the first step to becoming a Volunteer Minister. To help you become more proficient applying the principles herein, your local Scientology church or mission offers two courses based upon this handbook: one which can be studied at home and another delivered in the classroom.*

Following this, one must gain practical experience in helping others and do further training in order to become a fully certified Volunteer Minister. Complete details about this program are available from your local church or mission. (A listing of churches, missions and other groups is at the back of the book.)

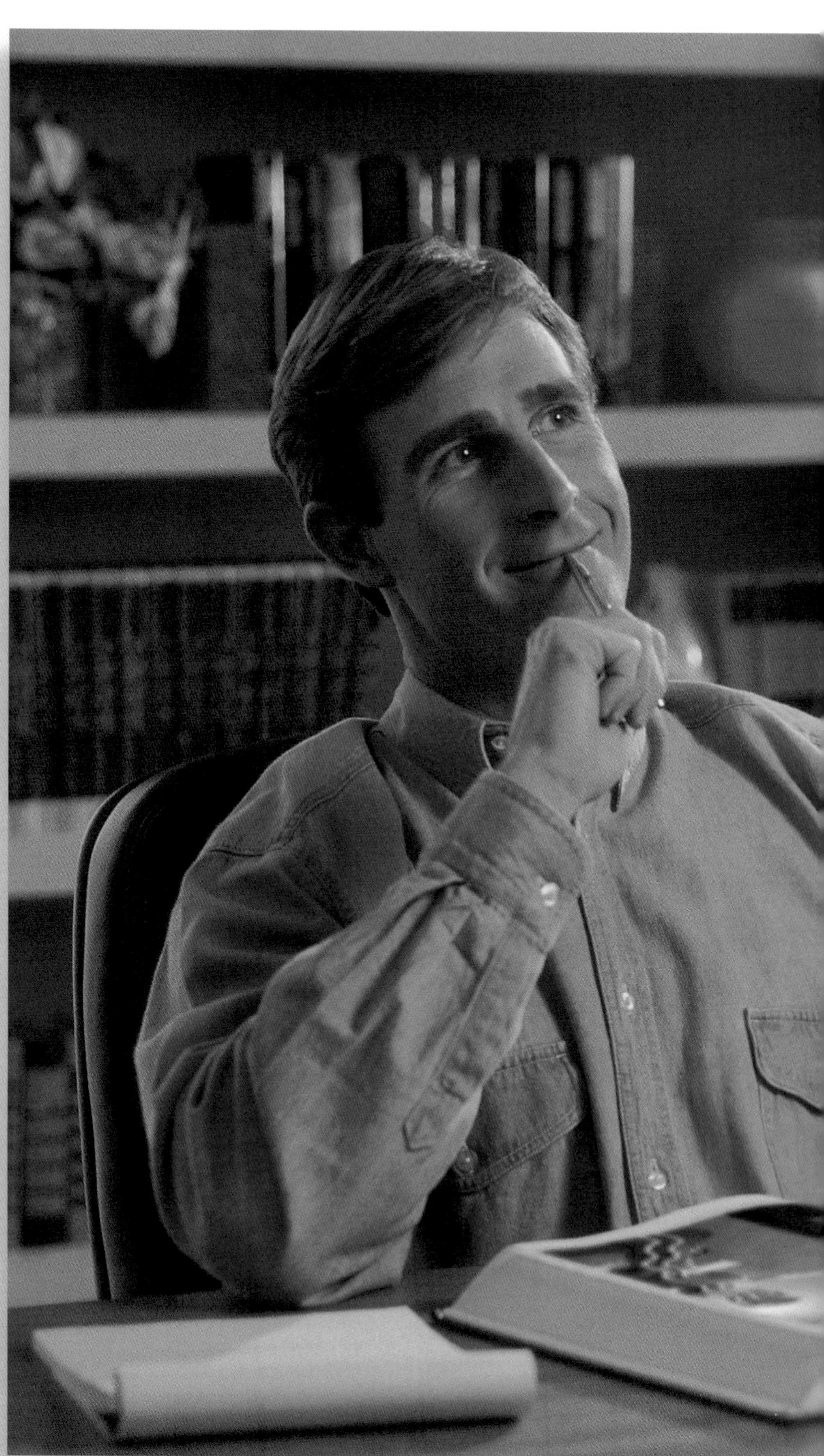

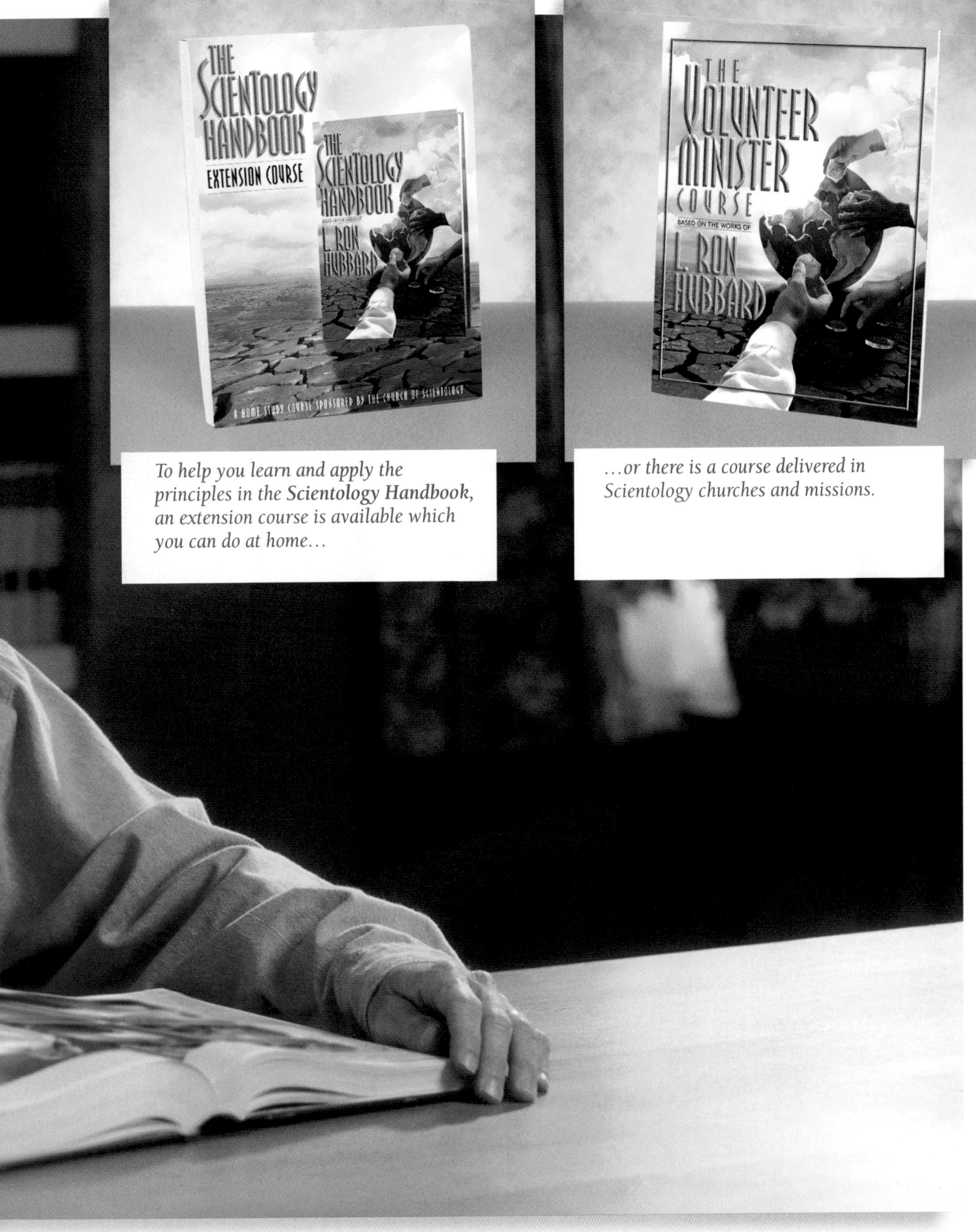

To help you learn and apply the principles in the ***Scientology Handbook****, an extension course is available which you can do at home…*

…or there is a course delivered in Scientology churches and missions.

Making Help Broadly Available

To help you help others, nineteen booklets are available, each one containing the contents of a chapter in this handbook. These valuable tools can be given singly or in bulk to groups, friends, associates or people you meet and want to help.

Their usefulness is virtually limitless. For instance, the booklet on communication will help anyone who has problems with this vital part of life. Or, if you were counseling someone who had difficulty getting along with others, you would have him study the booklet dealing with affinity, reality and communication. Whatever the problem or need, whether it involves assists, organization, personal goals or marriages, the appropriate booklet will provide workable solutions.

To get copies of these booklets, simply contact your nearest church or mission or the publisher directly.

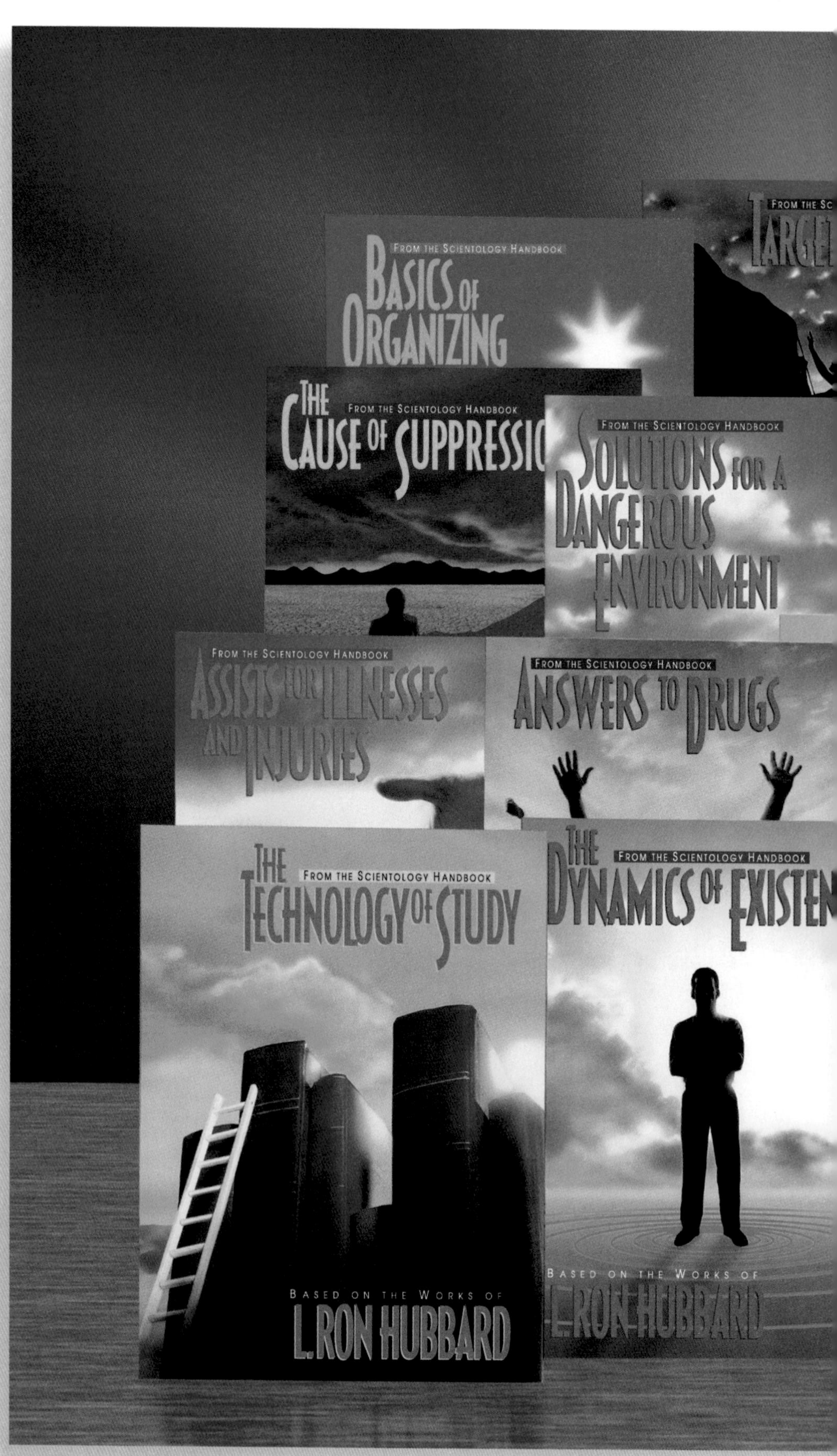

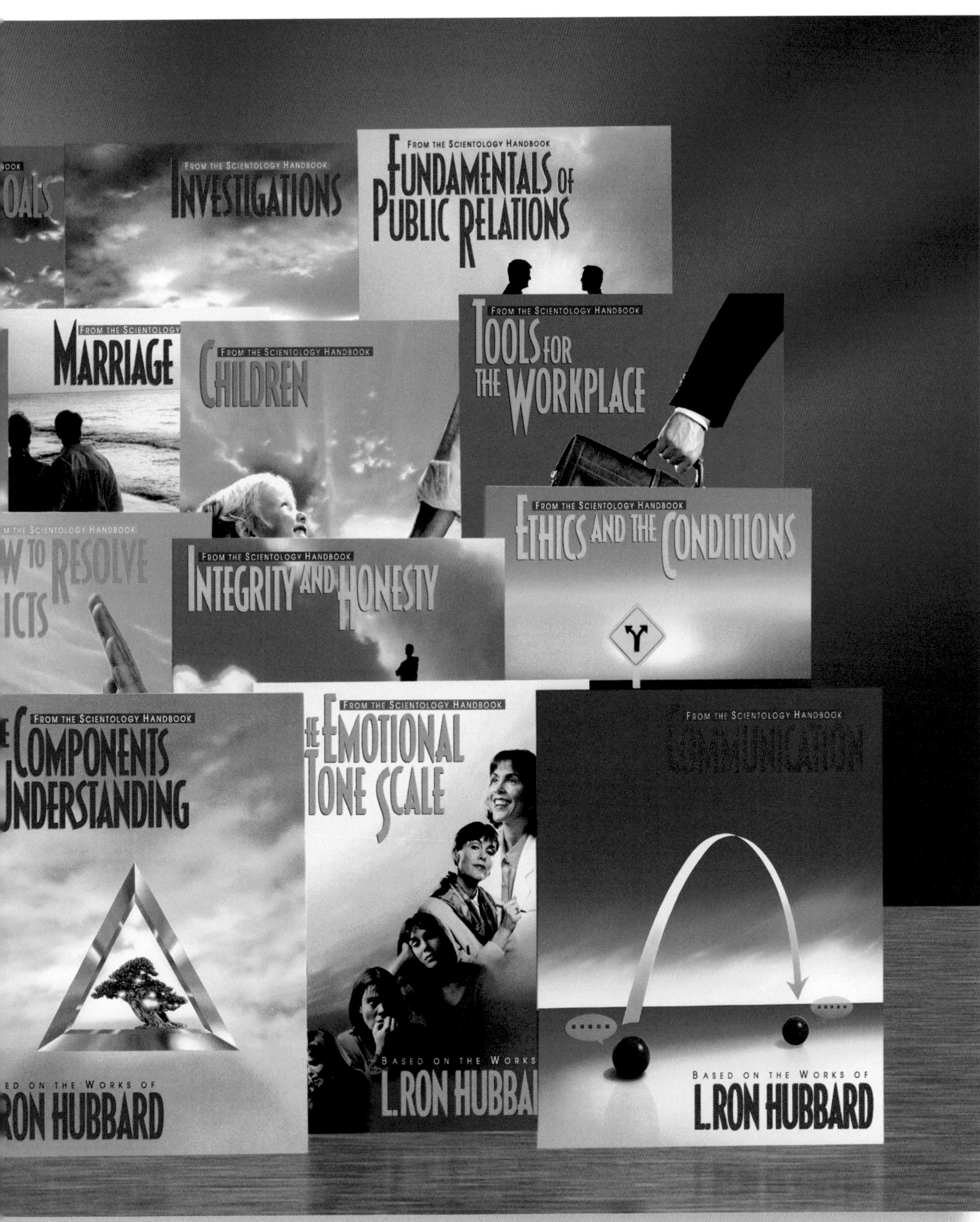
FROM THE SCIENTOLOGY HANDBOOK
INVESTIGATIONS
FROM THE SCIENTOLOGY HANDBOOK
FUNDAMENTALS OF PUBLIC RELATIONS
MARRIAGE
FROM THE SCIENTOLOGY HANDBOOK
CHILDREN
FROM THE SCIENTOLOGY HANDBOOK
TOOLS FOR THE WORKPLACE
FROM THE SCIENTOLOGY HANDBOOK
ETHICS AND THE CONDITIONS
FROM THE SCIENTOLOGY HANDBOOK
INTEGRITY AND HONESTY
FROM THE SCIENTOLOGY HANDBOOK
COMPONENTS
UNDERSTANDING
FROM THE SCIENTOLOGY HANDBOOK
EMOTIONAL
TONE SCALE
BASED ON THE WORKS
FROM THE SCIENTOLOGY HANDBOOK
COMMUNICATION
BASED ON THE WORKS OF
L. RON HUBBARD

Volunteer Ministers in Action

Today, people all over the world apply the technology in this handbook. Singly and in groups, Scientologists can be found in many areas helping others deal more successfully with situations in their lives.

Scientologists assist people in hospitals recover from illness or injury, they help the underprivileged secure a valuable education by improving their ability to study, they heal troubled marriages, they salvage lives from drug abuse, they are active in criminal rehabilitation, in raising society's moral standards and they are on the scene to bring relief to those victimized by disaster.

And what they are doing is changing lives, some actions profoundly affecting communities and the society at large, but most going quietly unheralded. All, however, are contributions to the hope of a better world.

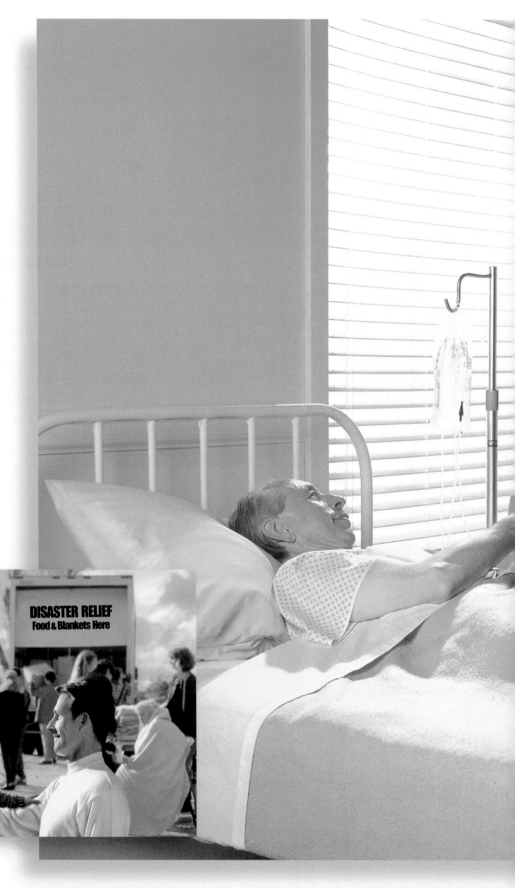

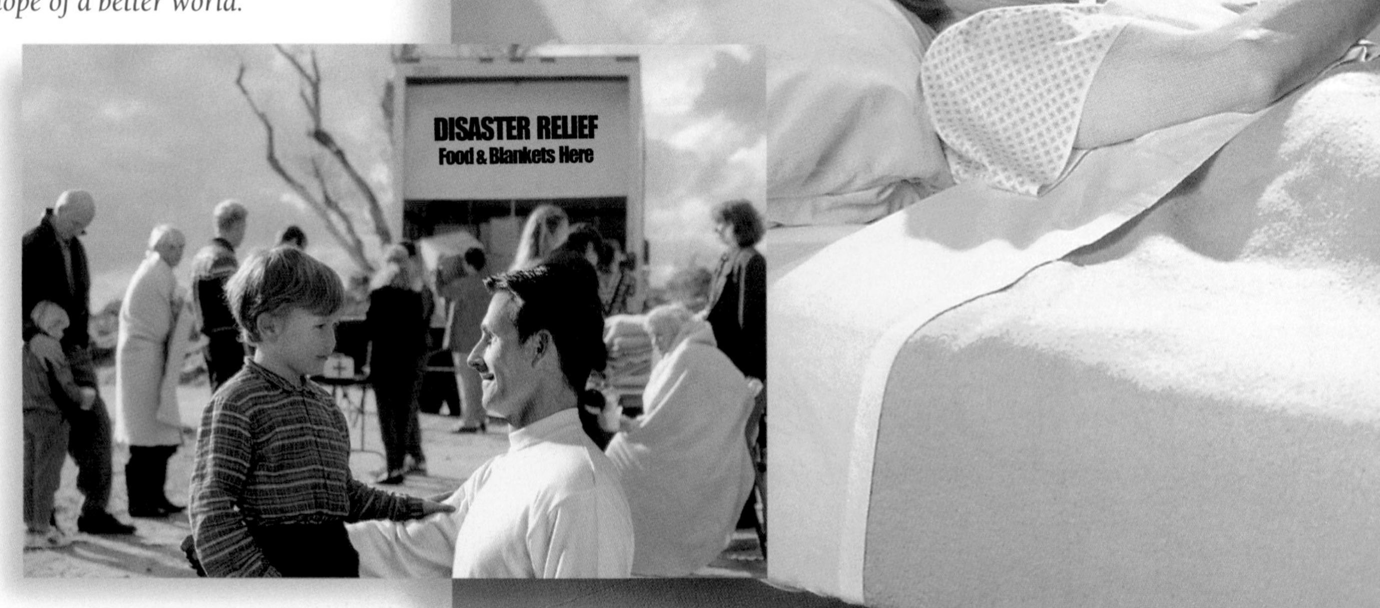

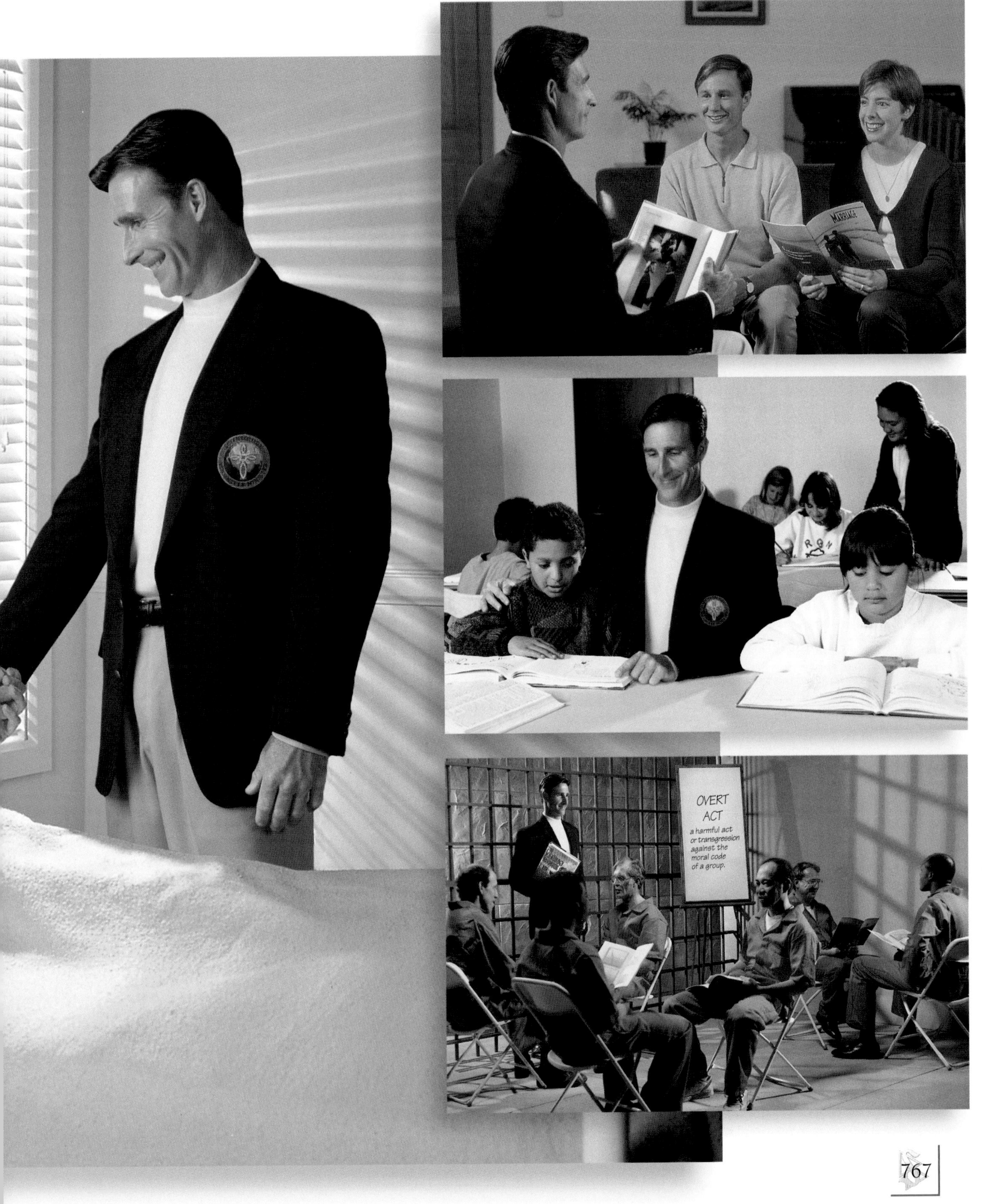
OVERT
ACT
a harmful act or transgression against the moral code of a group.

The Benefits of Further Training

The data in this handbook enables you to do more for people than was ever possible before. It is, however, just a start.

The more skills a Volunteer Minister develops, the more effective he will be. There is much to learn in Scientology and, although it is true that a little goes an astonishingly long way, the more knowledge one has the more one can do.

There are many courses available in churches of Scientology which will enable you to further study these and other more advanced principles and procedures. But the wisest action you can take is professional auditor training, for by learning to help another regain his spiritual abilities and rid himself of the shadows that restrain him, you have the ability to create the most basic yet profound changes possible. This training will give you an unshakeable understanding of life in its entirety. Fully versed in all that the religious philosophy of Scientology has to offer, and unhindered by the complexities and mysteries that cloud our thoughts and actions, you will become more effective in life and more able to assist your fellows.

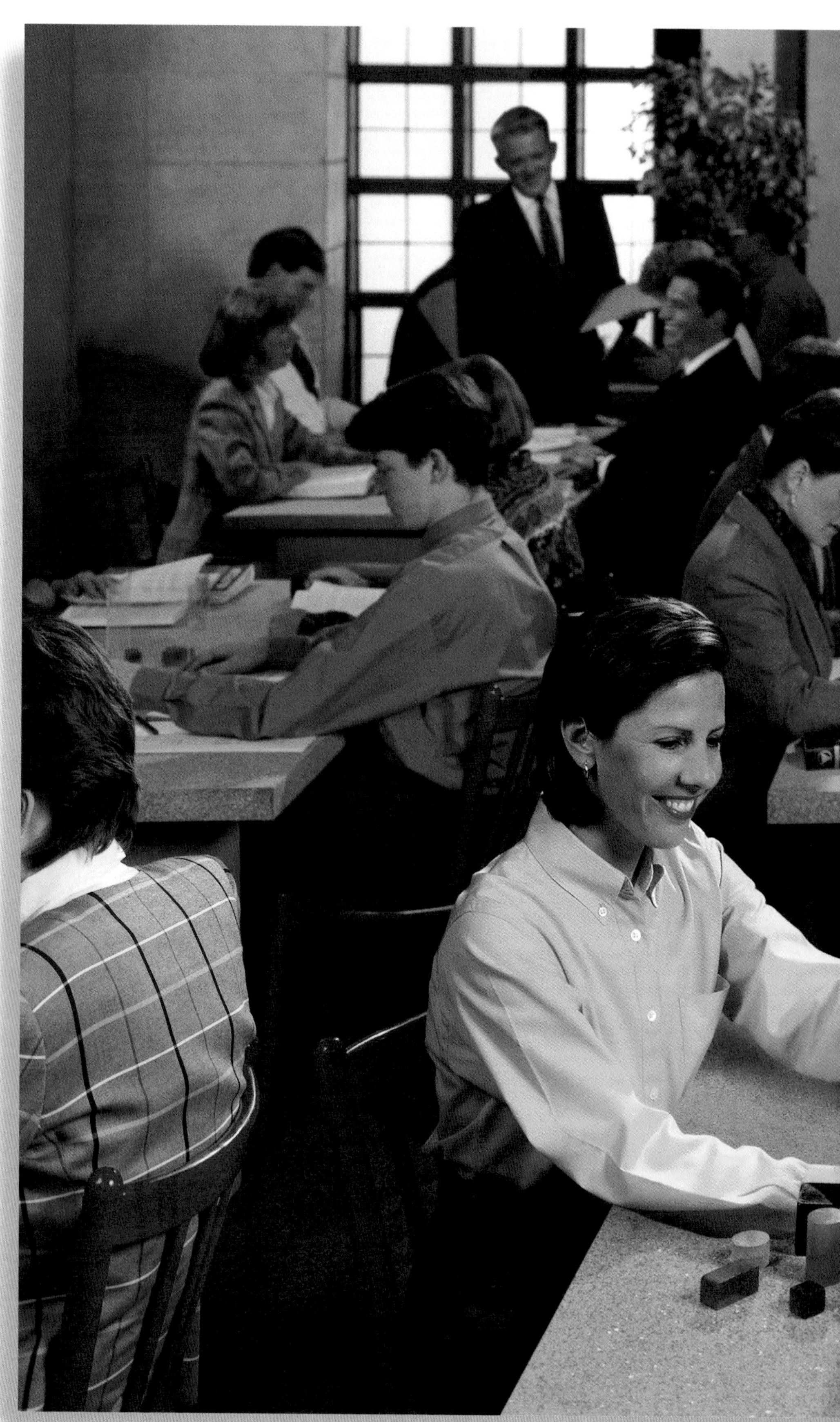

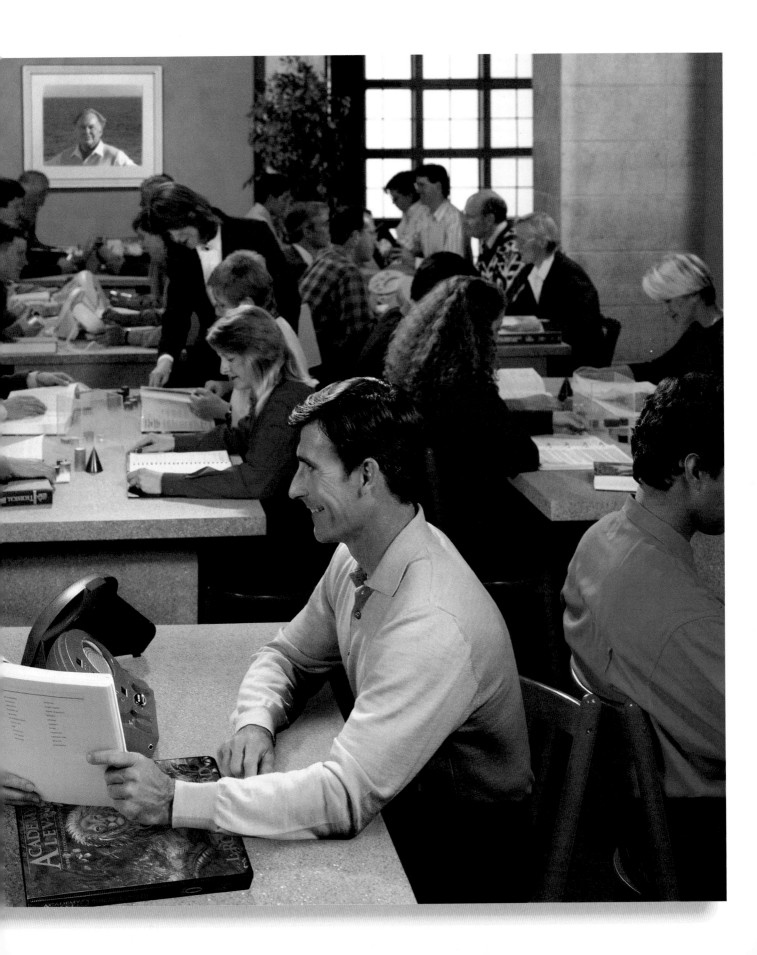

Building a Better World

Every age and religion has had its own technology. The technology of today and tomorrow is Scientology.

While science has wrought marvels to enhance our physical existence, man's lack of progress in the humanities could bring it all to naught. In fact, science has proven itself unable to keep up with the mushrooming crises we face today. The Scientology religion, however, contains an exact technology which fully resolves this dilemma. It not only provides man with the route to spiritual freedom, but also the wisdom to live responsibly.

Because of the broad application of Mr. Hubbard's discoveries, Scientology has long been concerned with society's decline, knowing full well that use of its technology will reverse this trend. And countless people are proving this to be true—in their own lives and in the lives of others who need help. They know that Scientology results in effective change. And they use it to improve life for themselves, their families and neighbors, groups and communities.

L. Ron Hubbard wrote,

"A civilization without insanity, without criminals and without war, where the able can prosper and honest beings can have rights, and where man is free to rise to greater heights, are the aims of Scientology."

Volunteer Ministers everywhere work to achieve these aims. And day by day, their efforts are succeeding.

We welcome you to the growing ranks of those who are creating a better world.

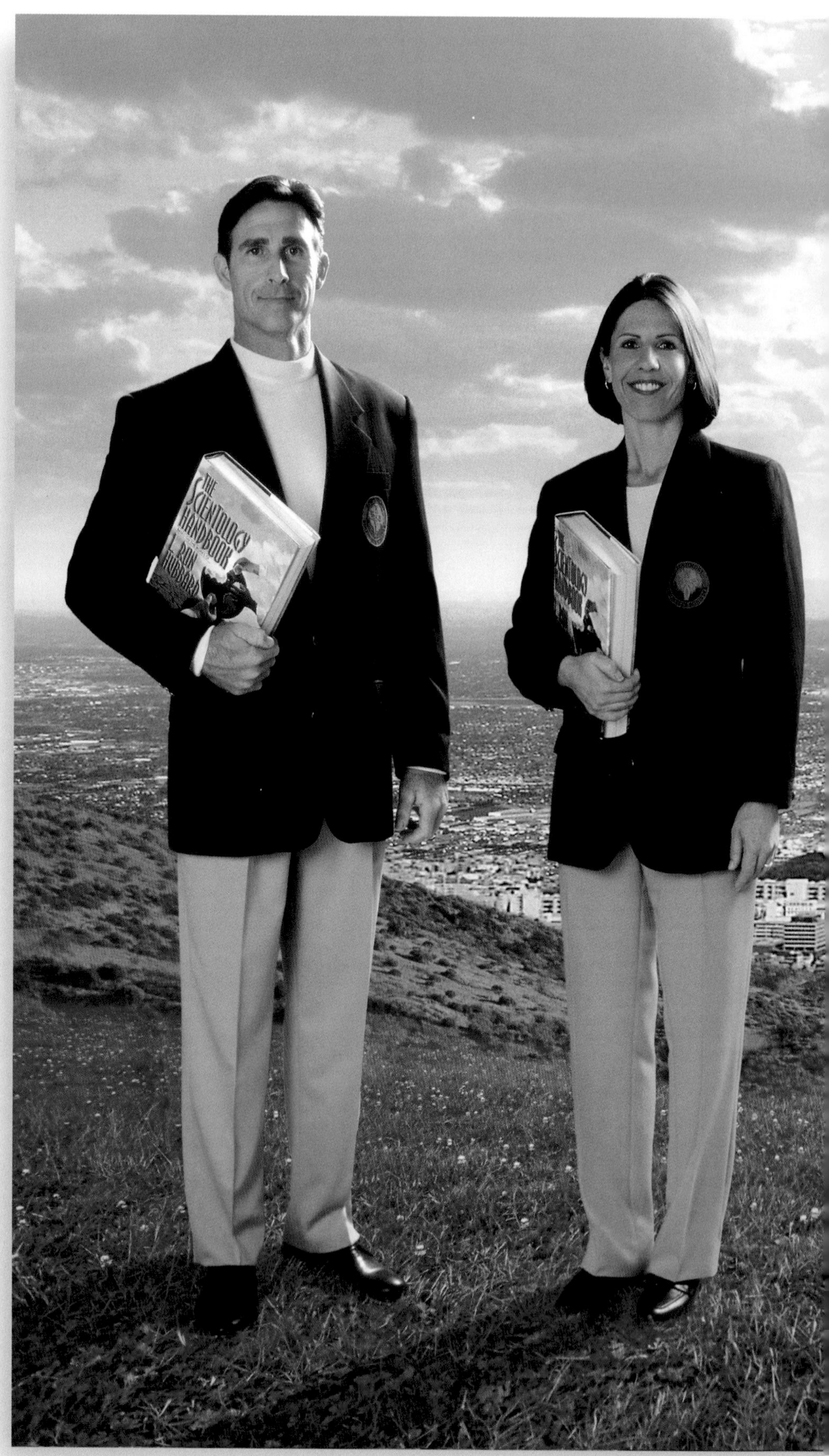

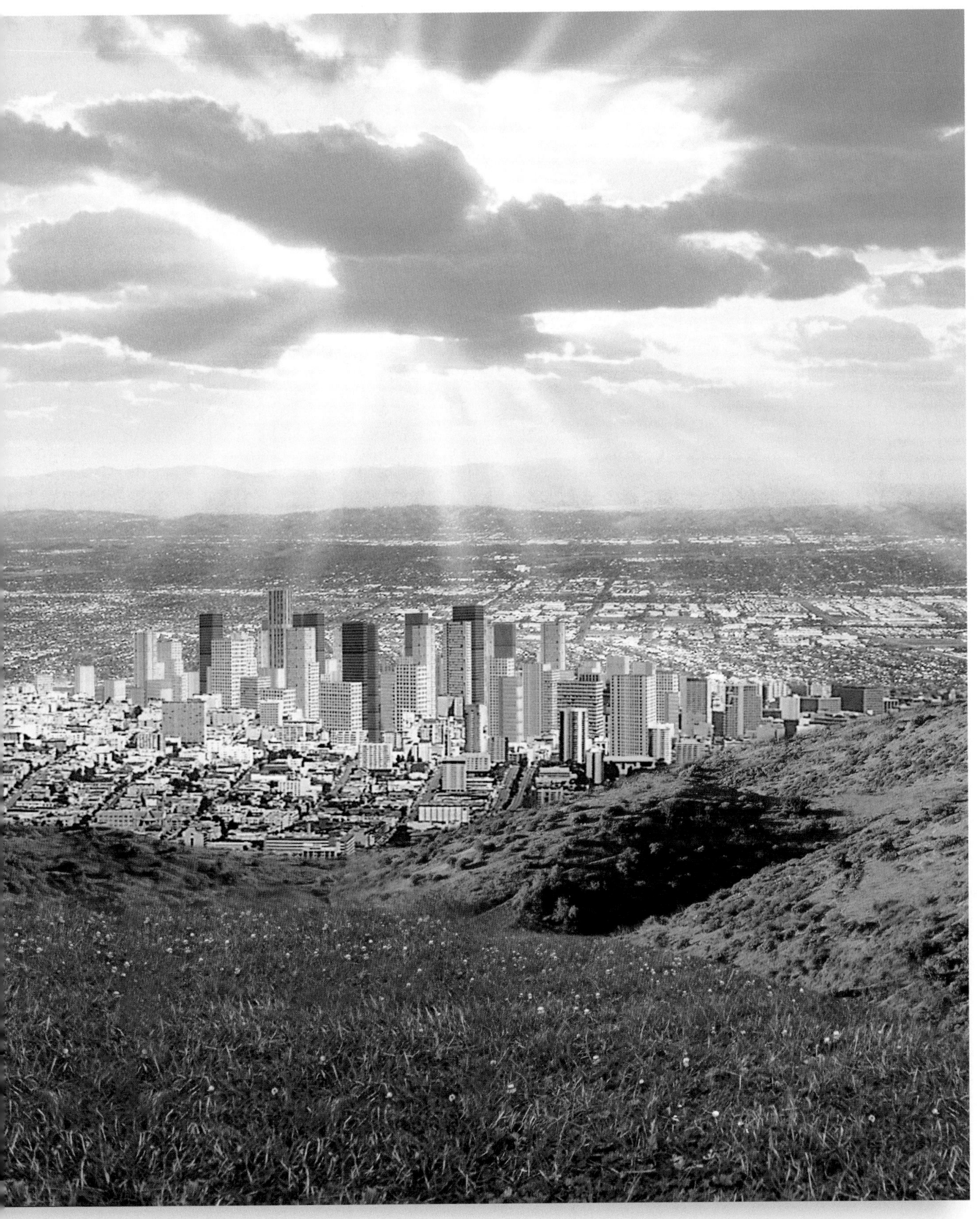

EPILOGUE

In today's climate of powerful centralized governments, divisive politics and hidden financial powers, where self-interest seems to rule and a relentless media churns out the bad news hourly, there is ample excuse to do nothing, to feel that one cannot make a difference anyway. After all, one is merely an individual among billions.

Yet this is not the truth. As is being proven daily around the globe through the actions of dedicated Scientologists, one individual acting in concert with another individual, and then another and another, constitutes the wave that will turn the tide.

Today individuals have tools they have never had before. The task is to make them known and get them used. And that is the purpose of this handbook.

It is a purpose that you have helped fulfill by reading this book. These tools are now yours. And what you do with them is in your hands.

Nothing happens without being caused. And the future has yet to be created.

With these tools, you can help create it.

The choice is yours.

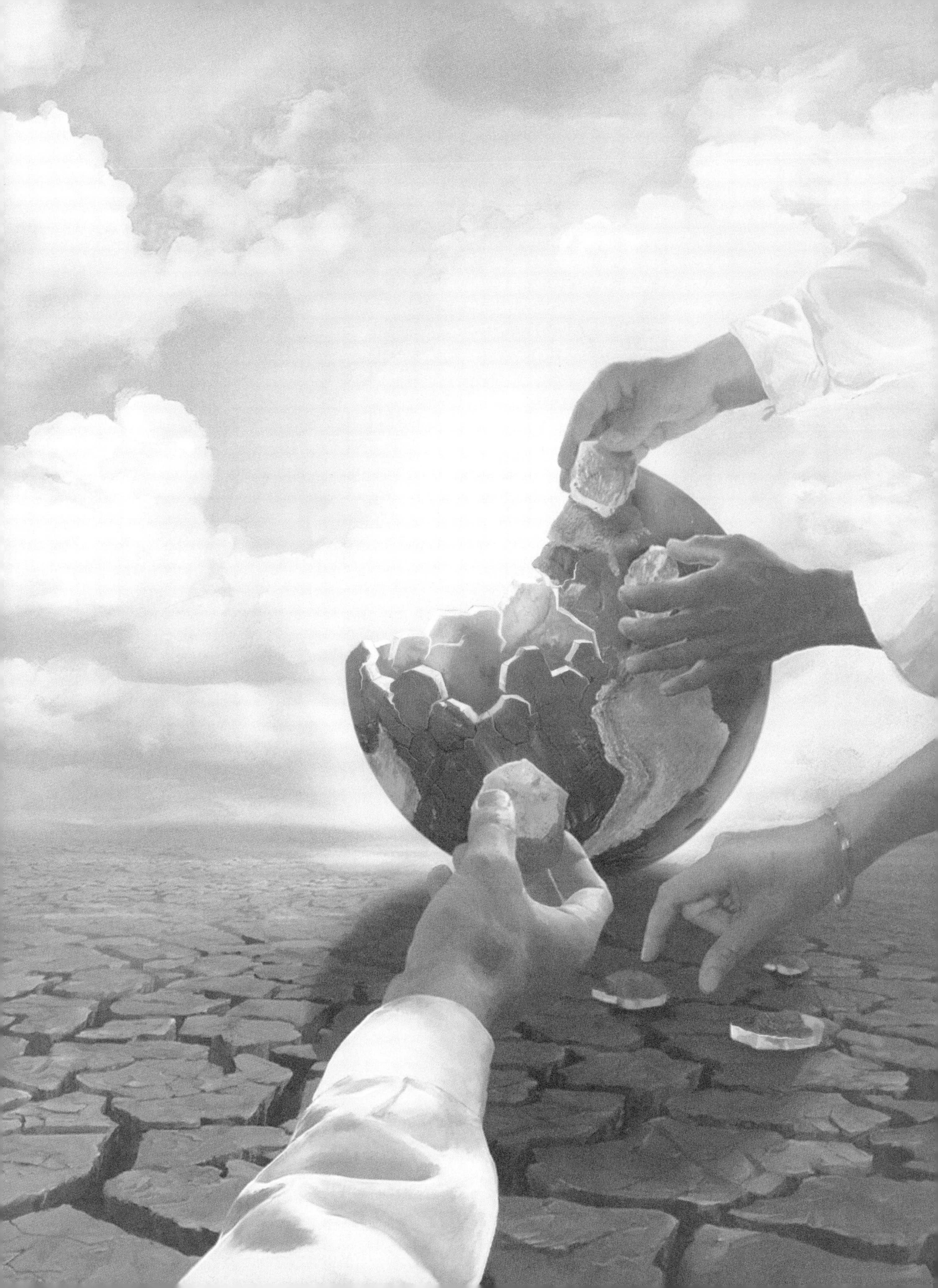

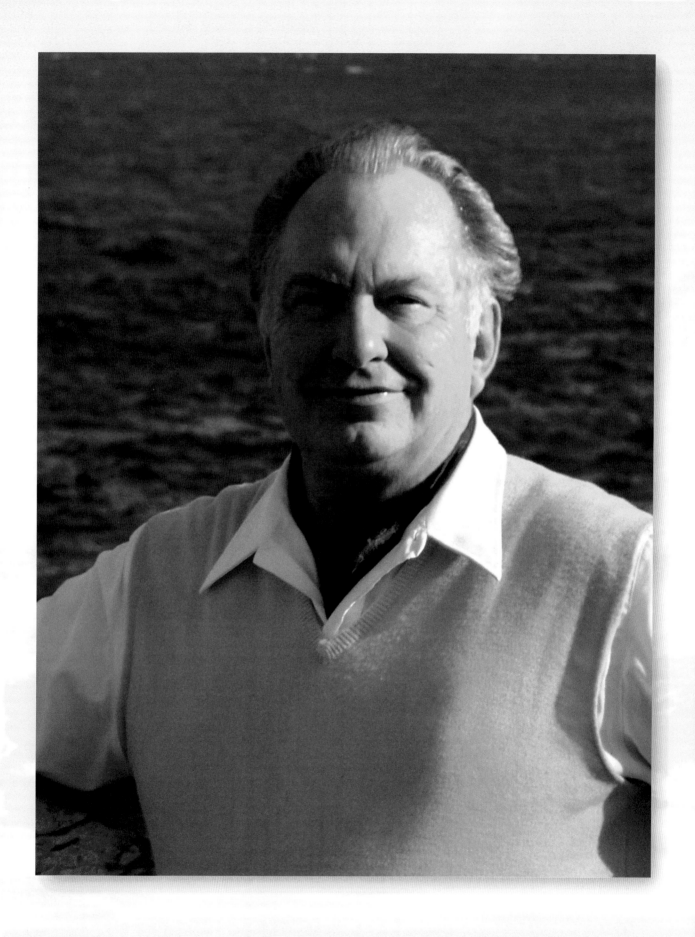

About L. Ron Hubbard

No more fitting statement typifies the life of L. Ron Hubbard than his simple declaration: "I like to help others and count it as my greatest pleasure in life to see a person free himself from the shadows which darken his days." Behind these pivotal words stands a lifetime of service to mankind and a legacy of wisdom that enables anyone to attain long-cherished dreams of happiness and spiritual freedom.

Born in Tilden, Nebraska on March 13, 1911, his road of discovery and dedication to his fellows began at an early age. "I wanted other people to be happy, and could not understand why they weren't," he wrote of his youth; and therein lay the sentiments that would long guide his steps. Under the tutelage of his mother, a thoroughly educated woman, he was reading well beyond his years—Shakespeare, Greek philosophy and later classics—all in an attempt to satisfy an insatiable curiosity. Yet his life was by no means bookish. Having moved with his family to the rugged plains of Helena, Montana, he was also riding by the age of three-and-a-half, and, later, breaking broncos with the best local wranglers.

It was additionally in Helena that Ron (as he wished to be known to his friends) first encountered the deeply spiritual heritage of the Blackfeet Indians, then still living in isolated settlements on the outskirts of town. His particular friend was a tribal medicine man, locally known as "Old Tom." Establishing a unique friendship with the usually taciturn shaman, Ron was eventually honored with the rare status of blood brother and thus entrusted with the various tribal secrets, lore and wisdom.

It was no less than a student of Sigmund Freud's who opened the next door of discovery to a young L. Ron Hubbard. Moving with his family to Seattle, Washington and then on to the nation's capital, Ron was befriended by Commander Joseph C. Thompson, the first American officer to study under Freud in Vienna. Recognizing an unusually keen intelligence in the twelve-year-old, the Commander spent several months passing on the substance of Freud's theories. Although genuinely fascinated with the premise of unconscious behavior, Ron was also left with many unanswered questions.

His father's naval career provided the next avenue of inquiry. Following an assignment to the island of Guam, the Hubbard family ventured East, and Ron was soon pursuing answers to very fundamental questions in what was then a remote Asia. By the age of nineteen, he had traveled more than a quarter of a million miles, examining the cultures of Java, Japan, India and the Philippines. With the same determination, he had even gained access to forbidden Buddhist lamaseries in the western hills of China. Yet for all the celebrated traditions of the East, he found much that troubled him: ignorance, poverty and wanton disregard for suffering. "And amongst this poverty and degradation," he later wrote, "I found holy places where wisdom was great, but where it was carefully hidden and given out only as superstition."

Returning to the United States in 1929, Ron resumed his formal education and enrolled in George Washington University the following year. There, he studied mathematics, engineering and the then new field of nuclear physics—all providing vital tools for continued research. After examining modern psychology, however, he came to another critical realization: Although the West may have possessed the methodology of investigation, it had never applied that methodology to basic questions relating to man's nature, his mind and life. In fact, as he wrote, "It was very obvious to me that I was dealing with and living in a culture which knew less about the mind than the lowest primitive tribe I had ever come in contact with. Knowing also that people in the East were not able to reach as deeply and predictably into the riddles of the mind as I had been led to expect, I knew I would have to do a lot of research."

To finance that research, Ron embarked upon a literary career in the early 1930s, and soon became one of the most widely read authors of popular fiction. His stories spanned all genres—adventure, mystery, western, science fiction and fantasy—and earned him worldwide recognition. He also scripted screenplays for Hollywood and instructive essays for fellow writers. Yet never losing sight of his primary goal, he continued his mainline research through extensive travel and expeditions to then remote islands in the Caribbean, and off British Columbia and Alaska where he studied among the Tlingit, Haida and Aleut tribes. In all, he examined twenty-one races and cultures while searching for underlying truths of human existence. In recognition of this work, he was awarded membership in the famed Explorers Club where he was known as a foremost ethnologist. And throughout all subsequent expeditions he would carry the coveted Explorers Club flag.

With the advent of World War II, he entered the United States Navy as a lieutenant (junior grade) and served as commander of antisubmarine corvettes. Although highly decorated, he was deeply saddened by the inhumanity of that conflict and so more resolved than ever to discover some workable means to better the human condition. To that end, he continued his research even through the darkest years of conflict.

Left partially blind and lame from injuries sustained during combat, he was diagnosed as permanently disabled by 1945 and hospitalized in Oakland, California. By this point, however, he had already formulated his first theories on the human mind and, through application of those theories, was not only able to help fellow servicemen, but also regain his own health. In short, he found that by relieving the mental trauma attendant to injuries, one could effect truly miraculous improvements.

After several more years of intensive work, wherein he applied his techniques to some four hundred individuals, Ron compiled his sixteen years of research into *The Original Thesis* (known today as *The Dynamics of Life*). Although not immediately published, this work inspired so much enthusiasm among scientific and professional circles that he was soon called upon to further explain the techniques he now termed *Dianetics*.

The first published article on the subject, entitled "Terra Incognita: The Mind," appeared in the Winter/Spring issue of the Explorers Club Journal, generating still greater enthusiasm and hundreds of inquiring letters. L. Ron Hubbard then commenced the writing of *Dianetics: The Modern Science of Mental Health,* the first popular handbook on the human mind expressly written for the man in the street. Dianetics was published on May 9, 1950 and became an immediate bestseller. Moreover, because it offered techniques for self-betterment that anyone could learn and apply, the book soon sparked what newspapers described as "The Fastest Growing Movement in America."

The publication of *Dianetics* ushered in a new era of hope for mankind and a new phase of life for its author. In constant demand, L. Ron Hubbard was soon crisscrossing the country to meet requests for public lectures and personal instruction in the application of Dianetics. Yet even through that intensely busy summer and autumn of 1950, he did not cease his research—first to perfect the technology with which he had resolved problems of the human mind, and then to examine an even more elusive question: What exactly is life? For as he wrote, "The further one investigated, the more one came to understand that here, in this creature, *Homo sapiens,* were entirely too many unknowns."

Although still applying a wholly scientific methodology, the research that followed soon led him into an entirely spiritual realm. In particular, he was examining what he had termed the life source and later described as the *thetan;* and as breakthrough after breakthrough was carefully codified through late 1951, the applied religious philosophy of Scientology was born. Offering man a route to new levels of awareness and ability, the first Church of Scientology was established in 1954.

Because Scientology explains the whole of life, there is no aspect of man's existence that L. Ron Hubbard's subsequent work did not address. Residing variously in the United States and England, his continued research brought forth solutions to such social ills as declining educational standards and the disintegrating family. Also utilizing the basic tenets of Scientology, he was able to discover remarkable methods of assisting the ill, repairing marriages, bettering relations and, in short, resolving any problem or conflict. And because an understanding of individuals ultimately provides an understanding of groups, he was soon employing Scientology truths to evolve a sane means of administering organizations—work which brought about the expansion of Scientology into a worldwide network.

On September 1, 1966, with Scientology now spanning the globe, L. Ron Hubbard resigned his position as Executive Director of the Church and stepped down from the boards of all Church corporations in order to fully devote himself to researches into the highest levels of spiritual awareness and ability. On the threshold of breakthroughs into such levels, he returned to sea aboard a 3,200-ton research vessel, *Apollo.* For the next seven years, he again traveled extensively, while devoting his attention to increasingly grave societal problems. Of special note from this period is his Scientology Drug Rehabilitation program, recognized by government studies as the world's most effective. He also developed and refined his revolutionary Study Technology, which has factually led to increased literacy for millions.

Moving to shore in 1975, Ron continued his travels—first from Florida to Washington, DC and Los Angeles before finally settling in a southern California desert community near Palm Springs, his home until 1979. There, as part of a larger program to bring Scientology and Dianetics to increasing numbers of people, he wrote and directed training films while also continuing to search out solutions to the world's most pressing problems.

In 1980, as part of his long-standing effort to reverse late-twentieth-century moral decay, he wrote the nonreligious moral code, *The Way to Happiness.* Applauded by community and political leaders, and civic groups, *The Way to Happiness* subsequently spawned a worldwide grass-roots movement to uplift the decency and integrity of man. To date, some fifty million copies are in circulation. Effective in many sectors of society, the booklet has also been described as the single most effective means of rehabilitating inmates of criminal institutions.

Resuming his travels in the early 1980s, he finally took up residence in the central California community of Creston, near San Luis Obispo. Here, he completed his research into advanced levels of Scientology and finalized the technical materials he had spent his life developing.

All told, L. Ron Hubbard's works on Scientology and Dianetics total forty million words of recorded lectures, books and writing. Together, these works constitute the legacy of a lifetime that ended on January 24, 1986. Yet the passing of L. Ron Hubbard in no way constituted an end; for with more than a hundred million of his books in circulation and millions of people daily applying his technologies for betterment, it can truly be said the world still has no greater friend. ■

My Philosophy

The subject of philosophy is very ancient. The word means: "The love, study or pursuit of wisdom, or of knowledge of things and their causes, whether theoretical or practical."

All we know of science or of religion comes from philosophy. It lies behind and above all other knowledge we have or use.

For long regarded as a subject reserved for halls of learning and the intellectual, the subject to a remarkable degree has been denied the man in the street.

Surrounded by protective coatings of impenetrable scholarliness, philosophy has been reserved to the privileged few.

The first principle of my own philosophy is that wisdom is meant for anyone who wishes to reach for it. It is the servant of the commoner and king alike and should never be regarded with awe.

Selfish scholars seldom forgive anyone who seeks to break down the walls of mystery and let the people in. Will Durant, the modern American philosopher, was relegated to the scrapheap by his fellow scholars when he wrote a popular book on the subject, **The Outline of Philosophy.** *Thus brickbats come the way of any who seek to bring wisdom to the people over the objections of the "inner circle."*

The second principle of my own philosophy is that it must be capable of being applied.

Learning locked in mildewed books is of little use to anyone and therefore of no value unless it can be used.

The third principle is that any philosophic knowledge is only valuable if it is true or if it works.

These three principles are so strange to the field of philosophy that I have given my philosophy a name: SCIENTOLOGY. This means only "knowing how to know."

A philosophy can only be a **route** *to knowledge. It cannot be knowledge crammed down one's throat. If one has a route he can then find what is true for him. And that is Scientology.*

Know thyself — and the truth shall set you free.

Therefore in Scientology we are not concerned with individual actions and differences. We are only concerned with how to show man how he can set himself or herself free.

This of course is not very popular with those who depend upon the slavery of others for their living or power. But it happens to be the only way I have found that really improves an individual's life.

Suppression and oppression are the basic causes of depression. If you relieve those, a person can lift his head, become well, become happy with life.

And though it may be unpopular with the slave master, it is very popular with the people. Common man likes to be happy and well. He likes to be able to understand things. And he knows his route to freedom lies through knowledge.

Therefore, since 1950 I have had mankind knocking on my door. It has not mattered where I have lived or how remote, since I first published a book on the subject my life has no longer been my own.

I like to help others and count it as my greatest pleasure in life to see a person free himself of the shadows which darken his days.

These shadows look so thick to him and weigh him down so that when he finds they are *shadows and that he can see through them, walk through them and be again in the sun, he is enormously delighted. And I am afraid I am just as delighted as he is.*

I have seen much human misery. As a very young man I wandered through Asia and saw the agony and misery of overpopulated and undereducated lands. I have seen people uncaring and stepping over dying men in the streets. I have seen children less than rags and bones. And amongst this poverty and degradation I found holy places where wisdom was great but where it was carefully hidden and given out only as superstition. Later in Western universities I saw man obsessed with materiality and with all his cunning, I saw him hide what little wisdom he really had in forbidding halls and make it inaccessible to the common and less favored man. I have been through a terrible war and saw its terror and pain uneased by a single word of decency or humanity.

I have lived no cloistered life and hold in contempt the wise man who has not **lived** *and the scholar who will not share.*

There have been many wiser men than I but few have traveled as much road.

I have seen life from the top down and the bottom up. I know how it looks both ways. And I know there **is** *wisdom and that there is hope.*

Blinded with injured optic nerves and lame with physical injuries to hip and back at the end of World War II, I faced an almost nonexistent future. My service record states: "This officer has no neurotic or psychotic tendencies of any kind whatsoever," but it also states "permanently disabled physically."

And so there came a further blow—I was abandoned by family and friends as a supposedly hopeless cripple and a probable burden upon them for the rest of my days. I yet worked my way back to fitness and strength in less than two years using only what I knew and could determine about man and his relationship to the universe. I had no one to help me; what I had to know I had to find out. And it's quite a trick studying when you cannot see.

I became used to being told it was all impossible, that there was no way, no hope. Yet I came to see again and walk again and I built an entirely new life. It is a happy life, a busy one and I hope a useful one. My only moments of sadness are those which come when bigoted men tell others all is bad and there is no route anywhere, no hope anywhere, nothing but sadness and sameness and desolation and that every effort to help others is false. I know it is not true.

So my own philosophy is that one should share what wisdom he has, one should help others to help themselves and one should keep going despite heavy weather for there is always a calm ahead. One should also ignore catcalls from the selfish intellectual who cries: "Don't expose the mystery. Keep it all for ourselves. The people cannot understand."

But as I have never seen wisdom do any good kept to oneself, and as I like to see others happy, and as I find the vast majority of the people can and do *understand, I will keep on writing and working and teaching so long as I exist.*

For I know no man who has any monopoly upon the wisdom of this universe. It belongs to those who can use it to help themselves and others.

If things were a little better known and understood, we would all lead happier lives.

And there is a way to know them and there is a way to freedom.

The old must give way to the new, falsehood must become exposed by truth, and truth though fought always in the end prevails.

L. Ron Hubbard

The Creed of the Church of Scientology

We of the Church believe:

That all men of whatever race, color or creed were created with equal rights;

That all men have inalienable rights to their own religious practices and their performance;

That all men have inalienable rights to their own lives;

That all men have inalienable rights to their sanity;

That all men have inalienable rights to their own defense;

That all men have inalienable rights to conceive, choose, assist or support their own organizations, churches and governments;

That all men have inalienable rights to think freely, to talk freely, to write freely their own opinions and to counter or utter or write upon the opinions of others;

That all men have inalienable rights to the creation of their own kind;

That the souls of men have the rights of men;

That the study of the mind and the healing of mentally caused ills should not be alienated from religion or condoned in nonreligious fields;

And that no agency less than God has the power to suspend or set aside these rights, overtly or covertly.

And we of the Church believe:

That man is basically good;

That he is seeking to survive;

That his survival depends upon himself and upon his fellows and his attainment of brotherhood with the universe.

And we of the Church believe that the laws of God forbid man:

To destroy his own kind;

To destroy the sanity of another;

To destroy or enslave another's soul;

To destroy or reduce the survival of one's companions or one's group.

And we of the Church believe:

That the spirit can be saved and

That the spirit alone may save or heal the body.

WHO TO CONTACT

I HELP

(INTERNATIONAL
HUBBARD ECCLESIASTICAL LEAGUE OF PASTORS)

The International Hubbard Ecclesiastical League of Pastors (I HELP) was created to provide guidance and assistance to people helping others using Scientology technology outside organized churches and missions. It aids all those applying Scientology out in the world by providing them with materials, publications and consultation services. It also offers assistance with any administrative or technical difficulties they may encounter.

INTERNATIONAL HUBBARD ECCLESIASTICAL LEAGUE OF PASTORS

6331 Hollywood Boulevard, Suite 702 Los Angeles, California 90028
VM Internet Site address: http: //www.volunteerministers.org

WESTERN UNITED STATES

▲ International Hubbard
Ecclesiastical League of Pastors
Western United States Office
1308 L. Ron Hubbard Way
Los Angeles, California 90027

EASTERN UNITED STATES

▲ International Hubbard
Ecclesiastical League of Pastors
Eastern United States Office
349 W. 48th Street
New York, New York 10036

▲ I HELP Representative
Flag Land Base
210 S. Fort Harrison Avenue
Clearwater, Florida 33756

UNITED KINGDOM

▲ International Hubbard
Ecclesiastical League of Pastors
United Kingdom Office
Saint Hill Manor
East Grinstead, West Sussex
England RH19 4JY

AFRICA

▲ International Hubbard
Ecclesiastical League of Pastors
African Office
6th Floor, Budget House
130 Main Street
Johannesburg 2001
South Africa

AUSTRALIA

▲ International Hubbard
Ecclesiastical League of Pastors
Australian, New Zealand and
Oceanian Office
201 Castlereagh Street
3rd Floor
Sydney, New South Wales
Australia 2000

CANADA

▲ International Hubbard
Ecclesiastical League of Pastors
Canadian Office
696 Yonge Street
Toronto, Ontario
Canada M4Y 2A7

COMMONWEALTH OF INDEPENDENT STATES

▲ International Hubbard
Ecclesiastical League of Pastors
CIS Office
c/o Hubbard Humanitarian
Center
129301 Moscow
Ul. Borisa Galushkina 19A
129301 Moscow, Russia

EUROPE

▲ International Hubbard
Ecclesiastical League of Pastors
European Office
Store Kongensgade 55
1264 Copenhagen K, Denmark

CENTRAL EUROPE

▲ International Hubbard
Ecclesiastical League of Pastors
Central European Office
1438 Budapest
Pf. 351
Hungary

ITALY

▲ International Hubbard
Ecclesiastical League of Pastors
Italian Office
Via Cadorna, 61
20090 Vimodrone, Milano, Italy

LATIN AMERICA

▲ International Hubbard
Ecclesiastical League of Pastors
Latin American Office
Puebla #31
Colonia Roma, C.P. 06700
Mexico, D.F.

TAIWAN

▲ International Hubbard
Ecclesiastical League of Pastors
Taiwanese Office
2nd Floor, 65, Sec. 4
Min-Sheng East Road
Taipei, Taiwan ROC

International Church Organizations

Church of Scientology International

Mother church of the Scientology religion
6331 Hollywood Boulevard, Suite 1200
Los Angeles, California 90028-6329

Religious Technology Center

Holder of the Dianetics and Scientology trademarks
1710 Ivar Avenue, Suite 1100
Los Angeles, California 90028

INTERNATIONAL ASSOCIATION OF SCIENTOLOGISTS

The International Association of Scientologists is a membership organization which unites individuals around the world in achieving the Aims of Scientology. Anyone in agreement with these aims may become a member.

For information concerning the activities of the IAS, to become a member or renew membership in the Association, you can write to:

INTERNATIONAL ASSOCIATION
OF SCIENTOLOGISTS
c/o Saint Hill Manor
East Grinstead, West Sussex
England RH19 4JY

or

US IAS Members Trust
1311 N. New Hampshire Avenue
Los Angeles, California 90027

LIST OF ORGANIZATIONS

CHURCHES OF SCIENTOLOGY

FOUNDATION CHURCH OF SCIENTOLOGY FLAG SHIP SERVICE ORGANIZATION

c/o *Freewinds* Relay Office
118 N. Fort Harrison Avenue
Clearwater, Florida 33755-4013

CHURCH OF SCIENTOLOGY FLAG SERVICE ORGANIZATION

210 S. Fort Harrison Avenue
Clearwater, Florida 34616

UNITED STATES

Continental Liaison Office
Western United States
1308 L. Ron Hubbard Way
Los Angeles, CA 90027

Continental Liaison Office
Eastern United States
349 W. 48th Street
New York, New York 10036

◆ Church of Scientology
American Saint Hill Organization
1413 L. Ron Hubbard Way
Los Angeles, California 90027

◆ Church of Scientology
American Saint Hill Foundation
1413 L. Ron Hubbard Way
Los Angeles, California 90027

◆ Church of Scientology
Advanced Organization of Los Angeles
1306 L. Ron Hubbard Way
Los Angeles, California 90027

Church of Scientology of Albuquerque
8106 Menaul Boulevard NE
Albuquerque, New Mexico 87110

Church of Scientology of Ann Arbor
2355 West Stadium Boulevard
Ann Arbor, Michigan 48103

Church of Scientology of Atlanta
1611 Mt. Vernon Road
Dunwoody, Georgia 30338

Church of Scientology of Austin
2200 Guadalupe
Austin, Texas 78705

Church of Scientology of Boston
448 Beacon Street
Boston, Massachusetts 02115

Church of Scientology of Buffalo
47 West Huron Street
Buffalo, New York 14202

Church of Scientology of Chicago
3011 North Lincoln Avenue
Chicago, Illinois 60657-4207

Church of Scientology of Cincinnati
215 West 4th Street, 5th Floor
Cincinnati, Ohio 45202-2670

Church of Scientology of Columbus
30 North High Street
Columbus, Ohio 43215

Church of Scientology of Denver
3385 South Bannock Street
Englewood, Colorado 80110

Church of Scientology of Detroit
28000 Middlebelt Road
Farmington Hills, Michigan 48334

Church of Scientology of Honolulu
1146 Bethel Street
Honolulu, Hawaii 96813

Church of Scientology of Kansas City
3619 Broadway
Kansas City, Missouri 64111

Church of Scientology of Las Vegas
846 East Sahara Avenue
Las Vegas, Nevada 89104

Church of Scientology of Long Island
99 Railroad Station Plaza
Hicksville, New York 11801-2850

LOS ANGELES AND VICINITY

Church of Scientology of Los Angeles
4810 Sunset Boulevard
Los Angeles, California 90027

Church of Scientology
of Orange County
1451 Irvine Boulevard
Tustin, California 92680

Church of Scientology of Pasadena
1277 East Colorado Boulevard
Pasadena, California 91106

Church of Scientology
of the Valley
15643 Sherman Way
Van Nuys, California 91406

Church of Scientology
of Los Gatos
2155 South Bascom Avenue,
Suite 120
Campbell, California 95008

Church of Scientology of Miami
120 Giralda Avenue
Coral Gables, Florida 33134

Church of Scientology
of Minneapolis
Twin Cities
1011 Nicollet Mall
Minneapolis, Minnesota 55403

Church of Scientology
of Mountain View
2483 Old Middlefield Way
Mountain View, California 94043

Church of Scientology
of New Haven
909 Whalley Avenue
New Haven, Connecticut 06515-1728

Church of Scientology
of New York City
227 West 46th Street
New York, New York 10036-1409

Church of Scientology of Orlando
1830 East Colonial Drive
Orlando, Florida 32803-4729

Church of Scientology
of Philadelphia
1315 Race Street
Philadelphia, Pennsylvania 19107

Church of Scientology of Phoenix
2111 West University Drive
Mesa, Arizona 85201

Church of Scientology of Portland
2636 NE Sandy Boulevard
Portland, Oregon 97232-2342

Church of Scientology
of Sacramento
825 15th Street
Sacramento, California 95814-2096

Church of Scientology
of Salt Lake City
1931 South 1100 East
Salt Lake City, Utah 84106

Church of Scientology
of San Diego
1330 4th Avenue
San Diego, California 92101

Church of Scientology
of San Francisco
83 McAllister Street
San Francisco, California 94102

Church of Scientology of San Jose
80 East Rosemary Street
San Jose, California 95112

Church of Scientology
of Santa Barbara
524 State Street
Santa Barbara, California 93101

Church of Scientology of Seattle
2226 3rd Avenue
Seattle, Washington 98121

Church of Scientology of St. Louis
6901 Delmar Boulevard
University City, Missouri 63130

Church of Scientology of Tampa
3617 Henderson Boulevard
Tampa, Florida 33609-4501

Founding Church of Scientology
of Washington, DC
1701 20th Street NW
Washington, DC 20009

Puerto Rico

Dianetics Center of Puerto Rico
272 JT Piñero Avenue
Hyde Park
San Juan, Puerto Rico 00918

Canada

Continental Liaison Office
Canada
696 Yonge Street
Toronto, Ontario
Canada M4Y 2A7

Church of Scientology
of Edmonton
10206 106th Street NW
Edmonton, Alberta
Canada T5J 1H7

Church of Scientology
of Kitchener
104 King Street West, 2nd Floor
Kitchener, Ontario
Canada N2G 1A6

Church of Scientology of Montreal
4489 Papineau Street
Montreal, Quebec
Canada H2H 1T7

Church of Scientology of Ottawa
150 Rideau Street, 2nd Floor
Ottawa, Ontario
Canada K1N 5X6

Church of Scientology of Quebec
350 Bd Chareste Est
Quebec, Quebec
Canada G1K 3H5

Church of Scientology of Toronto
696 Yonge Street, 2nd Floor
Toronto, Ontario
Canada M4Y 2A7

Church of Scientology
of Vancouver
401 West Hastings Street
Vancouver, British Columbia
Canada V6B 1L5

Church of Scientology
of Winnipeg
315 Garry Street, Suite 210
Winnipeg, Manitoba
Canada R3B 2G7

United Kingdom

Continental Liaison Office
United Kingdom
Saint Hill Manor
East Grinstead, West Sussex
England RH19 4JY

◆ Advanced Organization
Saint Hill
Saint Hill Manor
East Grinstead, West Sussex
England RH19 4JY

Church of Scientology
of Birmingham
8 Ethel Street
Winston Churchill House
Birmingham, England B2 4BG

Church of Scientology of Brighton
Third Floor, 79-83 North Street
Brighton, Sussex
England BN1 1ZA

Church of Scientology
Saint Hill Foundation
Saint Hill Manor
East Grinstead, West Sussex
England RH19 4JY

Hubbard Academy of Personal
Independence
20 Southbridge
Edinburgh, Scotland EH1 1LL

Church of Scientology of London
68 Tottenham Court Road
London, England W1P 0BB

Church of Scientology
of Manchester
258 Deansgate
Manchester, England M3 4BG

Church of Scientology
of Plymouth
41 Ebrington Street
Plymouth, Devon
England PL4 9AA

Church of Scientology
of Sunderland
51 Fawcett Street
Sunderland, Tyne and Wear
England SR1 1RS

Europe

Continental Liaison Office
Europe
Store Kongensgade 55
1264 Copenhagen K, Denmark

◆ Church of Scientology
Advanced Organization Saint
Hill for Europe and Africa
Jernbanegade 6
1608 Copenhagen V, Denmark

Austria

Church of Scientology of Vienna
Schottenfeldgasse 13/15
1070 Vienna, Austria

Belgium

Church of Scientology of Brussels
rue General MacArthur, 9
1180 Brussels, Belgium

Denmark

Church of Scientology of Aarhus
Vester Alle 26
8000 Aarhus C, Denmark

Church of Scientology
of Copenhagen
Store Kongensgade 55
1264 Copenhagen K, Denmark

Church of Scientology of Denmark
Gammel Kongevej 3–5, 1
1610 Copenhagen V, Denmark

France

Church of Scientology of Angers
28B, avenue Mendès
49240 Avrille, France

Church of Scientology
of Clermont-Ferrand
6, rue Dulaure
63000 Clermont-Ferrand
France

Church of Scientology of Lyon
3, place des Capucins
69001 Lyon, France

Church of Scientology of Paris
7, rue Jules César
75012 Paris, France

Church of Scientology
of Saint-Étienne
24, rue Marengo
42000 Saint-Étienne, France

GERMANY

Church of Scientology of Berlin
Sponholzstraße 51–52
12159 Berlin 41
Germany

Church of Scientology
of Düsseldorf
Friedrichstraße 28B
40217 Düsseldorf, Germany

Church of Scientology
of Frankfurt
Kaiserstraße 49
60329 Frankfurt 70
Germany

Church of Scientology of Hamburg
Domstraße 9
20095 Hamburg, Germany

Church of Scientology
of Eppendorf
Brennerstraße 12
20099 Hamburg, Germany

Church of Scientology of Hanover
Odeonstraße 17
30159 Hanover, Germany

Church of Scientology of Munich
Beichstraße 12
80802 Munich 40
Germany

Church of Scientology of Stuttgart
Hohenheimerstraße 9
70184 Stuttgart, Germany

HUNGARY

Church of Scientology of Budapest
1399 Budapest
1073 Erzsébet krt. 5. I. em.
Pf. 701/215. Hungary

ISRAEL

Scientology Center of Tel Aviv
12 Shontzino Street
PO Box 57478
61573 Tel Aviv, Israel

ITALY

Church of Scientology of Brescia
Via Fratelli Bronzetti, 20
25125 Brescia, Italy

Church of Scientology of Catania
Via Garibaldi, 9
95121 Catania, Italy

Church of Scientology of Milan
Via Lepontina, 4
20159 Milan, Italy

Church of Scientology of Monza
Largomolinetto, 1
20052 Monza (MI), Italy

Church of Scientology of Novara
Corso Milano, 28
28100 Novara, Italy

Church of Scientology of Nuoro
Via Lamarmora, 102
08100 Nuoro, Italy

Church of Scientology of Padua
Via Ugo Foscolo, 5
35131 Padua, Italy

Church of Scientology
of Pordenone
Via Dogana, 19
Zona Fiera
33170 Pordenone, Italy

Church of Scientology of Rome
Via del Caravita, 5
00186 Rome, Italy

Church of Scientology of Turin
Via Bersezio, 7
10152 Turin, Italy

Church of Scientology of Verona
Corso Milano, 84
37138 Verona, Italy

NETHERLANDS

Church of Scientology
of Amsterdam
Nieuwezijds Voorburgwal
116–118 1012 SH
Amsterdam, Netherlands

NORWAY

Church of Scientology of Oslo
Storgata 17
0184 Oslo, Norway

PORTUGAL

Church of Scientology of Lisbon
Rua dos Correiros N 205, 3°
Andar
1100 Lisbon, Portugal

RUSSIA

Hubbard Humanitarian Center
of Moscow
Ul. Boris Galushkina 19A
129301 Moscow, Russia

SPAIN

Dianetics Civil Association
of Barcelona
Pasaje Domingo, 11–13 Bahos
08007 Barcelona, Spain

Dianetics Civil Association
of Madrid
Villa Maria
C/ Montera 20, Piso 1° dcha.
28013 Madrid, Spain

Sweden

Church of Scientology of Göteborg
Värmlandsgatan 16, 1 tr.
413 28 Göteborg, Sweden

Church of Scientology of Malmö
Porslinsgatan 3
211 32 Malmö, Sweden

Church of Scientology of Stockholm
Götgatan 105
116 62 Stockholm, Sweden

Switzerland

Church of Scientology of Basel
Herrengrabenweg 56
4054 Basel, Switzerland

Church of Scientology of Bern
Muhlemattstrasse 31
Postfach 384
3000 Bern 14, Switzerland

Church of Scientology of Geneva
12, rue des Acacias
1227 Carouge
Geneva, Switzerland

Church of Scientology of Lausanne
10, rue de la Madeleine
1003 Lausanne, Switzerland

Church of Scientology of Zurich
Freilagerstrasse 11
8047 Zurich, Switzerland

Australia

Continental Liaison Office Australia, New Zealand and Oceania
201 Castlereagh Street, 3rd Floor
Sydney, New South Wales
Australia 2000

◆ Church of Scientology Advanced Organization Saint Hill Australia, New Zealand and Oceania
19–37 Greek Street
Glebe, New South Wales
Australia 2037

Church of Scientology of Adelaide
24–28 Waymouth Street
Adelaide, South Australia
Australia 5000

Church of Scientology of Brisbane
106 Edward Street, 2nd Floor
Brisbane, Queensland
Australia 4000

Church of Scientology of Canberra
43–45 East Row
Canberra City, ACT
Australia 2601

Church of Scientology of Melbourne
42–44 Russell Street
Melbourne, Victoria
Australia 3000

Church of Scientology of Perth
108 Murray Street, 1st Floor
Perth, Western Australia
Australia 6000

Church of Scientology of Sydney
201 Castlereagh Street
Sydney, New South Wales
Australia 2000

Japan

Scientology Tokyo
2-11-7, Kita-otsuka
Toshima-ku
Tokyo, Japan 170-0004

New Zealand

Church of Scientology of Auckland
159 Queen Street, 3rd Floor
Auckland 1, New Zealand

Africa

Continental Liaison Office Africa
6th Floor Budget House
130 Main Street
Johannesburg, 2001, South Africa

Church of Scientology of Bulawayo
Southampton House, Suite 202
Main Street and 9th Avenue
Bulawayo, Zimbabwe

Church of Scientology of Cape Town
Ground Floor, Dorlane House
39 Roeland Street
Cape Town 8001, South Africa

Church of Scientology of Durban
20 Buckingham Terrace
Westville, Durban 3630
South Africa

Church of Scientology of Harare
404-409 Pockets Building
50 Jason Moyo Avenue
Harare, Zimbabwe

Church of Scientology of Johannesburg
4th Floor, Budget House
130 Main Street
Johannesburg 2001
South Africa

Church of Scientology
No. 108 1st Floor, Bordeaux Centre
Gordon Road, Corner Jan Smuts Avenue
Blairgowrie, Randburg 2125
South Africa

Church of Scientology of Port Elizabeth
2 St. Christopher's
27 Westbourne Road Central
Port Elizabeth 6001
South Africa

Church of Scientology of Pretoria
307 Ancore Building
Corner Jeppe and Esselen Streets
Sunnyside, Pretoria 0002
South Africa

Latin America

Continental Liaison Office
Federacion Mexicana de Dianetica
Calle Puebla #31
Colonia Roma,
C.P. 06700, Mexico, D.F.

Argentina

Dianetics Association of Argentina
2169 Bartolomé Mitre
Capital Federal
Buenos Aires 1039, Argentina

Colombia

Dianetics Cultural Center of Bogotá
Carrera 30 #91–96
Bogotá, Colombia

Mexico

Dianetics Cultural Organization, A.C.
Avenida de la Paz 2787
Fracc. Arcos Sur
Sector Juárez, Guadalajara Jalisco
C.P. 44500, Mexico

Dianetics Cultural Association, A.C.
Belisario Domínguez #17-1
Villa Coyoacán
Colonia Coyoacán
C.P. 04000, Mexico, D.F.

Institute of Applied Philosophy, A.C.
Municipio Libre No. 40
Esq. Mira Flores
Colonia Portales
Mexico, D.F.

Latin American Cultural Center, A.C.
Rio Amazonas 11
Colonia Cuahutemoc
C.P. 06500, Mexico, D.F.

Dianetics Technological Institute, A.C.
Avenida Chapultepec 540, 6° Piso
Colonia Roma, Metro
Chapultepec
C.P. 06700, Mexico, D.F.

Dianetics Development Organization, A.C.
Avenida Xola #1113 Esq. Pitágoras
Colonia Narvarte
C.P. 03220, Mexico, D.F.

Dianetics Cultural Organization, A.C.
Calle Monterrey #402
Colonia Narvarte
C.P. 03020, Mexico, D.F.

Venezuela

Dianetics Cultural Organization, A.C.
Calle Yumare Cuinta Shangai
Entre Ave. Stanz y Ave. Casiquare
Caracas, Venezuela

Dianetics Cultural Association, A.C.
M.1 Refugio
Ave.Bolívar 141-45
Sector El Viñedo
Valencia, Edo. Carabobo
Venezuela

Celebrity Centres

Church of Scientology
Celebrity Centre International
5930 Franklin Avenue
Hollywood, California 90028

Church of Scientology
Celebrity Centre Dallas
1850 North Buckner Boulevard
Dallas, Texas 75228

Church of Scientology
Celebrity Centre Las Vegas
4850 W. Flamingo Road, Ste. 10
Las Vegas, Nevada 89103

Church of Scientology
Celebrity Centre Nashville
1204 16th Avenue South
Nashville, Tennessee 37212

Church of Scientology
Celebrity Centre New York
65 East 82nd Street
New York, New York 10028

Church of Scientology
Celebrity Centre Portland
708 SW Salmon Street
Portland, Oregon 97205

Church of Scientology
Celebrity Centre London
42 Leinster Gardens
London, England W2 3AN

Church of Scientology
Celebrity Centre Vienna
Senefeldergasse 11/5
1100 Vienna, Austria

Church of Scientology
Celebrity Centre Paris
69, rue Legendre
75017 Paris, France

Church of Scientology
Celebrity Centre Düsseldorf
Rheinland e. V.
Luisenstraße 23
40215 Düsseldorf, Germany

Church of Scientology
Celebrity Centre Munich
Lanshutter Allee 42
80637 Munich, Germany

Church of Scientology
Celebrity Centre Florence
Via Silvestrina 12
50100 Florence, Italy

Scientology Missions

International Office

Scientology Missions International
6331 Hollywood Boulevard
Suite 501
Los Angeles, California
90028-6314

United States

- ▲ Scientology Missions International
  Western United States Office
  1308 L. Ron Hubbard Way
  Los Angeles, California 90027
- ▲ Scientology Missions International
  Eastern United States Office
  349 W. 48th Street
  New York, New York 10036
- ▲ Scientology Missions International
  Flag Land Base Office
  210 South Fort Harrison
  Clearwater, Florida 33756

Missions and Dianetics Centers

Alaska

Church of Scientology
Mission of Anchorage
1300 East 68th Avenue
Suite 208A
Anchorage, Alaska 99502

California

Church of Scientology
Mission of Antelope Valley
22924 Lyons Avenue
Suite 204, 205
Newhall, California 91322

Church of Scientology
Mission of Auburn
17740 Crother Hills Road
Meadow Vista, California 95722

Church of Scientology
Mission of Berkeley (Bay Cities)
2975 Treat Boulevard, Suite D-4
Concord, California 94518

Church of Scientology
Mission of Beverly Hills
9885 Charleville Boulevard
Beverly Hills, California 90212

Church of Scientology
Mission of Brand Boulevard
143 South Glendale Avenue
Suite 103
Glendale, California 91205

Church of Scientology
Mission of Buenaventura
180 North Ashwood Avenue
Ventura, California 93003

Church of Scientology
Mission of Burbank
6623 Irvine Avenue
North Hollywood, California 91606

Church of Scientology
Mission of Capitol
9915 Fair Oaks Boulevard, Suite A
Fair Oaks, California 95628

Church of Scientology
Mission of Costa Mesa
4706 E. Bond Avenue
Orange, California 92869

Church of Scientology
Mission of the Diablo Valley
610 West 4th Street
Antioch, California 94509

Church of Scientology
Mission of Escondido
326 South Kalmia Street
Escondido, California 92025

Church of Scientology
Mission of the Foothills
2254 Honolulu Avenue
Montrose, California 91020

Church of Scientology
Mission of Inglewood
133 N. Prairie Avenue
Inglewood, California 90301

Church of Scientology
Mission of Los Angeles (Russian)
13059 Oxnard Street, Apt. #208
Van Nuys, California 91401

Church of Scientology
Mission of Malibu
6959 Dune Drive
Malibu, California 90263

Church of Scientology
Mission of Los Angeles
5408 Carpenter Avenue #204
North Hollywood, California 91607

Church of Scientology
Mission of Marin
1930 4th Street
San Rafael, California 94901

Church of Scientology
Mission of Montebello
(Spanish LA)
17904 Hurley Street
La Puente, California 91744

Church of Scientology
Mission of Newport Beach
3905 Channel Place
Newport Beach, California 92663

Church of Scientology
Mission of Orange
415 N. Tustin Avenue
Orange, California 92867

Church of Scientology
Mission of Palo Alto
3505 El Camino Real
Palo Alto, California 94306

Church of Scientology
Mission of Redondo Beach
413 Anita Street
Redondo Beach, California 94063

Church of Scientology
Mission of Redwood City
617 Veterans Boulevard, #205
Redwood City, California 94063

Church of Scientology
Mission of River Park
1010 Hurley Way, Suite 505
Sacramento, California 95825

Church of Scientology
Mission of San Bernardino
5 East Citrus Avenue, Suite 105
Redlands, California 92373

Church of Scientology
Mission of San Francisco
701 Sutter Street, 3rd Floor
San Francisco, California 94109

Church of Scientology
Mission of San Jose
826 North Winchester Boulevard,
Suite 1
San Jose, California 95128

Church of Scientology
Mission of Santa Clara Valley
3596 Calico Avenue
San Jose, California 95124

Church of Scientology
Mission of Santa Monica
1337 Ocean Avenue #C
Santa Monica, California 90410

Church of Scientology
Mission of Santa Rosa
850 2nd Street, Suite F
Santa Rosa, California 95404

Church of Scientology
Mission of Sherman Oaks
13517 Ventura Boulevard, Suite 7
Sherman Oaks, California 91423

Church of Scientology
Mission of Soma
966 Mission Street
San Francisco, California 94102

Church of Scientology
Mission of Temecula
30695 Lolita Road
Temecula, California 92592

Church of Scientology
Mission of Thousand Oaks
c/o 21010 Devonshire Street
Chatsworth, California 91311

Church of Scientology
Mission of Torrance
3620 Pacific Coast Highway
Torrance, California 90505

Church of Scientology
Mission of West Valley
21010 Devonshire Street
Chatsworth, California 91311

Church of Scientology
Mission of Westwood
12617 Mitchell Avenue #4
Los Angeles, California 90066

Colorado

Church of Scientology
Mission of Alamosa
511 Main Street, Suite #6
Alamosa, Colorado 81101

Church of Scientology
Mission of Boulder
1021 Pearl Street
Boulder, Colorado 80302

Church of Scientology
Mission of Roaring Fork
827 Bennett Avenue
Glenwood Springs, Colorado 81601

Delaware

Church of Scientology
Mission of Collingswood
PO Box 730
Claymont, Delaware 19703-0730

Florida

Church of Scientology
Mission of Belleair
2907 West Bay Drive
Belleair Bluffs, Florida 33756

Church of Scientology
Mission of Clearwater
100 North Belcher Road
Clearwater, Florida 33765

Church of Scientology
Mission of Fort Lauderdale
660 South Federal Highway
Suite 200
Pompano Beach, Florida 33062

Church of Scientology
Mission of Palm Harbor
565 Hammock Drive
Palm Harbor, Florida 34683

Church of Scientology
Mission of West Palm Beach
1966 South Congress Avenue
West Palm Beach, Florida 33406

Hawaii

Church of Scientology
Mission of Honolulu
6172 May Way
Honolulu, Hawaii 96821

Illinois

Church of Scientology
Mission of Champaign-Urbana
312 West John Street
Champaign, Illinois 61820

Church of Scientology
Mission of Chicago
6580 North NW Highway
Chicago, Illinois 60631

Church of Scientology
Mission of Peoria
2020 North Wisconsin
Peoria, Illinois 61603

Kansas

Church of Scientology
Mission of Wichita
3705 East Douglas
Wichita, Kansas 67218

Louisiana

Church of Scientology
Mission of Baton Rouge
9432 Common Street
Baton Rouge, Louisiana 70806

Church of Scientology
Mission of Lafayette
104 Westmark Boulevard, Suite 2A
Lafayette, Louisiana 70506

Maine

Church of Scientology
Mission of Brunswick
2 Lincoln Street
Brunswick, Maine 04011

Massachusetts

Church of Scientology
Mission of Merrimack Valley
142 Primrose Street
Haverhill, Massachusetts 01830

Church of Scientology
Mission of Watertown
313 Common Street #2
Watertown, Massachusetts 02472

Michigan

Church of Scientology
Mission of Genesee County
423 North Saginaw
Holly, Michigan 48442

Church of Scientology
Mission of Rochester Hills
850 Lakewood Drive
Rochester Hills, Michigan 48309

Nebraska

Church of Scientology
Mission of Omaha
843 Hidden Hills Drive
Bellevue, Nebraska 68005

Nevada

Church of Scientology
Mission of Las Vegas
2923 Schaffer Circle
Las Vegas, Nevada 89121

Church of Scientology
Mission of Sierra Nevada
1539 Vassar Street, Suite 201
Reno, Nevada 89502-2745

Church of Scientology
Mission of Vegas Valley
7545 Bermuda Road
Las Vegas, Nevada 89123

New Hampshire

Church of Scientology
Mission of Greater Concord
Suite 3C-4 Bicentennial Square
Concord, New Hampshire 03301

New Jersey

Church of Scientology
Mission of Elizabeth
339 Morris Avenue
Elizabeth, New Jersey 07208-3616

Church of Scientology
Mission of New Jersey
1029 Teaneck Road
Teaneck, New Jersey 07666

New York

Church of Scientology
Mission of Middletown
21 Mill Street
Liberty, New York 12754

Church of Scientology
Mission of Queens
56-03 214th Street
Bayside, New York 11364

Church of Scientology
Mission of Rochester
4178 Holley Byron Road
Holley, New York 14470

Church of Scientology
Mission of Rockland
11 Holland Avenue, White Plains
Westchester, New York 10603

Pennsylvania

Church of Scientology
Mission of Pittsburgh
220 Nazareth Drive
Belle Vernon
Pennsylvania 15012

SOUTH CAROLINA

Church of Scientology
Mission of Charleston
PO Box 606
Santee, South Carolina 29142

TENNESSEE

Church of Scientology
Mission of Memphis
1440 Central Avenue
Memphis, Tennessee 38104

TEXAS

Church of Scientology
Mission of El Paso
1120 North El Paso Street
El Paso, Texas 79902

Church of Scientology
Mission of Harlingen
1214 Dixieland Road, Suite 4
Harlingen, Texas 78552

Church of Scientology
Mission of Houston
2727 Fondren, Suite 1-A
Houston, Texas 77063

Church of Scientology
Mission of San Antonio
5119 Fort Clark Drive
Austin, Texas 78745

VIRGINIA

Church of Scientology
Mission of Piedmont
Sage Building, Box 15
115 Jefferson Highway
Louisa, Virginia 23093

WASHINGTON

Church of Scientology
Mission of Bellevue
15424 Bellevue-Redmond Road
Redmond, Washington 98052

Church of Scientology
Mission of Bellingham
722 N. State Street
Bellingham, Washington 98225

Church of Scientology
Mission of Burien
15216 2nd Avenue SW
Seattle, Washington 98166

Church of Scientology
Mission of Seattle
1234 NE 145th Street
Seattle, Washington 98155

Dianetics Center
Mission of Spokane
1810 North Ruby
Spokane, Washington 99207

WISCONSIN

Church of Scientology
Mission of Milwaukee
710 East Silver Spring Drive,
Suite E
Whitefish Bay, Wisconsin 53217

AFRICA

▲ Scientology Missions
International
African Office
6th Floor, Budget House
130 Main Street
Johannesburg 2001, South Africa

Missions and Dianetics Centers

Church of Scientology
Mission of Kinshasa
BP 1444
7, rue de Fele
Kinshasa/Limete, Zaire

Church of Scientology
Mission of Lagos
16 Moor Road
Off University Road, Yaba
Lagos, Nigeria
West Africa

Church of Scientology
Mission of Norwood
18 Trilby Street
Oaklands, Johannesburg 2192
Republic of South Africa

Church of Scientology
Mission of Soweto
PO Box 496 Kwa-Xuma
1868 Soweto
Republic of South Africa

AUSTRALIA, NEW ZEALAND AND OCEANIA

▲ Scientology Missions
International
Australian, New Zealand
and Oceanian Office
3rd Floor, 201
Castlereagh Street
Sydney, New South Wales,
Australia 2000

Missions and Dianetics Centers

AUSTRALIA

Church of Scientology
Mission of Inner West Sydney
4 Wangal Place
Five Dock, New South Wales
Australia 2046

Church of Scientology
Mission of Melbourne
55 Glenferrie Road
Malvern, Victoria
Australia 3144

New Zealand

Church of Scientology
Mission of Christchurch
PO Box 1843
Christchurch
New Zealand

Canada

▲ Scientology Missions International
Canadian Office
696 Yonge Street
Toronto, Ontario
M4Y 2A7, Canada

Church of Scientology
Mission of Beauce
11925, le avenue
Ville de St-Georges
Beauce, Quebec
Canada G5Y 2C9

Church of Scientology
Mission of Calgary
Box 22
Site 2 RR1
Millerville, Alberta
Canada T0L 1K0

Church of Scientology
Mission of Halifax
2589 Windsor Street
Halifax, Nova Scotia
Canada B3K 5C4

Church of Scientology
Mission of Montreal
1690 A, avenue de l'Église
Montreal, Quebec
Canada H4E 1G5

Church of Scientology
Mission of Toronto
2007 Danforth Avenue
Toronto, Ontario M4C 1J7
Canada

Church of Scientology
Mission of Vancouver
2860 West 4th Avenue
Vancouver, British Columbia
Canada V6K 1R2

Church of Scientology
Chinese Mission of Vancouver
304-7260 Lindsay Road
Richmond, British Columbia
Canada V7G 3M6

Church of Scientology
Mission of Victoria
2624 Quadra Street
Victoria, British Columbia
Canada V8T 4E4

Europe

▲ Scientology Missions International
European Office
Store Kongensgade 53
1264 Copenhagen K
Denmark

Missions and Dianetics Centers

Albania

Church of Scientology
Mission of Tirana
Rr "Bardhyl" PL. 18 shk: 2
AP: 3
Tirana, Albania

Austria

Scientology Mission Salzburg
Rupertgasse 21
5020 Salzburg, Austria

Scientology Mission Wolfsberg
Am Weiher 10
9400 Wolfsberg, Austria

Croatia

Church of Scientology
Mission of Zagreb
Tkalciceva 76
10000 Zagreb
Croatia

Czech Republic

Dianetics Center
Jindriska 7
110 00 Prague 10
Czech Republic

Denmark

Church of Scientology
Mission of Aalborg
Boulevarden 39 st.
9000 Aalborg, Denmark

Church of Scientology
Mission of Copenhagen City
Rathsacksvej 1, 4th floor
1862 Frederiksberg C
Denmark

Church of Scientology
Mission of Fyn
Ove Gjeddes Vej. 27
5220 Odense
Denmark

Church of Scientology
Mission of Lyngby
Sorgenfrivej 3
2800 Lyngby, Denmark

Church of Scientology
Mission of Silkeborg
Virklundvej 5, Virklund
8600 Silkeborg, Denmark

Finland

Church of Scientology
Mission of Helsinki
Peltolantie 2 B
01300 Vantaa, Finland

Church of Scientology
Dianetiikka-keskus
Hämeenkatu 11 D
15110 Lahti, Finland

France

Church of Scientology
Mission of Bordeaux
41, rue de Cheverus
33000 Bordeaux, France

Church of Scientology
Mission of Marseille
2, rue Devilliers
13005 Marseille, France

Church of Scientology
Mission of Nice
28, rue Gioffredo
06000 Nice, France

Church of Scientology
Mission of Toulouse
9, rue Edmond de Planet
31000 Toulouse, France

Germany

Scientology Mission Augsburg
Frauentorstr. 40
86152 Augsburg, Germany

Scientology Mission Bremen e.V.
Stolzenauer Str. 36
28207 Bremen, Germany

Dianetik Göppingen e.V.
Scientology Mission
Geislingerstraße 21
73033 Göppingen, Germany

Scientology Heilbronn
Mission der Scientology
Kirche e.V.
Am Wollhaus 8
74072 Heilbronn, Germany

Mission der Scientology Kirche
Karlstraße 46
76133 Karlsruhe, Germany

Scientology Mission Pasing
Landsbergstraße 416
81241 Munich, Germany

Scientology Kirche Bayern e.V.
Gemeinde Nuremberg
Färberstraße 5
90402 Nuremberg, Germany

Scientology Mission e.V.
Heinestraße 9
72762 Reutlingen, Germany

Scientology Mission Ulm e.V.
Eythstraße 2
89075 Ulm, Germany

Greece

Greek Dianetics and
Scientology Centre
Patision 200
11256 Athens, Greece

Italy

▲ Scientology Missions
International
Italian Office
Via Cadorna, 61
20090 Milano, Italy

Missions and Dianetics Centers

Church of Scientology
Mission of Aosta
Corso Battaglione, 13/B
11100 Aosta, Italy

Church of Scientology
Mission of Assemini
Via Sardegna 117
09032 Assemini (CA) Cagliari

Church of Scientology
Mission of Asti
Corso Alfieri, 51
14100 Asti, Italy

Church of Scientology
Mission of Avellino
Via Fratelli Bisogno, 5
83100 Avellino, Italy

Church of Scientology
Mission of Barletta
Via Cialdini, 67/B
70051 Barletta (BA), Italy

Church of Scientology
Mission of Bergamo
Via Roma, 85
24020 Gorle (BG), Italy

Church of Scientology
Mission of Bologna
Via delle Fragole, 14
40127 Bologna, Italy

Church of Scientology
Mission of Bolzano
Via Al Boschetto, 7
39100 Bolzano, Italy

Church of Scientology
Mission of Cagliari
Via Sonnino, 177
09127 Cagliari, Italy

Church of Scientology
Mission of Cantù
Via G. da Fossano, 40
22063 Cantù (CO), Italy

Church of Scientology
Mission of Carpi
Via Trento Trieste, 59
41012 Carpi (MO), Italy

Church of Scientology
Mission of Castelfranco
Piazza Serenissima, 40
31033 Castelfranco Veneto (TV), Italy

Church of Scientology
Mission of Como
Via Torno, 12
22100 Como, Italy

Church of Scientology
Mission of Conegliano
Via Manin, 9
31015 Conegliano (TV), Italy

Church of Scientology
Mission of Cosenza
Via Duca degli Abruzzi, 6
87100 Cosenza, Italy

Church of Scientology
Mission of Franciacorta
Via de Gasperi, 6
25040 Nigoline di Cortefranca (BS), Italy

Church of Scientology
Mission of Lecco
Via Mascari, 78
23900 Lecco, Italy

Church of Scientology
Mission of Lucca
Viale G. Puccini, 425/B
55100 Lucca, Italy

Church of Scientology
Mission of Macerata
Via Moretti, 1
62010 Piediripa (MC), Italy

Church of Scientology
Mission of Mantova
Via Alberto Mario, 21
46100 Mantova, Italy

Church of Scientology
Mission of Merate
Via Paolo Arlati (Ang. via Roma)
23807 Merate, (LC), Italy

Church of Scientology
Mission of Milano
Via Vannucci, 13
20135 Milano, Italy

Church of Scientology
Mission of Modena
Via Giardini, 468/C
41100 Modena, Italy

Church of Scientology
Mission of Olbia
Via Gabriele D'Annunzio, 13
c/o Martini
07026 Olbia (SS), Italy

Church of Scientology
Mission of Palermo
Via Mariano Stabile, 139
90100 Palermo, Italy

Church of Scientology
Mission of Ragusa
Via Caporale degli Zuavi, 67
97019 Vittoria (RG), Italy

Church of Scientology
Mission of Romano (Clusone)
Via G. Rubini, 12
24045 Romano di Lombardia (BG), Italy

Church of Scientology
Mission of Roncadelle
Vicolo del Mattino, 3
25030 Roncadelle (BS), Italy

Church of Scientology
Mission of Treviglio
Via Bicetti, 8A
24047 Treviglio (BG), Italy

Church of Scientology
Mission of Trieste
Via Gatteri, 28
34129 Trieste, Italy

Church of Scientology
Mission of Vicenza Centro
Via Contra Manin, 20
36100 Vicenza, Italy

MACEDONIA

Hubbard Center for Dianetics and Scientology
Bul. Partizanski Odredi 21/1
Deloven Kompleks "Porta Bunjakovec"
Mezzanine A 3/2
1000 Skopje
Republic of Macedonia

ROMANIA

Dianetics Center of Nagyvarad
3700 Oradea
Str. Progresului nr. 40,
BL B-19-20. ap. 5
Romania

Dianetics Center of Székelyudvarhely
4150 Odorheiu Secuiesc
Str. M. Sadoveanu 13
CP: 28
Romania

SLOVENIA

Dianetics Centre of Koper
Za Gradom, 21
6000 Koper
Slovenia

SPAIN

Centro de Eficiencia
Personal Dianética
C/Hermanos Rivas, 22-1-1A
46018 Valencia, Spain

Centro de Mejoramiento
Personal
C/Viera y Clavijo, 33-2 Planta
35002 Las Palmas de Gran Canaria
Spain

Centro de Mejoramiento
Personal
Urbanización Los Mirtos, 65
41020 Sevilla, Spain

Centro de Mejoramiento
Personal de Cercedilla
Cambrils, 19
28034 Madrid, Spain

Misión de la Moraleja
Cuesta Blanca, 213
28100 Madrid, Spain

SWEDEN

Dianetik Huset
Finnbodavägen 2, 4th
13131 Nacka, Sweden

SWITZERLAND

Church of Scientology
Mission of Lugano
Via Campagna, 30A
6982 Serocca D'Agno
Switzerland

Dianetik and Scientology
Luzern Mission
Zentrum für
Angewandte Philosophie
Sentimattstrasse 7
6011 Luzern, Switzerland

Mission der Scientology Kirche
Regensbergstrasse 89
8050 Zürich, Switzerland

CENTRAL EUROPE

▲ Scientology Missions
International
Central European Office
1438 Budapest
Pf. 351
Hungary

Missions and Dianetics Centers

Church of Scientology
Mission of Baja
6500 Baja
Galamb u. 13.
Hungary

Church of Scientology
Mission of Belváros
1052 Budapest
Károly krt. 4. III/10.
Hungary

Church of Scientology
Mission of Bonyhád
7150 Bonyhád
Bartók Béla u. 56/A
Hungary

Church of Scientology
Mission of Debrecen
4031 Debrecen
Derék u. 181. 4/12
Hungary

Church of Scientology
Mission of Dunaújváros
2404 Dunaújváros
Pf. 435
Hungary

Church of Scientology
Mission of Eger
3300 Eger
Pf. 215
Hungary

Church of Scientology
Mission of Esztergom
2500 Esztergom
Budapesti út 30.
Hungary

Church of Scientology
Mission of Győr
9026 Győr
Dózsa György rakpart 1/4.
Hungary

Church of Scientology
Mission of Kalocsa
6300 Kalocsa
Alkotás u. 20. II/7
Hungary

Church of Scientology
Mission of Kaposvár
7400 Kaposvár
Űrhajós u. 38. 1/1
Hungary

Church of Scientology
Mission of Kazincbarcika
3700 Kazincbarcika
Ságvári tér 3.
Hungary

Church of Scientology
Mission of Keszthely
8360 Keszthely
Sopron u. 41.
Hungary

Church of Scientology
Mission of Kiskunfélegyháza
6101 Kiskunfélegyháza
Pf. 23
Hungary

Church of Scientology
Mission of Mez kövesd
3400 Mez kövesd
Dr. Lukács Gáspár u. 5.
Hungary

Church of Scientology
Mission of Miskolc
3530 Miskolc
Széchenyi u. 34. I. em.
Hungary

Church of Scientology
Mission of Nyíregyháza
4400 Nyíregyháza
Vasvári Pál út 14.
Hungary

Church of Scientology
Mission of Ózd
3600 Ózd
Sárlitelep
Hungary

Church of Scientology
Mission of Paks
7030 Paks
Kodály Zoltán u. 30
Pf. 10
Hungary

Church of Scientology
Mission of Pécs
7621 Pécs
Király u. 8.
7602 Pécs 2
Pf. 41
Hungary

Church of Scientology
Mission of Sopron
9401 Sopron
Pf. 111
Hungary

Church of Scientology
Mission of Százhalombatta
2440 Százhalombatta
Pf. 69
Hungary

Church of Scientology
Mission of Szeged
6722 Szeged
Pf. 1258
Hungary

Church of Scientology
Mission of Székesfehérvár
8001 Székesfehérvár
Pf. 176
Hungary

Church of Scientology
Mission of Szekszárd
7100 Szekszárd
Pf. 165
Hungary

Church of Scientology
Mission of Tatabánya
2800 Tatabánya
Pf. 1372
Hungary

Church of Scientology
Mission of Tiszaújváros
3580 Tiszaújváros
Teleki Blanka u. 2.
Hungary

Church of Scientology
Mission of Veszprém
8200 Veszprém
Völgyhíd tér 3.
Hungary

Commonwealth Of Independent States

▲ Scientology Missions International
CIS Office
Hubbard Humanitarian Center,
Ul. Borisa Galushkina 19A
129301 Moscow, Russia

Missions and Dianetics Centers

Belarus

Borisov Dianetics Center
Borisov
2nd pereulok Turgeneva 19
Belarus

Dianetics Center of Minsk
Minsk 220017
AB Box 4
Belarus

Scientology Mission of Mogilev
212011 Mogilev
Ul. 8th March 54
Belarus

Georgia

Dianetics Mission of Tbilisi
Tbilisi
Ul. Ushangi Tchkheidze 8
Georgia

Kazakhstan

Dianetics Center of Almaty
480000, Kazakhstan, Almaty
AB Box 219
Kazakhstan

Dianetics Center of Aktau
466200 Kazakhstan
Aktau 6-21-58
Kazakhstan

Dianetics Center of Astana
Ul. Manasa 1412-16
Kazakhstan

Scientology Mission of Ekibastuz
Ekibastuz, Lenina 55-97
Kazakhstan

Dianetics Center of Karaganda
Karaganda
Erzhanova 10/2
Kazakhstan

Mission of Medeo (Almaty II)
Ul. Mate-Zalki 90-48
Almaty
Kazakhstan

Scientology Mission of Pavlodar II
Ul. Moscovskaya 93
Pavlodar
Kazakhstan

Scientology Mission of Semipalatinsk
Semipalatinsk
Naimanbayeva 10-311
Kazakhstan

Mission of Shymkent
Norimanova St. 2627
Shymkent
Kazakhstan

Mission of Ust-Kamenogorsk
c/o Olga Fominskaya
Scientology Mission of Semipalatinsk
490035 Pogranichnaya 44-11
Kazakhstan

Mission of Yugozapandnaya
Orbita – 1 Microregion 29-352
Karaogovorda
Kazakhstan

KYRGYZSTAN

Scientology Mission of Bishkek
Bishkek, Pr. Chuy, 34-77
Kyrgyzstan

MOLDOVA

Kishinev Dianetics Center
MD 2028, Kishinev
AB Box 1145
Moldova

RUSSIA

Scientology Mission of Arbat
Moscow
Tzvetnoy Blvd. 26
Russia

Scientology Mission of Arbat
107258 Moscow
Ul. 2nd Progonnaya 10, ap 159
Russia

Scientology Mission of Barnaul
Barnaul
Malakhova 85-183
Russia

Scientology Mission of Barnaul
656014 Barnaul
Ul. Vodoprovodnaja, 95
Russia

Scientology Mission of Bryansk
241037 Bryansk
Ul. Dokuchaeva 15-72
Russia

Scientology Mission of Chelny
423823 Naberezhny Chelny
Ul. Pushkina 6-464
Russia

Scientology Mission of Chelyabinsk
454136 Chelyabinsk
Ul. Molodogvardeitsev 70-16
Russia

Dianetics Center of Dimitrovgrad
Ulyanovskaja Obl.,
433510 Dimitrovgrad-12
AB Box 189
Russia

Mission of Dzerzhinsk
N. Novgorod M. Voronova 16-97
Russia

Scientology Mission of Ekaterinburg
610066 Ekaterinburg
Ul. Mira, 8-24
Ekaterinburg
Russia

Scientology Mission of Habarovsk
680021 Habarovsk
Ul. Pankova 13-332
Russia

Dianetics Center of Ivanovo
153000 Ivanovo
Ul. 3rd Internationala 41-11
Russia

Scientology Mission of Izhevsk
Izhevsk
Ul. Militsionnaya, 3
Izhevsk, Russia

Scientology Mission of Kaliningrad MR
141070 Kaliningrad MR
Moscow Region, Korolev MR
Ul. Frunze 24-13
Russia

Scientology Mission of
Kalininskaya
St. Petersburg
Ul. Vekeneeva 4-42
Russia

Dianetics Humanitarian Center
of Kaluga
248018 Kaluga
Ul. Marshala Zukova 18,
Russia

Scientology Mission of Kazan
420089 Kazan
Ul. Latyshskih Strelkov 33-171
Russia

Scientology Mission
of Kislovodsk
357746 Kislovodsk
Ul. Telmana 3-6
Russia

Scientology Mission
of Krasnoselskaya
Ul. Novoproletarskaya 52-3
Gatchina, St. Petersburg Region
188302
Russia

Dianetics Center of Krasnoyarsk
660077 Krasnoyarsk
Ul. Molokova 7, 323
Krasnoyarsk, Russia

Scientology Mission of Kursk
Kursk
Magistralny proezd 12-2
Russia

Scientology Mission of Kushva
624300 Kushva
Sverdlovsk Region
Krasnoarmeiskaya 13-18
Russia

Scientology Mission
of Ligovskaya
193036 St. Petersburg
Ligovskij Prospect, 33
Russia

Dianetics Center
of Magnitogorsk
455000 Magnitogorsk
AB Box 3008
Russia

Dianetics Center of Mitishi
141007 Moscovskaja Obl.
Mitishi
2-oj Shelkovsky proezd 5/1-62
Russia

Church of Scientology
of Moscovskaya
Ul. Plavnitskay 4-32
Krishi, Moscow
Russia

Scientology Mission of Moscow
103030 Moscow
Juzhnoportovaya proezd 27
Russia

Dianetics Center
of Moscow Central
Moscow
Ul. Argunovskaya 18-117
Russia

Dianetics Center of Murmansk
183766 Murmansk
Per. Rusanova 10-514
Russia

Mission of Nabarezny-Chelny
Nabarezny-Chelny 10/36
Flat 7
Russia

Dianetics Mission of Nazran
Grozny
Ul. Mozhayskogo 10
Russia

Mission of Nevinnomyssk
Ul. Partanskaya 11-122
Nevinnnomyssk
Russia

Scientology Mission
of Nizhnekamsk
423550 Tatarstan, Nizhnekamsk
Ul. Urmanche 3-3
Russia

Dianetics Center
of Nizhny-Novgorod
603074 Nizhny-Novgorod
Ul. Marshala Voronova 16-97
Russia

Scientology Mission of
Novgorod I+II
173001 Novgorod
AB Box 120
Russia

Scientology Mission
of Novokuznetsk
654917 Novokuznetsk Obl.
Kemerovo Region
Talzino
Ul. Sverdlova 15-3
Russia

Dianetics Center
of Novosibirsk
630104 Novosibirsk
Dostoevskogo 5-31
Russia

Scientology Mission
of Novy Urengoy
626718 Tiumenskaya Obl.
Novy Urengoy
Ul. Youbeleynaya 1-41
Russia

Hubbard Humanitarian Center
of Omsk
644043 Omsk
AB Box 3768
Russia

Dianetics Center of Omsk II
644099 Omsk, Glavpochtamt
AB Box 999
Russia

Dianetics Center of Orenburg
460024 Orenburg
Ul. Vystavochnaya 25-213
Russia

Scientology Mission of Oriol
302000, Oriol
Pl. Polikarpova 32
Russia

Scientology Mission of Penza
440034 Penza
Ul. Kalinina 108
Penza, Russia

Dianetics Center of Perm
614000 Perm
AB Box 7026
Russia

Scientology Mission of
Perovskaya
Moscow
Ul. 2nd Vladimirskaya 12-2-143
Russia

Scientology Mission of
Petrogradskaya
195176 St. Petersburg
Ul. Krasnodonskaja 19-9
Russia

Scientology Mission of
Petropavlovsk-Kamchatsky
683006 Petropavlovsk-
Kamchatsky
Ul. Kavkazskaja, 30/1-31
Russia

Scientology Mission of
Pushkinskaya
St. Petersburg, Pushkino,
Ul. Shishkova 32/15–241
Russia

Dianetics Center of Samara
443041 Samara
Leninskaya 22-1-3
Russia

Dianetics Center of Saratov
410601 Saratov
AB Box 1533
Russia

Scientology Mission of
Solnechnogorsk
141500 Solnechnogorsk
Ul. Podmoskavnaya 27-46
Russia

St. Petersburg Scientology
Center
193036 St. Petersburg
Ligovsky Prospect 33
Russia

St. Petersburg
Scientology Center II
St. Petersburg
Ul. Razezshaya 44
Russia

Scientology Mission
of Severnaya
St. Petersburg 6
Revolution Square 15-32
Russia

Scientology Mission
of Severomorsk
Murmansk, Ul. Marxa 32-64
Severomorsk
Russia

Dianetics Humanitarian
Center of Surgut
626400 Tumenskaya Obl., Surgut
Ul. Lermontova 6-1
Russia

Scientology Mission of Tambov
393724 Tambov Region
Pocrovo-Prigorodnoe Village
Ul. Sovetskaya 14
Russia

Dianetics Humanitarian
Center of Tolyatti
445050 Samarskaya Obl., Tolyatti
AB Box 14
Russia

Dianetics Center of Troitsk
142092 Troitsk
Sirenevaya 10-87
Russia

Scientology Mission of Tula
300000 Tula
Krasnoarmeysky prospect 7-127
Russia

Dianetics Center of Ufa
450076 Ufa
AB Box 7527
Russia

Scientology Mission of Ulan-Ude
670009 Ulan-Ude
Ul. Nevsky 11
Buryatia, Russia

Scientology Mission of Uljanovsk
Uljanovsk
Ul. Karbysheva L. 107
Russia

Scientology Mission
of Vladivostok
690001 Primorski Krai,
Vladivostok
AB Box 1-147
Russia

Dianetics Humanitarian
Center of Volgograd
400075 Volgograd
AB Box 6
Russia

Scientology Mission of Voronezh
394000 Voronezh
AB Box 146
Russia

Scientology Mission
of Zheleznogorsk
662990 Krasnoyarski Region
Zheleznogorsk-2
Ul. Komsomolskaya 37-19
Russia

UKRAINE

Hubbard Humanitarian Center
of Harkov
310052 Ukraine
Harkov
AB Box 53
Ukraine

Scientology Mission
of Kremenchug
315326 Kremenchug
Poltavskaya Obl., Mira 3-161
Ukraine

Scientology Mission
of Melitopol
Melitopol
Ul. Gorkorgo 1
Ukraine

Scientology Mission of Nikolayev
327038 Nikolayev
Karpenko 4-56
Ukraine

Dianetics Center of Uzgorod
294000 Uzgorod
Ul. Dobrianskogo 10-9
Ukraine

UNITED KINGDOM

▲ Scientology Missions
International
United Kingdom Office
Saint Hill Manor
East Grinstead
West Sussex, RH19 4JY
England

Missions and Dianetics Centers

Dianetics and Scientology
Mission of Bournemouth Ltd.
42 High Street
Poole, Dorset, England
BH15 1BT

Church of Scientology
Mission of Hove Ltd.
59A Coleridge Street
Hove, East Sussex, England
BN3 5AB

HONG KONG

Church of Scientology
Mission of Hong Kong
Flat E, 7/F, Tower 8
Laguna Verde,
Hung Hom, Kowloon
Central, Hong Kong

INDIA

Scientology Counseling Center
24 Sampooran Lodge
Ajit Nagar, Punjab 147001
India

Dianetics Center
of Ambala Cantt
6352 Punjabi Mohalla
Ambala Cantt 133001
India

Dianetics Center
of Calcutta
P404/2 Hemanta
Mukhopadhyay Sarani
Calcutta 700029
India

IRELAND

Church of Scientology
Mission of Dublin Ltd.
62/63 Middle Abbey Street
Dublin 1, Ireland

JAPAN

Church of Scientology
Dianetics Centre Akasaka
Akasaka-dori 50 Building, 5-5-11
Akasaka Minato-ku
Tokyo, Japan

Latvia

Dianetics Center of Riga
Latvia, Humanitarian Centrs "Dianetika"
Laspesa 27 of 4 Riga LV 1011
Latvia

Lithuania

Dianetics Center of Vilnius
Centrinis paštas 2000, p.d. 42
Vilnius, Lithuania

Latin America

▲ Scientology Missions International
Latin American Office
Puebla 31, Colonia roma
CP 06700 Mexico, D.F.

Missions and Dianetics Centers

Colombia

Asociación Dianética
Bogotá Norte
Avenida 13, No. 104-91
Bogotá, Colombia

Fundación para el Mejoramiento de la Vida
Calle 70A, No. 12-38
Bogotá, Colombia

Iglesia de Cienciología
Misión de Medellín
Carrera 13, No. 19-23
La Ceja, Antioquia, Colombia

Chile

Centro de Tecnología Hubbard
Jorge Washington, No. 338
Santiago de Chile
Chile

Centro Hubbard
Misión de Chile
Nuncio Laghi, 6558
La Reina, Santiago, Chile

Costa Rica

Instituto Tecnológico de Dianética
300 Mts. sur de auto mercado en Los Yoses C.R.
Apdo: 1245700-1000
San José, Costa Rica

Dominican Republic

Dianética Santo Domingo
Condominio Ambar Plaza II
Bloque II, Apto. 302
Avenida Núñez de Cáceres Esq. Sarasota
Santo Domingo
Dominican Republic

Ecuador

Iglesia de Cienciología
Misión de Guayaquil
Avenida Fco. de Orellana, No. 218
Guayaquil, Ecuador

Guatemala

Asociación de Cienciología Aplicada Dianética de Guatemala
21 Avenida "A," 32-28
Zona 5, Guatemala

Mexico

Centro de Dianética Hubbard de Aguascalientes A.C.
Hamburgo, No. 127
Fraccionamiento del Valle 1A Sec.
C.P. 20080 Aguascalientes, Ags.
Mexico

Instituto de Filosofía Aplicada de Bajío
Boulevard Adolfo López Mateos 507 Oriente
Zona Centro Entre Libertad y República
Leon Gto.
C.P. 37000, Mexico

Mission Chihuahua
Ortiz del Campo, 3309 Frace
Colonia San Felipe, Chihuahua
Chihuahua, Mexico

Centro Hubbard de Dianética Tecamachalco
#314 Prsdo. Norte
Lomas de Chapultepec
Mexico, D.F. Mexico

Instituto de Dianética Monterrey A.C.
Tulancingo, 1262, Col. Mitras
Monterrey
N.L., Mexico

Misión de Satelite
Calle Alamo, #93-3er Piso – Local B
Santa Monica, Tlalnepantla
Edo. de Mexico, 54040
Mexico

Misión de Tijuana
Calle Balboa, #5284
Lomas Hipódromo
Tijuana B.C.
C.P. 22480 Mexico

Misión de Valle
Juárez, 139
San Pedro Garza García
N.L. Monterrey, 66230 Mexico

Pakistan

Dianetics Center
A-3 Royal Avenue
(opposite Urdu College
Block 13C)
Gulshan-E-Iqbal
Karachi, Pakistan

Taiwan

▲ Scientology Missions
International
Taiwan Office
2F, No. 65, Sec. 4
Ming-Shung East Road
Taipei, Taiwan

Missions and Dianetics Centers

Church of Scientology
Mission of Capital
2F No. 28, Lane 63,
Liao-Ning Street
Taipei, Taiwan

Church of Scientology
Mission of Kaohsiung
No. 216, Fu-Jen Road
Ling-Ya District
Kaohsiung, Taiwan

Church of Scientology
Mission of Pingtung
No. 206, Pang-Chiu Road
Pingtung, Taiwan

Church of Scientology
Mission of Taichung
No. 82-2 Wu-Chuan-5th Street
Taichung, Taiwan

Church of Scientology
Mission of Tainan
3F, No. 70, Ching-Nien Road
Tainan, Taiwan

Church of Scientology
Mission of Taipei
No. 2, Lane 59, SEC. 2,
Sung-Chang North Road
Taipei, Taiwan

Thailand

Church of Scientology
Mission of Bangkok
Room B1, 2F, 339 Soi Pipat
Bangrak,
Bangkok, Thailand 10500

FREEDOM MAGAZINE

INTERNATIONAL OFFICE

Church of Scientology International
Freedom Magazine
6331 Hollywood Boulevard, Suite 1200
Los Angeles, California 90028-6329

Church of Scientology of Washington
Freedom Magazine
1701 20th Street, NW
Washington, DC 20009

AUSTRALIA

Church of Scientology of Sydney
Freedom Magazine
201 Castlereagh Street, Sydney
New South Wales, Australia 2000

AUSTRIA

Church of Scientology of Austria
Freedom Magazine
Schottenfeldgasse 13–15
1070 Vienna, Austria

BELGIUM

Church of Scientology of Belgium
Freedom Magazine
61, rue du Prince Royal
1050 Brussels, Belgium

DENMARK

Church of Scientology of Denmark
Frihed
Gammel Kongevej 3–5
1610 Copenhagen V, Denmark

FRANCE

Church of Scientology of Paris
Magazine *Éthique et Liberté*
7, rue Jules César
75012 Paris, France

GERMANY

Church of Scientology of Munich
Freiheit Magazine
Beichstraße 12
80802 Munich 40, Germany

GREECE

Dianetics and Scientology Center
Freedom Magazine
Patision 200, 11256 Athens, Greece

ITALY

Church of Scientology of Milano
Diritti dell'uomo
Via Abetone, 10
21037 Milano, Italy

JAPAN

Scientology Tokyo
Freedom Magazine
2-11-7, Kita-Otsuka, Toshima-ku
Tokyo, 170-0004, Japan

MEXICO

Federación Mexicana de Dianética A.C.
Freedom Magazine
Pomona, 53, Colonia Roma
C.P. 06700, Mexico, D.F.

NETHERLANDS

Church of Scientology of Amsterdam
Freedom Magazine
Nieuwezijds Voorburgwal 116-118
1012 SH Amsterdam, Netherlands

NEW ZEALAND

Church of Scientology of New Zealand
Freedom Magazine
159 Queen Street
Auckland 1, New Zealand

SOUTH AFRICA

Church of Scientology of Johannesburg
Freedom Magazine
6th Floor, Budget House
130 Main Street
Johannesburg 2001, South Africa

SPAIN

Church of Scientology of Spain
Ética y Libertad Magazine
C/ Montera 20, 1° dcha.
28013 Madrid, Spain

SWEDEN

Church of Scientology of Stockholm
Freedom Magazine
Götgatan 105
11662 Stockholm, Sweden

SWITZERLAND

Church of Scientology of Lausanne
Magazine *Éthique et Liberté*
10, rue de la Madeleine
1003 Lausanne, Switzerland

Church of Scientology of Zurich
Freiheit Magazine
Badenerstrasse 141
8004 Zurich, Switzerland

UNITED STATES

Church of Scientology Flag Service Organization
Freedom Magazine
503 Cleveland Street
Clearwater, Florida 33755

Church of Scientology of Los Angeles
Freedom Magazine
4810 Sunset Boulevard
Los Angeles, California 90027

Citizens Commission on Human Rights (CCHR)

INTERNATIONAL OFFICE

Citizens Commission on Human Rights International
6616 Sunset Boulevard
Los Angeles, California 90028

Australia

Citizens Commission on Human Rights
Australian National Office
201 Castlereagh Street, 2nd Floor
Sydney, New South Wales
Australia 2000

Citizens Commission on Human Rights Adelaide
24–28 Waymouth Street, 1st Floor
Adelaide, South Australia
Australia 5000

Citizens Commission on Human Rights Brisbane
PO Box 57
Lutwyche, Queensland
Australia 4030

Citizens Commission on Human Rights Perth
GPO Box N1709
Perth, Western Australia
Australia 6843

Citizens Commission on Human Rights Melbourne
42–44 Russell Street
Melbourne, Victoria
Australia 3000

Austria

Citizens Commission on Human Rights Austria
Postfach 133
Vienna 1072, Austria

Belgium

Citizens Commission on Human Rights Belgium
Boite Postale, 55
2800 Mechelen II, Belgium

Canada

Citizens Commission on Human Rights
Canadian National Office
27 Carlton Street, Suite 304
Toronto, Ontario
Canada M5B 1L2

Citizens Commission on Human Rights Montreal
4489 Avenue Papineau
Montreal, Quebec
Canada H2H 1T7

Citizens Commission on Human Rights Vancouver
401 West Hastings Street
Vancouver, British Columbia
Canada V6B 1L5

Commonwealth Of Independent States

Citizens Commission on Human Rights CIS
c/o Hubbard Humanitarian Center
Ul. Borisa Galushkina 19A
129301 Moscow, Russia

Czech Republic

Citizens Commission on Human Rights Czech Republic
PO Box 404
11121 Prague 1
Czech Republic

Denmark

Citizens Commission on Human Rights Copenhagen
Store Kongensgade 55
1264 Copenhagen K
Denmark

Citizens Commission on Human Rights Denmark
Lundegårdsvej 19
2900 Hellerup
Denmark

Finland

Citizens Commission on Human Rights Finland
PO Box 145
00511 Helsinki, Finland

France

Citizens Commission on Human Rights France
4, rue Burg
75018 Paris, France

Citizens Commission on Human Rights Angers
21, rue Marc Sagnier
49000 Angers, France

Citizens Commission on Human Rights Clermont-Ferrand
98, rue André Theuriet
63000 Clermont-Ferrand, France

Citizens Commission on Human Rights Lyon
11, rue Auguste Payant
69007 Lyon, France

GERMANY

Citizens Commission
on Human Rights National
Office
KVPM e. V.
Amalienstr. 49a
80799 Munich, Germany

Citizens Commission
on Human Rights Berlin
KVPM
Ahornstr. 14
14163 Berlin, Germany

Citizens Commission
on Human Rights Düsseldorf
KVPM
Kruppstr. 49
40227 Düsseldorf, Germany

Citizens Commission
on Human Rights Frankfurt
KVPM e. V.
Schopenhauerstr. 12
631510 Geusenstamm, Germany

Citizens Commission
on Human Rights Freiburg
KVPM e. V.
Im Grun 18
79395 Neuenburg, Germany

Citizens Commission
on Human Rights Hamburg
KVPM e. V.
Rostocker Straße 38
D-20099 Hamburg, Germany

Citizens Commission
on Human Rights Karlsruhe
KVPM e. V.
Baumeisterstr. 40
76137 Karlsruhe, Germany

Citizens Commission
on Human Rights Mannheim
KVPM e. V.
Heidebuckel 29
67319 Wattenheim, Germany

Citizens Commission
on Human Rights Nuremberg
KVPM e. V.
Dorfstr. 12
96132 Schlusselfeld, Germany

Citizens Commission
on Human Rights Stuttgart
KVPM e. V.
Azenbergaufgang 8
70192 Stuttgart, Germany

GREECE

Citizens Commission
on Human Rights Greece
65, Panepistimiou Str.
Athens 10564, Greece

HUNGARY

Citizens Commission
on Human Rights Hungary
1461 Budapest
PF 182
Hungary

ISRAEL

Citizens Commission
on Human Rights Israel
PO Box 37020
Tel Aviv, Israel

ITALY

Citizens Commission
on Human Rights
Italian National Office
Chiesa Scientology Nazionale
Via Cadorna, 16
20090 Vimodrone (MI), Italy

Citizens Commission
on Human Rights Brescia
c/o Luisa Lorini
Piazzale Spedali civili, 21
25123 Brescia, Italy

Citizens Commission
on Human Rights Garbagnate
and Arese
Via Montello, 18
20024 Garbagnate Milanese, Italy

Citizens Commission
on Human Rights Lucca
Corso Garibaldi, 91
55100 Lucca, Italy

Citizens Commission
on Human Rights Monza
Casella Postale 1
20048 Carate Brianza (MI), Italy

Citizens Commission
on Human Rights Novara
Corso Risorgimento, 24
28100 Novara, Italy

Citizens Commission
on Human Rights Padova
via Chiesotti, 16
35100 Padova, Italy

Citizens Commission
on Human Rights Pordenone
c/o Katia Pedroni
Via Castellana, 6
31010 Cimadolmo TV, Italy

Citizens Commission
on Human Rights Torino
Via Airasca, 3
10141 Torino, Italy

Citizens Commission
on Human Rights Verona
via A. Doria, 32
37138 Verona, Italy

JAPAN

Citizens Commission
on Human Rights Tokyo
2-11-7-7F, Kita-Otsuka,
Toshima-ku
Tokyo, 170-0004, Japan

Citizens Commission
on Human Rights Osaka
2-1-11 Higashi-imazato
Higashinari-ku
Osaka, Japan 537-0011

LATIN AMERICA

ARGENTINA

Citizens Commission
on Human Rights Argentina
Avenida Santa Fe 1769 2° Piso
1060 Capital Federal
Argentina

COLOMBIA

Citizens Commission
on Human Rights Colombia
A. A. 110463
Santa Fe de Bogotá
Colombia

COSTA RICA

Citizens Commission
on Human Rights Costa Rica
Instituto Tecnológico de Dianética
Los Yosos del auto mercado 100 Sur
Apdo 12470 1000
San José, Costa Rica

MEXICO

Citizens Commission
on Human Rights Mexico
Tuxpan 68
Colonia Roma
C.P. 06760, Mexico, D.F.

VENEZUELA

Citizens Commission
on Human Rights Venezuela
National Office
Urg. La Granja Res. Tenis Garden
Torre B piso 3 Apartamento 3-3
Valencia, Venezuela

Citizens Commission
on Human Rights Barquisimeto
c/o Associacion Cultural Dianetica
Carrera 26 A entre calles 8Y9
No 8-25
Barquisimeto Edo. Lara, Venezuela

NETHERLANDS

Citizens Commission
on Human Rights Netherlands
Postbus 3173
2001 DD Harlem, Netherlands

NEW ZEALAND

Citizens Commission
on Human Rights New Zealand
159 Queen Street, 1st Floor
Auckland 1, New Zealand

NORWAY

Citizens Commission
on Human Rights Norway
Postboks 8902
Youngstorget
0028 Oslo, Norway

PORTUGAL

Citizens Commission
on Human Rights Portugal
c/o Igreja de Cientologia
Rua da Prata 185, 2 Andar
1100 Lisbon, Portugal

SOUTH AFRICA

Citizens Commission
on Human Rights
South African National Office
PO Box 710
Johannesburg 2000, South Africa

Citizens Commission
on Human Rights Cape Town
PO Box 443
Green-Point
8051 Cape Town, South Africa

SWEDEN

Citizens Commission
on Human Rights Sweden
Johan Enbergs väg 36
171 61 Solna, Sweden

Citizens Commission
on Human Rights Göteborg
Box 7232
40235 Göteborg, Sweden

SWITZERLAND

Citizens Commission
on Human Rights Basel
Feldstrasse 10
4123 Allschwil, Switzerland

Citizens Commission
on Human Rights Bern
Postfach 338
3000 Bern 7, Switzerland

Citizens Commission
on Human Rights Geneva
Casella Postale 1282
1211 Geneva 1, Switzerland

Citizens Commission
on Human Rights Lausanne
Casella Postale 231
1000 Lausanne 17, Switzerland

Citizens Commission
on Human Rights Ticino
Casella Postale 613
6512 Giubiasco
Switzerland

Citizens Commission
on Human Rights Zurich
Postfach 1207
8026 Zurich, Switzerland

UNITED KINGDOM

Citizens Commission
on Human Rights
United Kingdom National Office
PO Box 188
East Grinstead, West Sussex RH19 4JF
England

Citizens Commission
on Human Rights Bournemouth
PO Box 1456
Wimborne
Dorset BH21 IYW, England

Citizens Commission
on Human Rights Brighton
PO Box 3277
Brighton, Sussex BN1 8RT,
England

Citizens Commission
on Human Rights Sunderland
9, The Crescent
Sunniside
Gateshead
Tyne and Wear NE16 5DH
England

Citizens Commission
on Human Rights Ireland
Ashton House, Casleknock
Dublin 15, Ireland

UNITED STATES

ARIZONA

Citizens Commission
on Human Rights Arizona
3021 E. Hubbell
Phoenix, Arizona 85008

CALIFORNIA

Citizens Commission
on Human Rights Los Angeles
PO Box 29754
Los Angeles, California
90029-0754

Citizens Commission
on Human Rights Mountain View
2483 Old Middlefield Way
Mountain View, California 94043

Citizens Commission
on Human Rights Orange County
PO Box 984
Tustin, California 92681

Citizens Commission
on Human Rights Riverside
17305 Santa Rosa Mine Road
Perris, California 92570

Citizens Commission
on Human Rights Sacramento
926 J Street Suite 519
Sacramento, California 95814

Citizens Commission
on Human Rights San Diego
222 Camino Vista Road
Chula Vista, California 91910

Citizens Commission
on Human Rights San Francisco
83 McAllister Street
San Francisco, California 94102

Citizens Commission
on Human Rights South Bay
80 East Rosemary Street
San Jose, California 95112

Citizens Commission
on Human Rights Temecula
30965 Lolita
Temecula, California 95112

Citizens Commission
on Human Rights Ventura County
8252 Tiara Street
Ventura, California 93004

Citizens Commission
on Human Rights West Valley
23056 Baltar Street
West Hills, California 91304

COLORADO

Citizens Commission
on Human Rights Colorado
c/o Church of Scientology
3385 S. Bannock Street
Englewood, Colorado 80110

CONNECTICUT

Citizens Commission
on Human Rights Connecticut
PO Box 17
Higganum, Connecticut 06441

Florida

Citizens Commission
on Human Rights Clearwater
305 North Fort Harrison Avenue
Clearwater, Florida 33755

Citizens Commission
on Human Rights Miami
PO Box 348173
Coral Gables, Florida 33234

Citizens Commission
on Human Rights Orlando
c/o Church of Scientology
Orlando, Florida 32803

Citizens Commission
on Human Rights Tampa
c/o Church of Scientology
3617 Henderson Blvd.
Tampa, Florida 33609

Georgia

Citizens Commission
on Human Rights Atlanta
5394 Valley Mist Trace
Norcross, Georgia 30092

Hawaii

Citizens Commission
on Human Rights Hawaii
1750 Kalakaua Avenue
Suite 103
PMB 3230
Honolulu, Hawaii 96826

Illinois

Citizens Commission
on Human Rights Chicago
PO Box 3422
Oak Brook, Illinois 60522

Indiana

Citizens Commission
on Human Rights Indiana
1312 Fairview Kingston Springs Rd.
Kingston Springs, Indiana 37082

Iowa

Citizens Commission
on Human Rights Iowa
17927 Allis Road
Council Bluffs, Iowa 51503

Maine

Citizens Commission
on Human Rights Maine
3 Brigham St.
Waterville, Maine 04901

Massachusetts

Citizens Commission
on Human Rights New England
c/o Church of Scientology
1112 Boylston Street, 213
Boston, Massachusetts 02215

Missouri

Citizens Commission
on Human Rights Kansas City
3619 Broadway
Kansas City, Missouri 64111

Citizens Commission
on Human Rights St. Louis
PO Box 24222
University City, Missouri 63130

Nebraska

Citizens Commission
on Human Rights Nebraska
PO Box 24291
Omaha, Nebraska 68124

New York

Citizens Commission
on Human Rights New York City
244 5th Avenue
New York, New York 10001

Oregon

Citizens Commission
on Human Rights Oregon
PO Box 8842
Portland, Oregon 97207

Pennsylvania

Citizens Commission
on Human Rights Philadelphia
PO Box 17313
Philadelphia, Pennsylvania 19105

Texas

Citizens Commission
on Human Rights Texas
403 E. Ben White
Austin, Texas 78704

Citizens Commission
on Human Rights Houston
50 Briar Hollowlane, Suite 300 East
Houston, Texas 77027

Utah

Citizens Commission
on Human Rights Utah
662 South State Street
Salt Lake City, Utah 84111

Washington

Citizens Commission
on Human Rights Seattle
300 Lendra Street B252
Seattle, Washington 98121

Washington, DC

Citizens Commission
on Human Rights DC
1701 20th Street NW
Washington, DC 20009

National Commission on Law Enforcement and Social Justice

National Commission on Law
Enforcement and Social Justice
9025 Fulbright Avenue
Chatsworth, California 91311

ASSOCIATION FOR BETTER LIVING AND EDUCATION

INTERNATIONAL OFFICES

Association for Better Living
and Education International
7065 Hollywood Boulevard
Suite 800
Los Angeles, California 90028

Association for Better Living
and Education
Expansion Office
210 South Fort Harrison Avenue
Clearwater, Florida 33756

AFRICA

Association for Better Living
and Education
African Office
6th Floor, Budget House
130 Main Street
Johannesburg 2001, South Africa

AUSTRALIA, NEW ZEALAND, OCEANIA

Association for Better Living
and Education
Australian, New Zealand and
Oceanian Office
201 Castlereagh Street
Sydney, New South Wales
Australia 2000

CANADA

Association for Better Living
and Education
Canadian Office
696 Yonge Street
Toronto, Ontario, Canada
M4Y 2A7

COMMONWEALTH OF INDEPENDENT STATES

Association for Better Living
and Education
CIS Office
c/o Hubbard Humanitarian Center
Ul. Borisa Galushkina 19A
129301 Moscow, Russia

EUROPE

Association for Better Living
and Education
European Office
Store Kongensgade 55
1264 Copenhagen K, Denmark

CENTRAL EUROPE

Association for Better Living
and Education
Central European Office
1438 Budapest
Pf. 351
Hungary

ITALY

Association for Better Living
and Education
Italian Office
Via Nerino, 8
20213 Milano
Milano, Italy

LATIN AMERICA

Association for Better Living
and Education
Latin American Office
Puebla #31
Colonia Roma, C.P. 06700
Mexico, D.F.

UNITED KINGDOM

Association for Better Living
and Education
United Kingdom Office
Saint Hill Manor
East Grinstead, West Sussex
England RH19 4JY

UNITED STATES

Association for Better Living
and Education
Eastern United States Office
349 W. 48th Street
New York, New York 10036

Association for Better Living
and Education
Western United States Office
1308 L. Ron Hubbard Way
Los Angeles, California 90027

Applied Scholastics

International Office

Applied Scholastics International
7060 Hollywood Boulevard
Suite 200
Los Angeles, California 90028

Africa

Education Alive Africa
6th Floor, Budget House
130 Main Street
Johannesburg 2001, South Africa

Australia

Applied Scholastics
National Office
44 Smith Street
Balmain, New South Wales
Australia 2041

Canada

Applied Scholastics
National Office
1680 Lakeshore Road West,
Unit 5a
Mississauga, Ontario
Canada L5J 1J4

Commonwealth Of Independent States

Applied Scholastics CIS
c/o Hubbard Humanitarian Center
129301 Moscow
Ul. Borisa Galushkina 19A
129301 Moscow, Russia

Europe

Applied Scholastics Europe
Nørregade 26, 1st floor
1165 Copenhagen K
Denmark

Hungary

Applied Scholastics Hungary
Alkalmazott Oktatástan
Magyarország
1085 Budapest
József Krt. 31/b
Hungary

United Kingdom

Applied Scholastics
United Kingdom
78 Northwood Road
Thornton Heath
Surrey CR7 8HR, England

United States

Applied Scholastics
Eastern United States
349 W. 48th Street
New York, New York 10036

Applied Scholastics
Western United States
17291 Irvine Boulevard, Suite 405
Tustin, California 92780

Criminon

International Office

Criminon International
7060 Hollywood Boulevard
Suite 220
Los Angeles, California 90028

Africa

Criminon Africa
6th Floor, Budget House
130 Main Street
Johannesburg 2001, South Africa

Australia, New Zealand, Oceania

Criminon ANZO
201 Castlereagh Street
Sydney, New South Wales
Australia 2000

Canada

Criminon Canada
696 Yonge Street
Toronto, Ontario, Canada
M4Y 2A7

Commonwealth Of Independent States

Criminon CIS
c/o Hubbard Humanitarian Center
129301 Moscow
Ul. Borisa Galushkina 19A
129301 Moscow, Russia

Europe

Criminon Europe
Store Kongensgade 55
1264 Copenhagen K
Denmark

Hungary

Criminon Hungary
1463 Budapest
Pf. 945
Hungary

LATIN AMERICA

Criminon Latin America
Pomona, 53, Colonia Roma
C.P. 06700
Mexico, D.F.

UNITED KINGDOM

Criminon United Kingdom
PO Box 128
East Grinstead, West Sussex
England RH19 4GB

UNITED STATES

Criminon Eastern United States
349 W. 48th Street
New York, New York 10036

Criminon Western United States
PO Box 9091
Glendale, California 91226

CRIMINON CENTERS

There are Criminon programs at the following locations:

COLOMBIA

Criminon Colombia
18a Street, 1646 South
Bogotá, Colombia

COMMONWEALTH OF INDEPENDENT STATES

Criminon Moscow
c/o Hubbard Humanitarian Center
129301 Moscow
Ul. Borisa Galushkina 19A
129301 Moscow, Russia

Criminon Oriol
302030 Oriol
Lenin Ul. 4, Apt. 39
Russia

FRANCE

Criminon France
6, avenue Hoche
Beauchamp 95250
France

ITALY

Criminon Italy
c/o Associazione per un Futuro Migliore
Via Cadamosto, 8
20129 Milano, Italy

SPAIN

Criminon Canary Islands
C/ Viera y Clavijo, 33-1
35002 Las Palmas de Gran Canaria
Spain

SWEDEN

Criminon Sweden
Finnbodavägen 2, 4 tr
13131 Nacka, Sweden

SWITZERLAND

Criminon Switzerland
Arbeitsgruppe Zurich
Postfach 8176
8036 Zurich, Switzerland

UNITED STATES

CALIFORNIA

Criminon Community Education Center
306 W. Compton Boulevard
Suite 203
Compton, California 90220

Criminon Community Education Center
1043 Glendora Avenue, Suite G
West Covina, California 91790

CONNECTICUT

Criminon Connecticut
PO Box 310202
Newington, Connecticut 06131

FLORIDA

Criminon Florida
PO Box 7727
Clearwater, Florida 34615

Criminon South Florida
PO Box 817211
Hollywood, Florida 33021

MINNESOTA

Criminon Minnesota
PO Box 82
Newport, Minnesota 55055

NEW YORK

Criminon Buffalo
2045 Niagara Street
Buffalo, New York 14207

OHIO

Criminon Ohio
PO Box 09579
Columbus, Ohio 43209

VENEZUELA

Criminon Fundación Auyantepuy
Dandoral Plaza, 122A
Avenida Sucre, Los Dos Caminos
Caracas, Venezuela

NARCONON

INTERNATIONAL OFFICE

Narconon International
7060 Hollywood Boulevard
Suite 220
Los Angeles, California 90028

AFRICA

Narconon Africa
6th Floor, Budget House
130 Main Street
Johannesburg 2001, South Africa

AUSTRALIA, NEW ZEALAND, OCEANIA

Narconon ANZO
PO Box 423, Leichhardt
Sydney, New South Wales
Australia 2040

CANADA

Narconon Canada
696 Yonge Street
Toronto, Ontario, Canada
M4Y 2A7

EUROPE

Narconon Europe
Nørregade 26, 1st floor
1165 Copenhagen
Denmark

CENTRAL EUROPE

Narconon Magyarorsazág
1245 Budapest
Pf. 1090
Hungary

ITALY

Narconon Italy
c/o Associazione per un
Futuro Migliore
Via Cadamosto, 8
20129 Milano, Italy

LATIN AMERICA

Narconon Latin America
Pomona, 53
Colonia Roma
C.P. 06700, Mexico, D.F.

THE WAY TO HAPPINESS

INTERNATIONAL OFFICE

The Way to Happiness Foundation International
7060 Hollywood Boulevard Suite 301
Los Angeles, California 90028

AFRICA

The Way to Happiness Foundation Africa
6th Floor, Budget House
130 Main Street
Johannesburg 2001, South Africa

AUSTRALIA, NEW ZEALAND, OCEANIA

The Way to Happiness Foundation ANZO
201 Castlereagh Street, 3rd Floor
Sydney, Australia 2000

CANADA

The Way to Happiness Foundation Canada
696 Yonge Street
Toronto, Ontario, Canada
M4Y 2A7

COMMONWEALTH OF INDEPENDENT STATES

The Way to Happiness Foundation CIS
c/o Hubbard Humanitarian Center
129301 Moscow
Ul. Borisa Galushkina 19A
129301 Moscow, Russia

EUROPE

The Way to Happiness Foundation Europe
Store Kongensgade 55
1264 Copenhagen K, Denmark

CENTRAL EUROPE

The Way to Happiness Foundation East Europe
Az Út A Boldogsághoz Alapítvány
1461 Budapest
Pf. 371
Hungary

LATIN AMERICA

The Way to Happiness Foundation Latin America
Pomona, 53
Colonia Roma
C.P. 06700
Mexico, D.F.

UNITED KINGDOM

The Way to Happiness Foundation United Kingdom
Saint Hill Manor
East Grinstead, West Sussex
England RH19 4JY

UNITED STATES

The Way to Happiness Foundation Eastern United States
349 W. 48th Street
New York, New York 10036

The Way to Happiness Foundation Western United States
1308 L. Ron Hubbard Way
Los Angeles, California 90027

World Institute of Scientology Enterprises

International Office

World Institute of Scientology Enterprises International
6331 Hollywood Boulevard Suite 701
Los Angeles, California 90028

Africa

World Institute of Scientology Enterprises—African Office
6th Floor, Budget House
130 Main Street
Johannesburg 2001, South Africa

ANZO

World Institute of Scientology Enterprises—Australian, New Zealand and Oceanian Office
201 Castlereagh Street
Sydney, New South Wales
Australia 2000

Canada

World Institute of Scientology Enterprises—Canadian Office
696 Yonge Street
Toronto, Ontario, Canada
M4Y 2A7

Commonwealth Of Independent States

World Institute of Scientology Enterprises—CIS Office c/o Hubbard Humanitarian Center
Ul. Borisa Galushkina 19A
129301 Moscow, Russia

Europe

World Institute of Scientology Enterprises—European Office
Store Kongensgade 55
1264 Copenhagen K, Denmark

Central Europe

World Institute of Scientology Enterprises—Central European Office
1082 Budapest
Leonardo da Vinci u. 8-12
Hungary

Italy

World Institute of Scientology Enterprises—Italian Office
Via Cadorna, 61
20090 Vimodrone, Milano, Italy

Latin America

World Institute of Scientology Enterprises—Latin American Office
Puebla #31, Colonia Roma
C.P. 06700, Mexico, D.F.

Taiwan

World Institute of Scientology Enterprises—Taiwanese Office
2F, 65, SEC.4,
Ming-Sheng EAST RD.
Taipei, Taiwan

United Kingdom

World Institute of Scientology Enterprises—United Kingdom Office
Saint Hill Manor, East Grinstead
West Sussex, England RH19 4JY

United States

World Institute of Scientology Enterprises—Eastern United States Office
349 W 48th Street
New York, New York 10036

World Institute of Scientology Enterprises—Flag Land Base Office
411 Cleveland Street, #283
Clearwater, Florida 33755

World Institute of Scientology Enterprises—Western United States Office
1308 L. Ron Hubbard Way
Los Angeles, California 90027

WISE Charter Committees

Australia

WISE Charter Committee Melbourne
10 Pratt Street, Ringwood
Victoria, Australia 3134

Canada

WISE Charter Committee Toronto
873 Broadview Avenue,
Lower Level
Toronto, Ontario
Canada M4K 2P9

France

WISE Charter Committee Paris
3, rue Bernoulli
75008 Paris, France

Germany

WISE Charter Committee Frankfurt
Johann-Peter-Bach Straße 10
61130 Nidderau, Germany

WISE Charter Committee Hamburg
Postfach 730404
22124 Hamburg, Germany

Publications Organizations

Bridge Publications, Inc.
4751 Fountain Avenue
Los Angeles, California 90029

Continental Publications
Liaison Office
696 Yonge Street
Toronto, Ontario
Canada M4Y 2A7

NEW ERA Publications
International ApS
Store Kongensgade 53
1264 Copenhagen K
Denmark

ERA DINÁMICA Editores,
S.A. de C.V.
Pablo Ucello #16
Colonia C.D. de los Deportes
Mexico, D.F.

NEW ERA Publications
UK Ltd.
Saint Hill Manor
East Grinstead, West Sussex
England RH19 4JY

NEW ERA Publications
Australia Pty Ltd.
Level 1, 61–65 Wentworth Avenue
Surry Hills, New South Wales
Australia 2000

Continental Publications
Pty Ltd.
6th Floor, Budget House
130 Main Street
Johannesburg 2001
South Africa

NEW ERA Publications
Italia S.r.l.
Via Cadorna, 61
20090 Vimodrone (MI), Italy

NEW ERA Publications
Deutschland GmbH
Hittfelder Kirchweg 5A
21220 Seevetal-Maschen
Germany

NEW ERA Publications
France E.U.R.L.
14, rue des Moulins
75001 Paris, France

NUEVA ERA DINÁMICA, S.A.
C/ Montera 20, 1° dcha.
28013 Madrid, Spain

NEW ERA Publications
Japan, Inc.
Sakai SS bldg 2F, 4-38-15
Higashi-Ikebukuro
Toshima-ku, Tokyo, Japan
170-0013

NEW ERA Publications
Group
Str. Kasatkina, 16, Building 1
129301 Moscow, Russia

NEW ERA Publications
Central European Office
1438 Budapest
Pf. 351
Hungary

All books and recorded lectures on Dianetics and Scientology may be obtained directly from the organizations listed above.

Recorded lectures by L. Ron Hubbard may be also obtained from:

Golden Era Productions

6331 Hollywood Boulevard
Suite 1305
Los Angeles, California
90028-6313

Subject Index

A

B

C

D

H

I

J

K

L

M

N

O

P

Q

R

S

T

U

V

W

X

Y

Z

Glossary

aberrated: not supported by reason, departing from rational thought or behavior. *See also* **aberration** in this glossary.

aberration: a departure from rational thought or behavior; irrational thought or conduct. It means basically to err, to make mistakes, or more specifically to have fixed ideas which are not true. The word is also used in its scientific sense. It means departure from a straight line. If a line should go from A to B, then if it is *aberrated* it would go from A to some other point, to some other point, to some other point, to some other point, to some other point, and finally arrive at B. Taken in this sense, it would also mean the lack of straightness or to see crookedly as, for example, a man sees a horse but thinks he sees an elephant. Aberrated conduct would be wrong conduct, or conduct not supported by reason. *Aberration* is opposed to sanity, which would be its opposite. From the Latin, *aberrare,* to wander from; Latin, *ab,* away, *errare,* to wander.

acknowledge: give (someone) an acknowledgment. *See also* **acknowledgment** in this glossary.

acknowledgment: something said or done to inform another that his statement or action has been noted, understood and received. See Chapter 5.

Admin Scale: short for *Administrative Scale,* a scale which gives a sequence (and relative seniority) of subjects relating to organization: goals, purposes, policy, plans, programs, projects, orders, ideal scenes, statistics, valuable final products. Each of these must operate in a coordinated manner to achieve success in the intended accomplishment of an envisioned goal. This scale is used to help one align them. See Chapter 17.

affinity: love, liking or any other emotional attitude; the degree of liking. The basic definition of affinity is the consideration of distance, whether good or bad. See Chapter 3.

alter-isness: an altered or changed reality of something. *See also* **reality** in this glossary.

analytical mind: that part of the mind which one consciously uses. It is the rational, conscious and aware part of the mind which thinks, observes data, remembers it and resolves problems.

ARC Straightwire: a type of processing in which a Scientology practitioner has a person recall moments when he actually felt he was receiving or giving affinity (A) or communication (C) or actually experiencing reality (R). It is called Straightwire because the practitioner directs the person's memory and in doing so is stringing wire, much on the order of a telephone line, between the person and the standard memory bank in the person's mind. *See also* **processing** in this glossary.

ARC triangle: a triangle which is a symbol of the fact that *affinity, reality* and *communication* act together to bring about understanding. No point of the triangle can be raised without also raising the other two points, and no point of it can be lowered without also lowering the other two points. See Chapter 3.

as-isness: the condition in which a person views anything exactly as it is, without any distortions or lies, at which moment it vanishes and ceases to exist. See Chapter 9.

assist: a process which can be done to alleviate a present time discomfort and help a person recover more rapidly from an accident, illness or upset. See Chapter 6.

auditing: same as *processing. See* **processing** in this glossary.

auditor: someone who is trained and qualified to apply Scientology processing to individuals for their benefit. The term comes from the Latin *audire,* "to listen." *See also* **processing** in this glossary.

battle plan: a series of exact doable targets for the coming day or week which forward the strategic planning of an individual or a group. See Chapter 17.

beingness: condition or state of being; existence. *Beingness* also refers to the assumption or choosing of a category of identity. Beingness can be assumed by oneself or given to oneself or attained. Examples of beingness would be one's own name, one's profession, one's physical characteristics, one's role in a game—each or all of these could be called one's beingness.

Bridge to Total Freedom: *See* **Classification, Gradation and Awareness Chart of Levels and Certificates** in this glossary.

bullbait: to find certain actions, words, phrases, mannerisms or subjects that cause the student doing a drill to become distracted by reacting to the coach. *Bullbaiting* is done by the coach in specific Training Routines. The word *bullbait* is derived from an English and Spanish sport of *baiting* which meant to set dogs upon a chained bull. *See also* **Training Routines** in this glossary.

button: (1) an item, word, phrase, subject or area that causes response or reaction in an individual. (2) in surveying, the subject, phrase or concept that is real to the majority of persons in a group and which can be used to get a response and gain agreement. The term comes from the early 1900s expression "press the button" which means, in a figurative sense, "to perform an action that automatically brings about the required state of affairs."

bypass: jump the proper person in a chain of command.

case: a general term for a person being treated or helped. It is also used to mean the entire accumulation of upsets, pain, failures, etc., residing in a person's reactive mind. *See also* **reactive mind** in this glossary.

charge: harmful energy or force contained in mental image pictures of experiences painful or upsetting to a person. *See also* **mental image pictures** in this glossary.

class: the level of classification of an auditor. Each level of classification is achieved through completion of an exactly laid out course of theory and practical learning. *See also* **auditor** in this glossary.

Classification, Gradation and Awareness Chart of Levels and Certificates: a chart which shows the proper step-by-step progression one takes in Scientology training or processing. Also called *The Bridge to Total Freedom* or *the Bridge.* See Introduction.

clay demonstration: a model made out of clay by a student to demonstrate an action, definition, object or principle. Also called a "clay demo." See Chapter 1.

Clear: a being who no longer has his own reactive mind. *See also* **reactive mind** in this glossary.

cognition: a new realization about life. It is a "What do you know, I..." statement; something a person suddenly understands or feels.

comm: short for *communication. See also* **communication** in this glossary.

communication: an interchange of ideas across space between two individuals. See Chapter 5.

communication lag: the length of time intervening between the asking of a question and the reply to that specific question by the person asked. See Chapter 5.

communication line: the route along which a communication travels from one person to another.

condition: one of the states of operation or existence which an organization, its parts or an individual passes through. Each condition has an exact sequence of steps, called a formula, which one can use to move from the current condition to another higher and more survival condition. See Chapter 10.

confront: to face without flinching or avoiding. The ability to confront is actually the ability to be there comfortably and perceive.

cycle of action: the sequence that an action goes through, wherein the action is begun, is continued for as long as is required and then is completed as planned.

demonstration kit: a kit composed of various small objects such as corks, caps, paper clips, pen tops, rubber bands, etc. A student uses these small objects to represent the various parts of something he is studying about. The objects can be moved about to show the mechanics and actions of a given concept and help the student understand it. Also called a "demo kit." See Chapter 1.

determinism: power of choice; power of decision; ability to decide or determine the course of one's actions.

Dianetics: comes from the Greek words *dia,* meaning "through" and *nous,* meaning "soul." Dianetics is a methodology developed by L. Ron Hubbard which can help alleviate such ailments as unwanted sensations and emotions, irrational fears and psychosomatic illnesses. It is most accurately described as *what the soul is doing to the body through the mind.*

doingness: the performance of some action or activity.

dope off: feel tired, sleepy or foggy as though doped or drugged.

drill: a method of learning or training whereby a person does a procedure over and over again in order to perfect that skill.

Drug Rundown: a series of processes that address the mental image pictures connected with having taken drugs. The result of the Drug Rundown is freedom from the harmful effects of drugs, alcohol and medicine, and freedom from the need to take them. See Chapter 7.

dub in: presume or have a false, delusory perception of.

duplication: the act of reproducing something exactly. See Chapter 5.

dynamic: an urge to survive along a certain course; an urge toward existence in an area of life. There are eight dynamics: first, self; second, sex and the family unit; third, groups; fourth, mankind; fifth, life forms; sixth, physical universe; seventh, spirits; and eighth, Supreme Being. See Chapter 2.

E-Meter: short for *electropsychometer,* a specially designed instrument used by a trained Scientology practitioner which helps locate long-hidden sources of travail. It does not diagnose or cure anything; it simply measures the mental state or change of state of an individual.

engram: a particular type of mental image picture which is a complete recording of every perception present in a moment of partial or full "unconsciousness." Engrams are stored in the reactive mind. *See also* **mental image pictures** and **reactive mind** in this glossary.

entheta: enturbulated theta; especially referring to communications, which, based on lies and confusions, are slanderous, choppy or destructive in an attempt to overwhelm or suppress a person or group. *See also* **enturbulate** and **theta** in this glossary.

enturbulate: put into a state of agitation or disturbance.

ethics: the actions an individual takes on himself to correct some conduct or situation in which he is involved which is contrary to the ideals and best interests of his group. It is a personal thing. When one is ethical or "has his ethics in," it is by his own determinism and is done by himself. See Chapter 10.

Expanded Dianetics: a branch of Dianetics which uses certain Dianetics techniques in special ways to address and handle such things as difficulties a person has in his environment, experiences of severe emotional stress, and points of his past from which he cannot free his attention. *See also* **Dianetics** in this glossary.

Grade: a series of processes done with the purpose of bringing a person to a particular state of Release. For example, Grade 0 consists of twenty-three processes, each of which is run in sequence to full end result. A person who completes Grade 0 is a Communications Release and has gained the ability to communicate freely with anyone on any subject. *See also* **process** and **Release** in this glossary.

gradient: a gradual approach to something taken step by step, level by level, each step or level being, of itself, easily attainable—so that finally, complicated and difficult activities can be achieved with relative ease. The term *gradient* also applies to each of the steps taken in such an approach.

hat: *(slang)* the title and work of a post in an organization. It is taken from the fact that in many professions such as railroading the type of hat worn is the badge of the job. For example, a train crew has a conductor who wears a conductor's hat—he has charge of the passengers and collects fares. To *hat* someone is to train him on the functions and specialties of his post, and when a person is fully trained to do these he is said to be *hatted.* See Chapter 16.

havingness: the feeling that one owns or possesses; it can also be described as the concept of being able to reach or not being prevented from reaching.

Hubbard Chart of Human Evaluation: a chart by which one can precisely evaluate human behavior and predict what a person will do. It displays the various characteristics that exist at different levels of the Tone Scale. See Chapter 4.

indicator: a condition or circumstance arising during a process which indicates (points out or shows) whether the process is going well or badly. For example, the person receiving the processing looking brighter or looking more cheerful would be good indicators. *See also* **process** in this glossary.

individuate: separate oneself from someone, a group, etc., and withdraw from involvement with it.

invalidate: refute, degrade, discredit or deny something someone else considers to be fact.

justice: the action taken on an individual by the group when he fails to take appropriate ethics actions himself. See Chapter 10.

justification: the attempt to lessen an overt act by explaining how it was not really an overt act. *See also* **overt act** in this glossary.

Locational Processing: a type of process which helps orient a person and puts him in communication with his environment. See Chapter 6.

major stable win: *See* **win** in this glossary.

mass: the actual physical objects, the things of life; as opposed to significance. *See also* **significance** in this glossary.

mental image pictures: three-dimensional color pictures with sound and smell and all other perceptions, plus the conclusions or speculations of the individual. They are mental copies of one's perceptions sometime in the past, although in cases of unconsciousness or lessened consciousness they exist *below* the individual's awareness.

misemotion: irrational or inappropriate emotion. It is a coined word taken from *mis-* (wrong) + *emotion.* To say that a person was *misemotional* would indicate that the person did not display the emotion called for by the actual circumstances of the situation. Being misemotional would be synonymous with being irrational. One can fairly judge the rationality of any individual by the correctness of the emotion he displays in a given set of circumstances. To be joyful and happy when circumstances call for joy and happiness would be rational. To display grief without sufficient present time cause would be irrational.

misunderstood word: a word which is *not* understood or *wrongly* understood. See Chapter 1.

motivator: an aggressive or destructive act received by the person or part of life. The reason it is called a "motivator" is because it tends to prompt that one pays it back—it "motivates" a new overt act. See Chapter 9.

New Era Dianetics: the technology which contains L. Ron Hubbard's ultimate refinements of Dianetics auditing, developed following discoveries he made in 1978. Using New Era Dianetics technology, a person can achieve the goals of Dianetics faster than ever before possible. *See also* **Dianetics** in this glossary.

New Era Dianetics for OTs: a series of advanced auditing actions developed by L. Ron Hubbard during his research into New Era Dianetics in the late 1970s. *See also* **OT** in this glossary.

Objective Process: a type of process which helps a person direct his attention off himself and onto his environment and the people and things in it. *Objective* refers to outward things, not the thoughts or feelings of the individual. *Objective Processes* deal with the real and observable. They call for the person to spot or find something exterior to himself. See Chapter 7.

obnosis: a coined word put together from "observing the obvious." It is the action of a person looking at another person or an object and seeing exactly what is there, not a deduction of what might be there from what he does see. See Chapter 4.

Operating Thetan: one who is knowing and willing cause over life, thought, matter, energy, space and time. See Introduction.

org board: short for *organizing board,* a board which displays the functions, duties, communication routes, sequences of action and authorities of an organization. It shows the pattern of organizing to obtain a product. See Chapter 16.

OT: abbreviation for *Operating Thetan. See* **Operating Thetan** in this glossary.

outness: a condition or instance of something being wrong, incorrect or missing.

outpoint: any one of several specific ways in which a relay of information or a situation can become illogical; any one datum offered as true that is in fact found to be illogical. See Chapter 18.

overt act: a harmful act or a transgression against the moral code of a group. An overt act is not just injuring someone or something, it is an act of *omission* or *commission* which does the least good for the least number of people or areas of life, or the most harm to the greatest number of people or areas of life. See Chapter 9.

pc: abbreviation for *preclear,* a person who is receiving processing on his way to becoming Clear, hence pre-Clear. Through processing he is finding out more about himself and life. *See also* **Clear** and **processing** in this glossary.

pluspoint: any one of several conditions which exist when a situation or circumstance is logical. Pluspoints show where logic exists and where things are going right or likely to. See Chapter 18.

postulate: (1) *(noun)* a conclusion, decision or resolution about something. (2) *(verb)* make something happen or bring something into being by making a postulate about it.

potential trouble source: a person who is in some way connected to and being adversely affected by a suppressive person. He is called a *potential* trouble source because he can be a lot of trouble to himself and to others. See Chapter 11.

present time: the time which is now and becomes the past as rapidly as it is observed. It is a term loosely applied to the environment existing in now.

process: an exact series of directions or sequence of actions taken to accomplish a desired result.

processing: a special form of personal counseling, unique in Scientology, which helps an individual look at his own existence and improves his ability to confront what he is and where he is. Processing is a precise, thoroughly codified activity with exact procedures.

PTS: abbreviation for *potential trouble source. See* **potential trouble source** in this glossary.

Purification Rundown: a program of exercise, sauna sweat-out, nutrition and properly ordered personal schedule. It cleans out and purifies one's system of all the accumulated impurities such as drugs, insecticides and pesticides, food preservatives, etc., which by their presence and restimulative effects could prevent or delay freeing the being spiritually through Scientology processing. See Chapter 7.

Q and A: short for *Question and Answer.* It means to not get an answer to one's question, to fail to complete something or to deviate from an intended course of action. Example: Question: "Do birds fly?" Answer: "I don't like birds." Question: "Why not?" Answer: "Because they're dirty." The original question has not been answered and has been dropped and the person who asked the question has deviated—this is Q and A. The person who deviates could be said to have "Q-and-Aed."

Reach and Withdraw: a method of getting a person familiarized and in communication with things so that he can be more in control of them. See Chapter 15.

reactive mind: that part of a person's mind which is not under his volitional control and which exerts force and the power of command over his awareness, purposes, thoughts, body and actions.

reality: that which appears to be. Reality is fundamentally agreement; the degree of agreement reached by people. What we agree to be real is real. See Chapter 3.

Release: the term for what occurs when a person separates from his reactive mind or some part of it. The degree and relative permanence of being pulled out of the reactive mind determines the state of Release. There are a number of states or stages of Release, and these are called Grades. *See also* **Grade** and **reactive mind** in this glossary.

restimulation: the reactivation of a memory of a past unpleasant experience due to similar circumstances in the present approximating circumstances of the past.

roller coaster: to better and worsen—a person gets better, gets worse, gets better, gets worse. The term was derived from the name of an amusement park ride that rises and then plunges steeply.

rundown: a series of steps designed to handle a specific aspect of a person's life or difficulties and which has a known end result.

Scientology: an applied religious philosophy developed by L. Ron Hubbard. It is the study and handling of the spirit in relationship to itself, universes and other life. The word *Scientology* comes from the Latin *scio,* which means "know" and the Greek word *logos,* meaning "the word or outward form by which the inward thought is expressed and made known." Thus, Scientology means knowing about knowing.

self-determinism: that state of being wherein the individual can or cannot be controlled by his environment according to his own choice. In that state the individual has self-confidence in his control of the material universe and other people.

session: the period of time during which processing occurs. *See also* **processing** in this glossary.

significance: the meaning or ideas or theory of something, as opposed to its mass. See Chapter 1.

Solo auditor: a person who has received special training so that he can audit himself—being at the same time the auditor and the person being audited—on certain of the upper levels of Scientology processing. *See also* **auditor** and **processing** in this glossary.

somatic: a word used in Scientology to designate any body sensation, illness, pain or discomfort. *Soma* means "body" in Greek.

SP: abbreviation for *suppressive person. See* **suppressive person** in this glossary.

Student Hat: a comprehensive course which contains *all* the Scientology technology on study. *See also* **hat** in this glossary.

suppressive person: a person who possesses a distinct set of characteristics and mental attitudes that cause him to suppress other people in his vicinity. This is the person whose behavior is calculated to be disastrous. Also called *antisocial personality.* See Chapter 11.

terminal: a person, point or position which can receive, relay or send a communication.

theta: thought or life. The term comes from the Greek letter *theta* (θ), which the Greeks used to represent *thought* or perhaps *spirit.* Something which is *theta* is characterized by reason, serenity, stability, happiness, cheerful emotion, persistence and the other factors which man ordinarily considers desirable.

thetan: the person himself—not his body or his name, the physical universe, his mind or anything else—it is that which is aware of being aware; the identity which *is* the individual. The term *thetan* was coined to eliminate any possible confusion with older, invalid concepts. It comes from the Greek letter *theta* which the Greeks used to represent *thought* or perhaps *spirit,* to which an *n* is added to make a noun in the modern style used to create words in engineering.

third party: one who by false reports creates trouble between two people, a person and a group, or a group and another group. See Chapter 8.

Third Party Law: a law which states that a third party must be present and unknown in every quarrel for a conflict to exist. See Chapter 8.

time track: the accumulated record of all one's mental image pictures. *See also* **mental image pictures** in this glossary.

Tone Scale: a scale which shows the successive emotional tones a person can experience. By "tone" is meant the momentary or continuing emotional state of a person. Emotions such as fear, anger, grief, enthusiasm and others which people experience are shown on this graduated scale. See Chapter 4.

TR: abbreviation for *Training Routine. See* **Training Routines** in this glossary.

Training Routines: training drills that enable a person to improve his level of communication skill. By doing these drills any person's ability to communicate with others can be vastly improved. See Chapter 5.

Why: reason or cause; the real reason for a positive or nonoptimum situation. See Chapter 18.

win: the accomplishment of any desired improvement. Examples of wins would be a person increasing his ability to communicate, experiencing an increased feeling of well-being or gaining more certainty about some area of his life. In Training Routines, when a student has reached the point where he can do a drill and his skill and ability to do it is stable, it is called a major stable win—a significant, lasting gain. *See also* **Training Routines** in this glossary.

withhold: an unspoken, unannounced transgression against a moral code by which a person is bound; an overt act that a person committed that he or she is not talking about. Any withhold comes *after* an overt act. See Chapter 9.

word clear: define, using a dictionary, any words not fully understood in the material a person is studying. See Chapter 1.

word clearer: a person who helps another person find and clear any misunderstood words.

Word Clearing: that body of Scientology procedures used to locate words a person has misunderstood in subjects he has studied and get the words defined by looking them up in a dictionary. See Chapter 1.

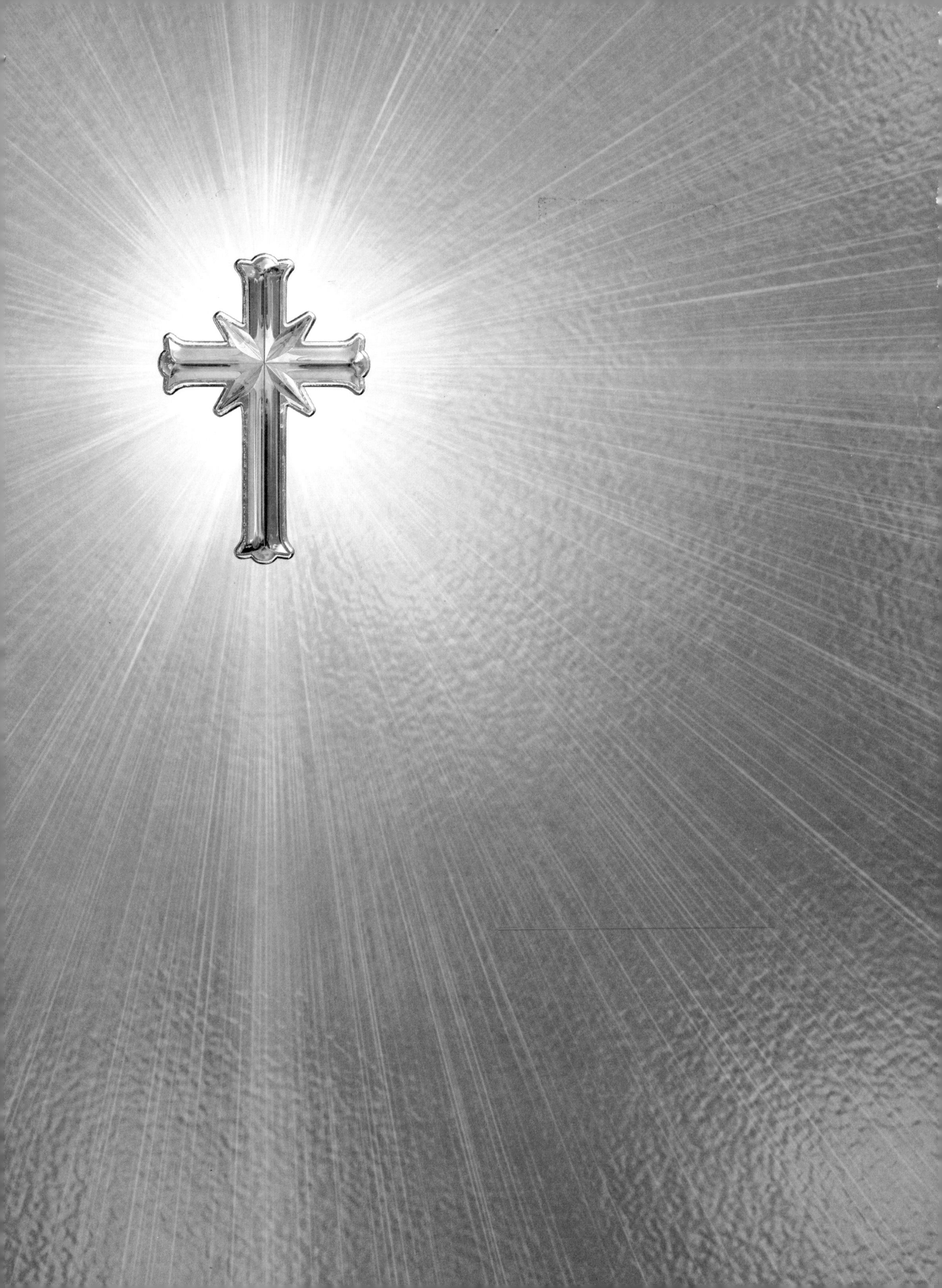